ERS|hand

Respiratory Medicine

2nd Edition

Editors
Paolo Palange
and Anita K. Simonds

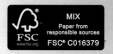

PUBLISHED BY
THE EUROPEAN RESPIRATORY SOCIETY

CHIEF EDITORS

Paolo Palange (Rome, Italy)

Anita K. Simonds (London, UK)

ERS STAFF

Alice Bartlett, Matt Broadhead, Neil Bullen, Alyson Cann, Jonathan Hansen,
Sarah Hill, Fiona Marks, Elin Reeves, David Sadler, Claire Turner

© 2013 European Respiratory Society

Design by Claire Turner and Lee Dodd, ERS
Typeset in China by Charlesworth Group
Printed by Charlesworth Press

CONTACT, PERMISSIONS AND SALES REQUESTS:
European Respiratory Society, 442 Glossop Road, Sheffield, S10 2PX, UK
Tel: +44 114 2672860 Fax: +44 114 2665064 e-mail: info@ersj.org.uk

ISBN 978-1-84984-040-8

Table of contents

Contributors

Chief Editors

Paolo Palange
Department of Public Health and
Infectious Diseases
Sapienza University of Rome
Rome, Italy
paolo.palange@uniroma1.it

Authors

Nicolino Ambrosino
Cardio-Thoracic Dept
University Hospital
Pisa, Italy
n.ambrosino@ao-pisa.toscana.it

Isabella Annesi-Maesano
Université Pierre et Marie Curie –
Paris 6
Medical School Saint-Antoine
UMR S 707: EPAR
Paris, France
isabella.annesi-maesano@inserm.fr

Andrea Antonelli
Allergologia e Fisiopatologia
Respiratoria, ASO S. Croce e Carle
Cuneo, Italy
andrea-antonelli@tiscali.it

Bruno Balbi
Fondazione Salvatore Maugeri
IRCCS
Veruno, Italy
bruno.balbi@fsm.it

Sandra Baldacci
Pulmonary Environmental
Epidemiology Unit, Institute of
Clinical Physiology National Research
Council
Pisa, Italy
baldas@ifc.cnr.it

Anita K. Simonds
NIHR Respiratory Disease Biomedical
Research Unit
Royal Brompton and Harefield NHS
Foundation Trust
London, UK
a.simonds@rbht.nhs.uk

Peter J. Barnes
National Heart and Lung Institute
Imperial College
London, UK
p.j.barnes@imperial.ac.uk

Bianca Beghé
Section of Respiratory Diseases
Department of Oncology
Haematology and Respiratory
Diseases
University Policlinic of Modena
University of Modena and Reggio
Emilia
Modena, Italy
bianca.beghe@unimore.it

Francesco Blasi
Respiratory Medicine Section
Dipartimento Toraco-Polmonare e
Cardiocircolatorio
Università degli Studi di Milano and
IRCCS Fondazione Cà Granda
Milan, Italy
francesco.blasi@unimi.it

Konrad E. Bloch
Pulmonary Division
University Hospital of Zurich
Zurich, Switzerland
konrad.bloch@usz.ch

Annette Boehler
University Hospital of Zurich
Zurich, Switzerland
capybara@compuserve.com

Chris T. Bolliger[†]

Philippe Bonniaud
Department of Pulmonary Medicine
and Intensive Care
CHU Dijon
Dijon, France
philippe.bonniaud@chu-dijon.fr

Aik Bossink
Diakonessenhuis
Utrecht, the Netherlands
aikbossink@mac.com

Julia Bott
Virgin Care
Chertsey, UK
Julia.Bott@virgincare.co.uk

Arnaud Bourdin
Department of Respiratory Disease
CHU Arnaud de Villeneuve
Montpellier, France
a-bourdin@chu-montpellier.fr

Thomas Brack
Cantonal Hospital Glarus
Glarus, Switzerland
thomas.brack@ksgl.ch

Barbara Burroni
Département de Pathologie
Pôle de Biologie et de Pathologie
Centre Hospitalier Universitaire A.
Michallon
INSERM U 823 – Institut A. Bonniot
Université J. Fourier
Grenoble, France
BBurroni@chu-grenble.fr

Andrew Bush
Imperial College and Royal Brompton
Hospital
London, UK
a.bush@rbht.nhs.uk

Philippe Camus
Department of Pulmonary Medicine
and Intensive Care
CHU Dijon
Dijon, France
ph.camus@chu-dijon.fr

Emilio Canalis
Thoracic Surgery Service
Hospital Universitari Joan XXIII
IISPV
URV
Tarragona, Spain
emilio.canalis@urv.cat

Kai-Håkon Carlsen
Institute of Clinical Medicine,
University of Oslo
Dept of Paediatrics, Oslo University
Hospital
Norwegian School of Sport Science
Oslo, Norway
k.h.carlsen@medisin.uio.no

Sonia Cerrai
Pulmonary Environmental
Epidemiology Unit
Institute of Clinical Physiology
National Research Council
Pisa, Italy
sonia.cerrai@ifc.cnr.it

Stefania Cerri
Centre for Rare Lung Disease
Dept of Medical and Surgical
Sciences
University of Modena and Reggio
Emilia
Modena, Italy
stefania.cerri@unimore.it

Pascal Chanez
Service de Pneumo-Allergologie et
Laboratoire d'Immunologie INSERM
U600
Université de la Méditerranée
AP-HM
Marseille, France
pascal.chanez@univmed.fr

Francesca Cherubino
Pneumology Unit, Fondazione
Salvatore Maugeri
IRCCS
Tradate, Italy
francesca.cherubino@fsm.it

Sara Chiesa
Department of Clinical and
Experimental Medicine
University of Parma
Parma, Italy
sara.chiesa@hotmail.it

Marco Chilosi
Department of Pathology
Università di Verona
Veronica, Italy
marco.chilosi@univr.it

Luke Clancy
TobaccoFree Research Institute
Ireland
Dublin, Ireland
lclancy@tri.ie

Amelia Clive
North Bristol Lung Centre
University of Bristol
Bristol, UK
Amelia.Clive@nbt.nhs.uk

Robert P. Coppes
Depts of Cell Biology and Radiation
Oncology
University Medical Center Groningen
University of Groningen
Groningen, the Netherlands
r.p.coppes@umcg.nl

Jean-François Cordier
Department of Respiratory Diseases
CHU de Lyon
Lyon, France
jean-francois.cordier@chu-lyon.fr

Ulrich Costabel
Dept of Pneumology and Allergy
Ruhrlandklinik
Essen
Germany
ulrich.costabel@ruhrlandklinik.uk-
essen.de

Vincent Cottin
Department of Respiratory Diseases
CHU de Lyon
Lyon, France
vincent.cottin@chu-lyon.fr

Jane C. Davies
Imperial College and Royal Brompton
Hospital
London, UK
j.c.davies@imperial.ac.uk

Wilfried De Backer
Dept of Pulmonary Medicine
University of Antwerp
Antwerp, Belgium
wilfried.debacker@ua.ac.be

Marc Decramer
Respiratory Rehabilitation and
Respiratory Division
University Hospital Leuven
Leuven, Belgium
marc.decramer@uzleuven.be

Giovanni Della Casa
Division of Radiology
Dept of Diagnostic and Imaging
Services
University of Modena and Reggio
Emilia
Modena, Italy
giodc@libero.it

Sabrina Della Patrona
Pneumology Unit
Fondazione Salvatore Maugeri
IRCCS
Tradate, Italy
sabrina.dellapatrona@fsm.it

Sofie Derijcke
Respiratory Oncology Unit
Dept of Pulmonology
University Hospital Leuven
Leuven, Belgium
sofie.derijcke@azgroeninge.be

Walter De Wever
University Hospitals Leuven
Leuven, Belgium
walter.dewever@uz.kuleuven.be

Maria Anna Digiulio
Dept of Clinical Medicine
Reference Centre for Primary
Immunodeficiencies
Sapienza University of Rome
Rome, Italy
mariaanna.digiulio@gmail.com

Antonino Di Stefano
Fondazione Salvatore Maugeri
IRCCS
Veruno, Italy
antonino.distefano@fsm.it

Lieven Dupont
Department of Respiratory Medicine
University Hospital Gasthuisberg
KU Leuven
Leuven, Belgium
lieven.dupont@uzleuven.be

Oliver Eickelberg
Comprehensive Pneumology Center,
Ludwig-Maximilians-University and
Helmholtz Zentrum München
Munich, Germany
oliver.eickelberg@helmholtz-
muenchen.de

Santiago Ewig
Thoraxzentrum Ruhrgebiet
Kliniken für Pneumologie und
Infektiologie
Evangelisches Krankenhaus Herne
und Augusta-Kranken-Anstalt
Bochum
Bochum, Germany
ewig@augusta-bochum.de

Leonardo M. Fabbri
Section of Respiratory Diseases
Department of Oncology
Haematology and Respiratory
Diseases
University Policlinic of Modena
University of Modena and Reggio
Emilia
Modena, Italy
fabbri.leonardo@unimo.it

Pierre-Emmanuel Falcoz
Université Louis Pasteur and
Hôpitaux Universitaires de
Strasbourg
Strasbourg, France
pierre-emmanuel.falcoz@wanadoo.fr

Ramon Farré
Unitat de Biofisica i Bioenginyeria,
Facultat de Medicina, Universitat de
Barcelona
CIBER Enfermedades Respiratorias
Institut de Investigacions
Biomèdiques August Pi Sunyer
Barcelona, Spain
rfarre@ub.edu

Alessandro Maria Ferrazza
Dept of Public Health and Infectious
Diseases
Sapienza University of Rome
Rome, Italy
ale.ferrazza@libero.it

Thomas Fuehner
Dept of Respiratory Medicine
Hanover Medical School
Hanover, Germany
fuehner.thomas@mh-hannover.de

Mina Gaga
Asthma Centre and 7th Respiratory
Medicine Dept
Athens Chest Hospital
Athens, Greece
minagaga@yahoo.com

Stefano Gasparini
Pulmonary Diseases Unit
Dept of Immunoallergic and
Respiratory Diseases
Azienda Ospedaliero-Universitaria
"Ospedali Riuniti"
Ancona, Italy
s.gasparini@fastnet.it

Mari Carmen Gilavert
Intensive Care Unit
Hospital Universitari Joan XXIII
IISPV
URV
Tarragona, Spain
mcgilavert.hj23.ics@gencat.cat

Rik Gosselink
Faculty of Kinesiology and
Rehabilitation Sciences
Dept of Rehabilitation Sciences
Katholieke Universiteit Leuven
Leuven, Belgium

Rik.Gosselink@faber.kuleuven.be
Jens Gottlieb
Dept of Respiratory Medicine
Hanover Medical School
Hanover, Germany
gottlieb.jens@mh-hannover.de

Mark Greer
Dept of Respiratory Medicine
Hanover Medical School
Hanover, Germany
greer.mark@mh-hannover.de

Fabio Guarracino
Cardio-Thoracic Dept
University Hospital
Pisa, Italy
f.guarracino@ao-pisa.toscana.it

Federico Gumiero
Department of Clinical and
Experimental Medicine
University of Insubria
Varese, Italy
federico.gumiero@fsm.it

Inge Hantson
Respiratory Oncology Unit
Dept of Pulmonology
University Hospital Leuven
Leuven, Belgium
inge.hantson@uzleuven.be

Sylvia Hartl
Dept of Respiratory and Critical Care
Otto Wagner Hospital
Vienna, Austria
sylvia.hartl@wienkav.at

Patricia L. Haslam
National Heart and Lung Institute
and Royal Brompton Hospital
Imperial College
London, UK
p.haslam@imperial.ac.uk

Allan F. Henderson
Norfolk and Norwich University
Hospital
Norwich, UK
afhenderson@live.com

Jeroen M. Hendriks
Department of Thoracic and Vascular
Surgery
Antwerp University Hospital
Antwerp, Belgium
jeroen.hendriks@uza.be

Matthew Hind
Royal Brompton Hospital
London, UK
M.Hind@rbht.nhs.uk

Clare Hooper
Worcestershire Royal Hospital
Worcester, UK
clarehooper@doctors.org.uk

Rudolf M. Huber
Division of Respiratory Medicine
and Thoracic Oncology, Hospitals
of Ludwig-Maximilians-University –
Campus Innenstadt, and Thoracic
Oncology Centre of Munich
Munich, Germany
huber@med.uni-muenchen.de

J. Mike Hughes
National Heart and Lung Institute
Imperial College
London, UK
mike.hughes@imperial.ac.uk

Marc Humbert
Université Paris-Sud
INSERM U999
Assistance Publique-Hôpitaux de
Paris
Service de Pneumologie
Hôpital Bicêtre
Paris, France
marc.humbert@bct.aphp.fr

Magareta Ieven
Laboratory of Medical Microbiology,
University Hospital Antwerp,and
Dept of Medical Microbiology,
Vaccine and Infectious Disease
Institute, Faculty of Medicine,
University of Antwerp
Antwerp, Belgium
Greet.Ieven@uza.be

Zubair Kabir
TobaccoFree Research Institute
Ireland
Dublin, Ireland
zkabir@tri.ie

Christian Karagiannidis
Abteilung für Pneumologie und
Internistische Intensivmedizin
Krankenhaus Oststadt-Heidehaus
Klinikum Region Hannover
Hanover, Germany
KaragiannidisC@kliniken-koeln.de

Coenraad F.N. Koegelenberg
Division of Pulmonology
Dept of Medicine
University of Stellenbosch and
Tygerberg Academic Hospital
Cape Town, South Africa
coeniefn@sun.ac.za

Melanie Königshoff
Comprehensive Pneumology Center
Ludwig-Maximilians-University and
Helmholtz Zentrum München
Munich, Germany
melanie.koenigshoff@helmholtz-
muenchen.de

Helen J. Lachmann
UK National Amyloidosis Centre
Division of Medicine
University College London Medical
School
London, UK
h.lachmann@ucl.ac.uk

Daniel Langer
Faculty of Kinesiology and
Rehabilitation Sciences
Dept of Rehabilitation Sciences
Katholieke Universiteit Leuven
Leuven, Belgium
Daniel.Langer@faber.kuleuven.be

Sylvie Lantuéjoul
Département de Pathologie
Pôle de Biologie et de Pathologie
Centre Hospitalier Universitaire A.
Michallon
INSERM U 823-Institut A.
Bonniot-Université J. Fourier
Grenoble, France
SLantuejoul@chu-grenoble.fr

Patrick Lauwers
Dept of Thoracic and Vascular
Surgery
Antwerp University Hospital
Antwerp, Belgium
patrick.lauwers@uza.be

Pierantonio Laveneziana
Equipe de Recherche ER 10 UPMC
Laboratoire de Physio-Pathologie
Respiratoire
Faculté de Médecine Pierre et Marie
Curie
Université Pierre et Marie Curie
(Paris VI)
Paris, France
pier_lav@yahoo.it

Romain Lazor
Interstitial and Rare Lung Disease
Unit
Lausanne University Hospital
Lausanne, Switzerland
romain.lazor@huv.ch

Wei Shen Lim
Respiratory Medicine
Nottingham University Hospitals
NHS Trust
Nottingham, UK
WeiShen.Lim@nuh.nhs.uk

Marc C.I. Lipman
University College London Medical
School and Royal Free London NHS
Foundation Trust
London, UK
marclipman@nhs.net

Robert Loddenkemper
Dept of Pneumology II
Lungenklinik Heckeshorn
HELIOS Klinikum Emil von Behring
Berlin, Germany
rloddenkemper@dzk-tuberkulose.de

Maurizio Luisetti
University of Pavia
SC Pneumologia
Dip. di Medicina Molecolare
IRCCS Policlinico San Matteo
Pavia, Italy
m.luisetti@smatteo.pv.it

Alexander J. Mackay
Academic Unit of Respiratory
Medicine
UCL Medical School
London, UK
alexander.mackay@ucl.ac.uk

Sara Maio
Pulmonary Environmental
Epidemiology Unit
Institute of Clinical Physiology
National Research Council
Pisa, Italy
saramaio@ifc.cnr.it

Adel H. Mansur
Birmingham Heartlands Hospital
Birmingham, UK
adel.mansur@heartofengland.nhs.uk

Georgios Margaritopoulos
Interstitial Lung Disease Unit
Royal Brompton Hospital
London, UK
gmargaritop@yahoo.gr

Yves Martinet
University of Nancy Henri Poincaré
Nancy, France
y.martinet@chu-nancy.fr

Nick Maskell
North Bristol Lung Centre
University of Bristol
Bristol, UK
nick.maskell@bristol.ac.uk

Gilbert Massard
Dept of Thoracic Surgery
Hôpitaux Universitaires de
Strasbourg
Strasbourg, France
Gilbert.Massard@chru-strasbourg.fr

Anne McLeer-Florin
Plateforme de Génétique Moléculaire
des Cancers
Pôle de Biologie et de Pathologie
Centre Hospitalier Universitaire A.
Michallon
INSERM U 823-Institut A.
Bonniot-Université J. Fourier
Grenoble, France
AFlorin@chu-grenoble.fr

Andrew Menzies-Gow
Royal Brompton and Harefield NHS
Foundation Trust
London, UK
a.menzies-gow@rbht.nhs.uk

Lénaïg Mescam-Mancini
Département de Pathologie et
Plateforme de Génétique Moléculaire
des Cancers
Pôle de Biologie et de Pathologie
Centre Hospitalier Universitaire A.
Michallon
INSERM U 823-Institut A.
Bonniot-Université J. Fourier
Grenoble, France
LMescam@chu-grenoble.fr

Giovanni Battista Migliori
WHO Collaborating Centre for TB
and Lung Diseases
Fondazione S. Maugeri
Care and Research Institute
Tradate, Italy
giovannibattista.migliori@fsm.it

Cinzia Milito
Dept of Molecular Medicine
Reference Centre for Primary
Immunodeficiencies
Sapienza University of Rome
Rome, Italy
cinzia.milito@uniroma1.it

Rob F. Miller
University College London Medical
School, and London School of
Hygiene and Tropical Medicine
London, UK
robert.miller@ucl.ac.uk

Marc Miravitlles
Pneumology Dept
Hospital Universitari Vall d'Hebron
Barcelona, Spain
marcm@separ.es

Luigi Moretti
Dept of Radiation Oncology
Institut Jules Bordet
Université Libre de Bruxelles
Brussels, Belgium
luigi.moretti@bordet.be

Alyn H. Morice
Hull York Medical School
University of Hull
Hull, UK
a.h.morice@hull.ac.uk

Jean-François Muir
Respiratory Dept and Respiratory
Intensive Care Unit
Rouen University Hospital
Rouen, France
Jean-Francois.Muir@chu-rouen.fr

Bruno Murer
Surgical Pathology Unit
Department of Clinical Pathology
Ospedale dell'Angelo
Venice, Italy
bruno.murer@ulss12.ve.it

Daniel Navajas
Unitat de Biofisica i Bioenginyeria,
Facultat de Medicina, Universitat
de Barcelona, CIBER Enfermedades
Respiratorias, and Institut de
Bioenginyeria de Catalunya
Barcelona, Spain
dnavajas@ub.edu

Benoit Nemery
Research Unit of Lung Toxicology,
Occupational, Environmental and
Insurance Medicine
KU Leuven
Leuven, Belgium
Ben.Nemery@med.kuleuven.be

Marc Noppen
University Hospital Brussels
Brussels, Belgium
Marc.Noppen@uzbrussel.be

Yvonne Nussbaumer-Ochsner
University Hospital Zurich
Zurich, Switzerland
yvonne.nussbaumer@swissonline.ch

Dario Olivieri
Department of Clinical and
Experimental Medicine
University of Parma
Parma, Italy
dario.olivieri@unipr.it

Paolo Onorati
Department of Public Health and
Infectious Diseases
Sapienza University of Rome
Rome, Italy
paolo.onorati@fastwebnet.it

Antonio Palla
Cardiothoracic and Vascular Dept
University of Pisa
Pisa, Italy
a.palla@med.unipi.it

Martyn R. Partridge
Imperial College, London, UK and
Lee Kong Chian School of Medicine,
Singapore
m.partridge@imperial.ac.uk

Riccardo Pellegrino
Allergologia e Fisiopatologia
Respiratoria
ASO S. Croce e Carle
Cuneo, Italy
pellegrino.r@ospedale.cuneo.it

Claudio Piersimoni
Regional Reference Mycobacteriology
Unit
Clinical Pathology Laboratory
Azienda Ospedaliera-Universitaria
Ospedali Riuniti
Ancona, Italy
c.piersimoni@ospedaliriuniti.
marche.it

Patrizia Pignatti
Allergy and Immunology Unit
Fondazione Salvatore Maugeri
IRCCS
Pavia, Italy
patrizia.pignatti@fsm.it

Massimo Pistolesi
Section of Respiratory Medicine
Dept of Experimental and Clinical
Medicine
University of Florence
Florence, Italy
massimo.pistolesi@unifi.it

Riccardo Pistelli
Catholic University
Columbus Hospital
Rome, Italy
riccardopistelli@h-columbus.it

Alessandro Pitruzzella
Fondazione Salvatore Maugeri
IRCCS
Veruno, Italy
alexpitruzzella@libero.it

Giovanni Poletti
Hematology Laboratory Area Vasta
Romagna
Pievesestina, Italy
gpoletti1958@gmail.com

Venerino Poletti
Department of Diseases of the
Thorax
Ospedale GB Morgagni
Forlì, Italy
venerino.poletti@gmail.com

Federica Pulvirenti
Dept of Clinical Medicine
Reference Centre for Primary
Immunodeficiencies
Sapienza University of Rome
Rome, Italy
federica.pulvirenti@hotmail.it

Isabella Quinti
Dept of Molecular Medicine
Reference Centre for Primary
Immunodeficiencies
Sapienza University of Rome
Rome, Italy
isabella.quinti@uniroma1.it

Elisabeth Quoix
University of Strasbourg
University Hospital
Strasbourg, France
equoix@gmail.com

Klaus F. Rabe
Centre for Pneumology and Thoracic
Surgery
Grosshansdorf Hospital
Grosshansdorf, Germany
k.f.rabe@kh-grosshansdorf.de

Anna Rask-Anderson
Uppsala University
Uppsala, Sweden
anna.rask-andersen@medsci.uu.se

Luca Richeldi
Centre for Rare Lung Disease
Dept of Medical and Surgical
Sciences
University of Modena and Reggio
Emilia
Modena, Italy
luca.richeldi@unimore.it

Josep Roca
Hospital Clinic
IDIBAPS
CIBERES
University of Barcelona
Barcelona, Spain
jroca@clinic.ub.es

Gernot Rohde
Dept of Respiratory Medicine
Maastricht University Medical Centre
Maastricht, the Netherlands
g.rohde@mumc.nl

Nicola Santelmo
Université de Strasbourg and
Hôpitaux Universitaires de
Strasbourg
Strasbourg, France
Nicola.Santelmo@chru-strasbourg.fr

Giuseppe Sarno
Pulmonary Environmental
Epidemiology Unit
Institute of Clinical Physiology
National Research Council
Pisa, Italy
sarnogiu@ifc.cnr.it

Giorgio Scano
Dept of Internal Medicine
Section of Immunology and
Respiratory Medicine
University of Florence
Florence, Italy
gscano@unifi.it

Arnaud Scherpereel
Faculté de Médecine, Université de
Lille Nord de France, CHRU de Lille,
and INSERM unit 1019, CIIL, Institut
Pasteur de Lille
Lille, France
arnaud.scherpereel@chru-lille.fr

Paul Schneider
DRK Kliniken Berlin
Thoracic Surgery
Berlin, Germany
p.schneider@drk-kliniken-berlin.de

Bernd Schönhofer
Abteilung für Pneumologie und
Internistische Intensivmedizin
Krankenhaus Oststadt-Heidehaus
Klinikum Region Hannover
Hanover, Germany
Bernd.Schoenhofer@t-online.de

Macé M. Schuurmans
University Hospital
Zurich, Switzerland
mschuurmans@me.com

Martina Sester
Dept of Transplant and Infection
Immunology
Institute of Virology
University of the Saarland
Homburg, Germany
Martina.Sester@uniklinikum-
saarland.de

Pallav L. Shah
Royal Brompton Hospital
London, UK
pallav.shah@ic.ac.uk

Nikolaos M. Siafakas
Dept of Thoracic Medicine
Medical School
University of Crete
Heraklion, Greece
siafak@med.uoc.gr

Torben Sigsgaard
Aarhus University
Aarhus, Denmark
Sigsgaard@dadlnet.dk

Marzia Simoni
Pulmonary Environmental
Epidemiology Unit
Institute of Clinical Physiology
National Research Council
Pisa, Italy
marzia_simoni@libero.it

Gérald Simonneau
National Reference Center for
Pulmonary Hypertension Hôpital
Antoine Béclère
Paris, France
France
gerald.simonneau@abc.aphp.fr

Giovanni Sotgiu
Epidemiology and Medical Statistics
Unit
Department of Biomedical Sciences,
University of Sassari
Sassari, Italy
gsotgiu@uniss.it

Paolo Spagnolo
Centre for Rare Lung Disease
Dept of Medical and Surgical
Sciences
University of Modena and Reggio
Emilia
Modena, Italy
paolo.spagnolo@unimore.it

Antonio Spanevello
Pneumology Unit, Fondazione Sal-
vatore Maugeri, IRCCS Tradate, and
Dept of Clinical and
Experimental Medicine, University of
Insubria, Varese, Italy
antonio.spanevello@fsm.it

Nick ten Hacken
University Medical Center Groningen
Groningen, the Netherlands
n.h.t.ten.hacken@umcg.nl

Einar Thorsen
University of Bergen
Bergen, Norway
einar.thorsen@helse-bergen.no

Pietro Torricelli
Division of Radiology
Dept of Diagnostic and Imaging
Services
University of Modena and Reggio
Emilia
Modena, Italy
pietro.torricelli@unimore.it

Thierry Troosters
Respiratory Rehabilitation and
Respiratory division, University
Hospital Leuven, and Faculty of
Kinesiology and Rehabilitation
Sciences, Dept of Rehabilitation
Sciences, KU Leuven
Leuven, Belgium
Thierry.Troosters@med.kuleuven.be

Amanda Tufman
Division of Respiratory Medicine
and Thoracic Oncology, Hospitals of
Ludwig-Maximilians-University, and
Thoracic Oncology Centre of Munich
Munich, Germany
Amanda.Tufman@med.uni-
muenchen.de

Panagiota Tzani
Department of Experimental and
Clinical Medicine
University of Parma
Parma, Italy
panagiotat@yahoo.com

Eleni G. Tzortzaki
Dept of Thoracic Medicine
Medical School
University of Crete
Heraklion, Greece
tzortzaki@med.uoc.gr

Davide Vallese
Fondazione Salvatore Maugeri
IRCCS
Veruno, Italy
vallese.dav@gmail.com

Paul Van Houtte
Dept of Radiation Oncology
Institut Jules Bordet
Université Libre de Bruxelles
Brussels, Belgium
paul.vanhoutte@bordet.be

Peter van Luijk
University Medical Center Groningen
University of Groningen
Groningen, the Netherlands
p.van.luijk@umcg.nl

Hans Van Remoortel
Faculty of Kinesiology and
Rehabilitation Sciences
Dept of Rehabilitation Sciences
KU Leuven
Leuven, Belgium
hans.vanremoortel@faber.kuleuven.
be

Paul E. Van Schil
Dept of Thoracic and Vascular
Surgery
Antwerp University Hospital
Antwerp, Belgium
Paul.VanSchil@uza.be

Johan Vansteenkiste
Respiratory Oncology Unit
Dept of Pulmonology
University Hospital Leuven
Leuven, Belgium
johan.vansteenkiste@uzleuven.be

Johny A. Verschakelen
University Hospitals Leuven
Leuven, Belgium
Johny.Verschakelen@uzleuven.be

Andrea Vianello
Respiratory Pathophysiology and
Intensive Care Division
University City Hospital of Padua
Padua, Italy
avianello@qubisoft.it

Chiara Vicari
Fondazione Salvatore Maugeri
IRCCS
Veruno, Italy
chiaravicari@libero.it

Giovanni Viegi
Pulmonary Environmental
Epidemiology Unit, Institute of
Clinical Physiology, National
Research Council, Pisa and
A. Monroy Institute of Biomedicine
and Molecular Immunology, National
Research Council, Palermo, Italy
viegig@ifc.cnr.it

Duccio Volterrani
Nuclear Medicine
University of Pisa
Pisa, Italy
duccio.volterrani@med.unipi.it

Florian von Groote-Bidlingmaier
Division of Pulmonology
Dept of Medicine
University of Stellenbosch and
Tygerberg Academic Hospital
Cape Town, South Africa
florianv@sun.ac.za

Susan A. Ward
Human Bio-Energetics Research
Centre
Crickhowell, UK
saward@dsl.pipex.com

Jadwiga A. Wedzicha
Academic Unit of Respiratory
Medicine
University College London
London, UK
w.wedzicha@ucl.ac.uk

Athol U. Wells
Interstitial Lung Disease Unit
Royal Brompton Hospital
London, UK
Athol.Wells@rbht.nhs.uk

Tobias Welte
Dept of Respiratory Medicine
Hannover Medical School
Hanover, Germany
Welte.Tobias@mh-hannover.de

Brian J. Whipp[†]

Nathalie Wirth
University of Nancy Henri Poincaré
Nancy, France
n.wirth@chu-nancy.fr

Mark Woodhead
Dept of Respiratory Medicine
Manchester Royal Infirmary
Manchester, UK
mark.woodhead@cmft.nhs.uk

Andrea Zanini
Pneumology Unit, Fondazione
Salvatore Maugeri, IRCCS, Tradate,
Italy and Dept of Clinical and
Experimental Medicine, University of
Insubria, Varese, Italy
andrea.zanini@fsm.it

Jean-Pierre Zellweger
Swiss Lung Association
Berne, Switzerland
zellwegerjp@swissonline.ch

Eleftherios Zervas
7th Pulmonary Dept
Athens Chest Hospital
Athens, Greece
lefzervas@yahoo.gr

Gernot Zissel
Dept of Pneumology
University Medical Centre Freiburg
Freiburg, Germany
gernot.zissel@uniklinik-freiburg.de

Preface

'To study the phenomenon of disease without books is to sail an uncharted sea, while to study books without patients is not to go to sea at all.' 'Too many men slip early out of the habit of studious reading, and yet that is essential.'

William Osler

Eight years ago, the ERS School started a very ambitious project to harmonise education in respiratory medicine for European specialists (HERMES). A preliminary survey among 29 European countries showed considerable variation in postgraduate training. Based on these findings, the ERS School developed a range of consensus documents: a core syllabus describing the competencies required, a curriculum of recommendations indicating how competencies should be taught and learned, an accreditation methodology for training centres, and a voluntary European examination to assess whether specialists have acquired the knowledge-based component of competence. The *Handbook*, together with a vast array of educational material, such as lectures, articles published in *Breathe* and the *European Respiratory Monograph*, and other lectures and courses, all available on the ERS School website, together comprise an unrivalled educational resource for anyone preparing for the European Examination in Adult Respiratory Medicine.

The first edition of the *ERS Handbook of Respiratory Medicine* was published in 2010 with the aim of providing state-of-the-art summaries in all areas of respiratory medicine. This second edition of the *Handbook* has been extensively peer review and revisited, and includes new sections on

- cytology of the lung
- HRCT of the chest
- long-term ventilation
- opportunistic infections in the immunocompromised host
- the pharmacology of asthma and COPD
- HRCT in the diagnosis of interstitial lung disease
- pathology and molecular biology of lung cancer
- palliative care

The *Handbook* is a comprehensive, easily accessible source of the essentials of respiratory medicine for senior medical staff requiring revalidation, and nursing and allied healthcare professionals at all levels who wish to keep their knowledge up to date. All readers can be assured that as they set sail to manage patients across the spectrum of respiratory disorders, they are armed with the best information, access to multiple-choice questions to check their knowledge, and a source guide for more in-depth study.

We are particularly indebted to the ERS School Committee, the ERS Publications Office who curated the entire contents of the *Handbook*, and all the contributors.

Paolo Palange, Anita K. Simonds
Chief Editors

Get more from this Handbook

By buying the *ERS Handbook of Respiratory Medicine*, you also gain access to the electronic version of the book, as well as an accredited online CME test.

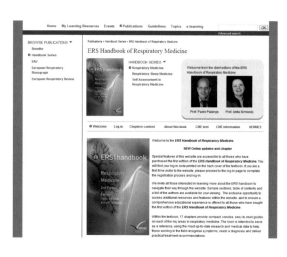

To log in, simply visit **www.ersnet.org/handbook** and enter the unique code printed on inside of the front cover of the book. Once logged in, you'll be able to download the entire book in PDF or EPUB format, to read on your computer or mobile device.

You'll also be able to take the online CME test. This handbook has been accredited by the European Board for Accreditation in Pneumology (EBAP) for 18 CME credits.

Also available from the ERS

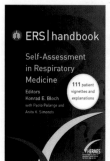

ERS Handbook: Self-Assessment in Respiratory Medicine
Edited by Konrad E. Bloch, Paolo Palange and Anita K. Simonds

Self-Assessment in Respiratory Medicine is an invaluable tool for any practitioner of adult respiratory medicine. The 111 multiple-choice questions cover the full breadth of the specialty, using clinical vignettes that test not only readers' knowledge but their ability to apply it in daily practice.

To buy a copy of this *Handbook* for €50 (€40 for ERS members) plus postage, please contact **sales@ersj.org.uk**

List of abbreviations

(C)HF	(Congestive) heart failure
AHI	Apnoea–hypopnoea index
AIDS	Acquired immunodeficiency syndrome
BMI	Body mass index
CF	Cystic fibrosis
COPD	Chronic obstructive pulmonary disease
CPAP	Continuous positive airway pressure
CT	Computed tomography
ECG	Electrocardiogram
ENT	Ear, nose and throat
FEV_1	Forced expiratory volume in 1 s
FVC	Forced vital capacity
Hb	Haemoglobin
HIV	Human immunodeficiency virus
HRCT	High-resolution computed tomography
K_{CO}	Transfer coefficient of the lung for carbon monoxide
MRI	Magnetic resonance imaging
NIV	Noninvasive ventilation
OSA(S)	Obstructive sleep apnoea (syndrome)
P_aCO_2	Arterial carbon dioxide tension
P_aO_2	Arterial oxygen tension
PCR	Polymerase chain reaction
$P_{tc}CO_2$	Transcutaneous carbon dioxide tension
S_aO_2	Arterial oxygen saturation
S_pO_2	Arterial oxygen saturation measured by pulse oximetry
TB	Tuberculosis
TLC	Total lung capacity
T_{LCO}	Transfer factor for the lung for carbon monoxide
V'_E	Minute ventilation

Genetics

Gernot Zissel

Genetics addresses the composition, function and transmission of inherited entities (genes) summing up to the genome of an individual. Generally, the term 'gene' is understood as a unit coding for a single RNA that gives rise to a single and specific protein. However, due to alternative splicing, one gene may code for different proteins. There are also genes not coding for proteins but for catalytic RNAs (tRNA, rRNA) or regulatory RNAs (microRNA (miRNA)). The genotype is the specific composition of genes of an individual that influences its phenotype. However, in contrast to the genotype, which is simply inherited, a phenotype is shaped by epigenetic phenomena, environment, climate, nutrition and other external factors.

Key points

- A few respiratory diseases, such as CF and α1-Pi deficiency, are single-gene conditions.

- A large range of respiratory diseases, including asthma, COPD, sarcoidosis, IPF and primary pulmonary hypertension, may have a genetic background.

- Non-harmful gene variants can nonetheless confer susceptibility to conditions such as chronic beryllium disease.

- The role of epigenetic regulatory mechanisms in respiratory disease is likely to be very significant.

Genes are transcribed to RNA and subsequently translated into proteins. Genes do not code for 'diseases'. Every genetic disease is based on an altered or missing protein. Because we are all equipped with a double set of chromosomes, in the vast majority of cases, a dysfunctional gene is corrected by its counterpart with normal function. A deficiency occurs only when the respective gene is dysfunctional on both chromosomes, or the gene product is either missing or does not perform its task.

Diseases caused by the alteration of a single gene with relevance for pulmonologists are CF and α1-proteinase inhibitor (PI) deficiency (formerly α1-antitrypsin (AT) deficiency). In other diseases such a clear-cut relationship between a gene and a disease is not evident, although facts, such as geographical distribution or familial clusters, indicate a genetic background. This is the case in asthma, sarcoidosis, pulmonary fibrosis and primary pulmonary hypertension. Table 1 shows examples of mutated genes involved in respiratory disorders.

There are also numbers of gene variations that are regarded as neutral variations of the human gene pool. These variations are not harmful per se, but together with distinct external stimuli they foster the development of certain diseases. Glutamine at position 69 in the human leukocyte antigen (HLA)-DPB1 gene does not cause an illness; however, when in contact with beryllium dust, carriers of Glu69+ HLA-DPB1 are at an increased risk of developing chronic beryllium disease (CBD). Up to 97% of CBD patients are Glu69+ HLA-DPB1 positive. Another example is the lack of functional

Table 1. Examples of mutated genes involved in respiratory disorders

Disease	Gene	Gene product	Mutation(s)
CF	CFTR	Cystic fibrosis transmembrane conductance regulator	>1500
Emphysema	SERPINA1	Serpin peptidase inhibitor, clade A (α-1 antiproteinase, antitrypsin)	SNP G-342A >90% of cases
Chronic beryllium disease	HLA-DPB1	Histocompatibility antigen, DP(W2) β-chain	Glutamine at position 69
Sarcoidosis	BTNL2	Butyrophilin-like 2	rs2076530 SNP G-11084A causing premature stop codon
	ANXA11	Annexin A11	rs1049550 SNP C→T, arginine to cysteine
	TNF	TNF	SNP G-308A
	TLR	TLR	SNPs in various TLR genes influence disease course
Cancer		c-Myc	Promoter translocation
	Ras	Family of GTPases	Various SNPs induce permanent activation
	EGFR	Epidermal growth factor receptor	Deletions, SNPs leading to over expression and permanent activation

SNP: single-nucleotide polymorphism.

receptors for interferon-γ or interleukin-12. In these cases the individuals grow up normally and reach adolescence; however, after the BCG (Bacillus Calmette–Guérin) vaccination or when they encounter environmental mycobacteria (e.g. Mycobacterium fortuitum, Mycobacterium chelonae), these individuals develop severe and sometimes fatal disease.

Epigenetics and regulatory genes

The genome is not a static blueprint of the phenotype as it was regarded in the past. Several mechanisms of genetic regulation, epigenetics and regulatory genes, have been discovered in recent years. The term epigenetics describes a wide field of DNA and histone modifications that contribute to the regulation of gene transcription. One of these modifications is the methylation of the nucleobase cytosine. Cytosine is methylated only in CG 'islands'; single cytosines are not methylated. Cytosine methylation inhibits binding of RNA polymerases to the gene,

which is subsequently not translated. Cytosine methylation is important in promoter silencing and inactivation of the X chromosome.

Histone modifications are an additional form of epigenetic regulation. Histones are protein spheres that bind DNA. There are four different histones, two of each histone together with the bound DNA build a nucleosome, the core of a chromosome. Histones can be modified, mainly by acetylation, methylation and various other mechanisms. Generally, acetylation of histones opens the nucleosome structure and the gene becomes accessible for transcription. In contrast, histone methylation leads to the accumulation of additional histone proteins in turn leading to a compacted nucleosome and subsequently inhibiting gene transcription.

The miRNAs are short, highly conserved, noncoding RNAs that bind to 3′-untranslated regions (3′-UTR) of mRNAs.

Incomplete binding leads to silencing and complete binding to degradation of the RNA. In fact, miRNAs are powerful regulators. Activation of transcription factors, such as nuclear factor (NF)-κB leads to the transcription of a variety of immune mediator genes. Simultaneous activation of miRNAs suppresses certain mediators, giving rise to a specific pattern of mediator activation. miRNAs are of strong importance in cancer and pulmonary fibrosis; however, one might expect that transcriptional regulation by miRNAs is also important in other diseases. The pattern of miRNAs expressed in several diseases and tumours is highly specific and might be used as a biomarker.

Genetics in CF

CF is caused by the dysfunction of the cystic fibrosis transmembrane conductance regulator (CFTR) gene, which codes for a chloride channel. However, although in all CF patients the CFTR is dysfunctional, there are >1500 different mutations known to affect CFTR and lead to a dysfunctional chloride channel. CF inheritance follows an autosomal recessive heredity, *i.e.* the disease becomes manifest only when CFTR genes on both chromosomes are mutated, albeit not necessarily by the same mutation. The most common defect is the deletion of a phenylalanine at position 508 (ΔF508), which is responsible for up to 70% of all CF cases. Interestingly, there is a marked difference in the frequency of this disease in different populations. It is most common in Caucasians (1:2000 being highest in Scotland and the Faroe Islands (1:500)) but lower in descendants from Africa (1:15 000); and lowest in Asians (1:30 000). CFTR mutations can be grouped into classes based on their functional consequences on the CFTR within the cell: CFTR is either not synthesised, inadequately processed, not regulated, shows abnormal conductance, discloses partially defective production or shows accelerated degradation.

Genetics of proteinase inhibitors

The PI α1-antitrypsin belongs to a family of serine PIs (serpins) and blocks serine proteases, such as neutrophil elastase, cathepsin G and proteinase 3, all released by neutrophils and is, therefore, renamed as α1-PI. The lack of α1-PI leads to an incomplete or absent containment of proteinases resulting in severe organ damage (e.g. emphysema), mostly in the lung.

There are several known mutations in the α1-PI gene, such as base substitutions, in-frame deletions, frame-shift mutations and exon deletions. More than 90% of cases are caused by single amino acid exchange at position 342 (glycine to lysine), which is called Z mutation. The Z mutation results in a structural alteration that inhibits post-translational modifications and secretion. Patients bearing the Z allele demonstrate <15% of the normal α1-PI level in serum, which additionally seems to be non-functional.

The gene frequency of the Z allele is rather common in Europe, with up to 4% of the population being heterozygotic. However, the frequency declines to <1% in southern Europe. The lowest frequency is found in African–Americans (0.4%).

Genetics in interstitial lung diseases

There is some indication that interstitial lung diseases, such as sarcoidosis, CBD or idiopathic pulmonary fibrosis (IPF), are based on a specific genetic background. Familial clusters are seen in sarcoidosis and IPF. In Europe, sarcoidosis frequency increases from South to North. This might also be a matter of climate, as the same distribution is seen in Japan. However, the Swedish population encounters the highest prevalence in Europe (55–64 per 100 000). In contrast, in the Finnish population living at the same latitude, the prevalence is just half of the Swedish (28 per 100 000). This difference points to a strong genetic background in the pathogenesis of sarcoidosis.

An inherited pre-disposition for sarcoidosis is also indicated by an increased risk of sarcoidosis in close relatives of patients. The percentage of patients with a positive family history ranges from 2.7% in Spain to 17% in African–Americans. Analysis of familial sarcoidosis suggests that multiple small or moderate genetic effects cause a predisposition for sarcoidosis.

Genes of high interest are the HLA class II antigens. Although some of these linkages are largely dependent on the population investigated, several associations seem to be preserved, e.g. HLA-DRB1*03 associates with spontaneous resolution and mild disease, as demonstrated in Swedish, Polish, Croatian and Czech populations.

Using different methods, a variety of candidate genes were identified and found to be associated with the susceptibility or the natural course of the disease. This included genes for co-stimulatory molecules (e.g. butyrophilin-like 2 (BTNL2)), genes involved in cell cycle (e.g. annexin A11 (ANXA11)), and genes involved in immune regulation (e.g. CD40), mediators (e.g. tumour necrosis factor (TNF)-α (TNFA2) or Toll-like receptors (TLR)). These genes may alter the reactivity of the respective cells to external stimuli which subsequently initiate an inadequate immune response.

Angiotensin-converting enzyme (ACE) is often used in the diagnosis and clinical monitoring of sarcoidosis. However, serum levels of ACE (sACE) are highly variable, which impairs the clinical use of ACE as a marker. The variability of sACE is based on a deletion/insertion in intron 16 of the ACE gene. The homozygote deletion variant is associated with higher sACE, whereas homozygote insertion is associated with lower levels. Heterozygotes exhibit intermediate values. Therefore, in populations of Caucasian origin, the knowledge of the zygosity of the deletion/insertion variants allows the application of genotype-corrected reference values of sACE, which leads to an improvement of the clinical application of this marker. However, this is not applicable in populations of African origin; the ACE gene in these populations is much more polymorphic and sACE levels are not linked with the deletion/insertion polymorphism.

Familial pulmonary fibrosis is frequently linked with two mutations in the surfactant protein C (SP-C) gene resulting either in a splice deletion of exon 4 in a SP-C variant that cannot be processed and accumulates as pro-SP-C in the cell causing cell stress and apoptosis. The pathological pattern of fibrosis is in both forms consistent with non-specific interstitial pneumonitis in younger patients and usual interstitial pneumonia in the elderly. A recent report points to a mutation in the telomerase reverse transcriptase (TERT) causing short ends in the telomeres and bone marrow hypocellularity. But also mutations in genes regulating cell cycle like TP53 and CDKN1A are found to influence survival times in IPF.

Genetics in asthma

There is a plethora of work related to the genetics of asthma. The idea of a genetic basis for asthma is supported by the fact that there are familial clusters of asthma and differences of asthma frequency in different populations (highest at the South Atlantic island Tristan da Cunha affecting >20% of the population). However, no single gene is responsible for the development or the clinical course of asthma; instead, several genes are regarded as risk genes for developing asthma. The gene products of these genes are involved in T-cell activation, cytokine release and balance, epithelial function and repair or smooth muscle contractility. Again, new genes involved in asthma susceptibility might be expected.

Nevertheless, although there are predisposing genes in asthma, the influence of lifestyle on the development of asthma is also evident. There is a clear increase in asthma incidences in developing countries. Therefore, asthma might be an elucidating example for the complex genotype/phenotype relationship.

4

Genetics in cancer

Mutations and epigenetic modifications are passed to the offspring as far as the germ cells are concerned. However, there are also mutations outside the germ line: so-called somatic mutations. As these mutations accumulate over years, a growing organism resembles merely a genetic mosaic rather than a unique clone of the germ cell it is derived from.

Most of these somatic mutations are silent and either do not cause any defect or are corrected by its respective counterpart. However, there is a variety of somatic mutations that finally cause tumour genesis. An example of such a somatic mutation involved in cancer is a mutation in the MYC gene, leading to the over-expression of c-Myc. The regulatory protein c-Myc binds to enhancer boxes in regulatory gene sequences inducing enhanced gene expression. In addition, it recruits histone acetylases leading to histone hyperacetylation. Approximately 15% of the human genes are affected by c-Myc regulation. Over-expression of c-Myc is an important factor in the pathogenesis genesis of small cell lung cancer (SCLC). However, no single event, like the mutation of c-Myc, is responsible for tumour genesis. In general, tumours like SCLC or nonsmall cell lung cancer present with a large variety of genetic alterations, like DNA methylation, alternative splicing, histone modifications or altered miRNA patterns, which all might be involved in oncogenesis.

As genetic tools become more common, the analysis of the individual pathways involved in the individual cancer pathogenesis might help to develop individual targets for therapy.

Conclusion

Genetic aspects have to be considered in all areas of pulmonary medicine. As physicians are faced with phenotypes, the underlying degree of genetic influence is not always obvious. The knowledge of the genotype causing a respective phenotype might be a promising tool to predict outcome or therapeutic options, and would enable individual genotype/phenotype-based therapies.

Further reading

- Al-Muhsen S, et al. (2008). The genetic heterogeneity of mendelian susceptibility to mycobacterial diseases. *J Allergy Clin Immunol*; 122: 1043–1051.
- Biller H, et al. (2006). Genotype-corrected reference values for serum angiotensin-converting enzyme. *Eur Respir J*; 28: 1085–1090.
- Blumenthal MN (2012). Genetic epigenetic, and environmental factors in asthma and allergy. *Ann Allergy Asthma Immunol*; 108: 69–73.
- Bogunia-Kubik K, et al. (2001). HLA-DRB1*03, DRB1*11 or DRB1*12 and their respective DRB3 specificities in clinical variants of sarcoidosis. *Tissue Antigens*; 57: 87–90.
- Coakley RJ, et al. (2001). α1-antitrypsin deficiency: biological answers to clinical questions. *Am J Med Sci*; 321: 33–41.
- Cottle LE (2011). Mendelian susceptibility to mycobacterial diseases. *Clin Genet*; 79: 17–22.
- Gooptu B, et al. (2009). Mechanisms of emphysema in α1-antitrypsin deficiency. *molecular and cellular insights. Eur Respir J*; 34: 475–488.
- Grunewald J. (2010). Review role of genetics in susceptibility and outcome of sarcoidosis. *Semin Respir Crit Care Med*; 31: 380–389.
- Kass DJ (2011). Evolving genomic approaches to idiopathic pulmonary fibrosis: moving beyond gene. *Clin Transl Sci*; 4: 372–379.
- Lommatzsch ST (2009). Genetics of cystic fibrosis. *Semin Respir Crit Care Med*; 30: 531–538.
- Maier LA, et al. (2003). Influence of MHC class II in susceptibility to beryllium sensitization and chronic beryllium disease. *J Immunol*; 171: 6910–6918.
- Müller-Quernheim J, et al. (2008). Genetics of sarcoidosis. *Clin Chest Med*; 29: 391–414.
- Postma DS (2009). Genetics of asthma where are we and where do we go? *Proc Am Thorac Soc*; 6: 283–287.
- Rowe SM, et al. (2005). Cystic fibrosis. *N Engl J Med*; 352: 1992–2001.
- Selroos O. Differences in sarcoidosis around the world: what they tell us. *In*: Baughman RP, ed. Sarcoidosis. New York, Informa, 2006; pp. 47–64.

- Thomas AQ, *et al.* (2002). Heterozygosity for a surfactant protein C gene mutation associated with usual interstitial pneumonitis and cellular nonspecific interstitial pneumonitis in one kindred. *Am J Respir Crit Care Med*; 165: 1322–1328.

- Turcios NL (2005). Cystic fibrosis an overview. *J Clin Gastroenterol*; 39: 307–317.
- Wen J, *et al.* (2011). Genetic and epigenetic changes in lung carcinoma and their clinical implications. *Mod Pathol*; 24: 932–943.

Molecular biology of the lung

Melanie Königshoff and Oliver Eickelberg

Understanding lung disease at the cellular and molecular level is crucial to developing new approaches for the diagnosis, treatment and prevention of lung disease. Although our knowledge at the molecular level is steadily increasing, we still have a limited understanding of the molecular events underlying lung diseases, which is reflected by very few therapies targeting specific defects.

The field of molecular biology focuses on the interactions between various systems of a cell and between cells, and particularly includes:

- gene structure, expression, replication and recombination
- structure, function, modification, and processing of proteins and nucleic acids
- cellular and developmental biology
- genetics, structure and growth cycles of viruses, bacteria and bacteriophages

The following paragraphs focus on selected (signalling) molecules and structures, all of which are altered in various lung disease and are important topics in the field of molecular biological research in respiratory medicine.

Key points

Major features of lung diseases are:

- altered deposition of extracellular matrix,
- impaired surfactant metabolism,
- Distorted endogenous defence mechanisms.

The extracellular matrix

Components of the extracellular matrix (ECM) surround and support the cell and cell–cell interaction. In the lung, the ECM around the conducting airways, alveolar and interstitial cells, and the vascular system has a major impact on lung architecture and function, particularly gas exchange. All lung cell types interact and signal through the ECM *via* adhesion molecules, surface receptors or growth factors (Suki *et al.*, 2008).

The lung fibroblast is the main producer of pulmonary ECM, which consists of:

- collagens
- elastins
- proteoglycans

The interstitium of the lung parenchyma contains mostly collagen types I and III, which are mainly responsible for tensile strength.

The pulmonary ECM is subjected to a continuous turnover of >10% of the total ECM per day. Thus, a dynamic equilibrium between synthesis and degradation of the pulmonary ECM maintains a physiological balance. This balance is tightly controlled by three regulatory mechanisms: 1) *de novo* synthesis and deposition of ECM components such as collagens, mainly by interstitial fibroblasts; 2) proteolytic degradation of existing ECM by matrix metalloproteinases (MMPs), a family of zinc-dependent enzymes; and 3) inhibition of MMP activity by specific endogenous antiproteases, the tissue inhibitors of metalloproteinases (TIMPs) (Mocchegiani *et al.*, 2011).

Excessive or inappropriate expression of MMPs and impaired expression of TIMPs are related to the pathogenesis of many chronic lung diseases, such as MMP-12 in emphysema or MMP-7 in lung fibrosis (Churg et al., 2011).

The impact of the altered matrix or cell–matrix interaction within the diseased lung represents an active area of investigation. While most research in the past focused on the effect of signalling molecules and pathways on matrix deposition and turnover, recent studies aimed to understand how the lung matrix influences cell differentiation and behaviour, and, subsequently, signal transduction (Fernandéz et al., 2012).

The surfactant system

The maintenance of normal lung function throughout the life of an organism is ensured largely by alveolar epithelial cells, which form a tight functional barrier essential for gas exchange. The alveolar epithelium is composed of alveolar type I (ATI) and type II (ATII) cells. These cells produce and secrete components of the ECM and growth factors thereof, which facilitates restoration of the interstitium and, subsequently, functional alveolar structure. ATII cells serve as progenitor cells for ATI cells, which largely cover the alveolus and are the primary cell responsible for gas exchange. ATII cells are cuboidal secretory cells mainly responsible for surfactant secretion (Herzog et al., 2008). Pulmonary surfactant is a complex mixture of phospholipids and proteins, with surfactant protein (SP)-A, SP-B and SP-C constituting 10% of surfactant. Its main role is to reduce surface tension in the alveoli following the onset of breathing, thereby leading to lung expansion. Mechanical stretch of the lung forces the secretion of lamellar bodies, the intracellular storage granules of surfactant, which form tubular myelin. The surfactant film stabilises the alveolar–air interface with low surface tension and prevents lung collapse. SP-B and SP-C are the main protein components. Following secretion, both surfactant proteins and lipids are recycled by the respiratory epithelium (Marraro et al., 2008).

Surfactant abnormalities have been described in many infant and adult lung diseases, such as respiratory distress syndrome, bronchiolitis, COPD and interstitial lung disease.

Defense and clearance mechanisms

SP-A and SP-D are involved in innate host defence of the lung. In addition, antimicrobial peptides, such as defensins, cathelicidins and or lactoferrin, are present in the airway and prevent infection. Moreover, cellular defense mechanisms include macrophage- and neutrophil-mediated cytokine release, such as interleukin (IL)-1, IL-8, tumour necrosis factor (TNF)-α and granulocyte-macrophage colony-stimulating factor (GM-CSF) (Suzuki et al., 2008).

Pulmonary alveolar proteinosis is caused by disruption of GM-CSF signalling. Loss of GM-CSF signalling in macrophages results in an impaired ability to catabolise surfactant proteins. Abnormal surfactant accumulation leads to respiratory insufficiency.

Mucociliary clearance represents the primary physiological defense mechanism. The ciliated airway cells clear mucus, which is produced by secretory cells, by forcing the mucus toward the larynx for elimination. Impaired mucociliary clearance is the main feature of CF.

The transforming growth factor-β pathway

The transforming growth factor (TGF)-β superfamily is critically involved in embryonic development, organogenesis and tissue homeostasis (Bartram et al., 2004). TGF-β superfamily members act as multifunctional regulators of cell growth and differentiation. The TGF-β superfamily includes >40 members, including the various isoforms of TGF-β itself. Three different TGF-β isoforms have been characterised so far: TGF-β1, TGF-β2 and TGF-β3. TGF-β1 is the most important isoform in the cardiopulmonary system, as it is ubiquitously expressed and secreted by several cell types, such as endothelial, epithelial and smooth muscle cells, as well as fibroblasts and most cells of the immune system. TGF-β is secreted in covalent association with the latent TGF-β binding protein, thus providing a reservoir in the ECM.

8

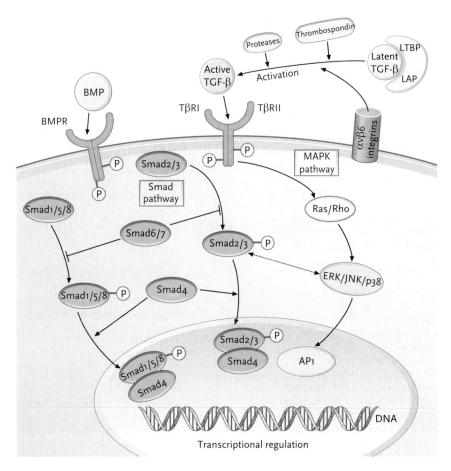

Figure 1. The TGF-β pathway. LTBP: latent TGF-β binding protein; LAP: latency-associated peptide; TβR: TGF-β receptor; P: phosphoryl group; MAPK: mitogen-activated protein kinase; ERK: extracellular signal-regulated kinase; JNK: Janus kinase; AP: activator protein; BMP: bone morphogenetic protein; BMPR: BMP receptor. Reproduced and modified from Königshoff M et al. (2009) with permission from the publisher.

For active signalling, TGF-β needs to be cleaved from the complex by a mechanism that involves various proteases, such as plasmin or MMPs, as well as interaction with integrins. Active TGF-β ligands bind to the type II TGF-β receptor, which subsequently forms heterotetrameric complexes with the type I TGF-β receptor. Subsequent transphosphorylation of the type I receptor results in recruitment of specific intracellular signal mediators called Smad proteins. Smad2 and Smad3 have been shown to be phosphorylated by the type I receptor, followed by complex formation with Smad4 and, finally,

nuclear translocation and regulation of gene transcription. These receptor-regulated Smads (Smad2 and Smad3), in combination with the co-Smad Smad4, positively regulate TGF-β-induced effects, while the inhibitory Smads (Smad6 and Smad7) negatively regulate TGF-β signalling (fig. 1).

Increased TGF-β signalling is the key pathophysiological mechanism that leads to fibrotic lung disease, which is characterised by an increase in activated (myo)fibroblasts and excessive deposition of ECM.

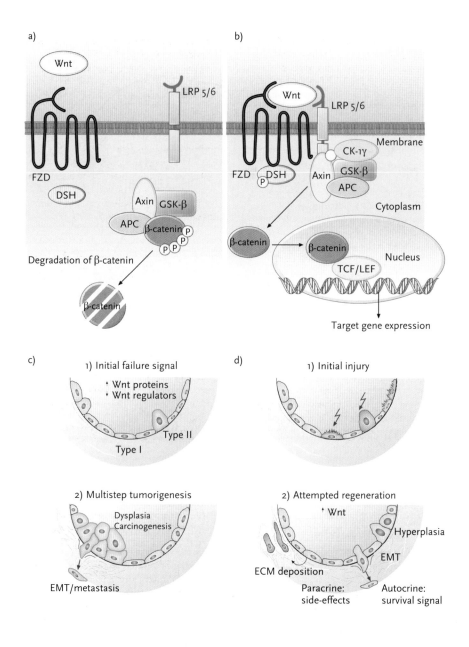

Figure 2. The Wnt/β-catenin pathway. The pathway is shown in the a) 'off' and b) 'on' states, and in lung c) cancer and d) fibrosis. DSH: Dishevelled; GSK: glycogen synthase kinase; APC: adenomatous polyposis coli protein; P: phosphoryl group; CK: casein kinase; TCF: T-cell-specific transcription factor; LEF: lymphoid enhancer-binding factor family protein; EMT: epithelial–mesenchymal transition. Reproduced and modified from Königshoff M et al. (2010) with permission from the publisher.

Furthermore, there is emerging interest in the role of TGF-β in the pathogenesis of COPD, particularly since genetic studies have demonstrated an association of gene polymorphisms of the TGF-β superfamily with COPD. In addition, increased expression of TGF-β1 in COPD was reported, suggesting an impact of TGF-β signalling in the development and progression of COPD (Königshoff et al., 2009).

The Wnt/β-catenin pathway

The Wnt/β-catenin signalling pathway was originally identified as a developmental signalling pathway. It constitutes a large family of secreted glycoproteins that signal via a variety of membrane-bound receptors. Wnt ligands bind to the membrane receptors Frizzled (FZD) and low-density lipoprotein receptor-related protein (LRP)5/6, resulting in the phosphorylation of LRP6, which subsequently leads to the recruitment of cytosolic proteins that are part of the so-called β-catenin destruction complex. Subsequently, the central mediator β-catenin is dephosphorylated and its degradation attenuated. Accumulated β-catenin then undergoes nuclear translocation and regulates target gene expression via interaction with members of the T-cell-specific transcription factor/lymphoid enhancer-binding factor family (fig. 2) (Moon et al., 2004).

Impaired Wnt/β-catenin signalling has been implicated in a variety of chronic lung diseases, such lung cancer, fibrosis and COPD/emphysema. In particular, active Wnt/β-catenin signalling has been linked to lung epithelial cell repair and survival mechanisms.

Importantly, Wnt/β-catenin signalling is tightly regulated during lung homeostasis. Several Wnt inhibitors, such as Dickkopf and secreted FZD-related proteins, are differentially expressed during chronic lung disease, thereby impacting proper Wnt/β-catenin signalling (Königshoff et al., 2009).

Nuclear factor-κB

Nuclear factor (NF)-κB is a ubiquitous transcription factor present in all cell types. In its resting stage, this factor resides in the cytoplasm as a heterotrimer consisting of p50, p65 and the inhibitory protein IκBα. Upon activation, the IκBα protein undergoes phosphorylation, ubiquitination and degradation. p50 and p65 are then released for translocation to the nucleus, bind specific DNA sequences present in the promoters of target genes and initiate transcription. IκBα kinase (IKK) is responsible for the initial phosphorylation. Several different kinases have been shown to activate IKK, such as Akt, MEKK1 and protein kinase C. In the nucleus, NF-κB induces the expression of a variety of genes, particularly mediators of inflammation, cell proliferation, metastasis and angiogenesis (Sun et al., 2008).

Many potentially noxious substances related to lung disease, such as cigarette smoke, radiation, chemotherapeutic agents, cytokines and growth factors, activate NF-κB, and increased NF-κB signalling has been associated with COPD and asthma (Edwards et al., 2009).

Further reading

- Bartram U, et al. (2004). The role of transforming growth factor beta in lung development and disease. Chest; 125: 754–765.
- Churg A, et al. (2012). Matrix metalloproteinases in COPD. Eur Respir J; 39: 197–209.
- Edwards MR, et al. (2009). Targeting the NF-κB pathway in asthma and chronic obstructive pulmonary disease. Pharmacol Ther; 121: 1–13.
- Fernandez IE, et al. (2012). New cellular and molecular mechanisms of lung injury and fibrosis in idiopathic pulmonary fibrosis. Lancet; 380: 680–688.
- Herzog EL, et al. (2008). Knowns and unknowns of the alveolus. Proc Am Thorac Soc; 5: 778–782.
- Königshoff M, et al. (2009). TGF-β signaling in COPD: deciphering genetic and cellular susceptibilities for future therapeutic regimen. Swiss Med Wkly; 139: 554–563.
- Konigshoff M, et al. (2010). WNT signaling in lung disease: a failure or a regeneration signal? Am J Respir Cell Mol Biol; 42: 21–31.

- Marraro GA (2008). Surfactant in child and adult pathology: is it time to review our acquisitions? *Pediatr Crit Care Med*; 9: 537–538.
- Mocchegiani E, *et al.* (2011). Metalloproteases/anti-metalloproteases imbalance in chronic obstructive pulmonary disease: genetic factors and treatment implications. *Curr Opin Pulm Med*; 17: Suppl. 1, S11–S19.
- Moon RT, *et al.* (2004). WNT and β-catenin signalling: diseases and therapies. *Nat Rev Genet*; 5: 691–701.
- Suki B, *et al.* (2008). Extracellular matrix mechanics in lung parenchymal diseases. *Respir Physiol Neurobiol*; 163: 33–43.
- Sun SC, *et al.* (2008). New insights into NF-κB regulation and function. *Trends Immunol*; 29: 469–478.
- Suzuki T, *et al.* (2008). Role of innate immune cells and their products in lung immunopathology. *Int J Biochem Cell Biol*; 40: 1348–1361.

Anatomy of the respiratory system

Pallav L. Shah

Pleura

The lungs are covered by a fine membrane known as the pleura. The parietal pleura is the outer layer and the visceral pleura is adherent to the lungs. The two are in continuity with each other and there is a very fine space between the two, the pleural cavity. The parietal pleura is described according to the surface that it is adjacent to: costovertebral, diaphragmatic, cervical and mediastinal. There are also pleural recesses where the two different pleural surfaces are situated next to each other without any intervening lung in normal respiration. The costodiaphragmatic recesses are a thin area between the costal and diaphragmatic pleura. The costomediastinal recess is between the

---

Key points

- The anatomy of the thorax can be divided broadly into the pleura, lungs, mediastinum, diaphragm and heart.

- The lungs can be further subdivided into lobes, segments, trachea and bronchi.

- The mediastinal space contains structures including the thymus gland, thoracic lymph nodes, thoracic duct, vagus nerve and autonomic nerve plexus.

- The thoracic structures include the vital organs for respiration and circulation. This section will focus on the pleura, lungs, mediastinum and diaphragm. The anatomy of the heart is not discussed.

---

costal and mediastinal pleura, and is found behind the sternum and costal cartilages.

The pleura is supplied by its regional blood vessels. Hence, the cervical pleura is supplied by branches of the subclavian artery, the costovertebral pleura by the intercostal arteries and the diaphragmatic pleura from the vascular plexus from the surface of the diaphragm. The venous drainage occurs into the corresponding veins, which then drain into the vena cava. The lymphatic drainage is into the corresponding lymph nodes, *e.g.* the intercostal lymphatics drain into the posterior lymph nodes and then into the thoracic duct. The visceral pleura is supplied by the bronchial vessels and the lymphatics drain into the intercostal and peribronchial lymphatics. The parietal pleura is supplied by the regional nerves and contains the pain fibres. The costal and peripheral aspects of the diaphragmatic pleura are supplied by the corresponding intercostal nerves, whereas the diaphragmatic and mediastinal pleura are supplied by the phrenic nerves.

Lungs

The apex of the lung extends into the thoracic inlet and on the anterior aspect lies above the first costal cartilage. On the posterior aspect, the apex of the lung is level with the neck of the first rib. At its highest position it is ~2.5 cm above the clavicle. The base of the lung is a concave structure and lies over the diaphragm. The main surface of the lung is the costal surface, which is smooth and shaped according to the chest wall. The medial surface of the lung is shaped posteriorly according to the vertebral column and medially by the heart.

The lungs are also indented by the numerous vascular structures, such as the aorta, that are in contact with them.

The right lung consists of upper, middle and lower lobes (fig. 1a). The left lung is composed of an upper and lower lobe (fig. 1b). In the right lung there are two fissures. The oblique fissure separates the lower lobe from the upper and middle lobes. The smaller horizontal fissure separates the upper and middle lobes. In the left lung, the oblique fissure separates the upper lobe from the lower lobe.

Bronchopulmonary segments

The main bronchi divide into lobar bronchi that, in turn, divide into segmental bronchi. Each divides into a structurally and functionally independent unit of tissue. The right lung consists of 10 bronchopulmonary segments: three in the upper lobe, two in the middle lobe and five in the lower lobe.

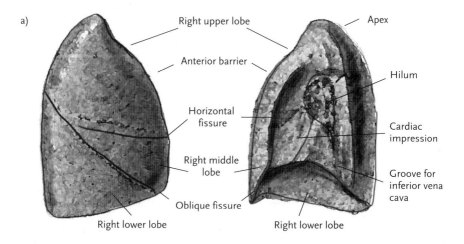

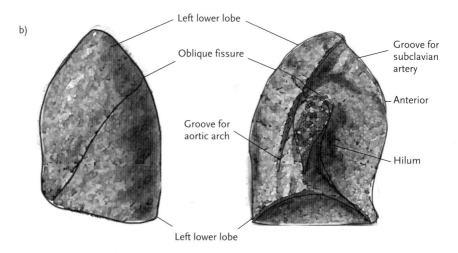

Figure 1. Medial aspect of a) right and b) left lung. © P.L. Shah.

The left lung comprises nine segments: five in the upper lobe, including two within the lingula, and four in the lower lobes. There is no true medial segment in the left lower lobe as this area is occupied by the heart.

Each bronchus continues to subdivide into smaller, narrower airways until they finally form terminal bronchioles and then respiratory bronchioles, which are devoid of cartilage. These in turn lead to several alveolar ducts, which in turn end in several alveoli. The collective structure is termed an acinus. The secondary pulmonary lobule is the smallest part of the peripheral lung bounded by connective tissue, and usually consists of three to six pulmonary acini forming a hexagonal pattern with a central artery, lymphatic and peripheral veins.

Trachea and bronchi

The trachea (figure 2) is 100 mm long and made up of anterolateral cartilage rings with a fibromuscular posterior wall. The trachea divides at the level of the fourth vertebral body (level with the aortic arch) into the right and left bronchi. The right main bronchus is ~25 mm long and divides into the right upper lobe at the level of the fifth thoracic vertebra. It then continues as the bronchus intermedius, which is ~20 mm in length. The right main bronchus is wider, shorter and more vertical than the left main bronchus and, hence, foreign bodies tend to lodge more frequently into the right main bronchus. The bronchus intermedius then branches into the middle and lower lobes. The right middle lobe is formed on the anterior aspect of the bronchus intermedius. The right lower lobe bronchus gives off a branch to the superior segment and continues to descend posterolaterally, giving off branches to the medial, anterior, lateral and posterior segments of the lower lobe.

The left main bronchus is longer, measuring ~40 mm in length, and enters the hilum of the left lung at approximately the level of the sixth thoracic vertebra. It divides into the left upper lobe and left lower lobe bronchus; the left upper lobe bronchus in turn gives off the superior division and supplies the apical posterior and anterior branches of the left

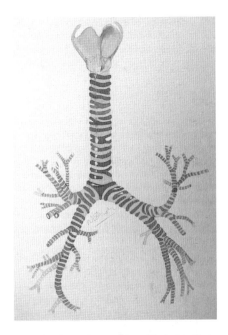

Figure 2. The trachea and bronchi. © P.L. Shah.

upper lobe and the inferior division, which supplies the superior segment of the lingula and inferior segment of the lingula. The left lower lobe descends posterolaterally and first gives off a posteriorly located branch to the apical segment of the lower lobe and then gives branches to anteromedial, lateral and posterior basal bronchi.

The trachea is supplied superiorly by branches of the inferior thyroid arteries and more inferiorly by branches of the bronchial arteries. The venous drainage tends to be towards the inferior thyroid venous plexus and the lymphatic drainage to the pre-tracheal and para-tracheal lymph nodes. The bronchi and the airways are supplied by the bronchial arteries, which originate from the systemic circulation and arise either directly from the descending thoracic aorta or indirectly *via* the intercostal arteries. The venous drainage of the airways is more complicated and consists of deep bronchial veins that communicate with pulmonary veins that drain back into the left atrium. There are also superficial bronchial veins that drain into the azygos or the intercostal veins.

The innervation of the endobronchial tree is *via* the anterior and posterior pulmonary plexus, which include branches from the vagus, recurrent laryngeal and sympathetic nerves.

Hila

The pulmonary hila join the medial aspect of the lung to the heart and the trachea. In each hilum, there are a number of structures either entering or leaving the structure. They include the main bronchi, pulmonary artery, superior pulmonary vein, inferior pulmonary vein, bronchial artery, bronchial vein, pulmonary autonomic neural plexus, lymphatics and loose connective tissue.

Pulmonary vasculature and lymphatic drainage

The pulmonary artery carries deoxygenated blood to the alveoli and the oxygenated blood then returns *via* the pulmonary veins to the left atrium. The pulmonary arteries lie anterior to the carina and the corresponding main bronchi. The artery then enters the lung *via* the hilum. On the right side, the upper lobe branch of the pulmonary arteries is anterior and lateral to the right upper lobe whereas the inferior branch of the pulmonary artery passes laterally and posterior to the lower lobe bronchus. On the left side, both upper and lower lobe pulmonary artery branches are lateral and posterior to the corresponding airways. The descending branch of the left pulmonary artery passes behind the left upper lobe and travels laterally and inferior to the left lower lobe bronchi.

There are two pulmonary veins on each side (superior and inferior pulmonary veins) that pass anterior and inferior to the pulmonary artery and bronchi. The lymphatic vessels drain into the hilar and subsequently into the tracheobronchial lymph nodes.

Mediastinum

The mediastinum is the space between the two lungs. The superior extent of the mediastinum is the thoracic inlet and the inferior extent the diaphragm. The anterior border is the sternum and the posterior border is the vertebral column. It is divided into the superior, anterior, middle and posterior mediastinum. The mediastinum contains numerous structures, such as the thymus gland, thoracic lymph nodes, thoracic duct, vagus nerve and autonomic nerve plexus.

The thymus gland lies in the superior and anterior mediastinum. The lower border is down to the fourth costal cartilage. Its blood supply is derived from a branch of the internal thoracic artery and the inferior thyroid artery. The thymic veins drain into the left brachial cephalic vein and internal thoracic veins. The lymphatic drainage is into the tracheobronchial lymph nodes.

The mediastinum lymph nodes have special significance in the staging of lung cancer. They are found in the pre-tracheal, para-tracheal, subcarinal and para-oesophageal positions. They are classified according to the International Association for the Study of Lung Cancer (IASLC) lymph node map into lymph node stations (*e.g.* station 4 is the right paratracheal lymph node). The thoracic duct starts at the lower level of the 12th thoracic vertebra and enters the mediastinum through the aortic opening of the diaphragm. It runs in the posterior aspect of the mediastinum just right of the midline between the aorta and the azygos vein. In the superior mediastinum, it ascends onto the left side adjacent to the oesophagus. It finally terminates into one of the subclavian veins or the internal jugular vein.

The vagus nerve on the right side is found lateral to the trachea and posterior medial to the right brachiocephalic vein and super vena cava. It then passes behind the right main bronchus and continues to the posterior aspect of the right atrium. Here it divides into braches, which form the pulmonary autonomic plexus. The left vagus nerve is found between the left common carotid and subclavian artery and behind the left brachiocephalic vein. It crosses the aortic arch and passes behind the left hilum. Here, it divides and forms the pulmonary plexus. The autonomic nervous plexus in the mediastinum is formed from the vagus nerve, thoracic sympathetic chain and the autonomic plexus (cardiac, oesophageal and pulmonary plexus).

The right phrenic nerve descends laterally to the super vena cava anterior to the pulmonary hilar and then along the pericardium (over the right atrium) before reaching the diaphragm. The left phrenic nerve runs anteromedially to the vagus nerve above the aortic arch and then anteriorly to the left hilum. It then runs along the pericardium (covering the left ventricle) before supplying the diaphragm.

Diaphragm

The diaphragm is a musculofibrous sheet that separates the thorax and abdomen. It has an important role in the mechanism of breathing and coughing. It has a convex upper surface and is circumferentially attached to the lower aspect of the thorax by muscle fibres that converge to a central tendon. The diaphragm has three openings within it through which pass the inferior vena cava (at the level of eighth thoracic vertebra, T8), the oesophagus (T10) and the aorta (T12). Its blood supply is from the lower five intercostal arteries, the subcostal artery and the phrenic arteries. The venous drainage is from the phrenic veins, which drain into the inferior vena cava. The diaphragm is supplied by the phrenic nerve, which primarily originates from the C4, C5

and C6 cervical nerve root (the course of which is described previously).

Development

The development of the respiratory system occurs at ~26 days of gestation with proliferation of a diverticulum that originates from the foregut. The laryngotracheal tube and main bronchi are formed first. Over the next 10 weeks, the lower conducting airways develop and, finally, the acinar structures develop. The alveoli and interstitial tissue are then formed. Alveolar development occurs from 28 weeks gestation and continues during early childhood.

Further reading

- Shah PL. Pleura, lungs, trachea and bronchi. *In:* Standring S, ed. Gray's Anatomy. 40th Edn. London, Churchill Livingstone, 2008; pp. 989–1006.
- Shah PL. Diaphragm and phrenic nerve. *In:* Standring S, ed. Gray's Anatomy. 40th Edn. London, Churchill Livingstone, 2008; pp. 1007–1012.
- Shah PL, *et al.* Mediastinum. *In:* Standring S, ed. Gray's Anatomy. 40th Edn. London, Churchill Livingstone, 2008; pp. 939–957.

Respiratory physiology

Susan A. Ward

The appropriateness of the ventilatory ($V'E$) response to challenges, such as hypoxia or altered metabolic rate, depends on $V'E$ and on whether the pulmonary gas-exchange and acid–base requirements are achieved: *i.e.* regulation of $PaCO_2$, arterial pH (pHa) and PaO_2 within the relatively narrow range for optimal functioning. This involves a cascade of mechanisms: airflow and volume generation; pulmonary oxygen uptake ($V'O_2$) and carbon dioxide output ($V'CO_2$); and $V'E$ control with its associated respiratory perceptions. Each of these mechanisms can be adversely affected in pulmonary disease, with impaired respiratory-mechanical and gas-exchange function increasing the $V'E$ demands of the task and, in turn, the costs of meeting these demands in terms of respiratory-muscle work, perfusion and oxygen consumption.

Key points

- The mechanical work of breathing comprises elastic (volume-related) and resistive (flow-related) components.

- With expiratory efforts causing PIP to become positive, an EPP is created that results in expiratory flow limitation.

- Arterial hypoxaemia can result from alveolar hypoventilation, diffusion limitation, $V'A/Q'$ mismatch and/or right-to-left shunt. Only the latter three mechanisms also lead to a widened $PA{-}aO_2$ (*i.e.* inefficient pulmonary oxygen exchange).

Ventilatory requirements

Alveolar, and hence arterial, carbon dioxide and oxygen tensions ($PACO_2$, PAO_2, $PaCO_2$ and PaO_2, respectively) can only be regulated if alveolar ventilation ($V'A$) increases in an appropriate proportion to $V'CO_2$ and $V'O_2$, respectively. For carbon dioxide exchange (Fick's principle):

$$V'A = 863 \cdot V'CO_2 / PACO_2 \tag{1}$$

where 863 is the constant that corrects for the different conditions of reporting gas volumes (*i.e.* standard temperature and pressure, dry; body temperature and pressure, saturated) and the transformation of fractional concentration to gas tension.

Similarly, for oxygen:

$$V'A = 863 \cdot V'O_2 / (PI*O_2 - PAO_2) \tag{2}$$

where PIO_2 is inspiratory oxygen tension (PO_2) and $*$ is a relatively small correction factor (FAN_2/FIN_2, where FAN_2 and FIN_2 are alveolar and inspiratory nitrogen fractions, respectively) that takes account of inspired ventilation normally being slightly greater than the expired. This reflects the body's metabolic processes releasing less carbon dioxide relative to the oxygen used for a normal western diet, with a respiratory quotient (RQ=metabolic carbon dioxide production/metabolic oxygen consumption) of ~0.8.

As $V'A$ is common to equations 1 and 2, then:

$$(863 \cdot V'CO_2)/PACO_2 \leftarrow V'A \rightarrow (863 \cdot V'O_2)/(PI*O_2 - PAO_2) \tag{3}$$

If $V'CO_2$ and $V'O_2$ are equal (*i.e.* respiratory exchange ratio (R)=1), both $PACO_2$ and PAO_2

can be regulated. However, both cannot be regulated if $V'CO_2$ and $V'O_2$ differ, *e.g.* when:

1) RQ changes as a result of dietary- or activity-related alterations in metabolic substrate utilisation; or

2) there are transient variations in body gas stores (particularly the carbon dioxide stores) as metabolic rate changes.

Under such conditions, $V'A$ changes in closer proportion to $V'CO_2$ than to $V'O_2$, with $PACO_2$ consequently being more closely regulated than PAO_2; as these associated PO_2 changes normally occur over the relatively flat region of the oxygen dissociation curve, arterial oxygen content (CaO_2) is not greatly affected. However, the regulatory outcome is more complex if, for example:

1) significant arterial hypoxaemia develops, causing $V'A$ to increase out of proportion to $V'CO_2$ (hyperventilation) so as to constrain the fall in PAO_2; or

2) with metabolic acid–base disturbances that evoke compensatory respiratory responses to ameliorate the pHa change.

Importantly, it is the total $V'E$, rather than $V'A$, that is controlled to effect these regulatory functions. Substituting $V'E \cdot (1\text{-}VD/VT)$ for $V'A$ in equation 1 (where VD is the physiological dead space volume, VT is the tidal volume and VD/VT is the physiological dead space fraction of the breath), and assuming $PACO_2$ to equal to $PaCO_2$ yields:

$$V'E = (863 \cdot V'CO_2)/(PaCO_2 \cdot (1\text{-}VD/VT)) \qquad (4)$$

Thus, the $V'E$ requirement is determined by $PaCO_2$, $V'CO_2$ and VD/VT. Furthermore, the influence of metabolic acid–base disturbances can be accommodated by substituting $PaCO_2$ from equation 4 into the Henderson–Hasselbalch equation, *i.e.*

$$pHa = pK' + \log([HCO_3^-]a/\alpha \cdot PaCO_2) \qquad (5)$$

where $[HCO_3^-]a$ is the arterial bicarbonate concentration and α is the carbon dioxide solubility coefficient relating $PaCO_2$ to carbon dioxide content. This yields:

$$pHa = pK' + (\log([HCO_3^-]a/25.6)) \cdot (V'E/V'CO_2) \cdot (1\text{-}VD/VT) \qquad (6)$$

Thus, $\log[HCO_3^-]a/25.6$ represents the set point, $V'E/V'CO_2$ the 'control' term and $1\text{-}VD/VT$ represents gas exchange efficiency.

Respiratory mechanics

A particular $V'E$ requirement can, in theory, be accomplished with an infinite combination of VT and respiratory frequency (fR). The VT–fR combination, in turn, influences the inspiratory-muscle pressure ($Pmus$) needed to effect inspiration:

$$Pmus = E \cdot V + R \cdot v' + I \cdot v'' \qquad (7)$$

where V, v' and v'' are volume, air (and pulmonary tissue) flow and acceleration, and E, R and I are the pulmonary elastance, resistance and inertance, respectively. Normally, the inertance-related term makes an insignificant contribution, *i.e.* although the acceleration of the air can be large, its mass is small, and while the mass of the thorax is relatively large, its acceleration is small (*c.f.* conditions such as obesity having an abnormally increased thoracic mass). Thus, $Pmus$ has static (volume-related, with no associated air flow) and resistive (flow-related) components.

The static component of $Pmus$ equals the increment in transpulmonary pressure (Ptp) required to effect the required degree of lung distension under static conditions:

$$Ptp = Palv\text{-}PIP = V/CL \qquad (8)$$

where $Palv$ and PIP are alveolar and intrapleural pressures, respectively, and CL is lung compliance. CL is determined by the elastic properties of the lung parenchyma and the surface-active forces operating at the alveolar air–liquid interface, which are constrained by the influence of surfactant.

The normal static V–Ptp relationship (line 2 in fig. 1) shows CL to be largely independent of V over the tidal range but to decline as TLC is approached. When CL is decreased (*e.g.* restrictive lung disease), a greater than normal increase in Ptp is required to effect a given lung inflation (line 1 in fig. 1); an increased CL (*e.g.* emphysema) requires a smaller Ptp increment (line 3 in fig. 1). Also, as functional residual capacity (FRC) and the associated PIP are determined by the

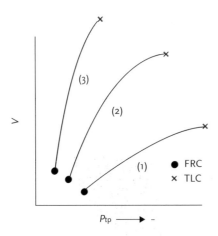

Figure 1. *C_L curve between FRC and TLC for increased (1) and decreased (3) lung recoil relative to normal (2). The slope at any point represents C_L, i.e. change in V induced by change in P_{tp}.*

magnitude of the opposing chest wall and lung recoil forces, FRC is smaller and P_{IP} more subatmospheric under conditions of increased recoil (line 1 in fig. 1) than when recoil is reduced (line 3 in fig. 1).

The resistive component of P_{mus} is the increment in 'driving' pressure required to effect air flow, i.e. the difference between P_{alv} and pressure at the airway opening (atmospheric pressure (P_{atm})):

$$P_{alv}-P_{atm}=v'\cdot R=k_1\cdot v'+k_2\cdot v'^2 \qquad (9)$$

The major site of this resistance lies in the segmental bronchi and larger-sized small bronchi. The bronchioles, although individually constituting sites of high resistance because of their very small radius, collectively contribute relatively little to the overall resistance as they are very numerous (only around 10–20% of the airway resistance being related to airways <2 mm in diameter). The term $k_1\cdot v'$ reflects the 'laminar' component of airflow, with $k_1=8\eta l/r^4$, where l is airway length, r is airway radius and η is gas viscosity. The term $k_2\cdot v'^2$ reflects the 'turbulent' component, which imposes a greater demand on pressure generation because of the squaring of the v' term. Turbulent flow develops when the Reynolds

number (Re) exceeds a value of ~2000. As $Re=v\cdot 2r\cdot\rho/\eta$, where v is the linear velocity and ρ is gas density, turbulent flow will predominate when v is high, at branch points or across constricted regions. Hence, reducing ρ, for example by breathing high concentrations of helium instead of nitrogen (heliox), makes turbulence less likely.

The thoracic expansion that occurs during inspiration causes P_{alv} to become negative (i.e. below P_{atm}) and flow to occur, until the end of inspiration, when P_{alv} again equals P_{atm} (fig. 2a). Thus, the pressure requirements for inspiratory flow and volume generation are reflected in P_{IP}: under static conditions, volume changes are simply related to changes in P_{IP} through the static C_L relationship (as P_{alv} is zero), while, during a normal inspiration, the additional muscular force needed to overcome R causes a greater negativity of P_{IP} at any given lung volume. The difference between the P_{IP} change needed to provide v' and that required to distend the lung statically is represented by the blue area in figure 2a, and is consequently greatest when v' is greatest. The respiratory-muscle work (W) performed in producing the inspiration can thus be calculated as: $\Delta V\cdot\Delta P_{IP}$ (fig. 2b), where Δ represents a change, i.e. the sum of the elastic work required to overcome the static lung recoil forces (red area) and the resistive work (blue area). When breathing is stimulated (e.g. in exercise), the greater P_{alv} required to generate the increased v' amplifies the dynamic component of the V–P relationship (right-hand panels of fig. 2a) and, therefore, increases W. A similar effect is seen in patients with an abnormally increased R, in whom a greater P_{alv} is required to achieve a particular v'. Expressing W relative to time yields the power output (W') of the inspiratory muscles that, when related to their oxygen consumption (Q'_{O_2}), allows considerations of overall respiratory muscle efficiency. It is only at very high levels of V'_E (e.g. at peak exercise in very fit endurance athletes) or when respiratory impedance is abnormally high (as in pulmonary disease) that W, W' and Q'_{O_2} can become significant, predisposing to respiratory muscle fatigue.

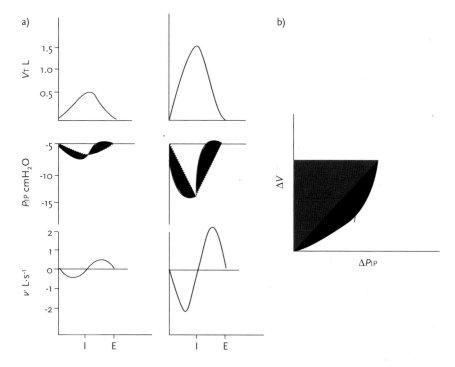

Figure 2. a) VT, PIP and v' changes for normal resting and exercising breaths. The dashed line on the PIP curve represents pressure needed to produce lung inflation statically. The blue area is the extra PIP required to generate flow. b) Dynamic inspiratory V–PIP curve. The red area represents static inspiratory work of breathing; the blue area is the dynamic component. I: inspiration; E: expiration.

When V'_E is low, expiration can be achieved entirely through the recoil pressure (PREC) generated in the elastic structures of the lungs during the previous inspiration, i.e. providing the necessary driving pressure by increasing P_{alv} (left-hand panels of fig. 2a):

$$P_{tp} = PREC = P_{alv}\text{-}PIP = R \cdot v' \qquad (10)$$

Flow at any point in expiration is thus determined by the interplay between static lung recoil, PIP and R:

$$v' = PREC + PIP/R \qquad (11)$$

Furthermore, the equality for PREC deriving from equations 8 and 9 yields:

$$V/CL = R \cdot v' \qquad (12)$$

which can be rearranged as:

$$v'/V = 1/R \cdot CL \qquad (13)$$

The term $R \cdot CL$ is the mechanical time constant (τ) of the respiratory system, and has the unit of time, i.e. $(cmH_2O \cdot L^{-1} \cdot s) \cdot (L \cdot cmH_2O^{-1}) = s$. Thus, if R or CL (or both) are large, then v' will be low for a given lung volume. Complete passive emptying (i.e. down to FRC) for a spontaneous expiration requires expiratory duration to be sufficiently long (i.e. effectively $4 \cdot \tau$ for an exponential process). With a normal τ of ~ 0.4 s (R and CL being $\sim 2\ cmH_2O \cdot L^{-1} \cdot s$ and $0.2\ L \cdot cmH_2O^{-1}$, respectively), this minimum period is ~ 1.6 s and translates to a total breath time (t_{tot}) of ~ 3 s, assuming an inspiratory duty cycle (t_I/t_{tot}, where t_I is inspiratory time) of ~ 0.4. Thus, if f_R exceeds ~ 20 breaths·min^{-1}, complete emptying requires expiratory flow to be augmented by expiratory muscle action; without this, end-expiratory lung volume will be greater than FRC. Such

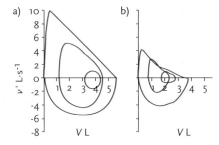

Figure 3. Inspiratory (downwards) and expiratory (upwards) flow–volume curves at rest, maximal exercise and with maximal volitional effort for a) a normal subject and b) a patient with COPD. Reproduced from Klas et al. (1989), with permission from the publisher.

dynamic hyperinflation is a hallmark of the exercising COPD patient (fig. 3b), where disease-related increases in R and/or C_L can lower this limiting f_R quite considerably.

That the maximal volitionally generated expiratory v' is greater at high than at low lung volumes (fig. 3) is, of course, implicit in equation 11. That is, R and P_{REC} are each volume-dependent: at high volumes, R is relatively low, reflecting a modest degree of airway distension (whose effect is amplified through the r^4 term) while P_{REC} is relatively high. Indeed, for a given τ, v' decreases as a linear function of V (equation 13), accounting for the descending limb of the maximal expiratory flow–volume curve normally being so linear (fig. 3a).

In COPD, however, the lower maximal v' at TLC, despite the higher absolute lung volume (line 3 in fig. 1), is indicative of an increased R and, for emphysema, decreased P_{REC} (fig. 3b), and thus v' at a particular lung volume is lower than normal. In contrast, for restrictive lung disease, while maximal v' at TLC is low owing to poor distensibility (line 1 in fig. 1), v' at a particular lung volume can even be slightly higher than normal owing to an increased P_{REC}. Furthermore, when there is regional nonuniformity of τ, for example, as in COPD, this can contribute to the typically 'scooped' maximal expiratory v' profile (fig. 3b).

However, the effects of P_{IP} on expiratory v' are not quite as straightforward as those of R and P_{REC} (equation 13). P_{IP} is an index of the effort transmitted from the respiratory muscles to the lungs via the chest wall. During expiration, P_{IP} can become positive as a function of the applied expiratory effort, i.e. the chest wall volume decreases faster than the lungs' intrinsic recoil. This results in a compressive force being applied to the intrapleural space. As $P_{alv}=P_{IP}+P_{REC}$ (equation 10), P_{alv} will be more positive than P_{IP} by an amount equal to P_{REC}. Airway pressure (P_{aw}) declines from the alveolar value down to zero at the mouth as a result of frictional losses along the airways. At the point where $P_{aw}=P_{IP}$ (i.e. the transmural pressure across the airway is zero) (fig. 4), an equal pressure point (EPP) results.

In normal subjects, the EPP occurs in the large airways (lower trachea or main stem bronchi), which, despite the tendency to become compressed, are prevented from collapsing by their cartilaginous support. Thus, the EPP becomes the limiting point for expiratory flow generation, dictating the maximum expiratory flow (v'_{max}):

$$v'_{max}=P_{REC}/R_{us} \qquad (14)$$

where R_{us} is the resistance of the upstream segment of the airways (between the alveolus and the EPP) (fig. 4). This explains why progressively greater expiratory efforts,

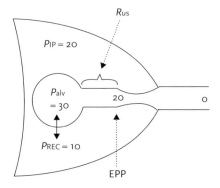

Figure 4. Airflow limitation in expiration. An EPP results when P_{aw} declines to a value equal to P_{REC}. Values are expressed in cmH_2O.

although leading to a progressively more positive P_{IP}, do not lead to a progressively greater v'; greater expiratory effort simply compresses the airways more, raising downstream R in proportion to the increased effort. Therefore, v' becomes maximised at a constant value (at that lung volume), independent of effort.

With the loss of lung recoil and/or increases in small airway resistance, however, the EPP migrates upstream. If it encroaches into the small unsupported airways, airways collapse occurs – with profound effects on v'_{max} (equation 14).

Pulmonary gas exchange

The effectiveness of pulmonary oxygen exchange is conventionally judged by the magnitude of the alveolar–arterial oxygen tension difference (P_{A-aO_2}), using P_{AiO_2}, which is the P_{AO_2} of the 'ideal lung' (one that hypothetically exchanges gases ideally). P_{AiO_2} thus circumvents the difficulty of providing a single representative value for P_{AO_2} when there are regional variations in gas-exchange efficiency. It can be derived by re-arranging and amalgamating equations 1 and 2:

$$V'_{CO_2}/V'_{O_2} = R = (V'_A \cdot ((P_{IO_2} \cdot F_{AN_2}/F_{IN_2}) - P_{AiO_2}))/(V'_A \cdot P_{ACO_2}) \quad (15)$$

$$P_{AiO_2} = P_{IO_2} - P_{ACO_2}/R + (P_{ACO_2} \cdot F_{IO_2} \cdot (1-R)/R) \quad (16)$$

where F_{IO_2} is the inspiratory oxygen fraction. It is common practice to neglect the term $P_{ACO_2} \cdot F_{IO_2} \cdot (1-R)/R$, as it is zero when $R=1$, and only contributes a few mmHg or so when $R \neq 1$. Therefore:

$$P_{AiO_2} = P_{IO_2} - P_{ACO_2}/R \quad (17)$$

Impairments of pulmonary gas exchange typically result in arterial hypoxaemia and, in some instances, arterial hypercapnia. Six mechanisms can be identified as independent causes of arterial hypoxaemia: three of these affect P_{AO_2} (ambient hypoxia as with ascent to altitude, reduced RQ and alveolar hypoventilation) and three affect P_{A-aO_2} (diffusion limitation, increased right-to-left shunt and V'_A/perfusion (Q') maldistribution).

Reduced RQ Recalling that V'_E operates to regulate P_{ACO_2} by responding in a proportional fashion to V'_{CO_2}, when the RQ of the dietary substrate is reduced (*i.e.* by ingestion of a high-fat diet), the associated reduction in metabolic carbon dioxide production requires less ventilation to maintain a stable P_{ACO_2} (equation 3). This leads to hypoventilation relative to oxygen, *i.e.* V'_E is normal relative to V'_{CO_2} but low relative to V'_{O_2}. Thus, P_{AO_2} and P_{aO_2} will fall.

Alveolar hypoventilation can occur in diseases or with drugs that affect the medullary respiratory-integrating centres or respiratory neuromuscular function and, therefore, reduce the level of respiratory motor output. It may also be seen in severe COPD, consequent to increased small airway resistance and a high resistive work of breathing. Arterial hypoxaemia and hypercapnia result (equations 2 and 1, respectively), with the fall of P_{aO_2} being related to the rise of P_{aCO_2} through R (equation 17). When $R=1$, the increase in P_{ACO_2} and fall in P_{AO_2} that result from a reduction in V'_A are equal, as notionally are the corresponding changes in P_{aCO_2} and P_{aO_2}. However, as R is normally ~0.8 at rest, for each 10-mmHg decrease in P_{aO_2} that results from a fall of V'_A, P_{aCO_2} will increase by only 8 mmHg. It should be noted that the hypoxaemia can be offset by administration of supplementary oxygen.

Diffusion impairment Fick's law indicates that impairments in the pulmonary diffusive flux of oxygen (or carbon dioxide) can result from

1) a reduction in the driving pressure (for oxygen, ΔP_{O_2}),

2) a reduction in the available surface area for diffusion (A) and/or

3) an increased path length for diffusion (l):

$$V'_{O_2} = A/l \cdot d \cdot \Delta P_{O_2} \quad (18)$$

where d, the diffusion coefficient for oxygen, is inversely proportional to gas molecular weight (MW) in the gas phase ($d = 1/\sqrt{MW}$), while directly proportional also to gas solubility (s) in the blood phase ($d = s/\sqrt{MW}$). Hence, as oxygen is lighter than carbon dioxide, it diffuses 18% more rapidly in the gas phase for the same gas tension gradient. In the blood phase, however, carbon dioxide is 20 times more diffusible than oxygen, owing to its greater solubility.

During inspiration, oxygen is transported down the tracheobronchial tree by convective or bulk flow. At the level of the alveolar ducts, owing to the large overall cross-sectional area of the airways and the resulting reduction in linear velocity of the inspired gas, movement to the alveolar–capillary membrane relies on diffusion. Diffusion through the alveolar gas space does not normally limit gas transfer into pulmonary capillary blood. Thus, as the average alveolar diameter is normally only $\sim$100 µm, diffusion equilibrium (i.e. ΔP_{O_2}=0) throughout the alveolus is attained rapidly: this is normally 80% complete within $\sim$0.002 s, which is several orders of magnitude less than the time for which pulmonary capillary blood is exposed to the alveolar gas-exchange surface (i.e. the pulmonary–capillary transit time (t_{TR}), which is $\sim$0.8 s at rest). In conditions such as emphysema, air-sac enlargement increases intra-alveolar diffusion distances, predisposing to less efficient oxygen and carbon dioxide exchange.

More commonly, however, diffusion limitation reflects exchange impairments between alveolar gas and pulmonary capillary blood. The rate of diffusive uptake of oxygen into blood is given by:

$$V'_{O_2}=A/l \cdot d \cdot (P_{AO_2}\text{-}P_{cO_2}) \qquad (19)$$

where A is the alveolar surface area in contact with perfused pulmonary capillaries; l is the diffusion path length between the alveolar surface fluid lining and the erythrocyte interior that includes alveolar epithelium, interstitial space, capillary endothelial cells, plasma, erythrocyte cell membrane and, for a reactive gas species such as oxygen, its chemical combination with haemoglobin; and P_{cO_2} is mean pulmonary capillary P_{O_2}. It is conventional to combine A, l and d into a single term, the transfer factor of the lung for oxygen (T_{LO_2}):

$$V'_{O_2}=T_{LO_2} \cdot (P_{AO_2}\text{-}P_{cO_2}) \qquad (20)$$

T_{LO_2} can be usefully subdivided into its functional components: the 'membrane' component (T_{MO_2}) and that due to chemical combination:

$$1/T_{LO_2}=1/T_{MO_2}+1/\theta \cdot V_c \qquad (21)$$

where θ is the reaction rate coefficient for chemical combination of oxygen with haemoglobin and V_c is pulmonary capillary blood volume. Because of technical limitations associated with estimating P_{cO_2}, it is conventional to determine transfer factors of the lung and membrane for carbon monoxide (T_{LCO} and T_{MCO}, respectively), as the high affinity of haemoglobin for carbon monoxide ensures that the pulmonary capillary carbon monoxide tension (P_{CO}) is effectively zero.

The initial driving pressure across the alveolar–capillary membrane (i.e. at the entrance to the capillary bed) is given by the difference between P_{AO_2} (normally $\sim$100 mmHg) and mixed venous P_{O_2} (P_{vO_2}) (normally $\sim$40 mmHg at rest, although decreasing in exercise). The rate at which oxygen is taken up into the blood as it traverses the capillary declines, reflecting the increasing P_{cO_2} (and consequent decrease in P_{AO_2}), which in turn reduces the instantaneous ΔP_{O_2}. Diffusion equilibrium is normally reached within 0.25–0.3 s (i.e. well before blood reaches the end of the capillary); thus, pulmonary end-capillary P_{O_2} ($P_{c'O_2}$)=P_{AO_2}. This large safety margin becomes compromised, however, when t_{TR} is shortened to such a degree that there is insufficient time for the attainment of diffusion equilibrium, i.e. $P_{c'O_2}$<P_{AO_2}. As t_{TR}=V_c/Q', an increase in Q' (e.g. high-intensity exercise) can compromise diffusion equilibrium, resulting in arterial hypoxaemia. However, the decrease in t_{TR} with increases in Q' is less than expected, because the capillary blood volume (Q_c) actually increases with Q', consequent to distension of already-perfused capillaries and recruitment of previously unperfused capillaries; this serves to protect against diffusion disequilibrium.

A lowered P_{AO_2}, as occurs with ascent to high altitude, when a subject breathes an hypoxic inspirate or with hypoventilation, slows the P_cO_2 rise time. This is because the initial driving pressure (P_AO_2-P_vO_2) is smaller, as the operating slope of the oxygen dissociation curve (β) is steeper, with the arteriovenous oxygen content difference expressing a smaller arteriovenous P_{O_2} difference.

A useful expression relating to the interplay of factors that dictate whether or not diffusion equilibrium will actually be attained (*i.e.* whether $P_c',O_2 = P_AO_2$) is:

$$(P_AO_2\text{-}P_cO_2) = (P_AO_2\text{-}P_vO_2) \cdot e^{-T_LO_2/Q' \cdot \beta} \quad (22)$$

The term $T_LO_2/Q' \cdot \beta$ has been termed the 'equilibrium coefficient' by Piiper *et al.* (1980) and the 'diffusive–perfusive conductance' ratio by West *et al.* (1998). Thus, diffusion equilibrium is less likely to be attained if T_LO_2 is low and/or Q' and β are high. For example, an increased path length (*e.g.* alveolar proteinosis or pulmonary oedema) and/or a reduced surface area for exchange (*e.g.* pulmonary embolism or restrictive lung disease) slow the diffusive flux of oxygen because of their effects on T_LO_2. With very high levels of Q' (*e.g.* very fit endurance athletes exercising at or close to maximum) or very high linear capillary-blood velocities (*e.g.* pulmonary embolism, where there are fewer participating capillaries), the reduction in tTR can lead to a widened P_A-aO_2 and arterial hypoxaemia. Supplemental oxygen can, through its effects on P_AO_2 and, therefore, driving pressure, speed the increase of P_cO_2 and thus ameliorate the degree of gas-exchange impairment.

However, although severe degrees of arterial hypoxaemia can result from diffusion impairment, carbon dioxide retention is rarely a problem. This is because any increase in P_aCO_2 that might occur tends to be corrected by ventilatory control mechanisms, which are considered to be exquisitely sensitive to carbon dioxide (*i.e.* central and carotid body chemoreflexes); in contrast, hypoxic ventilatory stimulation only becomes appreciable when P_aO_2 falls below ~60 mmHg. Hence, moderate diffusion impairment is accompanied by a decreased P_aO_2, a widened P_A-aO_2 and a relatively normal P_aCO_2; with more severe impairment, which leads to hypoxic ventilatory stimulation, there will be a more marked arterial hypoxaemia, greater widening of the P_A-a,O_2 and a low P_aCO_2.

Right-to-left shunt A right-to-left shunt ($Q's$) occurs when venous blood bypasses the pulmonary capillary circulation, thus providing a degree of venous admixture with blood from exchanging alveolar units. It normally reflects venous drainage from the larger airways (which enters the pulmonary veins) and from coronary vessels (which enters the left ventricles *via* the Thebesian veins). This represents only a small percentage of Q' and, therefore, amounts to a reduction in P_aO_2 of only a few mmHg below P_c',O_2. However, $Q's/Q'$ can be markedly increased in congenital heart disease (*e.g.* atrial or ventricular septal defects, and pulmonary arteriovenous fistulae), leading to significant arterial hypoxaemia and widening of the P_A-a,O_2.

The $Q's/Q'$ relationship derives from the recognition that the rate of oxygen delivery into the systemic arterial circulation can be viewed as being made up of a homogeneous 'ideal' pulmonary capillary component and a 'pure' shunt component. Reverting again to the Fick principle, but now for the 'blood' side, and using the simple equality $Q' = Q'c + Q's$:

$$Q' \cdot CaO_2 = Q'c \cdot Cc'O_2 + Q's \cdot CvO_2 \quad (23)$$

were $Cc'O_2$ is the end-capillary oxygen content and CvO_2 is the mixed-venous oxygen content, which rearranges to yield:

$$Q's/Q' = (Cc'O_2\text{-}CaO_2)/(Cc'O_2\text{-}CvO_2) \quad (24)$$

CaO_2 and CvO_2 can be measured directly from blood samples, while $Cc'O_2$ is derived through the standard oxygen dissociation curve, assuming $Pc'O_2 = P_AiO_2$ (equation 17). It should be noted that this equation also assumes that all the shunted blood is of mixed-venous composition, which may not necessarily be the case for bronchial venous blood. This estimate of $Q's/Q'$ thus provides an overestimate of the true shunt, as it incorporates a fraction of the perfusion draining from alveolar units having poorly functional capillaries (with low $V'A/Q'$ values), *i.e.* creating a 'shunt-like' effect.

A right-to-left shunt must therefore result in arterial hypoxaemia, *i.e.* even a small contribution from nonarterialised blood will depress the resulting CaO_2, owing to the influence of the nonlinear oxygen dissociation curve. The severity of the hypoxaemia will depend both on $Q's/Q'$ and CvO_2, being more marked when the former is larger and the latter is lower. A hallmark feature of a pure right-to-left shunt is that the elevation of PaO_2 in response to administration of 100% oxygen is appreciably less than expected. This is because the shunt flow cannot 'see' the elevated PAO_2 in the exchanging alveoli, and also that further increases in PAO_2 will have little effect on $Cc'O_2$ because the blood is already essentially fully saturated; it is only the dissolved component of the oxygen content that can be increased, and this will be relatively small because of the low solubility of oxygen in plasma.

A right-to-left shunt also has the potential to cause carbon dioxide retention but this is rarely observed owing to the normally small mixed venous-to-arterial carbon dioxide tension (PCO_2) difference (~ 6 mmHg at rest *versus* ~ 60 mmHg for oxygen) and also (see earlier) the mechanisms of ventilatory control that normally restore an increased $PaCO_2$ to normal. Again, however, should PaO_2 fall sufficiently to cause hypoxic stimulation of the carotid chemoreceptors, then $PaCO_2$ will fall; but, without this, $PaCO_2$ will rise. Thus, a moderate right-to-left shunt leads to a reduced PaO_2 and a widened $PA{-}aO_2$, but a relatively normal $PaCO_2$. Severe right-to-left shunts cause a markedly reduced PaO_2 and a markedly widened $PA{-}aO_2$, with the possibility of a lowered $PaCO_2$.

$V'A/Q'$ **maldistribution** Although overall $V'A$ may be approximately equal to overall Q' in the lung, there may nonetheless be regions with high, normal and low $V'A/Q'$ ratios. This has important implications for regional alveolar gas and pulmonary end-capillary blood composition, and therefore for overall arterial blood-gas status. That is, gas and blood from low $V'A/Q'$ regions will reflect

hypoventilation (*i.e.* low PO_2 and high PCO_2) and, in the extreme, alveolar shunt ($V'A/Q'=0$) (see previously); gas and blood from normal $V'A/Q'$ regions will have a normal PO_2 and PCO_2; and gas and blood from high $V'A/Q'$ regions will reflect hyperventilation (*i.e.* high PO_2 and PCO_2) with, in the extreme, alveolar dead space ($V'A/Q'=\infty$).

An analogous formulation to that for estimation of $Q's/Q'$ can be applied to the estimation of VD/VT (recalling that VD reflects the sum of the anatomical and alveolar dead spaces). That is, the assumption is made that the volume of carbon dioxide cleared in exhalation originates solely from a homogeneous exchanging alveolar compartment (Bohr technique):

$$VT \cdot FECO_2 = VA \cdot FACO_2 \qquad (25)$$

where $FECO_2$ is mixed expired carbon dioxide fraction and VA is the volume of exchanging alveoli. Substituting $VT{-}VD$ for VA, converting fractional concentrations to gas tensions, making the reasonable assumption that $PACO_2 = PaCO_2$ (attributable to Enghoff) and rearranging yields:

$$VD/VT = (PaCO_2 {-} PECO_2)/PaCO_2 \qquad (26)$$

Even in the normal lung, there is evidence of mild $V'A/Q'$ mismatch. Owing to the influence of gravity, Q' is distributed preferentially to the dependent regions of the lung (*i.e.* towards the base in the upright posture). A similar, gravitationally induced effect is also seen for $V'A$, though it is less striking. Thus, the alveoli in the dependent regions of the lung are smaller, as the hydrostatic pressure in the surrounding interstitium is greater. They are therefore constrained to operate over the steeper, lower portion of the CL curve, in contrast to the larger apical units. Thus, the smaller basal units undergo a greater expansion for a given increase of PTP during inspiration and are therefore better ventilated than are the apical units. The apical units thus have a relatively high $V'A/Q'$ while the basal units have a low $V'A/Q'$. Naturally, the degree of $V'A/Q'$ mismatch is considerably greater in many pulmonary disease states (*e.g.* COPD, diffuse interstitial fibrosis and pulmonary vascular occlusive disease) and its topographical location is not predictable.

The overall (or mean) P_{AO_2} and P_{ACO_2} result from an averaging of the respective gas concentrations from each individual gas 'stream', in proportion to the local V'_A. Likewise, the overall (or mean) P_{aO_2} and P_{aCO_2} will result from a flow-weighted averaging of the respective gas contents from each individual blood 'stream'. However, it is important to recognise that account has also to be taken of the shape of the oxygen and carbon dioxide dissociation curves in order to derive these P_{aO_2} and P_{aCO_2} values (fig. 5).

Owing to the sigmoid shape of the oxygen dissociation curve, low V'_A/Q' regions lead both to low P_{O_2} and low oxygen content in pulmonary end-capillary blood; in contrast, while high V'_A/Q' regions lead to a high $P_{c'O_2}$, $C_{c'O_2}$ is only slightly increased above the normal value because the oxygen dissociation curve is relatively flat in this range (fig. 5). Mixing blood from low V'_A/Q' regions with blood from high V'_A/Q' regions will therefore result in a mean P_{aO_2} that is weighted towards low V'_A/Q' blood values (fig. 5). P_{aO_2} will also depend on the volumes of blood from each region contributing to the mixed arterial blood. Thus, the high

V'_A/Q' regions (even if haemoglobin is completely saturated) are unable to compensate for the low V'_A/Q' regions, as their perfusion is usually less. Consequently, even though the overall V'_A/Q' may be normal, V'_A/Q' mismatch results in arterial hypoxaemia, with mean P_{aO_2} being lower than the actual mean P_{AO_2} or its 'ideal' representation; i.e. P_{A-aO_2} is widened.

In contrast, the carbon dioxide dissociation curve is essentially linear in the physiological range (fig. 5). This therefore allows the hyperventilatory effects of the high V'_A/Q' regions to better counterbalance the hypoventilatory effects of the low V'_A/Q' regions on the resulting mean P_{aCO_2} (fig. 5). It should be noted, however, that the high V'_A/Q' regions exert a proportionally greater influence on mean P_{ACO_2} than do the low V'_A/Q' regions. Hence, $P_{ACO_2} < P_{aCO_2}$.

The pattern of arterial blood and alveolar gas tensions in V'_A/Q' mismatch is such that with mild or moderate mismatch, P_{aO_2} is low, P_{A-aO_2} is widened, with P_{aCO_2} being normal or low depending on the degree of ventilatory stimulation consequent to the hypoxaemia. In severe V'_A/Q' impairment associated with severe airway obstruction, hypoventilation can ensue owing to the increased work of breathing and, therefore,

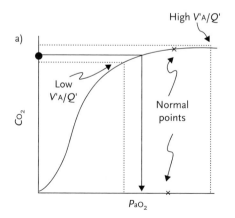
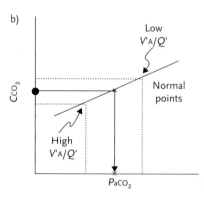

Figure 5. Influence of altered V'A/Q' on mean PaO₂ and PaCO₂ tensions. a) The sigmoid oxygen dissociation curve leads to arterial hypoxaemia (arrow) compared with 'normal' (×). b) This effect is not evident for carbon dioxide, because the carbon dioxide dissociation curve is linear. Reproduced from Whipp (2002) with permission from the publisher.

cause an increased $P_{a}CO_2$. This, of course, reduces P_{a,O_2} even more.

Further reading

- D'Angelo E (1999). Dynamics. *Eur Respir Monogr*; 12: 54–67.
- Farhi LE. Ventilation–perfusion relationships. *In:* Farhi LE, *et al.*, eds. Handbook of Physiology. The Respiratory System, Mechanics of Breathing, vol. IV. Bethesda, American Physiological Society, 1986; pp. 199–215.
- Hughes JMB. Diffusive gas exchange. *In:* Whipp BJ, *et al.*, eds. Pulmonary Physiology and Pathophysiology of Exercise. New York, Dekker, 1991; pp. 143–171.
- Klas JV, *et al.* (1989). Voluntary *versus* reflex regulation of maximal exercise flow: volume loops. *Am Rev Respir Dis*; 139: 150–156.
- Lumb AB. Nunn's Applied Respiratory Physiology. 7th Edn. London, Elsevier, 2010.
- Maina JN, *et al.* (2005). Thin and strong! The bioengineering dilemma in the structural and functional design of the blood–gas barrier. *Physiol Rev*; 85: 811–844.
- Mead J, *et al.* Dynamics of breathing. *In:* Fenn WO, *et al.*, eds. Handbook of Physiology, Respiration, vol. 1. Washington, American Physiological Society, 1964; pp. 411–427.
- Otis AB. The work of breathing. *In:* Fenn WO, *et al.*, eds. Handbook of Physiology, Respiration, vol. 1. Washington, American Physiological Society, 1964; pp. 592–607.
- Piiper J, *et al.* Blood gas equilibration in lungs. *In:* West JB, ed. Pulmonary Gas Exchange, Vol. II. New York, Academic Press, 1998: pp. 132–161.
- Pride NB, *et al.* Lung mechanics in disease. *In:* Macklem PT, *et al.*, eds. Handbook of Physiology. The Respiratory System, Mechanics of Breathing, vol. III, part 2. Bethesda, American Physiological Society, 1986; pp. 659–692.
- Riley RL, *et al.* (1949). "Ideal" alveolar air and the analysis of ventilation–perfusion relationships in the lung. *J Appl Physiol*; 1: 825–847.
- Rodarte JR, *et al.* Dynamics of respiration. *In:* Macklem PT, *et al.*, eds. Handbook of Physiology. The Respiratory System, Mechanics of Breathing, vol. III, part 1. Bethesda, American Physiological Society, 1986; pp. 131–144.
- Weibel ER. Pathway for Oxygen. Cambridge, Harvard University Press. 1984.
- West JB. Ventilation/Blood Flow and Gas Exchange. Oxford, Blackwell, 1990.
- West JB, *et al.* (1998). Pulmonary gas exchange. *Am J Respir Crit Care Med*; 157: S82–S87.
- Whipp BJ. The physiology and pathophysiology of gas exchange. *In:* Bittar EE, ed. Pulmonary Biology in Health and Disease. New York, Springer-Verlag, 2002; pp. 189–217.

Cytology of the lung

Venerino Poletti, Giovanni Poletti, Marco Chilosi and Bruno Murer

The role of cytological techniques for investigation of respiratory disorders has been recognised since the earliest days of clinical cytology. Improvement in sampling techniques, and in particular, the advent of fibreoptic bronchoscopy, transparietal fine-needle aspiration, cytological sampling assisted by echoendoscopy, the use of immunocytochemical and, more recently, molecular biology methods, recent advances in liquid-based cytology, and the use of cell block processing methods have increased the clinical impact of cytological diagnoses. Finally, the rapid, on-site analysis of cytological samples or of preparations obtained from bioptic samples (smears or touch imprints) has also improved the diagnostic yield of the investigative methods. A knowledge of 'basic cytology' should be part of the education for becoming a pulmonologist and this knowledge should be maintained in daily clinical practice.

Technical notes

The routine staining procedures that pulmonologists should be familiar with are Diff-Quik, May–Grünwald–Giemsa (MGG), Papanicolaou, haematoxylin–eosin and Gram staining, and a staining for acid-fast bacilli (Ziehl–Neelsen and/or Kinyoun). Papanicolaou stain is a polychrome stain: the nucleus stains deep blue, nuclear details are sharp, the nucleolus stains red, and the cytoplasm stains eosinophilic, cyanophilic or orange. Keratin stains deep orange. The slides must be wet-fixed swiftly and rapidly. Diff-Quik is a three step procedure requiring about 20–30 s to complete. The staining kit includes fixative solution A (trimethane dye and methyl alcohol, but 95% ethyl alcohol is valid), solution I that contains xanthene dye and solution II that contains a buffered solution of thiazine dyes. Slides are air dried and then fixed. Material obtained by fine-needle aspiration techniques should be used for smears and for cell-block preparations, cytofluorimetric analysis and genetic studies when deemed necessary. Summaries of the routine staining procedures, cytological preparations and genetic studies feasible on cytological material are presented in tables 1–3, respectively.

Key points

- BAL is an important source of cytological samples.

- Fine-needle aspiration has increased the impact of cytological diagnoses.

- Cell blocks are easy to prepare and useful for immunocytochemistry.

- Reactive cytological features in respiratory samples can be characteristic but nonspecific.

- Cytology can be used to diagnose respiratory infections.

- Lung carcinoma presents a variety of characteristic patterns.

- Lymphoproliferative disorders are more readily diagnosed in BAL fluid or fine-needle aspirates.

- Immunocytochemistry and molecular biology add to cytological diagnoses.

Table 1. Routine staining techniques

Stain	Advantages	Disadvantages

Papanicolaou	Very useful to:
	  detect and classify neoplastic
	    cells
	  identify vital inclusions
		Time consuming

Diff-Quik	Very easy to perform for rapid,
	  on-site examination
		Not precise in defining nuclear
		  details

MGG	The reference to classify
	  'haematologic' cells
	Very useful to identify viral
	  cytoplasmic inclusions
		Tends to overestimate 'dysplastic'
		  changes

Gram	To identify and classify bacteria	
Kinyoun	For weakly acid-fast bacilli	

General cytological findings in respiratory samples

Squamous cells are the most common cells in sputum but are less frequent in other specimens, being inconsistently found or absent. They appear as irregularly polygonal or rectangular cells with well-demarcated borders, small nuclei, abundant clear pale cyanophilic to eosinophilic cytoplasm in Papanicolaou preps. The intermediate-type cells have a small central nucleus with thready chromatin and a lack of nucleoli.

Bronchial epithelial cells are columnar or triangular in shape, and lie singly, in short ribbons or in flat sheets. They have a bluish grey cytoplasm with MGG or Diff-Quik stains, or cyanophilic in Papanicolaou preps, tapering at the point of previous anchorage.

Their nuclei vary considerably in size and shape but are usually basal, rounded or oval with open granular or condensed chromatin and a single small nucleolus. Cilia (red in Papanicolaou preparations) are often well preserved, arising from a dark-stained terminal bar at the end of the cell.

Goblet cells are columnar, with a basally placed nucleus and supranuclear cytoplasm distended by globules of mucin. Cilia are absent. These cells increase in number in bronchial irritation.

Reserve cells are small (slightly larger than lymphocytes), regular cells grouped to form sheets. Their nuclear/cytoplasmic ratio is high, the chromatin is coarse and there is a narrow rim of cytoplasm (green in Papanicolaou preps, or blue in Diff-Quik or MGG preps).

Table 2. Routine 'cytological' preparations

Smear	Used for:
	  fine-needle aspiration samples
	  rapid, on-site examination of bioptic material (squash or touch
	    preparations)

Cytospin	The standard for cytological analysis of BAL fluid
Thin preparations	The standard for bronchial washing or lavage and pleural fluid
Cell block preparations	Easy to prepare Very useful for immunocytochemical studies
Flow cytometry	The standard for lymphocyte subset identification, and for demonstration of B-cell monoclonality and characterisation of myeloid cells

Table 3. Molecular studies on cytological material

| EGFR mutations (exons 18–21) |
| ALK–EML4 fusion |
| BRAF^{V600E} mutation |
| MicroRNA profiles |
| Heavy chain monoclonal rearrangement |
| T-cell receptor monoclonal rearrangement |

Club cells (Clara cells), Feyrter cells and type II pneumocytes are prone to rapid degenerative changes and are not recognisable in respiratory samples unless hyperplastic/dysplastic.

Macrophages are round or oval cells, usually >10 μm in diameter, and possess generally abundant pale cytoplasm, with an oval or reniform nucleus showing a sharp nuclear membrane, finely granular, evenly dispersed chromatin, micronucleoli and sometimes also macronucleoli. Binucleation is common and giant cells with numerous nuclei are not uncommon. These cells are phagocytic and their cytoplasm may be vacuolated or may contain small particles coated by iron, coarse granules of haemosiderin or inhaled particles.

Inflammatory cells A variety of inflammatory cells may be recognisable in lung specimens:

- polymorphonuclear leukocytes
- lymphocytes
- eosinophils
- mast cells
- plasma cells

Megakaryocytes can be identified in pulmonary arterial samples and may be misinterpreted as malignant.

Mesothelium Tissue fragments of benign mesothelium are often collected during a transthoracic aspiration procedure. Most mesothelial tissue fragments appear as flat, two-dimensional sheets that present a honeycomb pattern. Mesothelial cells are, however, mainly found in pleural fluid. They are usually 15–30 μm in diameter but may be significantly larger. They may be present as solitary cells or in small cohesive clusters. The cytoplasm usually shows two zones: in Diff-Quik-stained smears, the endoplasm is lightly stained with peripheral darker ectoplasm. The peripheral cell border is ruffled with blebs. As mesothelial cells imbibe water from the surrounding fluid, their cytoplasm may acquire a foamy macrophage phenotype. Mesothelial cell nuclei have crisp, thin nuclear membranes, evenly distributed, finely granular chromatin, one or two micronucleoli, and occasionally grooves.

Other components of respiratory samples
Mucus appears as a pale, thin, translucent shroud or as strings stained with varying intensity and with enmeshed cellular elements. Inspissated mucus appears as darkly stained blobs. Coils of compressed mucus are known as Curschmann's spirals and represent casts of the small bronchioles. Charcot–Leyden crystals, derived from the breakdown products of eosinophil granules, appear as orange-, yellow- or pinkish-stained diamond- or needle-shaped crystals. They are mainly observed in conditions evoking pulmonary eosinophilia. Calcific blue bodies and corpora amylacea are similar in routine preps. The former consists largely of calcium carbonate and shows central birefringence. Corpora amylacea are noncalcified, rounded structures composed of pulmonary surfactant proteins, epithelial membrane antigen and glycoproteins including amyloid. They stain pale pink, are Congo red positive and exhibit birefringence. Psammoma bodies (calcipherites) are laminated, nonrefractile, calcified concretions sometimes found in the presence of malignancy. Ferruginous bodies are formed when filamentous dust particles such as asbestos become coated with protein and iron in the lung parenchyma. They vary from 5 to 200 μm in length and are golden brown in colour with a characteristic segmented or beaded bamboo shape with knobbed or bulbous ends and stain blue with Perl's stain for iron. Other noncellular entities that may be found in respiratory specimens are calcium oxalate crystals (frequently associated with

Aspergillus infection), Schaumann bodies, asteroid bodies, elastin fibres and amyloid.

Nonspecific reactive changes of the respiratory epithelium

Benign disorders of the respiratory tract may be manifested by characteristic but nonspecific abnormalities of the squamous epithelium, bronchial epithelium and alveolar epithelium. Reactive squamous cells from the upper respiratory tract have slightly enlarged hyperchromatic nuclei. Anucleate, keratinised squamous cells, if present in large numbers, suggest an area of hyperkeratosis. Squamous metaplasia is defined as the replacement of the respiratory mucosa by squamous epithelium, and is a common reaction to injury in the trachea and in the bronchial tree. Particularly severe squamous atypia has been described in the trachea of patients with prolonged tracheal intubation and patients with tracheitis sicca occurring in patients who have permanent tracheostomy or in patients with tracheal inflammatory conditions, bronchial and parenchymal tuberculotic or mycotic lesions. The loss of cilia and the terminal plate (ciliocytophthoria) is a common response of the respiratory epithelium to acute injury; this phenomenon is observed mainly in viral infections. Papillary hyperplasia of the respiratory epithelium is most commonly observed in chronic inflammatory bronchial disorders (bronchiectasis and bronchial asthma) and appears cytologically as characteristic pseudopapillary cell clusters (Creola bodies) showing well-preserved bronchial epithelial cells with cilia or terminal plates or goblet cells at the periphery and a central core containing small cells. Reserve cell hyperplasia is represented by clusters of tightly packed small cells with uniform, dark, round or oval nuclei. Nucleoli may be observed but are tiny. Nuclear moulding is not present or at least not prominent. Type II alveolar cell hyperplasia has been typically reported bronchoalveolar lavage (BAL) fluid obtained from patients with acute respiratory distress syndrome (ARDS) but it is the cytological hallmark of diffuse alveolar damage (DAD) observed in a variety of acute lung disorders. Pneumocytes appear singly, in flat plates or in rosette-like groups, are polygonal or rectangular in shape, have large nuclei with single or multiple prominent nucleoli and a pale or dense chromatin. The cytoplasm appears basophilic in Diff-Quik preps, often with vacuolation. Extracellular osmiophilic or metachromatic material representing fragments of hyaline membranes is sometimes surrounded by these reactive cells.

Cytological changes in pulmonary infections
Bacteria may be detected by specific stains, or by immunofluorescence or immunocytochemistry. Acid-fast mycobacteria are easily recognised when present in significant quantity in Ziehl–Neelsen preparations. *Nocardia*, a weakly acid fast, aerobic, branching filamentous bacterium, is seen better using the Kinyoun method. *Actinomyces*, anaerobic or microaerophilic Gram-positive bacteria form colonies of radiating, thin filamentous organisms better seen by silver staining. *Legionella* organisms are tiny Gram-negative bacilli that can be demonstrated by silver stains and by immunofluorescence. Numerous other cocci or bacilli may be recognised in Diff-Quik or MGG preps but are better identified using Gram staining. Granulomatous reaction, mainly associated with TB, is cytologically characterised by the presence, in fine-needle aspiration preparations, of pale histiocytes with elongated nuclei collected in nodular structures with poorly demarcated borders, surrounded by inflammatory cells (lymphocytes and neutrophils), necrosis and cellular debris. Malakoplakia due to *Rhodococcus equi* manifests cytologically with epitheloid macrophages with abundant foamy and granular cytoplasm, and intra- and extracytoplasmic, concentrically laminated bodies (Michaelis–Gutmann bodies).

Viral infections may determine cytopathic effects providing a background to the diagnosis. Furthermore, necrosis, inflammation, ciliocytophthoria, and bronchial and alveolar cell hyperplasia/

dysplasia may be associated with these cytopathic changes or may be the only cytological manifestation of these infections. The cellular alterations suggesting a herpes simplex infection are: cells with multiple nuclei, which may contain eosinophilic irregular inclusion bodies with a halo separating the inclusion from the nuclear membrane (Cowdry type A inclusions) (fig. 1) or exhibit a peculiar type of nuclear degeneration that appear as slate grey, homogenised contents (Cowdry type B inclusions). Cells infected by cytomegalovirus (CMV) are larger with large amphophilic, smooth, intranuclear inclusions, surrounded by very prominent halos and marked margination of chromatin on the inner surface of the nuclear membrane. Intracytoplasmic small inclusions well seen by Diff-Quik or MGG stains are also identifiable. Infection with adenovirus produces two types of intranuclear inclusions: the first consists of a small red body surrounded by a well-circumscribed clear halo and the second is a homogenous basophilic mass almost completely replacing the nucleus. The most characteristic cytological finding in measles pneumonia is the presence of multinucleated giant cells containing eosinophilic inclusions both within the nucleus and cytoplasm. Respiratory syncytial virus (RSV) also stimulates a proliferation of multinucleated giant cells with cytoplasmic basophilic inclusions surrounded by halos. Other viruses that may give characteristic inclusions in respiratory cells are: parainfluenza viruses, rubella, coronavirus, polyomavirus and human papillomavirus. Immunoreactivity using specific monoclonal antibodies increases the capacity to recognise virus elements in cytological specimens.

Fungal infections may also be documented cytologically; however, the distinction between colonisation and pneumonia requires clinical and radiological data. *Candida* species may appear as small, oval, 2–4-µm budding yeasts; occasionally, they may elongate into pseudohyphal forms with additional budding at the points of constriction. Filamentous fungal organisms

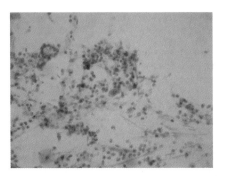

Figure 1. BAL sample showing a multinucleated cell with typical Cowdry A nuclear inclusions in herpes simplex pneumonitis in a transplanted patient. Papanicolaou staining.

are identified by routine stains but silver staining is more precise in identifying septation and the angle of branching. Fragmented hyphae usually identified in silver methenamine-stained preps along with numerous eosinophils, necrotic debris and neutrophils are the cytological hallmark of allergic bronchopulmonary aspergillosis. As angioinvasive mycoses are associated with parenchymal haemorrhage, iron-laden macrophages are usually found in the background. *Cryptococcus* may be identified also using a simple technique: adding some drops of India ink to the sample, the fungus appears as transparent oval or round microorganisms in a dark background. *Pneumocystis jiroveci* is easy to identify in BAL fluid using routine stains: finely vacuolated or foamy proteinaceous casts are typical. Diff-Quik or MGG preps are useful to recognise cysts and, within cysts, up to eight tiny, dot-like trophozoites or sporozoites, measuring 0.5–1 µm in diameter. The wall of the cyst is also stained by Grocott's methenamine silver stain. Numerous fungi are identifiable by routine staining procedures or using silver staining or immunocytochemistry using monoclonal antibodies.

Typical features may also be due to parasites (*Toxoplasma gondii, Entamoeba histolytica, Strongyloides stercoralis, Ancylostoma duodenale, Echinococcus, Paragonimus westermani*, *Microfilaria*, *Dirofilaria* and *Microsporidium*).

Benign non-neoplastic disorders with characteristic cytological findings Sarcoid granulomas have typical cytological features that are easy to recognise in fine-needle aspiration material and smears obtained by biopsy: nodular structures with sharp borders, consisting of epithelioid multinucleated cells in the central portion and of mature lymphocytes at the periphery. Alveolar proteinosis is the cause of a characteristic milky or opaque BAL fluid recovery: on microscopy, a dirty background consisting of amphophilic granules is associated with the presence of globules or chunks of amorphous, amphophilic, periodic acid–Schiff (PAS)-positive material. Foamy macrophages with PAS-positive cytoplasmic inclusions, cholesterol crystals, scattered hyperplastic type II pneumocytes and mature lymphocytes complete the pattern. Exogenous lipid pneumonia may be diagnosed when large macrophages with large cytoplasmic empty vacuoles (that may displace the nuclei at the periphery), or abundant bubbly or lacy, vacuolated cytoplasm are detected. Oil material is easy to detect using Oil Red O or other specific stains. In BAL, an increase of lymphocytes may be an ancillary finding. In individuals smoking 'crack' cocaine, BAL fluid contains alveolar macrophages that accumulate large quantities of carbonaceous material in their cytoplasm; the material is also present extracellularly, imparting black discolouration to the specimen. Organising pneumonia, hypersensitivity pneumonitis, eosinophilic pneumonia, DAD, chronic or acute alveolar haemorrhage, amiodarone lung injury, pulmonary fat embolism, and rarer disorders (Gaucher's disease and Neimann–Pick disease) present characteristic or specific cytological features in BAL fluid. Organising pneumonia also presents characteristic aspects in touch imprints: globules of metachromatic purple amorphous material (Masson bodies) mingled with lymphocytes and scattered mast cells (fig. 2). Cellular nonspecific pneumonitis, idiopathic or secondary and lymphocytic interstitial pneumonitis (LIP) are usually associated with lymphocytosis in BAL fluid. Alveolar macrophages in smokers or recently former smokers show small brown or dark particles in the cytoplasm; these particles are Perl's positive because they also contain iron. However, in desquamative interstitial pneumonitis (DIP), a smoking-related interstitial disease in most cases, BAL eosinophilia is a typical finding. Giant cell pneumonitis, a hard-metal pneumoconiosis, is characterised by numerous giant cells with multiple nuclei, with leukocytes in the cytoplasm (cannibalism); the metals may be documented by analytical electron microscopy. Cytotoxic effects of chemotherapy or radiation and chronic thermal injury determine alterations in nuclei and cytoplasm with aspects mimicking those observed in neoplastic cells (squamous metaplasia/dysplasia; multinucleation, nuclear enlargement with prominent nucleoli, and nuclear or cytoplasmic vacuolisation). Immunocytochemistry is needed to identify Langerhans' cells (monoclonal antibodies against CD1a or langerin).

Lung tumours

Squamous carcinoma The grading of squamous dysplasia is based on nuclear morphology, the amount of cytoplasm and

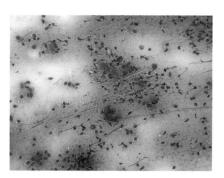

Figure 2. Touch imprint of a transbronchial lung biopsy showing balls of metachromatic, amorphous, extracellular material mingled with lymphocytes an scattered mast cells. Biopsy confirmed the diagnosis of organising pneumonia. Diff-Quick preparation, rapid on-site examination.

the nuclear/cytoplasmic ratio. Well-differentiated keratinising squamous carcinomas are characterised by a polymorphous population of neoplastic cells: very large squamous cells may appear next to very small cells; spindly cells and tadpole cells are quite characteristic. In Papanicolaou preparations, the keratin accumulation in cytoplasm is easy to detect; the nuclei are hyperchromatic with coarsely textured chromatin, and irregular. Nucleoli are evident in poorly differentiated tumours. In nonkeratinising cancer, cytoplasm appears basophilic or amphophilic. In fine-needle aspiration samples, neoplastic cells are more frequently grouped in sheets or smooth clusters. The background may be necrotic. Immunocytochemistry documents expression of p63/p40 protein in the nucleus. Thyroid transcription factor (TTF)-1 staining is negative.

Adenocarcinoma Cell aggregates are a characteristic feature. These clusters have a three-dimensional papillary or approximately spherical configuration. Sheets or rosettes of neoplastic cells are frequent in fine-needle aspiration preparations. The papillary or acinar clusters of cancer cells may resemble and must be distinguished from the so-called Creola bodies. Cancer cells are large, usually round or polygonal, but occasionally columnar or cuboidal. Nuclei are large, pleomorphic and eccentric, with a vesicular chromatin pattern and prominent nucleoli. Cytoplasm may contain mucin or appear vacuolated, mimicking that observed in foamy macrophages. The expression of TTF-1 is evident in nonmucinous adenocarcinoma cells. Immunocytochemistry (napsin positive and p63/p40 negative), and molecular biology investigations regarding *EGFR* (epidermal growth factor receptor) mutations, *ALK* (anaplastic large cell lymphoma kinase) rearrangement with *EML4* (echinoderm microtubule-associated protein like 4) gene and *BRAF*^{V600E} mutation are also feasible in cytological specimens.

Small cell lung cancer Here, the neoplastic cells are small and can be misinterpreted as lymphocytes in sputum. However, in samples obtained by fine-needle aspiration or in smears from bioptic specimens, the proportion of well-preserved viable cells is larger, and they appear two or three times larger than lymphocytes with nuclei showing a vesicular–granular chromatin pattern, inconspicuous nucleoli and a small rim of cytoplasm. The neoplastic cells are in short chains and the moulding of adjacent nuclei in clusters of tumour cells is very common (fig. 3). Hyperchromatic or pyknotic cells and a necrotic background are other elements useful to confirm the diagnosis. Small cell carcinomas are predominantly TTF-1 positive, CD 56 positive, chromogranin and/or synaptophysin positive, p63 negative, Cytokeratin 5 negative and Cytokeratin 8 positive. Tumour cells closely resembling small cell carcinoma may be observed in pulmonary cytology from children with lung metastases of neuroblastoma, embryonal rhabdo-myosarcoma, Ewing's sarcoma, desmoplastic small round cell tumours, lymphomas, and Wilms' tumours and from adults with metastases of Merkel cell carcinoma, poorly differentiated synovial sarcoma, mixoid/round cell chondrosarcoma.

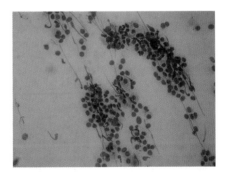

Figure 3. Touch imprint of a transbronchial biopsy showing cells two or three times larger than lymphocytes with nuclei showing a vesicular chromatin pattern, inconspicuous nucleoli and a small rim of cytoplasm. The neoplastic cells are in short chains and the moulding of adjacent nuclei in clusters of tumour cells is evident. The pattern is characteristic of small cell lung cancer.

Large cell carcinoma The cytological findings that suggest a diagnosis of large cell carcinoma are: disorganised groups of large pleomorphic cells or giant cells with clear malignant nuclear aspects (prominent nucleoli and coarse granulation of chromatin), intracytoplasmic neutrophils and a necrotic background. A neuroendocrine differentiation documented by immunocytochemistry (chromogranin, synaptophysin and CD56) is observed in a minority of cases.

Carcinoid tumours are cytologically usually diagnosed on fine-needle aspiration samples as they rarely, if ever, shed neoplastic cells into the sputum. Cells appear dispersed, isolated, in loosely cohesive groups or in syncytial tissue fragments, as cords, nests or anastomosing ribbons with occasional acinar pattern. They are small and round to cuboidal, with poorly defined cell borders and stippled chromatin. Some pleomorphic large cells with bizarre nuclei may also be detected. Spindle cells are more typical of the peripheral neoplasms. Markers such as chromogranin and synaptophysin are unequivocally positive; TTF-1 is negative. Necrosis and mitoses (or a significant positivity for Ki-67 (MIB-1)) suggest the diagnosis of atypical carcinoid.

Other malignant epithelial tumours may be recognised by cytological criteria: adenoid cystic carcinoma (the diagnostic features are the presence of hyaline globules of basement membrane material with intervening small hyperchromatic cells), mucoepidermoid carcinoma and metastases (in these cases, immunocytochemistry may be diriment).

Lymphoproliferative and myeloid disorders
Primary lymphoid tumours in the lung are rare while lymph node-based lymphomas frequently affect the lung during the course of the disease. Acute myeloid leukaemia (M4–M5) may clinically debut with acute respiratory failure. These malignancies are more readily diagnosed on BAL or fine-needle aspiration preparations. Flow cytometry of suspended cells or immunocytochemistry, mainly on cell block

preparations, are the usual ancillary studies required for a more precise definition of the lesions. Primary MALT (mucosa-associated lymphoid tissue) lymphomas in the lung are characterised by noncohesive lymphoid cells with centrocytic, monocytoid or plasmocytoid-like appearances. Flow cytometry is necessary to identify a light chain monoclonal restriction. In addition, other low-grade B-cell lymphomas/ leukaemias may be recognised by cytological and flow cytometry analysis. More sophisticated tools are promising regarding specificity and sensitivity; however, they are not yet included in clinical practice. Large B-cell lymphomas and highly malignant natural killer (NK) T-cell lymphomas may be captured by cytological/immunocytological analyses, and this may be sufficient to confirm lung recurrence but a cytological diagnosis in primary tumours is not feasible. Typical Reed–Sternberg (bilobed or multilobulated cells with distinct nucleoli and an abundant pale-grey cytoplasm on Diff-Quik or MGG preps) or Hodgkin cells (large mononuclear cells with prominent nucleolus and abundant cytoplasm), which are CD30 and CD15 positive, may be recognised in respiratory specimens associated with reactive, small CD3-positive lymphocytes and scattered eosinophils, and this may confirm the diagnosis of relapse of the tumour in the thorax. Myeloid neoplastic cells have been recognised in acute leukaemia, mainly M4 and M5, and in chronic myelomonocytic leukaemia, but also in other forms, either in BAL fluid or in fine-needle aspiration samples (fig. 4).

Thymomas, although rare, are the most common thymic tumours in adults. Cytological findings are: cohesive aggregates of epithelial cells with an associated variable lymphocytic infiltration. Tissue fragments composed of epithelial cell aggregates intimately associated with lymphocytes are called lymphoepithelial complexes, and their presence is generally diagnostic of thymoma. There are two epithelial cell types in thymoma.

1.   Spindle/oval type, which possesses oval or fusiform, normochromatic nuclei

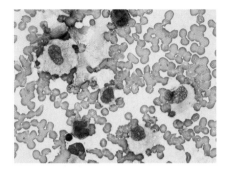

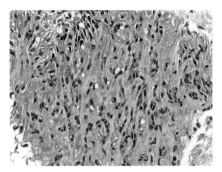

Figure 4. BAL sample showing myeloid blasts showing almost cerebriform nuclei, evident nucleoli and sparse granules in the cytoplasm. Scattred alveolar foamy macrophages are also present. The sample is from a patient with acute promyelocytic leukaemia (M3), microgranular variant. Diff-Quik staining.

Figure 5. Cell block preparation obtained by echoendoscopic transoesophageal fine-needle aspiration. Spindle cells with eosinophilic cytoplasm are embedded in a myxoid stroma. Immunocytochemistry corroborated the diagnosis of gastrointestinal stromal tumour. Haematoxylin and eosin staining.

with dispersed or unevenly distributed chromatin, indistinct or small nucleoli, and lightly stained or indistinct cytoplasm: type A or mixed (AB) thymoma.

2. Polygonal/round cells, which possess round, normochromatic, often clear nuclei, conspicuous round nuclei, and variable amounts of light green-stained cytoplasm: type B thymoma.

Malignant thymic carcinomas present clear-cut cytological features of malignancy. Immunocytochemistry is useful to highlight epithelial cells or mature and immature lymphocytes.

Germ cell tumours The mediastinum is the most common site for the development of extragonadal germ cell tumours. In seminoma, mixed inflammatory cells rich in lymphocytes surround cohesive malignant cells with delicate cytoplasm and a pale nucleus with prominent nucleoli. Embryonal carcinoma has a cytological aspect similar to adenocarcinoma. Yolk sac tumour (endodermal sinus tumour) is characterised by the presence of clusters of epithelial, highly malignant cells containing eosinophilic, PAS-positive, spherical hyaline bodies. Choriocarcinoma can be recognised in aspirates by the presence of large, multinucleated syncytiotrophoblastic cells

with eosinophilic cytoplasm. Immunocytochemistry is very useful to mark the β-subunit of human chorionic gonadotropin or α-fetoprotein. Germ cell tumours may be a cause, along with Hodgkin's disease, of sarcoid-like granulomas collected by fine-needle aspiration techniques.

Mesenchymal tumours Chondroid hamartochondromas may be easily recognised cytologically. In fine-needle aspiration samples, the combination of fibrillar myxoid connective tissue, hyaline cartilage, entrapped bronchiolar epithelium and fat are pathognomonic. The cytological features that are more or less distinctive of other benign or malignant neoplasm of mesenchymal origin (primary in the lung or metastatic) have been described for sclerosing haemangioma (pneumocytoma), granular cell tumour, solitary fibrous tumour, meningioma, schwannoma, gastrointestinal stromal tumour (fig. 5), neurofibroma, ganglioneuroma, glomus tumour, pulmonary blastoma, ganglioneuroblastoma, melanoma, glioblastoma and a wide variety of sarcomas. Cytology in malignant mesothelioma has been deeply investigated, as collection of pleural fluid is very easy during thoracentesis, and cytological features of malignancy and immunocytological markers (calretinin, *etc.*) indicating the origin of neoplastic cells are now well known.

Further reading

- Adams J, *et al.* (2012). The utility of fine-needle aspiration in the diagnosis of primary and metastatic tumors to the lung: a retrospective examination of 1,032 cases. *Acta Cytol*; 56: 590–595.
- Allen TC, *et al.* Mesenchymal and miscellaneous neoplasms. *In:* Hasleton P, *et al.*, eds. Spencer's Pathology of the Lung. Cambridge, Cambridge University Press, 2013; pp. 1224–1316.
- Borie R, *et al.* (2011). Clonality and phenotyping analysis of alveolar lymphocytes is suggestive of pulmonary MALT lymphoma. *Respir Med*; 105: 1231–1237.
- Chilosi M, *et al.* (2010). Mixed adenocarcinoma of the lung: place in new proposals in classification, mandatory for target therapy. *Arch Pathol Lab Med*; 134: 55–65.
- Giles TM, *et al.* Respiratory tract. *In:* Gray W, *et al.*, eds. Diagnostic Cytopathology. Philadelphia, Churchill Livingstone Elsevier, 2010; pp. 17–111.
- Kini SR. Color Atlas of Pulmonary Cytopathology. New York, Springer, 2002.
- Koss L, *et al.*, eds. Koss' Diagnostic Cytology. Philadelphia, Lippincott Williams & Wilkins, 2006.
- Linssen KC, *et al.* (2004). Reactive type II pneumocytes in bronchoalveolar lavage fluid. *Acta Cytol*; 48: 497–504.
- Murer B, *et al.* Metastases involving the lungs. *In:* Hasleton P, *et al.*, eds. Spencer's Pathology of the Lung. Cambridge, Cambridge University Press, 2013; pp. 1375–1407.
- Parham DM, *et al.* (1993). Cytologic diagnosis of respiratory syncytial virus infection in bronchoalveolar lavage specimen from a bone marrow transplant recipient. *Am J Clin Pathol*; 99: 588–592.
- Poletti V, *et al.* (2007). Bronchoalveolar lavage in malignancy. *Semin Respir Crit Care Med*; 28: 534–545.
- Ravaglia C, *et al.* (2012). Diagnostic role of rapid on-site cytologic examination (ROSE) of broncho-alveolar lavage in ALI/ARDS. *Pathologica*; 104: 65–69.
- Shidham VB, *et al.* Serous effusions. *In:* Gray W, *et al.*, eds. Diagnostic Cytopathology. Philadelphia, Churchill Livingstone Elsevier, 2010; pp. 115–175.
- Tabatowski K, *et al.* (1988). Giant cell interstitial pneumonia in a hard metal worker. Cytologic, histologic and analytic electron microscopic investigation. *Acta Cytol*; 32: 240–246.
- Travis WD, *et al.* Tumours of the Lung, Pleura, Thymus and Heart. Lyon, IARC Press, 2004.

Immunology and defence mechanisms

Bruno Balbi, Davide Vallese, Alessandro Pitruzzella, Chiara Vicari and Antonino Di Stefano

Each day, 10 000–15 000 L of air are inhaled by the respiratory system, air containing microorganisms and pollutants gases and particles. It is conceivable, therefore, that adequate and efficient immunological and defence mechanisms exist inside the respiratory system to avoid damage to its structure and to limit the number, extent and severity of upper and lower respiratory tract infections (Reynolds, 1997).

The first line of defence against pathogens is represented by the epithelial barrier of the airways. The epithelium is composed of several different cell types, the structural and functional features of which are described in table 1.

Between the epithelium and the lamina propria there is a thin basal membrane, formed by a lamina propria and a lamina reticularis; these two laminae have a different protein compositions, the basal being composed of connective proteins

(Bucchieri *et al.*, 2009). Additional protection comes from polypeptide mediators of the innate, non-antibody-mediated host defence, and professional phagocytes. Once innate host defense systems are activated by the cytokine and chemokine pathways, acquired, antibody-mediated immune responses and subsequent tissue repair and remodelling are orchestrated by immunocompetent cells and mediators.

Anatomical barriers

In the upper respiratory tract (URT), the density of microbes is greater than in the lower respiratory tract (LRT). In fact, it is usually considered that only a small number of bacteria are present in the LRT of healthy individuals. This process of cleaning the LRT of bacteria is due to mechanical barriers and reflex mechanisms. The nose itself can be considered a first-line barrier. The vibrissae present on the vestibular region of the nasal cavity are able to trap the largest particles contained in inhaled air. Nasal mucosa is a type of respiratory mucosa able to trap other smaller particles by means of its mucus layer. Nasal cilia are able to transport the mucus toward the oropharynx to be swallowed. LRT airways represent a difficult physical barrier system to overcome (Reynolds, 1997). Dichotomous branching and angulation of the airways favour the impact of inhaled particles on the bronchial mucosa surface. At points of impaction, bronchial-associated lymphoid tissue (BALT) is able to interact with inhaled airborne microbes and particles, and to start clearance by phagocytes and immune reactions by immunocompetent cells.

Key points

- The respiratory system is exposed to a variety of microbiological, physical and chemical insults through inhaled air.

- Innate, intrinsic and adaptive, acquired host immune defences cooperate in lowering the risk of damage to respiratory structures in an integrated host defence system.

- In disease states, one or more of these complex mechanisms can be impaired and/or dysfunctional.

Table 1. Main features of bronchial epithelium cells

Cell type	Ultrastructural features	Known roles	Putative roles
Ciliated cells: the most prevalent cell type	Cuboidal Each cell has ~250 cilia, each cilium is ~6 μm long	Transport of mucus stream Decreased in chronic inflammation	
Club cells (Clara cells): the second most prevalent cell type	Cuboidal/columnar, nonciliated, nonmucus-secreting cells Granules are present in apical cytoplasm	Secretory function Airway clearance Increased in chronic inflammation	Progenitors of type II pneumocytes Surfactant production
Basal cells: rare in bronchioles, unknown cell origin	Small round cells with numerous secretory granules	Precursors of other cell types Involved in carcinogenesis	Stem cells
Neuroendocrine (Kulchitsky) cells: rare in bronchioles	Cuboidal/columnar, mucus-secreting cells	Part of diffuse neuroendocrine system	Origin of small cell lung cancer
Goblet cells: rare in bronchioles	Cuboidal/columnar mucus secreting cells	Secretory function contributing to the cleaning of smallest airways Increased in chronic inflammation	
Lymphocytes: rare in bronchioles	Small, round cells with scarce cytoplasm Scattered among the other cell types or adjacent to the luminal surface of epithelium	Immune surveillance Increased in chronic inflammation	

Reflex mechanisms

A number of reflex mechanisms may help the defence of the respiratory tract (Reynolds, 1997). They are made possible by the presence of irritant and stretch receptors on the mucosa of the airways of the URT and of the largest LRT airways.

Sneezing is a complex reflex starting from the irritant receptors in the nose, usually stimulated by inhaled particles, followed by itching, mucus secretion and, ultimately, leading to a forceful and sudden expiration through the nose, preceded by a deep and fast inspiration, that is able to eliminate the potentially harmful inhaled particles.

Cough In the tracheobronchial tree, the cough reflex plays a similar role in eliminating foreign inhaled particles.

Dyspnoea can also be considered, at least under certain circumstances, a defence mechanism, as it can result from both hypersecretion of mucus and/or bronchospasm. By reducing the airway calibre, both are able to impair the ability of inhaled harmful particles to reach the LRT.

Mucociliary clearance and fluid homeostasis

The constant mechanical clearance of mucus from the airways is considered a primary airway defense mechanism (Knowles et al., 2002). Through ciliary function and mucus secretion with proper salt/water components, the airway epithelial surface is able to act to maintain the mucociliary clearance with a mucus 'escalator' from the lowest airways to the top. With a mucus layer distal to the epithelium containing different types of mucins and a largely prevalent aqueous layer beneath this, the airway secretions are, under normal conditions, able to entrap the vast majority of inhaled foreign particles and microbes on the mucus layer and to transport the mucus up to the larger airways to be swallowed or eliminated by coughing. More recent studies have emphasised the role of a 'chemical shield' from inhaled bacteria. This view underlies the importance of the production and secretion into the airway lumen of two components by the airway epithelia: salt-sensitive defensins and a low-salt liquid able to activate defensins.

Innate defence molecules

The epithelial lining fluid in the airways contains a myriad of peptides and proteins exerting innate antimicrobial activities, not only against bacteria and viruses but also, in some cases, against fungi and parasites. As a whole, these innate antimicrobial molecules, although with many differences in site and the cell types producing them,

Table 2. Key antimicrobial factors in epithelial lining fluid and their activities

Factor	Type of molecule	Cell origin	Antimicrobial activities	Main immunomodulatory activities
Defensins	Peptides	Phagocytic cells Lymphocytes Airway epithelial cells	BC BS AV AF AP	Mitogenic Chemotactic Degranulates MCs
Cathelicidins	Pro-peptides	Neutrophils Monocytes MCs Lymphocytes Airway epithelial cells	BC BS AV AF	Downregulation of TNF-α Chemotactic
SLPI	Protein	Macrophages Neutrophils Airway epithelial cells	BC BS AV AF	Antiprotease Anti-inflammatory
SP-A, SP-D	Lipoproteins	Alveolar type II cells Club cells (Clara cells)	BC BS AV AF	Opsonic Modulate leukocyte functions Structural barrier
Lactoferrin	Glycoprotein	Neutrophils Airway epithelial cells	BC BS AV AF	Antioxidant Binds LPS Inhibits biofilm formation
Lysozyme	Enzyme	Neutrophils Airway epithelial cells	BC BS	Unknown
Lactoperoxidase	Enzyme	Airway epithelial cells	BC AV AF	Antioxidant?

BC: bactericidal; BS: bacteriostatic; AV: antiviral; AF: antifungal; AP: antiparasitic; MC: mast cell; TNF: tumour necrosis factor; SLPI: secretory leukocyte peptidase inhibitor; SP: surfactant protein; LPS: lipopolysaccharide.

secretory stimuli, and direct and indirect activities (table 2), provide a highly evolutionarily conserved, powerful screen against infections in the naïve host. They also trigger more specific and targeted immune reactions taking place into the airways and in the alveolar structures. In addition, the same molecules have a role as immune modulators, antioxidants and antiproteases. Not surprisingly, attempts have been made to use some of these 'natural antibiotics' for therapeutic purposes.

Professional phagocytes

Microbial pathogens activate pattern recognition receptors (*e.g.* Toll-like receptors, NOD-like receptors, scavenger receptors, *etc.*) on phagocytes, namely macrophages and neutrophils, as well as on epithelial cells, mast cells, eosinophils and natural killer cells. This is followed by the release of several mediators and factors with effector functions and inflammatory cascades, such as the complement system, acute phase reactant proteins, oxidative and nitrosative stress molecules, prostaglandins, interferons, cytokines and chemokines. Macrophages are the resident respiratory phagocytes. Although they are present throughout the airways and interstitium, their major roles are played in the alveolar spaces, as alveolar macrophages. In the normal individual, the vast majority of cells recovered through bronchoalveolar lavage (BAL) are alveolar macrophages. These cells initiate and orchestrate the immune reactions against pathogens and chemicals inhaled by the host (*e.g.* mineral particles). In a hypothetical model of infection by a bacterial species, a pathogen that has reached the alveolar space, eluding URT and LRT first-line defences, represents a risk for the host as its replication and associated alveolar inflammation may damage respiratory structures. This invader microorganism will ultimately be enmeshed with the epithelial lining fluid and, thus, be coated with opsonins. These may be non-immune or immune, *i.e.* specific immunoglobulins originated by previous immunisation of the host against the pathogen. Opsonins facilitate alveolar macrophage phagocytosis and subsequent bacterial clearance by the intracellular killing systems. The size of the bacterial inoculum, virulence and resistance, and possibly deficits of local immunity mechanisms in the host, may cause the failure, at least in a first round, of host defences. This will cause recruitment of additional phagocytes, such as neutrophils, at sites of infection, and sustain an immune and inflammatory reaction.

Acquired immune reactions with immunoglobulin, cytokine and chemokine production

Lymphoid tissue is present in the respiratory tract in different forms:

- tonsils and adenoids in the URT
- lymph nodes in the mediastinum and hila
- submucosal aggregates in branching points of the airways (BALT)
- free immunocompetent cells on the airways and alveolar surface

BALT is also considered to be part of a lymphoid network common to other types of mucosa. In this model, immunisation can occur at a distant site (*e.g.* gastrointestinal mucosa) and, by the recirculation of lymphocytes, protection can be provided in the respiratory system. Acquired immune reactions start also in the lung with the interaction between antigens and antigen-presenting cells. In the lung, at least two types of antigen-presenting cell exist: macrophages and dendritic cells. Dendritic cells are present in the bronchi, representing roughly 1% of epithelial cells, in the alveolar septa and in the interstitium. Together with a phagocytic function, they share with alveolar macrophages the ability to process microbial proteins into small peptide fragments that are then transported on the cell surface together with major histocompatibility complex (MHC) molecules. The complex between the MHC and antigenic epitopes is then presented to T-cells. Antigen presentation is made through the T-cell receptor (TCR) on the T-cell surface.

Antigen presentation initiates the production of immunoenhancing cytokines and chemokines. A part from the interleukins (ILs) and other mediators associated with the

Intrinsic and innate host defences		Adaptive and acquired immune defences
Anatomic barriers Defence reflexes Mucociliary clearance Fluid homeostasis Innate defence molecules Nonimmune opsonins Professional phagocytes	Pathogens Particles	Secretory IgA and other immune opsonins Antigen recognition and presentation Cellular immunity T- and B- cells Cytokines/chemokine production and networking Chemotactic influx of inflammatory, immunoeffector cells

Figure 1. Integrated host defence systems in the respiratory tract.

T-helper (Th) type 1 or 2 immune reactions, IL-17 is a pro-inflammatory cytokine mainly produced by T-cells with an important role in induction of a neutrophil-mediated protective immune response against bacteria or fungal pathogens (Matsuzaki et al., 2007; Di Stefano et al., 2009). IL-17 seems to be an example of the crossroads between different host defense mechanisms, as it regulates cell-mediated immunity and induction of antimicrobial peptides, such as defensins.

This process of specific immune reaction also promotes adaptive B-cell proliferation and specific immunoglobulin production. The relative proportions of different immunoglobulins in the URT and LRT differ one from each other as well as compared with the blood. Immunoglobulins represent ~10% of total proteins in airway secretions. In the URT, IgA represent the vast majority of this immunoglobulin. Airway IgA is predominantly polymeric: secretory IgA comprises two IgA monomers held together by a joining chain and by another glycoprotein, the secretory component, which is produced by serous and epithelial cells. In contrast with the URT, in the LRT, as detected by BAL, IgG is predominant, representing ~5% of the total protein content in BAL fluid from normal individuals. IgM is present only in trace amounts, due to its large size.

Conclusions

The complex, integrated host defence system described and depicted in figure 1 represents a superb model of how the human body is able to interact efficiently with the external environment in order to preserve its structure and function.

Conversely, impairment and/or dysfunction of each of the different components of this system represent the pathogenetic basis for the development of many respiratory disorders. As an example, primary ciliary dyskinesia results in recurrent airway infections, CF is associated with dysfunction of mucociliary clearance and fluid homeostasis, and in chronic colonisation and/or infection of the airways and in inflammatory airway disorders, many different mechanisms undergo changes, enhancement or impairment (Di Stefano et al., 2009; Pignatti et al., 2009).

Further reading

- Balamayooran T, et al. (2010). Toll-like receptors and NOD-like receptors in pulmonary antibacterial immunity. Innate Immun; 16: 201–210.
- Bals R, et al. (2004). Innate immunity in the lung: how epithelial cells fight against respiratory pathogens. Eur Respir J; 23: 327–333.

- Bucchieri F, *et al.* (2009). Stem cell populations and regenerative potential in chronic inflammatory lung diseases. *J Tissue Eng Regen Med*; 2: 34–39.
- Di Stefano A, *et al.* (2009). T helper type 17-related cytokine expression is increased in the bronchial mucosa of stable chronic obstructive pulmonary disease patients. *Clin Exp Immunol*; 157: 316–324.
- Knowles MR, *et al.* (2002). Mucus clearance as a primary innate defense mechanism for mammalian airways. *J Clin Invest*; 109: 571–577.
- Martin TR, *et al.* (2005). Innate immunity in the lungs. *Proc Am Thor Soc*; 2: 403–411.
- Matsuzaki G, *et al.* (2007). Interleukin-17 as an effector molecule of innate and acquired immunity against infections. *Microbiol Immunol*; 51: 1139–1147.
- McCormack FX, *et al.* (2002). The pulmonary collectins, SP-A and SP-D, orchestrate innate immunity in the lung. *J Clin Invest*; 109: 707–712.
- Oppenheim JJ, *et al.* (2003). Roles of antimicrobial peptides such as defensins in innate and adaptive immunity. *Ann Rheum Dis*; 26: Suppl. 2, ii17–ii21.
- Pignatti P, *et al.* (2009). Tracheostomy and related host-pathogen interaction are associated with airway inflammation as characterised by tracheal aspirate analysis. *Respir Med*; 103: 201–208.
- Reynolds HY. Integrated host defense against infections. *In:* Crystal RG, *et al.*, eds. The Lung: Scientific Foundation. Philadelphia, Lippincott-Raven Publishers, 1997: pp. 2353–2365.
- Rogan MP, *et al.* (2006). Antimicrobial proteins and polypeptides in pulmonary innate defence. *Respir Res*; 7: 29–40.
- Sallenave JM (2010). Secretory leukocyte protease inhibitor and elafin/trappin-2: versatile mucosal antimicrobials and regulators of immunity. *Am J Respir Cell Mol Biol*; 42: 635–643.
- Whitsett JA (2002). Intrinsic and innate defenses in the lung: intersection of pathways regulating lung morphogenesis, host defense, and repair. *J Clin Invest*; 109: 565–569.
- Yang D, *et al.* (2001). Participation of mammalian defensins and cathelicidins in antimicrobial immunity: receptors and activities of human defensins and cathelicidin (LL-37). *J Leuk Biol*; 69: 691–697.
- Zanetti M (2005). The role of cathelicidins in the innate host defenses of mammals. *Curr Issues Mol Biol*; 7: 179–196.

Cough and sputum

Alyn H. Morice

Cough is a vital protective mechanism defending the airways from inhalation and aspiration. Patients with a defective cough reflex, such as those with stroke or Parkinson's disease, have an increase in mortality and morbidity caused by the increased propensity for aspiration. However, in lung disease, cough is often not helpful. Thus, in the commonest form of cough, that due to upper respiratory tract infection, coughing serves no useful purpose from the sufferer's point of view, but aids viral transmission. In chronic cough, the frequency and severity of coughing bouts may cause serious disruption to the patient's life. Quality-of-life instruments have indicated that patients with chronic cough may have a similar decrement to that seen with conditions such as cancer and severe COPD. Cough may also have significant comorbidity. 50% of the females attending cough clinics are incontinent and cough syncope is thought to be responsible for a number of driving fatalities.

Acute cough

Acute cough due to one of the myriad upper respiratory tract viruses places an enormous demand on the healthcare community. It is the commonest new presentation to primary care, accounting for 50% of consultations. In temperate regions there is a marked seasonal variation with autumn and winter epidemics. Viral transmission requires person-to-person contact, either through airborne droplet infection or the manual passage of secretions. Superimposed on this seasonal pattern are peaks caused by socialisation, e.g. return to school for the autumn term and Christmas family

> **Key points**
>
> - Cough is characterised by irritant receptor hypersensitivity.
> - Nonacid reflux into the airways frequently precipitates cough.
> - Clinical history followed by therapeutic trials is the management strategy of choice.

gatherings. Apart from general health measures, such as hand washing and avoidance of contact, there is no specific treatment for upper respiratory tract infection-induced cough. The demonstrable effect of the many cough remedies is likely to be due to a physicochemical (demulcent) effect rather than through a specific pharmacological action of any particular agent.

Chronic cough

Chronic cough is one of the commonest presentations to the respiratory physician. A survey in Yorkshire, UK, indicated that 12% of the normal population complain of a chronic cough and 7% of these thought it interfered with activities of daily living. Many reports from specialist cough clinics point to a particular syndrome in patients with chronic cough. The typical patient is middle-aged and female. The cough appears to have no pattern to it but a careful history will often reveal many common features of the presenting complaint. It has been traditional to divide these patients without radiographic abnormalities and no obvious other lung disease into a triad of diagnoses, namely asthmatic cough, post-nasal drip syndrome (rhinitis) and reflux cough (table 1). These subdivisions have recently been called into question. For example, asthmatic cough is unlike classic atopic asthma in that it is usually of late onset without obvious precipitants and often without evidence of bronchoconstriction. In the form known as eosinophilic bronchitis there is even an absence of bronchial hyperreactivity. Similar caveats apply to post-nasal drip syndrome and reflux cough. Thus, the latter frequently does not conform to the criteria for peptic gastro-oesophageal reflux disease. Because of the commonality of the clinical history in chronic cough (table 2), it has been suggested that there is a single unifying diagnosis of cough hypersensitivity syndrome, with the other diagnoses representing different phenotypes of the condition. The risk factors for chronic cough suggest that nonacid reflux may be an important precipitant (table 3).

Virtually all patients presenting with a chronic cough complain of increased sensitivity to a wide range of environmental stimuli. This hypersensitivity can be objectively demonstrated in the laboratory using cough challenge. Thus, patients cough with ethanol inhalation, whereas normal subjects do not. There is a wide variation in cough reflex sensitivity in normal subjects, with females being more sensitive than males. Sensitivity is accentuated in cough patients. Inhalation of capsaicin, the pungent extract of peppers, is typically used to demonstrate cough reflex responsiveness (fig. 1). Capsaicin works by stimulating one of a family of nociceptors of the transient receptor potential (TRP) group (fig. 2). The capsaicin-sensitive 'hot' receptor (TRPV1) is upregulated in patients with cough. This is due to pro-inflammatory mediators increasing expression of TRPV1, either in neurones or in other airway tissues. Rather than directly causing a cough, angiotensin-converting enzyme inhibitors alter cough sensitivity by a TRPV1-dependent mechanism, thus explaining the continued irritation long after drug withdrawal. Another TRP receptor, TRPA1, is highly reactive to a

Table 1. Early reports from cough clinics illustrating the variety of cough diagnosis dependent on criteria used

	Mean age years	Patients (females) n	Diagnosis % total		
			Asthma syndrome	GOR	Rhinitis
Irwin et al. (1981)	50.3	49 (27)	25	10	29
Poe et al. (1982)		109 (68)	36	0	8
Poe et al. (1989)	44.8	139 (84)	35	5	26
Irwin et al. (1990)	51	102 (59)	24	21	41
Hoffstein et al. (1994)	47	228 (139)	25	24	26
O'Connell et al. (1994)	49	87 (63)	6	10	13
Smyrnios et al. (1995)	58	71 (32)	24	15	40
Mello et al. (1996)	53.1	88 (64)	14	40	38
Marchesani et al. (1998)	51	92 (72)	14	5	56
McGarvey et al. (1998)	47.5	43 (29)	23	19	21
Palombini et al. (1999)	57	78 (51)	59	41	58
Brightling et al. (1999)		91 (0)	31	8	24

The typical patient is a middle-aged female. These diagnoses are now thought to represent phenotypes of the cough hypersensitivity syndrome. GOR: gastro-oesophageal reflux. Studies can be found in Morice et al. (2004).

Table 2. Areas of enquiry in chronic cough

Hoarseness or a problem with your voice
Clearing your throat
The feeling of something dripping down the back of your nose or throat
Retching or vomiting when you cough
Cough on first lying down or bending over
Chest tightness or wheeze when coughing
Heartburn, indigestion or stomach acid coming up, or do you take medications for this?
A tickle or a lump in your throat
Cough with eating (during or soon after meals)
Cough with certain foods
Cough when you get out of bed in the morning
Cough brought on by singing or speaking (*e.g.* on the telephone)
Coughing more when awake than asleep
A strange taste in your mouth

Responses may either lead to further questioning or be scored 0–5 and used as a diagnostic tool to demonstrate the presence of cough hypersensitivity syndrome. A questionnaire version in various languages is available at www.issc.info

Table 3. Risk factors for chronic cough

Variable	With cough n/N (%)	Unadjusted OR (95% CI)	p-value
Sex			
Male	78/1704 (4.6)	1.0	
Female	135/2179 (6.2)	1.38 (1.03–1.86)	0.028
Heartburn			
No	148/2990 (4.9)	1.0	
Yes	65/889 (7.3)	1.51 (1.10–2.06)	0.009
Regurgitation			
No	158/3314 (4.8)	1.0	
Yes	54/568 (9.5)	2.10 (1.49–2.92)	<0.0001
IBS			
No	111/2914 (3.8)	1.0	<0.0001
Yes	98/909 (10.8)	3.05 (2.27–4.09)	
BMI category			
Normal	74/1547 (4.8)	1.0	
Overweight	72/1448 (5.0)	1.04 (0.74–1.47)	0.86
Obese	60/776 (7.7)	1.67 (1.15–2.41)	0.006

Nonacid reflux symptoms in the form of regurgitation are more closely associated with cough than acid reflux. IBS: irritable bowel syndrome.

wide range of environmental irritants and causes cough in humans. Upregulation of this receptor provides a mechanism for the exquisite hypersensitivity complained of by patients to agonists such as acrolein, the pro-tussive ingredient in smoke.

Management of chronic cough

All patients presenting with chronic cough should have a chest radiograph. The clinical history should indicate the most likely treatment options. The European Respiratory Society guidelines recommend therapeutic trials based on clinical judgement. Thus, in patients with episodes of wheezing and evidence of eosinophilic inflammation, a trial of asthmatic medication may well be beneficial (fig. 3). Where available, exhaled nitric oxide fraction may be a useful screening tool. Bronchoconstriction may not be a major component of this phenotype of cough hypersensitivity syndrome and, consequently, long-acting β-agonists may be less effective than anti-eosinophilic medication such as leukotriene antagonists. Reflux disease may be very problematical, as much airway reflux is nonacidic and, therefore, not amenable to blockade by proton pump inhibitors. Pro-motility agents, such as metoclopramide and domperidone, may be used. Other motility agents, such as erythromycin, azithromycin and magnesium, have also been advocated. Operative treatment *via* Nissen fundoplication can be effective in intractable coughing. An alternative strategy is to treat the hypersensitivity component with agents such as gabapentin. Finally, the use of central cough suppression in the form of antitussive agents, such as low-dose morphine, can ameliorate cough in a third of patients with otherwise intractable symptoms.

Sputum

In subjects with chronic cough, production of moderate amounts of sputum does not alter the diagnostic profile. The separation from individuals with excessive sputum production is arbitrary, but is generally regarded as a cup of sputum per day. Above this limit, a diagnosis of bronchiectasis becomes increasingly likely. The presence of sputum purulence indicates a greater likelihood but does not seem to predict the degree of anatomical damage to the airway. Indeed, the diagnosis of bronchiectasis, relying as it does on the dilation and destruction of the airways, will not include many patients with functional abnormalities of the bronchi.

In conditions characterised by sputum hypersecretion, there is usually a change in the composition of the mucus. Several mechanisms are responsible for this change. Thus, in CF, the increase in sodium reabsorption leads to a reduction in the sol phase of the airway surface liquid. Airway inflammation, particularly that caused by release of enzymes such as myeloperoxidase (which produces the characteristic green colour) and neutral endopeptidase, and by polymorphs, causes alteration of mucin (*MUC*) gene expression through proteinase-activated receptors. The death of inflammatory cells and bacteria lead to a soup of DNA that cross-links with filamentous actin, producing gelatinous plugs that increase ventilation/perfusion ratio mismatch with resulting systemic hypoxia.

The treatment of mucus hypersecretion may be challenging. In the presence of purulent sputum, every effort should be made to identify the causative organism. Eradication with appropriate high-dose antibiotic therapy may lead to sustained remission. More frequently, there is rapid relapse, indicating the need for maintenance antibiotics either orally or *via* the nebulised route.

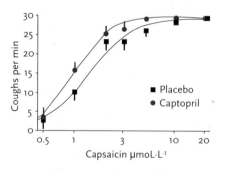

Figure 1. Capsaicin cough challenge in normal subjects, the effect of captopril enhancing cough reflex sensitivity.

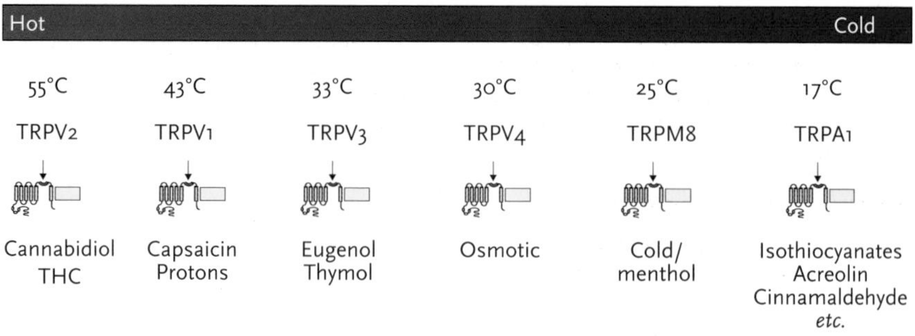

Hot					Cold
55°C	43°C	33°C	30°C	25°C	17°C
TRPV2	TRPV1	TRPV3	TRPV4	TRPM8	TRPA1
Cannabidiol THC	Capsaicin Protons	Eugenol Thymol	Osmotic	Cold/ menthol	Isothiocyanates Acreolin Cinnamaldehyde etc.

Figure 2. *The thermosensitive transient receptor potential (TRP) channels that are important in cough reflex sensitivity. Typical 'natural' agonists are listed below each channel. THC: tetrahydrocannabinol.*

The advantage of this latter strategy is that side-effects may be minimised by using agents with high local potency but poor oral bioavailability, such as colomycin or tobramycin. Antioxidant mucolytics are widely prescribed but evidence of efficacy is limited. The largest study of N-acetylcysteine over 3 years showed no effect on decline in lung function or exacerbation rate. In COPD, two agents, azithromycin and roflumilast, have been shown to be efficacious in those with exacerbations of chronic bronchitis.

Perhaps because of the paucity of specific agents for mucus hypersecretion, nonpharmacological therapy in the form of airway clearance techniques is frequently advocated. However, a recent Cochrane review found the quality of randomised studies to be poor and concluded that any benefits achieved may be small (Osadnik *et al.*, 2012).

Haemoptysis

Haemoptysis presents in two clinical scenarios. First, the patient may present with *de novo* haemoptysis without pre-existing lung disease. Any mucosal lesion may cause haemoptysis of small amounts of blood mixed with sputum. Since this is a common presentation of lung cancer, chest radiography is obligatory in patients when presenting with haemoptysis and, in heavy smokers, CT or bronchoscopy is also required. Aspergilloma and TB may similarly cause blood-stained bronchitis. More peripheral lung pathology, such as lobar pneumonia, gives rise to sputum that is frequently described as 'rusty'. Haemoptysis of frank blood is a common sign of pulmonary embolism or infarction.

Obviously, recurrent haemoptysis initially presents with acute haemoptysis. Typically, bronchiectasis leads to recurrent, sometimes massive and occasionally fatal haemoptysis. The bronchial blood supply arises from the aorta and, in contrast to the pulmonary circulation, is at systemic pressure. In bronchiectasis, there is hypertrophy of the bronchial arteries as a consequence of recurrent infection. When the patient presents with life-threatening haemoptysis,

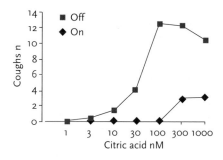

Figure 3. *Cough challenge with citric acid in eosinophilic bronchitis and the response to inhaled steroids. Number of coughs off and on budesonide is shown.*

radiographic percutaneous bronchial artery embolisation is the treatment of choice. Vasculitis is a common and frequently missed cause of recurrent haemoptysis and diffuse alveolar haemorrhage. While the systemic connective tissue diseases, such as systemic lupus erythematosus, may produce small-vessel haemoptysis, the commonest cause is microscopic polyangiitis. The perinuclear anti-neutrophil cytoplasmic antibody (MPO ANCA) is positive in ~70% of cases. Finally, haemoptysis may be the result of alveolar haemorrhage. Disease of the vascular or alveolar wall, such as Goodpasture's syndrome or alveolar haemosiderosis, may present with recurrent haemoptysis. Clearly, disorders of coagulation, both congenital and acquired, and including warfarin therapy or thrombocytopenia, will predispose to haemoptysis.

Further reading

- Birrell MA, et al. (2009). TRPA1 agonists evoke coughing in guinea-pig and human volunteers. Am J Respir Crit Care Med; 180: 1042–1047.
- Decramer M, et al. (2005). Effects of N-acetylcysteine on outcomes in chronic obstructive pulmonary disease (Bronchitis Randomized on NAC Cost-Utility Study, BRONCUS): a randomised placebo-controlled trial. Lancet; 365: 1552–1560.
- Ford AC, et al. (2006). Cough in the community: a cross sectional survey and the relationship to gastrointestinal symptoms. Thorax; 61: 975–979.
- Millqvist E, et al. (2008). Inhaled ethanol potentiates the cough response to capsaicin in patients with airway sensory hyperreactivity. Pulm Pharmacol Ther; 21: 794–797.
- Mitchell JE, et al. (2005). Expression and characterization of the intracellular vanilloid receptor (TRPV1) in bronchi from patients with chronic cough. Exp Lung Res; 31: 295–306.
- Morice AH (2010). The cough hypersensitivity syndrome: a novel paradigm for understanding cough. Lung; 188: 87–90.
- Morice AH, et al. (2004). The diagnosis and management of chronic cough. Eur Respir J; 24: 481–492.
- Morice AH, et al. (2007). Opiate therapy in chronic cough. Am J Respir Crit Care Med; 175: 312–315.
- Osadnik CR, et al. (2012). Airway clearance techniques for chronic obstructive pulmonary disease. Cochrane Database Syst Rev; 3: CD008328.
- Palombini BC, et al. (1999). A pathogenic triad in chronic cough: asthma, postnasal drip syndrome, and gastroesophageal reflux disease. Chest; 116: 279–284.
- Rogers DF (2007). Physiology of airway mucus secretion and pathophysiology of hypersecretion. Respir Care; 52: 1134–1146.

Dyspnoea

Pierantonio Laveneziana and Giorgio Scano

Dyspnoea is the major reason for referral for pharmacological treatment and respiratory rehabilitation programmes in patients with COPD. Dyspnoea is a subjective experience of breathing difficulty that consists of qualitatively distinct sensations that vary in intensity. This definition underlines the importance of the different qualities (cluster descriptors) covered by the term dyspnoea, the involvement of integration of multiple sources of neural information about breathing and the physiological consequences. More specifically, it has been postulated that dyspnoea arises when there is a conscious awareness of a mismatch between what the brain expects and what it receives in terms of afferent information from the lungs, airways and receptors in the tendons and muscles of the chest wall (fig. 1 and table 1).

Evaluation of dyspnoea during physical tasks

Exertional dyspnoea can be easily defined as 'the perception of respiratory discomfort that occurs for an activity level that does not normally lead to breathing difficulty' (Killian et al., 1995). It follows that the intensity of dyspnoea can be determined by assessing the activity level required to produce dyspnoea (i.e. dyspnoea at rest is more severe than dyspnoea only when climbing stairs). The Medical Research Council (MRC) dyspnoea scale can be used for this purpose (table 2), as well as other scales such as the Baseline Dyspnoea Index. Dyspnoea can also be evaluated during a physical task, such as cardiopulmonary exercise testing (CPET). For this purpose, the 10-point Borg scale can be used (table 2). In the Borg scale, the end-points are anchored such that zero represents 'no breathlessness at all' and 10 is 'the most severe breathlessness that one had ever experienced or could imagine experiencing'. Using the Borg scale, subjects rate the magnitude of their perceived breathing discomfort during exercise. Though

Key points

- Dyspnoea is a subjective experience of breathing discomfort that consists of qualitatively distinct sensations that vary in intensity.

- The mechanisms of dyspnoea are complex and multifactorial: there is no unique central or peripheral source of this symptom.

- The sense of heightened inspiratory effort is an integral component of exertional dyspnoea and is pervasive across health and disease.

- The NVD theory of dyspnoea states that the symptom arises when there is a disparity between the central reflex drive (efferent discharge) and the simultaneous afferent feedback from a multitude of peripheral sensory receptors throughout the respiratory system. The feedback system provides information about the extent and appropriateness of the mechanical response to central drive.

- Despite the diversity of causes, the similarity of described experiences of dyspnoea suggests common underlying mechanisms.

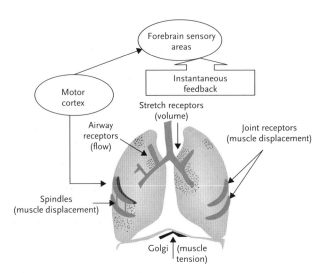

Figure 1. Schematic representation of the neurophysiological underpinnings of perceived dyspnoea during exercise in healthy humans. During a voluntary increase in ventilation, the motor cortex increases the outgoing motor signal to the respiratory muscles and conveys a copy (central corollary discharge) through cortical interneurons to the sensory/association cortex, which is informed of the increased motor drive to increase ventilation. Volitional respiratory effort in healthy subjects is harmoniously matched with the appropriate increase in flow or volume displacement via concurrent afferent proprioceptive information transmitted via vagal, glossopharyngeal, spinal and phrenic nerves. This information is conveyed to the medulla and central cortex, where it is integrated. The result is a harmonious neuromechanical coupling with avoidance of respiratory discomfort or distress. Reproduced and modified from Scano et al. (2010) with permission from the publisher.

somewhat less popular, the visual analogue scale (VAS) is another dyspnoea measuring instrument with proven construct validity during CPET. Both the VAS and Borg scale have been shown to provide similar scores during CPET, and to be reliable and reproducible over time in healthy subjects, and in patients with asthma and COPD undergoing CPET.

Physiology

The recent American Thoracic Society statement has emphasised the multidimensional nature of dyspnoea in the sensory–perceptual (intensity and quality), affective distress and impact domains. To gain more insight into our understanding of dyspnoea, a case can be made for answering the following questions.

1) What is the role of mechanical factors and ventilatory constraints in dyspnoea?

2) What are the neurophysiological underpinnings of the most selected cluster descriptors that define the qualitative dimension of dyspnoea in patients?

3) Do obstructive and restrictive lung diseases share some common underlying mechanisms?

Dyspnoea is perceived as a sense of effort

During voluntary increase in ventilation, the motor cortex increases the outgoing motor signal to respiratory muscles and conveys a copy (central corollary discharge) through cortical interneurones to the sensory/ association cortex, which is informed of the voluntary effort to increase ventilation. It is also likely that the sense of the respiratory effort arises from the simultaneous activation of the sensory cortex and muscle contraction: a variety of muscle receptors provides feedback to the central nervous

Table 1. Putative neurophysiological basis of exertional dyspnoea

Central (corollary discharge)	↑ motor drive (inspiratory effort): cortical ↑ reflex drive (chemical, neural): medullary
Peripheral (afferent activity)	Airway/lung receptors (pulmonary stretch receptors, C-fibres, J-receptors) Ventilatory muscle receptors (muscle spindles, Golgi tendon organs, joint receptors, type III and IV mechano- and metaboreceptors in the diaphragm and chest wall muscles) Peripheral chemoreceptors Locomotor muscles receptors (type III and IV afferents)

The most important receptors (afferences) and efferences to respiratory and locomotor muscles involved in the putative pathogenesis of exertional dyspnoea in cardiopulmonary disease. Please see the main text for more details.

system about force and tension, and information from these receptors may conceivably underlie the sense of effort. For clinical purposes, the perceived magnitude of respiratory effort is expressed by the ratio of the tidal oesophageal pressure (P_{oes}) to the maximal pressure generation capacity of the respiratory muscles (P_{Imax}). In healthy subjects, volitional respiratory effort is matched by lung/chest wall displacement (*i.e.* change in tidal volume (V_T) as percentage of vital capacity (VC)) *via* concurrent afferent proprioceptive information, transmitted *via* vagal, glossopharyngeal, spinal and phrenic nerves, that monitors displacement, and is processed and integrated in the sensory cortex. The result is a harmonious neuromechanical coupling with avoidance of respiratory discomfort or distress (fig. 1 and table 1).

Dyspnoea is perceived as a sense of air hunger

Under some clinical and experimental circumstances, the relationship between dyspnoea and effort is less apparent. If normal subjects suppress their ventilation to a level below that dictated by chemical drive (carbon dioxide), dyspnoea increases without corresponding increases in indices of respiratory effort. Likewise, in experimental and clinical conditions where peripheral stretch receptors are inhibited, the sensory cortex is not informed of the ventilatory response. In these circumstances, dyspnoea is perceived as a sensation of air hunger, the intensity of which depends on a mismatching between the level of chemically stimulated drive and ongoing inhibition from pulmonary mechanosensors signalling the current level of ventilation. In turn, dyspnoea arises and may qualitatively change when peripheral afferent feedback is altered and inspiratory motor output either increases or stabilises.

Pathophysiology

COPD Two qualitative descriptor clusters of dyspnoea are commonly selected by patients with COPD during physical activity.

The descriptor cluster that alludes to increased respiratory work/effort ('breathing requires more effort or work') is commonly selected by patients with COPD. Increased sense of work/effort is related to the increased motor drive to the respiratory muscles and increased central neural drive (due to chemostimulation) as a consequence of progressive metabolic and ventilation/perfusion disruptions during exercise. Therefore, increased perceived work/effort during physical activity, in part, reflects the greater ventilatory demand for a given task compared with health. In addition, contractile muscle effort is increased for any given ventilation because of:

Table 2. *The MRC dyspnoea scale and the Borg scale*

Grade	Description
MRC dyspnoea scale	
1	Not troubled by breathlessness except with strenuous exercise
2	Troubled by shortness of breath when hurrying on the level or walking up a slight hill
3	Walks slower than people of the same age on the level because of breathlessness or has to stop for breath when walking at own pace on the level
4	Stops for breath after walking ~90 m or after a few minutes on the level
5	Too breathless to leave the house or breathlessness when dressing or undressing
Borg scale	
0	No breathlessness at all
0.5	Very, very slight (just noticeable)
1	Very slight
2	Slight breathlessness
3	Moderate
4	Somewhat severe
5	Severe breathlessness
6	
7	Very severe breathlessness
8	
9	Very, very severe (almost maximum)
10	Maximum

1) the acutely increased intrinsic mechanical (elastic/threshold) loading; and

2) functional respiratory muscle weakness.

These respiratory mechanical/muscular abnormalities are, in part, related to resting and dynamic hyperinflation during exercise, and may lead to either a decrease in P_{Imax} or a further increase in P_{oes} as percentage of P_{Imax}. Because of these effects, greater neural drive or electrical activation of the respiratory muscle is required to generate a given force. Furthermore, because of limbic system activation, the corollary discharge may be sensed as abnormal, thus evoking a sensation of distress (fig. 1 and table 1).

The other descriptor cluster alludes to unsatisfied inspiration. Structural abnormalities (chronic bronchitis and emphysema), *via* their negative physiological consequences, *i.e.* expiratory flow limitation and dynamic hyperinflation, result in dyspnoea. A patient's physical activity is indeed characterised by a growing mismatch between increase in central neural output to the respiratory muscles and the blunted respiratory mechanical/muscular response (lung/chest wall displacement). This mismatch, which we call neuroventilatory dissociation (NVD), has been proposed to be, at least in part, the neurophysiological basis of the perceived unsatisfied inspiration. In a clinical setting, the slope that defines NVD (*i.e.* effort *versus* displacement) is steeper and shifted upward compared with healthy subjects. The steeper the slope, the greater the intensity of dyspnoea (fig. 2). In particular, patients experience intolerable dyspnoea during exercise because V_T expansion is constrained from below (by the effects of dynamic lung hyperinflation or the already critically reduced resting inspiratory capacity), as there is no space to breathe. This so-called dyspnoea threshold seems to be at the level at which the inspiratory reserve volume (IRV) critically approaches 0.5 L. Once this critical IRV is achieved, further expansion in V_T is negated, the effort–volume displacement ratio (P_{oes}/P_{Imax} divided by V_T/VC) increases sharply and dyspnoea intensity rises steeply to intolerable levels. The data support the central importance of mechanical restriction in causing dyspnoea in COPD patients.

Neuromuscular disorders Patients with neuromuscular disorders (NMD) exhibit heightened neuromotor output, which is sensed as increased respiratory muscle effort and, as such, is likely to be the principal mechanism of dyspnoea in NMD. Nonetheless, a significant positive relationship between increased dyspnoea per unit increase in ventilation and dynamic elastance affects the coupling between respiratory effort and displacement (fig. 3).

Interstitial lung disease As in COPD, restrictive dynamic respiratory mechanics limits the ability of patients with interstitial lung disease (ILD) to increase ventilation in

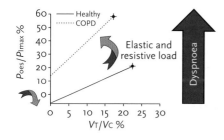

Figure 2. NVD. The slope that defines the mismatch between increase in neural output (inspiratory effort, i.e. P_{oes}/P_{Imax}) and lung/chest wall displacement (V_T/VC) is steeper and shifted upwards in patients with COPD compared with healthy subjects.

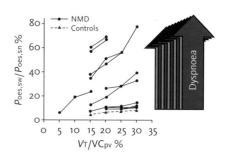

Figure 3. A mismatch between inspiratory effort (swing in oesophageal pressure ($P_{oes,sw}$) as a percentage of oesophageal pressure during a sniff manoeuvre ($P_{oes,sn}$)) and lung/chest wall displacement (V_T as a percentage of the predicted value of the vital capacity (VC_{pv})) in patients with NMD compared with average data from controls. The steeper the slope, the greater the perception of dyspnoea.

response to the increased metabolic demands of physical tasks. One of the characteristic features of ILD is a reduction in lung compliance and lung volumes. This has two major consequences.

1. Greater pressure generation is required by the inspiratory muscles for a given V_T.

2. The resting TLC and IRV are often diminished compared with health.

Therefore, V_T expansion is constrained from above early in exercise (reflecting the reduced TLC and IRV), which results in greater reliance on increasing breathing frequency to increase ventilation. Differences in dynamic ventilatory mechanics, including possible expiratory flow limitation in some patients, account for distinct qualitative perception in ILD patients, namely inspiratory difficulty/unsatisfied inspiration and rapid shallow breathing. Because of increases in both dynamic elastance and efferent respiratory drive, inspiratory difficulty/unsatisfied inspiration may have its neurophysiological basis in the conscious awareness of a dissociation between the increased drive to breathe (and concurrent increased respiratory effort, *i.e.* P_{oes}/P_{Imax}) and the restricted mechanical response of the respiratory system (*i.e.* V_T/VC), *i.e.* the inability to expand V_T appropriately in the face of an increased drive to breathe. In turn, the possibility has also been put forward that intensity of exertional dyspnoea in ILD is more closely linked to mechanical constraints on volume expansion than to indexes of inspiratory effort *per se*.

Chronic heart failure The key message that has emerged from therapeutic intervention studies in patients with CHF is that exertional dyspnoea alleviation is consistently associated with reduced excessive ventilatory demand (secondary to reduced central neural drive), improved respiratory mechanics and muscle function and, consequently, enhanced neuromechanical coupling of the respiratory system during exercise. Pressure support is reported to reduce the tidal inspiratory pleural pressure–time slope without affecting submaximal dyspnoea ratings but allows patients to exercise for additional time without experiencing any significant rise in dyspnoea. The available data suggest that increased ventilatory demand, abnormal dynamic ventilatory mechanics and respiratory muscle dysfunction are instrumental in causing exertional dyspnoea in patients with severe cardiac impairment.

Obesity An increase in respiratory neural drive is deemed to be the reason for the similar increase in dyspnoea in obese and lean subjects. However, different underlying mechanisms may affect dyspnoea in obese subjects. Exercise performance is impaired compared with healthy, normal-weight subjects when corrected for the increased lean body mass, but normal when expressed as a percentage of predicted for ideal body weight in subjects who hyperinflate their lungs to the same extent as those obese subjects who deflate their lungs, with both volume subgroups reaching similar dyspnoea scores. In 'hyperinflators', dynamic hyperinflation, along with a decrease in IRV, increases respiratory muscle loading, respiratory drive and

perception of respiratory discomfort. In contrast, 'deflators' exhibit a negative relationship between resting end-expiratory lung volume (EELV) and perceptual respiratory response during exercise: the lower the EELV, the greater the Borg score. A low EELV has three important consequences linked together during exercise:

1) Decrease in expiratory reserve volume

2) Dynamic airway compression

3) Changes in transmural airway pressure resulting in airway dynamic compression

Thus, an alteration in the central drive to the respiratory muscles in response to afferent activity from upper airway mechanoreceptors may also contribute to the unpleasant respiratory sensation in obese subjects.

Effects of interventions on dyspnoea

Effective improvement in exertional dyspnoea represents one of the most challenging targets of management in patients with cardiopulmonary disease. Traditionally, the approach to improving exertional dyspnoea in all of the major cardiopulmonary diseases involves interventions that:

1) reduce ventilatory demand (by reducing the drive to breathe);

2) improve ventilatory capacity;

3) improve respiratory mechanics (by reducing the mechanical load);

4) increase the functional strength of weakened ventilatory muscles;

5) address the affective dimension of dyspnoea; and

6) any combination of the above.

It is of note that interventions should be selected based on the underlying pathophysiological background of the specific disease under examination and may differ from one disease to another. However, multiple interventions are generally required and appear to have additive or synergistic effects.

Some of these interventions include the following.

- Bronchodilators
- Oxygen
- Heliox
- Exercise training
- Biventricular pacing (specific for CHF patients)
- Biofeedback techniques
- NIV
- Lung volume reduction surgery and related endoscopic techniques
- Various combinations of these

All of the above strategies have proven to provide beneficial sensory consequences in a variety of patients with cardiopulmonary diseases.

In selected patients, interventions such as opiates (oral and inhaled) reduce respiratory drive and alter affective components of dyspnoea. Recently, it has been shown that inhaled furosemide may modulate respiratory sensation by altering afferent inputs from vagal receptors within the lungs. Psychological counselling, cognitive/behavioural modification and anxiolytics can have favourable influences on the affective dimension of chronic dyspnoea.

Conclusions

We are still a long way from understanding the symptom of dyspnoea. Although mechanical factors are important contributors to dyspnoea, the precise mechanisms of dyspnoea remain obscure. One approach to the study of this symptom is to identify the major qualitative dimensions of the symptom in an attempt to uncover different underlying neurophysiological mechanisms. The remarkable similarity in choices of qualitative descriptors (work/effort, inspiratory difficulty/unsatisfied inspiration, air hunger and rapid breathing) for exertional dyspnoea in patients with restrictive and obstructive syndromes raises the intriguing possibility that they share some common underlying mechanisms.

Further reading

- DeLorey DS, et al. (2005). Mild to moderate obesity: implications for respiratory mechanics at rest and during exercise in young men. *Int J Obes (Lond)*; 29: 1039–1047.
- Guenette JA, et al. (2012). Does dynamic hyperinflation contribute to dyspnoea during exercise in patients with COPD? *Eur Respir J*; 40: 322–329.
- Killian KJ, et al. Dyspnoea. In: Roussos C, ed. The Thorax, part B. New York, Dekker, 1995; pp. 1709–174.
- Lanini B, et al. (2001). Perception of dyspnea in patients with neuromuscular disease. *Chest*; 120: 402–408.
- Laveneziana P, et al. (2009). Effect of biventricular pacing on ventilatory and perceptual responses to exercise in patients with stable chronic heart failure. *J Appl Physiol*; 106: 1574–1583.
- Laveneziana P, et al. (2011). Evolution of dyspnea during exercise in chronic obstructive pulmonary disease: impact of critical volume constraints. *Am J Respir Crit Care Med*; 184: 1367–1373.
- O'Donnell DE, et al. (1997). Qualitative aspects of exertional breathlessness in chronic airflow limitation: pathophysiologic mechanisms. *Am J Respir Crit Care Med*; 155: 109–115.
- O'Donnell DE, et al. (1998). Qualitative aspects of exertional dyspnoea in patients with interstitial lung disease. *J Appl Physiol*; 84: 2000–2009.
- O'Donnell DE, et al. (1999). Ventilatory assistance improves exercise endurance in stable congestive heart failure. *Am J Respir Crit Care Med*; 160: 1804–1811.
- O'Donnell DE, et al. (2006). Sensory-mechanical relationships during high intensity, constant-work-rate exercise in COPD. *J Appl Physiol*; 101: 1025–1035.
- Ofir D, et al. (2007). Ventilatory and perceptual responses to cycle exercise in obese females. *J Appl Physiol*; 102: 2217–2226.
- Parshall MB, et al. (2012). An official American Thoracic Society statement:

update on the mechanisms, assessment, and management of dyspnea. *Am J Respir Crit Care Med*; 185: 435–452.

- Romagnoli I, *et al.* (2008). Role of hyperinflation *vs* deflation on dyspnea in severely to extremely obese subjects. *Acta Physiol*; 193: 393–402.

- Scano G, *et al.* (2005). Understanding dyspnoea by its language. *Eur Respir J*; 25: 380–385.

- Scano G, *et al.* (2010). Do obstructive and restrictive lung diseases share common underlying mechanisms of breathlessness? *Respir Med*; 104: 925–933.

Chest pain

Matthew Hind

Chest pain is a frequent symptom of illness and a common reason for seeking medical attention. Rapid assessment is crucial so that life-threatening disease, such as cardiac chest pain, aortic dissection and oesophageal rupture, can be identified and managed appropriately. A basic history often points to the cause and is used in the triage of patients attending emergency rooms. Questions are typically asked about the character, location, radiation, severity, exacerbating and relieving factors, and relationship to movement such as breathing or coughing. Objective assessment using a questionnaire, such as the McGill Pain score (Melzack, 1975) can be useful. Occasionally, it is difficult to tease out differences between cardiac, gastrointestinal and respiratory causes of pain.

The pathophysiology of chest pain is complex and not completely understood but involves peripheral nociceptors, either small Aδ myelinated or unmyelinated C afferent fibres that project via sympathetic and parasympathetic nerves into the dorsal horn of the spinal cord. These neurons synapse with spinothalamic fibres that ascend, cross the spinal cord and terminate in the contralateral venteroposterior thalamic nucleus. Thalamocortical neurons project via the posterior limb of the internal capsule to the somatosensory cortex. The diaphragm has dual nociceptive sensory innervation from both the phrenic nerve and the lower six intercostal nerves; therefore, diaphragmatic irritation can present with pain referred to the shoulder or upper abdomen. The trachea and large airways have afferent fibres that project along the vagus nerve. Respiratory chest pain can therefore originate from the chest wall, pleura, large airways and mediastinum but visceral 'lung' pain is unusual.

Pleural pain is often described as sharp, stabbing and made worse with movement such deep respiration. The pain is often unilateral, reflecting the site of disease. A pleural rub may be heard. Pleuritic pain with sudden onset prompts a diagnosis of pulmonary emboli, infarction or pneumothorax, whereas pleuritic pain building over a few hours may suggest infection, such as pneumonia or pleurisy; onset over days suggests empyema, malignancy or tuberculosis.

Tracheobronchitis can present with a midline burning pain made worse with respiration. Massive mediastinal lymphadenopathy can cause an indistinct, heavy central chest pain. Similarly, chest pain associated with pulmonary hypertension can be difficult to distinguish from cardiac chest pain. Nondescript, heavy chest pain is quite common in exacerbations of bronchiectasis.

Chest wall pain is usually well localised, reproduced with movement and associated with tenderness. Costochondritis and Tietze's syndrome are inflammatory

Key points

- Chest pain can be a feature of a wide range of pathology.

- An accurate history is essential to direct appropriate investigation of patients presenting with chest pain.

disorders of thoracic joints that present with chest wall pain and tenderness. Bornholm disease (epidemic pleurodynia or devil's grip), often associated with Coxsackie B virus, can present with epidemics of chest wall pain of sudden onset.

Neuralgic pain can be sharp and knife-like or dull and heavy, and there may be associated sensory symptoms. Pain in a dermatomal distribution requires examination of overlying skin for the characteristic vesicular rash of herpes zoster.

ECG is essential for immediate assessment of cardiac chest pain. Further investigation may include exercise ECG, stress echocardiography or myocardial perfusion scanning. Angiography offers the opportunity for therapeutic angioplasty and stent insertion.

Chest radiographs are useful to identify consolidation, pneumothorax, pleural effusion and bony abnormalities such as vertebral or rib fractures. Contrast CT has made identification of pulmonary emboli, aortic dissection and oesophageal rupture straightforward, and can identify abnormalities often missed on plain radiographs. Nuclear medicine scans have a role in both diagnosis and management of pulmonary emboli. Bone scintigraphy is useful in the evaluation of 'bony' pain. MRI examination is of particular use in visualising nerve roots. Direct endoscopic visualisation of either the upper gastrointestinal tract (oesophagogastroduodenoscopy) or major airways (bronchoscopy) allows epithelial inspection and offers the opportunity for direct microbiological, cytological and histological sampling.

Management of chest pain is clearly influenced by the underlying disease. It is, however, essential to provide adequate analgesia not only to alleviate suffering but prevent secondary complications such as pneumonia. The use of a pain ladder, starting with simple analgesics such as paracetamol and nonsteroidal anti-inflammatory drugs escalating to mild then stronger opiates, follows guidance by the World Health Organisation (WHO) for management of cancer pain but is also extremely useful for noncancer pain. Topical analgesia, such as capsaicin creams or infiltration of local anaesthetic, are particularly useful following thoracic surgery. The use of adjuvants, to calm fear and anxiety, can be considered at each step of the pain ladder. Tricyclic antidepressants together with anticonvulsants can be particularly helpful in neuropathic pain. Nonpharmacological management, such as radiotherapy for painful bony metastasis, can also be extremely useful. It is essential drugs are given 'by the clock' rather than 'on demand'. The three-step approach advocated by WHO of administering the correct drug, at the correct dose, at the correct time is inexpensive and 80–90% effective.

Further reading

- Melzack R (1975). The McGill Pain Questionnaire: major properties and scoring methods. *Pain*; 1: 277–299.
- World Health Organization. WHO's Pain Ladder. www.who.int/cancer/palliative/painladder/en/

Physical examination

Martyn R. Partridge

Physical findings in the context of the history

The purpose of clinical assessment is to make an accurate diagnosis. Making an accurate diagnosis in cases of respiratory disease can be challenging not only because of the diversity of respiratory ill health but also because symptoms of respiratory disease are shared with disorders of other body systems.

Breathlessness (a sensation of difficult, laboured or uncomfortable breathing) may have a physiological or psychological explanation but it is extremely important that every time we are faced with a patient complaining of shortness of breath we consider the following.

Is this patient breathless because of:

- heart disease,
- lung disease,
- pulmonary vascular disease,
- a systemic disorder (anaemia, obesity or hyperthyroidism), or
- respiratory muscle weakness?

It is vital that we go through this checklist both with new presentations of the symptom of breathlessness as well as in those with established disease, and we need to bear this list in mind when examining the patient. The patient with COPD might this time be breathless not because of an exacerbation but because they have gone into atrial fibrillation, or the patient with known heart failure may this time be breathless because of a complicating pneumonia.

Asking specifically about the onset of the symptom of breathlessness can be helpful in

Key points
• It is essential to bear in mind that breathlessness can have a variety of causes.
• Physical examination should follow the taking of the medical history and differential diagnoses, and is an opportunity to confirm normality or discover abnormality.
• Physical examination comprises inspection, palpation, auscultation and percussion.
• The respiratory physician must not forget that disease of other systems may also be the cause of the symptoms and that comorbidity is common.

the differential diagnostic process and this is summarised in table 1.

Cough and breathlessness

A practical approach to the assessment of cough and breathlessness is summarised in figure 1.

Physical examination

In the vast majority of cases, the taking of the medical history should lead to the construction of a list of differential diagnoses. The examination is then an opportunity either to confirm normality or to discover abnormalities consistent with one or other of one's differential diagnoses. Key features, as with all clinical examination, depend upon inspection, palpation, auscultation and percussion.

Table 1. *Breathlessness: differential diagnosis according to onset*

Onset	Differential diagnosis
Within minutes	Pulmonary embolus Pneumothorax MI Cardiac rhythm disturbance Dissecting aneurysm Acute asthma
Over hours or days	Pneumonia Pleural effusion LVF (LV dysfunction or valve dysfunction or septal rupture post-MI) Asthma Blood loss Lobar collapse Respiratory muscle weakness (Guillain–Barré syndrome)
Over weeks	Infiltration (malignancy, sarcoidosis, fibrosing alveolitis, extrinsic allergic alveolitis, eosinophilic pneumonia) Respiratory muscle weakness (motor neurone disease) Main airway obstruction Anaemia Valvular dysfunction (SBE)
Over months	Same as for 'Over weeks' Obesity Muscular dystrophy Asbestos-related conditions
Over years	COPD Chest wall deformity Heart valve dysfunction Obesity

MI: myocardial infarction; LVF: left ventricular failure; LV: left ventricular; SBE: subacute bacterial endocarditis.

Inspection

On inspection, the key points to observe are as follows.

- General appearance (breathlessness or cachexia)
- Respiratory rate
- Appearances of the hand (finger clubbing (fig. 2), tremor, tobacco staining or flapping tremor suggestive of carbon dioxide retention)
- Does the chest wall move symmetrically?
- Are there any chest wall deformities (scoliosis or pectus excavatum) or scars (figs 3 and 4)?
- Are there any abnormal vessels suggestive of superior vena cava obstruction (fig. 5)?
- Nasal stuffiness or obstruction should be noted

- A note should be made of the neck/collar size and also of obvious jaw abnormalities and oropharyngeal abnormalities

Remember that inspection of relevance to the respiratory system involves more than inspection of the chest itself; for example, one should note erythema nodosum (fig. 6) or gynaecomastia (fig. 7).

Palpation

This involves the following.

- Assessment of chest expansion, where we may be able to elicit reduced expansion symmetrically, suggestive of hyperinflation, or reduced movement on one side, suggesting localised pathology on that side.

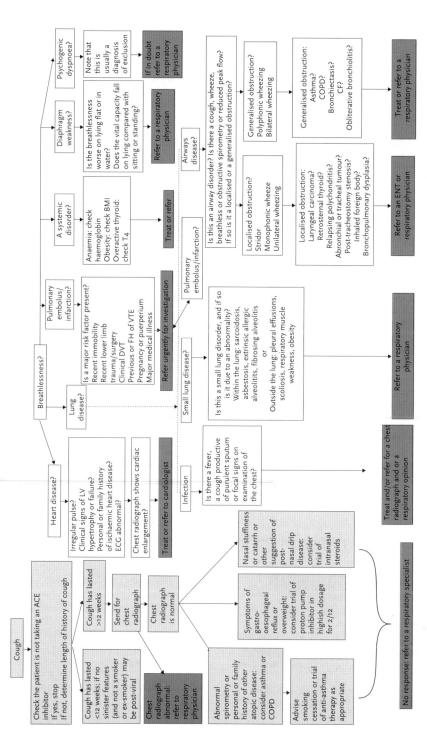

Figure 1. Diagnosis and management of respiratory disease. ACE: angiotensin-converting enzyme; LV: left ventricular; DVT: deep vein thrombosis; FH: family history; VTE: venous thromboembolism.

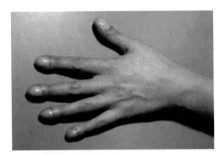

Figure 2. The presence of finger clubbing should obviously be noted and the patient asked if they are aware of how long it has been present or whether a doctor has commented upon it previously.

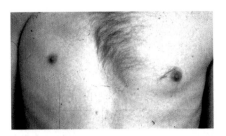

Figure 4. Chest wall abnormalities may be congenital or acquired. In a case of congenital absence of the pectoralis major, as seen here, the abnormality should be noted, for it will otherwise potentially lead to confusion in interpretation of the chest radiograph.

- Determining the position of the trachea by inserting the index and middle fingers in the suprasternal notch.
- Examining the cervical and supraclavicular lymph nodes for enlargement.
- Assessing vocal fremitus by asking the patient to loudly and deeply repeat the words 'ninety-nine' while you compare both sides of the chest. Voice sounds are better transmitted through consolidated lung than normal lung and poorly transmitted through pleural effusions.

Percussion

Percussion is often poorly undertaken and the key features are to:

- make the movement of your finger a stroke from the wrist;
- strike firmly at right angles upon the finger of the other hand, which lies along the intercostal space; and

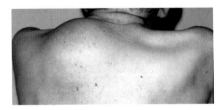

Figure 3. The chest wall should be carefully examined for clues as to underlying lung disease. In this case, an infiltrating lung tumour is invading the chest wall.

- do so in a symmetrical manner, systematically comparing both sides of the chest at a point equidistant from the midline.

The percussion note may be hyper-resonant symmetrically in patients with underlying hyperinflated lungs or asymmetrically in a large pneumothorax, or may be dull in cases of consolidation or pleural effusion.

Auscultation

Listening to the breath sounds involves the following.

- Checking for the presence of bronchial breathing, which is the presence of breath sounds that are similar to those heard over the large central airways in a more peripheral location. Bronchial breathing is classically heard over a consolidated lung (and in association with dullness to percussion) but is also sometimes heard over the upper aspect of a pleural effusion and sometimes over a collapsed lung.
- Determining whether there are any abnormal added sounds, which may be musical sounds (wheezing) or crackles. In cases of wheezing, it is important to determine whether the wheezing is polyphonic and bilateral, as in asthma or COPD, or monophonic and localised, as may be found in cases of lung cancer, bronchial stenosis or inhaled foreign bodies.
- Crackles may be fine and occur in cases of interstitial lung disease or acutely in

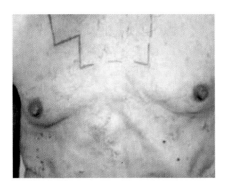

Figure 5. Dilated vessels over the anterior chest wall are often the most obvious sign of superior vena cava obstruction, with the other feature being a raised jugular venous pressure that is nonpulsatile.

cases of pulmonary oedema, or coarse, as often heard in patients with bronchiectasis.

- Pleural rubs sound like a squeaky noise, are usually localised and clearly vary in intensity with respiration. Care in

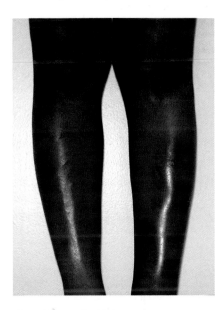

Figure 6. Inspection of the respiratory system involves more than inspection of the chest. In this example, the presence of erythema nodosum is likely to explain the pulmonary abnormalities.

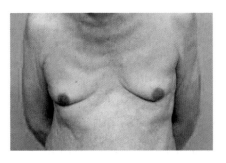

Figure 7. While gynaecomastia can occur for a number of reasons, its presence is always important to note and an important underlying cause to consider is lung cancer.

interpreting a noise as a pleural rub is necessary in very thin patients where the diaphragm of the stethoscope may move over the ribs.

- Vocal resonance is found under the same circumstances as vocal fremitus and, when found in conjunction with bronchial breathing, is highly suggestive of consolidation. Some physicians find detection of whispering pectoriloquy a more definite sign; to elicit this, one asks the patient to whisper 'ninety-nine' and, when it is present, such as in cases of consolidation, the whispered sound is heard clearly over the chest wall when transmitted through consolidated lung whereas a normally air-filled lung would muffle the whispered sound and make it indistinct.

Finally, one should remember that disorders of other systems may coexist and, while examining the chest, one should especially look for evidence of heart and pulmonary vascular disease, noting signs of peripheral oedema and elevation of the jugular venous pressure.

Further reading

- Gibson GJ, et al. Respiratory Medicine. Philadelphia, Saunders Elsevier Science Ltd, 2002.
- Partridge MR. Understanding Respiratory Medicine: a Problem-Orientated Approach. London, Manson Publishing Ltd, 2006.

Static and dynamic lung volumes

Riccardo Pellegrino and Andrea Antonelli

Ventilation is constrained by the mechanical properties of the airways, lung and chest wall. The latter two determine the volume at which the movement of gas is accomplished at rest and in daily activities such as exercise, phonation, laughing, changes in body posture, *etc.* However, when cardiopulmonary disease is present, lung volumes may also be modified as a result of dynamic mechanisms within the airways and changes in breathing pattern, in addition to static changes in lung and chest wall properties.

Determinants of lung volumes in health and disease

Tidal volume (V_T) is the volume of gas inspired during each breath (fig. 1) necessary to preserve gas exchange. In healthy subjects, inspiration is switched off by neural reflexes, whereas expiration is terminated near the relaxation volume as a result of static or dynamic mechanisms (see section dedicated to functional residual capacity). Except during exercise, when a lack of increase in V_T with ventilation is a functional marker of ventilatory limitation, and perhaps in patients undergoing assisted ventilation, V_T has little clinical usefulness in clinical practice.

Total lung capacity (TLC) is the volume of gas contained in the lungs after a deep breath. It is determined by the maximum force exerted by the inspiratory muscles to balance lung and chest wall elastic recoils (figs 1 and 2).

In healthy conditions, TLC tends to remain fairly stable with ageing, presumably because the natural decrease of the force of the inspiratory muscles and/or the increase in chest wall stiffness are balanced by the progressive loss of lung elastic recoil. Sports like swimming are associated with an increase in TLC as a result of an increase in inspiratory muscle force.

Key points

Measurement of lung volumes in clinical practice has been proven to be important to assist in the following:

- Diagnosis of pulmonary defects,

- Evaluation of candidates for lung volume resection surgery,

- Prognosis of COPD and interstitial lung diseases,

- Evaluation of the bronchomotor response to constrictor and dilator agents as well as to physical exercise.

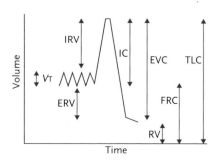

Figure 1. Lung volume plotted versus time. EVC: slow expiratory vital capacity; IRV and ERV: inspiratory and expiratory volume reserves, respectively.

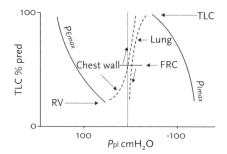

Figure 2. Quasi-static pressure–volume curves of the chest wall and the lung (dashed lines) related to pleural pressure (P_{pl}) generated during maximum inspiratory and expiratory static efforts (P_{Imax} and P_{Emax}, respectively; continuous lines). Volume is expressed as a percentage of TLC. TLC is the volume at which P_{Imax} equals the inward elastic recoils of both lung and chest wall. RV is the volume at which P_{Emax} overcomes the outward elastic recoil of the chest wall. FRC is the volume at which inward lung recoil equals outward chest wall recoil (arrows with opposite direction).

In contrast, TLC tends to increase in emphysema and, sometimes, in chronic bronchitis and severe asthma. Though the decrease in lung elastic recoil is presumably the most important mechanism of the increase in TLC under these conditions, an increased force of the inspiratory muscles and chest wall remodelling may also play a role. Surprisingly, for the same level of airflow obstruction, TLC tends to increase during spontaneous long-lasting but not acutely induced bronchospasm. This is presumably because of the different time course necessary to produce airflow obstruction and hyperinflation. That this may be so is shown by a study documenting that when a resistive valve was implanted in the dog trachea, it took time for TLC to increase. Thus it is possible that breathing at high lung volumes for long periods of time as a result of severe chronic airflow obstruction may also contribute to the increase in TLC.

TLC decreases in all conditions characterised by an increase in lung elastic recoil (e.g. pulmonary fibrosis and cardiac failure), chest wall stiffness (e.g. neuromuscular diseases, obesity, ascitis and pregnancy) or thoracic space competition (e.g. pleural effusions and pneumothorax).

Measuring TLC is of great importance in clinical practice, as it allows the identification of restrictive pulmonary defects. In addition, TLC is also useful in the evaluation of an emphysematous patient as a candidate for lung volume resection surgery, or for follow-up of interstitial lung diseases.

Residual volume (RV) is the volume of gas that remains in the lungs after a complete expiration. In young healthy individuals, RV is, for the most part, determined by the balance between the force of the expiratory muscles and the outward recoil of the chest wall (figs 1 and 2). In the elderly, it increases as a result of airway closure or reduced lung elastic recoil.

In restrictive diseases, RV decreases in proportion to the increase in lung elastic or chest wall recoils and/or loss of lung parenchyma.

In obstructive pulmonary diseases, RV is higher than predicted because of premature airway closure, loss of lung elastic recoil, and stiffness of the chest wall. Additional mechanisms may dynamically contribute to the elevation of RV in obstructive lung diseases. For instance, in patients with acutely induced or chronic airflow obstruction, RV achieved after a forced expiration is always higher than after a slow expiration. This is mainly because of two mechanisms. First, during forced expiration in airflow obstruction, expiratory flow limitation (EFL) occurs soon after initiation of the manoeuvre, especially within the airways that are already narrowed. In contrast, during a slow expiration, pleural pressure will not exceed the critical pressure necessary to generate maximal flow, thus allowing EFL to occur late in expiration and at a lower lung volume. Secondly, some airways could close near TLC early in expiration as a result of disease, thus preventing the subtending alveolar units from emptying and contributing to the increase in RV.

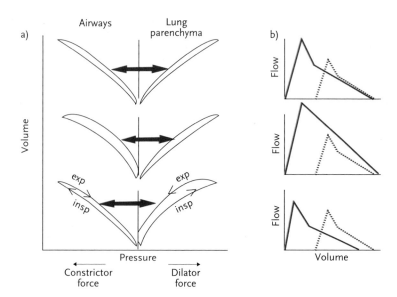

Figure 3. *Effects of deep breath on maximum expiratory flow and residual volume according to the relative hysteresis theory of Froeb et al. (1968). a) Pressure–volume loops of lung parenchyma and airways on inspiration (insp) and expiration (exp). The area inside the loop is called hysteresis. b) Partial and maximal flow–volume loops (dotted and continuous lines, respectively). Upper panels: both hystereses are similar, so that the constrictor and dilator forces after the deep breath remain equal compared to before inflation. As a result, forced flow and residual volume during the maximum forced expiratory manoeuvre are the same as the partial manoeuvre. Middle panels: airway hysteresis prevails over lung hysteresis, so that the constrictor force is reduced after the large inflation. Consequently, for a given lung volume, maximum flow will exceed partial flow and residual volume will decrease more after a maximal manoeuvre than after a partial manoeuvre. Lower panels: lung parenchyma hysteresis prevails over airway hysteresis, so that the dilator force will decrease after the deep breath. Under these conditions, forced expiratory flow and residual volume after a maximal manoeuvre will decrease and increase, respectively, compared to a partial manoeuvre.*

In addition, the effects of volume history of the manoeuvre preceding the expiration may affect RV. For instance, in healthy subjects or mild-to-moderate asthmatics exposed to a bronchoconstrictor agent, a manoeuvre initiated from TLC will generate greater flow and lower RV than a manoeuvre initiated from end-tidal inspiration. The opposite occurs in chronic airflow obstruction. This suggests that RV is also modulated through the changes in airway calibre caused by large lung inflations. How the deep inspiration manoeuvre affects lung and airway mechanics is still a matter of debate. When a deep breath is taken, the inflating stimulus is transmitted to the lung as well as the airways through the elastic network of lung parenchyma. According to Froeb *et al.* (1968), the effects of volume history on airway size depend on the mechanical characteristics of the lung parenchyma and airways. Both tissues may lose energy or pressure and deform with stretching, a phenomenon named hysteresis. Since lung elastic recoil and transmural pressure are the forces that determine airway size, any change relative to one of these will necessarily entail a change in flow and RV. As shown in figure 3, if airway hysteresis exceeds parenchymal hysteresis, airway volume will be greater during deflation than inflation, and RV will be achieved at a lower lung volume. This generally occurs when constriction is mostly limited to the airways and little affects lung parenchyma, such as with induced airway narrowing. In contrast, when lung parenchyma hysteresis is larger than airway hysteresis, airway volume will be reduced on expiration compared with inspiration and RV achieved at a higher volume. This is what presumably occurs in chronic airflow obstruction or severe asthma. Finally, when airway and lung parenchyma hystereses change by similar extent, airway size will be similar before and after a deep breath, and so will RV. The effects of volume history may be easily assessed *in vivo* by comparing forced expiratory manoeuvres initiated from total lung capacity and a volume below it (fig. 3b), or by changes in airflow resistance soon after taking a deep breath.

Vital capacity (VC) is the difference between TLC and RV. Because RV is dependent on volume and flow histories in addition to airway, parenchyma and/or chest wall components of the diseases, as discussed above, VC will depend on the type of respiratory manoeuvre from which it is taken and the underlying disease. In general, the largest VC is that obtained during a full inflation from RV (achieved after a slow expiration from end-tidal inspiration) to TLC (inspiratory vital capacity), followed by the slow expiratory vital capacity from TLC to RV, and the VC measured during a forced expiratory manoeuvre (FVC). A decrease of VC does not allow differentiation between restriction and obstruction, as it may be due to a decrease in TLC or an increase in RV, or both.

In clinical practice, VC is of central importance for the diagnosis of obstructive pulmonary defects.

Functional residual capacity (FRC) is the volume of gas remaining in the lungs at the end of a tidal expiration performed in a seated or upright position (fig. 1). Its mechanical determinants are the inward elastic recoil of the lung and the opposing outward recoil of the chest wall (fig. 2). In the supine position, the abdominal content is displaced towards the chest cavity, thus reducing FRC. Also, during speech, singing, laughing or exercise, FRC tends to decrease to favour these activities.

In obstructive pulmonary diseases, FRC tends to increase for a series of reasons. For instance, an increase in breathing frequency or in time constant of the respiratory system, as a result of either an increase in airflow resistance or a decrease in lung compliance, will lead to an expiratory time relatively too short to allow the respiratory system to empty fully. Presumably, the occurrence of EFL during tidal expiration may also contribute to an increase in FRC to a lung volume where EFL is minimal. Under these circumstances, the dynamic compression of the airways downstream from the flow limiting segment may evoke neural reflexes that prematurely activate the inspiratory muscles to avoid breathing for too long a time under EFL conditions. On the one hand the increase in FRC in airflow obstruction is beneficial as it allows breathing at a volume where the airways are larger, thus decreasing the resistive work of breathing. On the other hand, however, breathing at high lung volume is associated with an increase in the elastic work of breathing and causes dyspnoea.

A decrease in FRC occurs in restrictive respiratory diseases due to an increase in lung elastic recoil (*e.g.* in pulmonary fibrosis, atelectasis, lung resection, alveolar liquid filling and cardiac diseases) or in chest wall elastance (*e.g.* in chest wall and pleural diseases, respiratory muscle paralysis, and obesity). This is important, as reduced FRC is associated with hypoxaemia and, in obesity, with increased airway responsiveness.

Inspiratory capacity (IC) is the volume difference between TLC and FRC. In pulmonary diseases, it tends to decrease as a result of an increase in FRC (obstructive conditions) or a decrease in TLC (restrictive diseases), or both. In clinical practice, changes in IC with acute interventions on airway calibre, such as bronchoprovocation or reversibility tests, or during exercise, reflect mirror-like changes in FRC, assuming that TLC remains unmodified.

IC has no role in the diagnosis of ventilatory defects.

Expiratory and inspiratory reserve volumes allow V_T to expand when necessary (fig. 1). Though of little interest at rest, they play a critical role during exercise. For instance, in healthy subjects the increase in V_T with exercise is achieved at the expense of a decrease in end-expiratory lung volume (EELV) and an increase in end-inspiratory lung volume (EILV). In contrast, in airflow obstruction, the increase in V_T is limited by the premature and sustained increase in EELV that may eventually contribute to causing dyspnoea together with the increase in EILV near TLC.

Measurements of lung volumes in clinical practice: technical aspects

VC, V_T, IC, EILV and EELV can be measured by simple spirometry. In contrast, TLC, RV and FRC need to be measured with special techniques described below.

Gas dilution techniques (nitrogen washout and helium dilution) are based on the principle of the conservation of mass; that is, the amount of gas resident in the lungs at the beginning of the test can be calculated as the product of concentration and volume of eliminated nitrogen or diluted helium. Both methods yield measurements of lung volumes that communicate with open airways only. In severely obstructed patients, an underestimation of the true lung volume may be a result of some regions with long time constants.

Body plethysmography allows rapid and reproducible measurements of absolute lung volumes. The test is based on Boyle's law, in that lung volume can be calculated from the relationship between changes in mouth pressure (assumed equal to alveolar pressure) and box pressure (constant volume plethysmography) or volume (constant pressure plethysmography) during gentle panting manoeuvres against a closed shutter. As opposed to gas dilution techniques, plethysmography measures the whole intrathoracic gas, thus including nonventilated and/or poorly ventilated lung regions. This method may overestimate lung volumes in cases of severe airflow obstruction if the panting frequency is >1 Hz.

Conclusions

Measuring lung volumes is now an integrative part of lung function assessment. In addition to assisting in the diagnosis of the ventilatory defects, it helps explain the presence of respiratory symptoms and hypoxia in cardiopulmonary diseases, has clinical prognostic implications in both obstructive and restrictive diseases, and plays an integral role in the functional evaluation for lung volume reduction surgery in emphysema.

Further reading

- Agostoni E, et al. Static behaviour of the respiratory system. In: Macklem PT, et al., eds. Handbook of Physiology. The Respiratory System. Mechanics of breathing. Section 3, Vol. III, part 1. Bethesda, American Physiological Society, 1986; pp. 113–113.
- Brusasco V, et al. (1997). Vital capacities during acute and chronic bronchoconstriction. Dependence of flow and volume histories. Eur Respir J; 10: 1316–1320.
- Casanova C, et al. (2005). Inspiratory-to-total lung capacity ratio predicts mortality in patients with chronic obstructive pulmonary disease. Am J Respir Crit Care Med; 171: 591–597.
- Ceanton TL, et al. (1987). Effects of swim training on lung volumes and inspiratory muscle conditioning. J Appl Physiol; 62: 39–46.
- Criner GJ, et al. (2008). A clinician's guide to the use of lung volume reduction surgery. Proc Am Thorac Soc; 5: 461–467.
- Froeb HF, et al. (1968). Relative hysteresis of the dead space and lung in vivo. J Appl Physiol; 25: 244–248.
- King TE Jr, et al. (2001). Predicting survival in idiopathic pulmonary fibrosis. Scoring system and survival model. Am J Respir Crit Care Med; 164: 1171–1181.
- O'Donnell DE, et al. (2007). Pathophysiology of dyspnea in chronic obstructive pulmonary disease. Proc Am Thorac Soc; 4: 145–168.
- Olive JT, et al. (1972). Maximal expiratory flow and total respiratory resistance during induced bronchoconstriction in asthmatic subjects. Am Rev Respir Dis; 106: 366–376.

- Pellegrino R, *et al.* (1979). Expiratory flow limitation and regulation of end-expiratory lung volume during exercise. *J Appl Physiol*; 74: 2552–2558.
- Pellegrino R, *et al.* (1996). Lung mechanics during induced bronchoconstriction. *J Appl Physiol*; 81: 964–975.
- Pellegrino R, *et al.* (2005). Interpretative strategies for lung function tests. Official statement of the American Thoracic Society and the European Respiratory Society. *Eur Respir J*; 26: 948–968.
- Pride NB, *et al.* Lung mechanics in disease. *In*: Macklem PT, Mead J, eds. Handbook of Physiology. The Respiratory System. Mechanics of breathing. Section 3, Vol. III, part 2. Bethesda, American Physiological Society, 1986; pp. 659–669.
- Torchio R, *et al.* (2009). Mechanical effects of obesity on airway responsiveness in otherwise healthy humans. *J Appl Physiol*; 107: 408–416.
- Vinegar A, *et al.* (1979). Dynamic mechanisms determine functional residual capacity in mice, *Mus musculus*. *J Appl Physiol*; 46: 867–871.

Respiratory mechanics

Daniel Navajas and Ramon Farré

Pulmonary ventilation is determined by the resistive and elastic properties of the lungs and chest wall, and by the driving pressure of the respiratory muscles. Both the lungs and chest wall are elastic structures. The lungs have a very small resting volume. Above this volume, the lungs are distended, exerting an inward elastic recoil pressure (P_L) that rises markedly with lung volume (V_L). The chest wall has a much higher resting volume, exhibiting outward and inward elastic recoil pressure (P_{CW}) below and above its resting volume, respectively.

At end-expiratory volume during quiet breathing (functional residual capacity (FRC)) in a healthy subject, the respiratory muscles are relaxed and the lungs and chest wall reach the combined resting state (fig. 1).

In this situation, the inward P_L is counterbalanced by the outward P_{CW} and the alveolar pressure (P_{alv}) equals atmospheric pressure. Inspiration is produced by activation of inspiratory muscles. The outward muscular pressure (P_{mus}) expands the chest wall, thereby lowering pleural pressure (P_{pl}). This drop in P_{pl} expands the lung and decreases P_{alv} to subatmospheric values. The mouth–alveolar pressure gradient drives inspiratory flow. During quiet breathing in a normal subject, expiration is achieved by relaxing the inspiratory muscles. The net inward elastic recoil of the total respiratory system (P_{rs}), the sum of P_L and P_{CW}, tends to return the system to the overall equilibrium volume,

Key points

- P_{alv} is lower and higher than P_{ao} during inspiration and expiration, respectively.

- The lungs exert inward elastic recoil that increases with V_L.

- Body plethysmography allows the measurement of both R_{aw} and V_L.

- The FOT allows the measurement of respiratory resistance during spontaneous breathing with minimum patient collaboration.

- Respiratory mechanics can be monitored in sedated mechanically ventilated patients performing post-inspiratory and post-expiratory pauses.

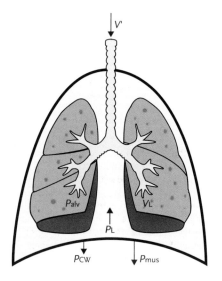

Figure 1. Mechanical behaviour of the respiratory system.

increasing P_{alv} to above mouth pressure (P_{mo}) and driving expiratory flow. The activation of the expiratory muscles results in a faster expiration.

Airway resistance

The airflow generated by the pressure gradient between the mouth and the alveoli is determined by airway resistance (R_{aw}), defined as

$$R_{aw} = \frac{P_{mo} - P_{alv}}{V'}$$

where V' is the gas flow. In healthy adults, R_{aw} measured at FRC is $\sim 2\,hPa \cdot s \cdot L^{-1}$. Intrathoracic airway calibre increases as lungs expand, resulting in a hyperbolic dependence of R_{aw} on lung volume. Therefore, an approximately linear relationship is obtained by computing airway conductance (G_{aw}):

$$G_{aw} = \frac{1}{R_{aw}}$$

Since large lungs have wider airways, the specific airway resistance (sR_{aw}) computed as

$$sR_{aw} = R_{aw} \cdot FRC$$

provides a resistance measurement normalised for differences in lung size. Similarly, specific airway conductance (sG_{aw}) is defined as

$$sG_{aw} = \frac{G_{aw}}{FRC}$$

Body plethysmography

Measurement of R_{aw} requires the recording of airflow and driving pressure. Airflow can be recorded with a pneumotachograph connected to the mouth. P_{mo} is simply atmospheric pressure or, alternatively, it can be readily measured with a pressure transducer. As the alveolar airspace is not directly accessible, P_{alv} can be estimated by means of a whole-body plethysmograph (fig. 2). This technique involves the subject sitting inside a closed cabin breathing the gas from the box. The mouth can be occluded with a shutter coupled to the

mouthpiece. First, the shutter is opened and the ratio between V' and the pressure within the box (P_{box}) is measured during breathing (V'/P_{box}).

During inspiration, air moves from the box to the lung. The inspired gas takes on a higher volume in the lungs than in the box due to the decrease in pressure ($P_{alv} < P_{box}$), the increase in temperature (37°C) and the addition of water vapour. The calibration ratio of the plethysmograph (k) is experimentally determined by closing the shutter at FRC and recording P_{mo} and P_{box} during gentle respiratory efforts against the occlusion. Under zero airflow conditions, $P_{alv} \approx P_{mo}$ and

$$k = \frac{P_{alv}}{P_{box}}$$

Therefore,

$$R_{aw} = \frac{P_{alv}}{V'} = \frac{k \cdot P_{box}}{V'}$$

Body plethysmography measurements of R_{aw} are usually computed at low respiratory flows ($<0.5\,L$) recorded during shallow panting to minimise the effects of temperature changes during inspiration and

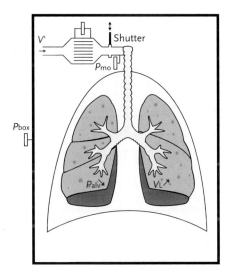

Figure 2. Measurement of R_{aw} by body plethysmography.

expiration. Alternatively, measurements can be made during quiet breathing after computer correction for changes in the physical conditions of the gas.

Whole-body plethysmography is the procedure most commonly used to measure R_{aw}. An added advantage of this technique is that it provides a FRC measurement for the computation of sR_{aw}. However, the device is bulky and expensive, and is not suited to measurement in supine patients.

Interrupter technique

R_{aw} can also be measured outside the box with a pneumotachograph–shutter system. The subject breathes at rest through the pneumotachograph. When airflow reaches a given threshold, the mouth is briefly (~0.1 s) occluded with the shutter. During flow interruption, the pressure is equilibrated within the different lung compartments. Therefore, R_{aw} can be computed as the ratio between the flow just before occlusion and the P_{mo} recorded during flow interruption. R_{aw} is usually computed as the mean of flow interruptions performed in several breathings.

The interrupter technique can be implemented in handheld devices and requires only minimal patient cooperation. However, due to progressive equilibration between P_{mo} and P_{alv}, the computed value of R_{aw} depends on the time lag between the start of occlusion and P_{mo} measurement. Slow pressure equilibration in patients with airflow obstruction results in an underestimation of R_{aw}.

Forced oscillation technique

In addition to R_{aw}, lung and chest wall tissues also exhibit resistive load because of internal frictional resistance to motion. Resistance of the total respiratory system (R_{rs}) is the sum of R_{aw} and tissue resistance. The tissue component of R_{rs} is generally small in comparison with R_{aw}.

R_{rs} can be measured during quiet breathing by the forced oscillation technique (FOT).

This technique is based on applying a small-amplitude (± 1 hPa) pressure oscillation to the patient's mouth or nose with a loudspeaker or a small pump. R_{rs} is computed as the ratio of forced pressure oscillation and in-phase flow. The ratio between forced pressure and the out-of-phase flow defines the reactance (X_{rs}) that provides a combined measurement of the inertial and elastic properties of the respiratory system. Forced oscillation is applied at frequencies (>4 Hz) higher than the breathing rate to facilitate the separation of forced oscillation from tidal breathing. The use of multifrequency oscillation (usually 4–32 Hz) provides a measurement of the frequency dependence of respiratory mechanics.

Current FOT devices are portable and easy to use. The technique does not require any special collaboration from the patient and measurements can be performed supine. Changes in R_{rs} during the breathing cycle can be precisely monitored. Moreover, FOT can be coupled to mechanical ventilators. Therefore, FOT is especially useful for epidemiological studies, measurements in infants, and monitoring respiratory mechanics in patients during sleep and mechanical ventilation.

Lung compliance

The elastic behaviour of the lung is described by the P_L–V_L relationship. Lung deformability is measured as lung compliance (C_L), defined as the change in volume divided by the change in pressure:

$$C_L = \frac{\Delta V_L}{\Delta P_L}$$

ΔV_L can readily be measured with a spirometer connected to the mouth. The measurement of ΔP_L requires the simultaneous recording of P_{pl} and P_{alv}. P_{pl} is usually estimated from the oesophageal pressure (P_{oes}) recorded with a small balloon attached to the tip of a catheter introduced through the nose into the lower oesophagus. P_{alv} is estimated in the mouth during brief flow interruptions. In practice, the subject performs a full inspiration followed by a very slow expiration to FRC. A shutter attached to the spirometer performs successive brief ($\sim$1 s) occlusions during expiration. The P_L–V_L relationship is curvilinear, with C_L decreasing markedly with volume. C_L is habitually computed in the range of tidal volume at rest (between FRC and FRC+0.5 L). In the normal adult, C_L is $\sim$0.2 L·hPa^{-1}. The elastic behaviour of the lung can also be characterised by lung elastance (E_L), defined as the reciprocal of C_L:

$$E_L = \frac{1}{C_L}$$

Chest wall compliance (C_{CW}) is computed as

$$C_{CW} = \frac{\Delta V_L}{\Delta P_{CW}}$$

In healthy subjects, the value of C_{CW} is comparable to that of C_L. Since the elastic pressure of the respiratory system is $P_{rs} = P_L + P_{CW}$, the compliance of the respiratory system (C_{rs}) is related to C_L and C_{CW} as

$$\frac{1}{C_{rs}} = \frac{1}{C_L} + \frac{1}{C_{CW}}$$

C_{rs} and C_{CW} can only be measured during complete respiratory muscle relaxation, which is extremely difficult to achieve in conscious patients.

Measurement of respiratory mechanics in mechanical ventilation

Respiratory mechanics can be measured in sedated mechanically ventilated patients by recording airflow and pressure at the airway opening (P_{ao}). The driving pressure required to overcome the elastic and resistive loads (E_{rs} and R_{rs}, respectively) of the respiratory system is

$$P_{ao} = R_{rs} \cdot V' + E_{rs} \cdot V$$

where V is volume. R_{rs} and E_{rs} can be computed by least-squares fitting of this equation to P_{ao}, V' and V recordings.

In patients ventilated with a constant flow waveform, R_{rs} and E_{rs} can also be measured by performing a post-inspiratory pause. Flow interruption results in a sharp drop in pressure from the peak value at end inspiration (P_{max}) to P_1, followed by a slow decay to a plateau (P_2). The sudden decrease in P_{ao} is associated with the resistive load of the airways. Therefore, R_{aw} is estimated as

$$R_{aw} = \frac{P_{max} - P_1}{V'}$$

A higher value of resistance due to the contribution of tissue viscoelasticity and gas redistribution within the lungs is computed from the pressure drop to the plateau ($P_{max} - P_2$).

The additional performance of a post-expiratory pause allows E_{rs} to be computed as the ratio of pressure and volume changes at the end of the post-inspiratory and post-expiratory pauses.

Respiratory muscle strength

Since direct measurements of muscular pressure are not clinically available, respiratory muscle performance is commonly assessed by measuring maximal pressures generated at the mouth during maximal inspiratory and expiratory efforts against an occluded airway (or occluded except for a small leak). Maximum expiratory pressure (P_{Emax}) is measured at TLC. Maximum inspiratory pressure measurements (P_{Imax}) are taken at either FRC or residual volume (RV). Alternatively, inspiratory muscle strength can be assessed during sniffing with one nostril occluded with a plug. Maximum pressure (sniff P_{di}) is recorded into the occluded nostril during a rapid, forceful inspiratory sniff performed at FRC.

The clinical testing of maximal respiratory pressures is quick and simple but measurement is dependent on effort. The test is useful for excluding significant respiratory muscle weakness.

Further reading

- American Thoracic Society, *et al.* *(2002)*. ATS/ERS statement on respiratory muscle testing. *Am J Respir Crit Care Med; 166:* *518–624*.
- Beydon N, *et al.* (2007). An official American Thoracic Society/European Respiratory Society statement: pulmonary function testing in preschool children. *Am J Respir Crit Care Med*; 175: 1304–1345.
- Farré R, *et al.* (2004). Noninvasive monitoring of respiratory mechanics during sleep. *Eur Respir J*; 24: 1052–1060.
- Gibson GJ. Clinical Tests of Respiratory Function. 3rd Edn. London, Hodder Arnold, 2009; pp. 3–5.
- Hyatt RE, *et al.* Interpretation of Pulmonary Function Tests. A Practical Guide. 3rd Edn. Philadelphia, Lippincott Williams & Wilkins, 2008; pp. 75–78.
- Lucangelo U, *et al.* (2007). Lung mechanics at the bedside: make it simple. *Curr Opin Crit Care*; 13: 64–72.
- Oostveen E, *et al.* (2003). The forced oscillation technique in clinical practice: methodology, recommendations and future developments. *Eur Respir J*; 22: 1026–1041.
- Pride NB. Airflow resistance. *In:* Hughes JMB, *et al.*, eds. Lung Function Tests: Physiological Principles and Clinical Applications. London, W.B. Saunders, 1999; pp. 27–24.

Gas transfer: T_{LCO} and T_{LNO}

J. Mike Hughes

Transfer factor of the lung for carbon monoxide

Apart from spirometry, the transfer factor of the lung for carbon monoxide (T_{LCO}) is the most frequently performed pulmonary function test. It focuses on the integrity of the alveolar (gas exchanging) part of the lung. T_{LCO} can detect abnormalities limited to the pulmonary microcirculation, the only routine test that can do so. It helps to think of T_{LCO} as a measure of the anatomy of the alveolar region, whereas blood gas measurements (P_{aO_2} and P_{aCO_2}) measure a physiological efficiency, which involves airways and larger blood vessels, as well as alveolar structures. For example, T_{LCO} is normal in asthma (alveoli are uninvolved), but the P_{aO_2} may be considerably reduced.

Definition

The transfer factor (called D_{LCO} in North America) measures the surface area available for gas exchange. It is closely related to the oxygen diffusing capacity. T_{LCO} is the quantity of inhaled carbon monoxide absorbed, per unit time and per unit carbon monoxide partial pressure. The pressure gradient is the alveolar–plasma carbon monoxide tension (P_{CO}) difference. Carbon monoxide is chosen for alveolar–capillary exchange because, after diffusing into capillary blood, carbon monoxide binds to Hb as carboxy-Hb (HbCO), but at an extremely low partial pressure (P_{CO}). Plasma P_{CO} is so low that it is not usually measured, but it may reach significant levels in current smokers. Carbon monoxide uptake is independent of blood flow, but it is dependent on the number of Hb-binding sites, $i.e.$ on capillary volume, as well as molecular diffusion across the alveolar–capillary membranes. 'Transfer' is the better term, because chemical reaction as well as 'diffusion' is involved.

Technique

Nearly all clinical laboratories use the single-breath technique of Ogilvie et $al.$ (1957). The T_{LCO} is measured during a 10-s breath-hold at maximal inspiration (this volume is the TLC).

Breath-holding at TLC optimises the distribution of the inhaled marker gases (helium (or another insoluble gas such as methane (CH_4)) and carbon monoxide), and makes T_{LCO} independent of ventilation distribution. The breathing manoeuvre is shown in figure 1. The subject is asked to:

- exhale slowly to residual volume;
- make a signal;
- inspire rapidly to full inflation;
- hold their breath.

The breath-hold is assisted by automatic closure of the inspiratory and expiratory valves for a pre-set time (9–11 s), after which

---

Key points

- T_{LCO} measures alveolar function.
- T_{LCO} is the product of K_{CO} and V_A.
- K_{CO} (or T_L/V_A) is the more specific index of alveolar integrity.
- K_{CO} is low in emphysema and fibrosis.
- K_{CO} is high in extrapulmonary restriction.

---

exhalation occurs rapidly (there is no need for a forced expiration) and an alveolar sample is taken, from which water vapour and carbon dioxide are absorbed before helium and carbon monoxide concentrations are analysed. The effective breath-hold time is calculated according to Jones et al. (1961) (fig. 1).

Calculation of the TLCO

The key point is that the TLCO is the product of two measurements, the alveolar volume (VA) and the rate of alveolar uptake of carbon monoxide, given by the slope (kCO) of alveolar uptake of CO (fig. 2), equivalent to the transfer coefficient of the lung for carbon monoxide (KCO). During the breath-hold at maximal inspiration, VA should equal TLC minus the anatomical dead space (97–98%

of the TLC). In practice, VA in normal subjects is 93.5% of TLC $\pm$ 6.6% (1SD) (Roberts et al., 1990). The 10-s breath-hold is insufficient time for complete gas mixing; in airflow obstruction, the measured VA may be much less than 80% of the actual TLC (measured by multi-breath gas dilution or plethysmography).

The kCO is the rate of alveolar uptake of carbon monoxide during the breath-hold (the slope in fig. 2). It is a rate constant with units of s^{-1} or min^{-1}. When normalised to barometric pressure (minus water vapour pressure) ($Pb*$), kCO/$Pb*$ = $k^{\dagger}$CO ($min^{-1} \cdot kPa^{-1}$). The final step in the calculation of TLCO is the multiplication of $k^{\dagger}$CO by VA (in mmol: 1 mmol=22.4 mL standard temperature, pressure and dry).

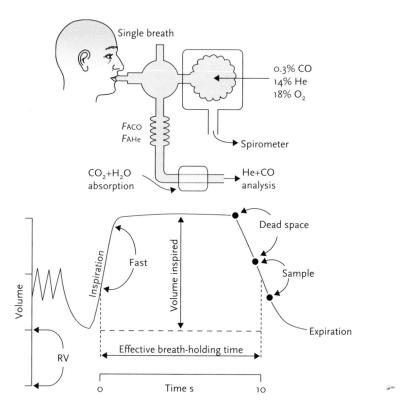

Figure 1. TLCO set-up and breathing protocol. The breath-hold time is set automatically, and is calculated from 0.33 × inspired time to the time after 1 L of expiration. FACO: alveolar carbon monoxide fraction; FAHe: alveolar helium fraction; RV: residual volume.

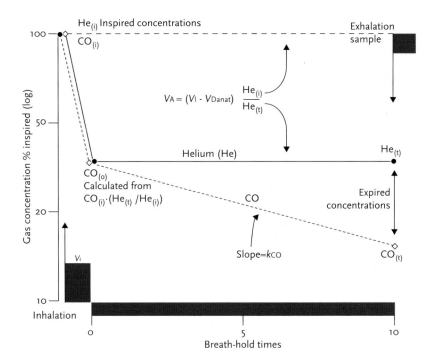

Figure 2. TLCO: carbon monoxide and helium analysis. Carbon monoxide and helium concentrations versus breath-hold time to illustrate the origin and calculation of the two components (slope of the transfer coefficient of the lung for CO (kCO) and alveolar volume (VA)) from which TLCO is derived. CO(i) and CO(t) are carbon monoxide concentrations inspired (i) and after exhalation (with dead space discard) at time t after breath-hold (the same for He(i) and He(t)). CO(o) is the calculated alveolar concentration at breath-hold start before alveolar uptake has begun. VI: inspired volume. VDanat: anatomic dead space.

$K_{CO} \times V_A = T_{LCO}$ (mmol·min⁻¹·kPa⁻¹)

The next step is the division of T_{LCO} by V_A in L (body temperature, pressure, saturated at 37°C, not mmol):

$T_{LCO}/V_A = K_{CO}$ (mmol·min⁻¹·kPa⁻¹·L⁻¹)

but the units only differ from $k^†_{CO}$ by a constant factor except for small variations in Pb*, ($K_{CO}/k^†_{CO} \sim 37$). Thus, T_{LCO}/V_A (=K_{CO}) remains, in essence, the rate constant for alveolar carbon monoxide uptake. This terminology is confusing (Hughes et al., 2012) because the impression is given that T_{LCO}/V_A (=K_{CO}) 'corrects' the T_{LCO} for variations in V_A. Unfortunately, this is not the case, and with normal lung structure K_{CO} at 50%, TLC predicted (as % of K_{CO} at predicted TLC) is

150% not the 100% required by an accurate volume 'correction'.

If V_A remains constant, T_{LCO} and K_{CO} will change equally (as % predicted). There are formulae to correct T_{LCO} for anaemia, so the Hb level should always be known. Smoking raises plasma P_{CO} (a 'back pressure' effect) and produces HbCO, displacing HbO_2 (an 'anaemia' effect), so smoking should be prohibited for 12–24 h before testing. Oxygen breathing with an increase in alveolar oxygen tension (P_{AO_2}) reduces T_{LCO} and K_{CO} by competitive antagonism between oxygen and carbon monoxide; it is the basis of the Roughton–Forster equation which partitions $1/T_{LCO}$ (transfer resistance) into $1/D_M$ (alveolar–capillary membrane diffusion resistance) and $1/\theta V_c$ (transfer resistance of red cells).

Table 1. Physiological influences on the T_{LCO} and the K_{CO}

	T_{LCO}	K_{CO}
Anaemia	↓	↓
Cardiac output increase	↑	↑
P_{AO_2} increase	↓	↓
V_A ↓ (reduced alveolar expansion)	↓	↑ ↑
V_A ↓ (reduction in no. of aerated units)	↓	↑

P_{AO_2}: alveolar oxygen tension.

When V_A is reduced and lung structure (or the remaining lung structure) is normal, T_{LCO} and K_{CO} change in opposite directions (table 1) if the cause is:

- reduced alveolar expansion, e.g. extrapulmonary restriction, or
- a reduction in aerated alveolar units, e.g. pneumonectomy or consolidation or atelectasis.

Other causes of a reduced V_A are: 1) diffuse alveolar damage (emphysema or fibrosis) (T_{LCO} and K_{CO} both reduced), and 2) airflow obstruction (V_A low due to poor gas mixing), where T_{LCO} and K_{CO} are variable, being low in emphysema and normal or high in asthma.

Implications of $K_{CO} \times V_A = T_{LCO}$

Transfer coefficient of the lung T_L/V_A does not correct T_{LCO} for a low V_A because T_L/V_A often rises when V_A falls. T_L/V_A is equivalent to K_{CO}, the rate constant for alveolar uptake of CO.

The same T_{LCO} (say 60% predicted) can arise from different combinations of K_{CO} and V_A, such as: 1) high K_{CO} and low V_A (extrapulmonary restriction); 2) low K_{CO} and normal V_A (pulmonary vasculopathy); or 3) low-ish K_{CO} and low-ish V_A (fibrosis) (table 2).

Transfer factor of the lung for nitric oxide

The transfer factor of the lung for nitric oxide (T_{LNO}) was introduced into clinical medicine by Guenard et al. (1987) and Borland et al. (1989). The methodology and calculations are the same as the T_{LCO}, and both tests can be performed simultaneously in one single-breath manoeuvre. The rate of alveolar uptake of nitric oxide (K_{NO}) is 4–5 times faster than K_{CO}, so the breath-hold time may have to be reduced to 5–6 s unless a very sensitive nitric oxide analyser is used. The faster uptake of

Table 2. Different combinations of K_{CO} and V_A but a similar T_{LCO}

Diagnosis	T_{LCO} % pred	K_{CO} % pred	V_A % pred	Comment
Inspiratory muscle weakness	59	120	50	Lack of alveolar expansion
Pneumonectomy	58	111	51	Localised loss of lung units
Diffuse interstitial lung disease	54	84	66	Alveolar capillary damage (±loss of units)
Emphysema	54	59	91	Alveolar capillary damage (FEV$_1$/FVC ratio reduced)
Idiopathic PH	56	58	96	Microvascular damage (FEV$_1$/FVC ratio normal)

% pred: % predicted; PH: pulmonary hypertension; FEV$_1$: forced expiratory volume in 1 s; FVC: forced vital capacity; Reproduced and modified from Hughes et al. (2012).

nitric oxide is due to a two-fold (*versus* carbon monoxide) increase in diffusivity through the alveolar–capillary membranes, and a faster reaction with red blood cell Hb than carbon monoxide. The T_{LNO}/T_{LCO} and K_{NO}/K_{CO} ratios (they are identical since V_A is common to both measurements) are 4.3–4.9 in normal subjects. The T_{LNO} is less sensitive to physiological changes in the pulmonary circulation than the T_{LCO}; the T_{LNO} is independent of changes in haematocrit and P_{AO_2}. The T_{LNO}/T_{LCO} ratio is reduced in alveolar under expansion and may be a marker of extrapulmonary restriction; it is expected to be reduced in chronic heart failure. Further research is needed to see whether the T_{LNO}/T_{LCO} ratio has a role in pulmonary function testing (Hughes *et al.* 2013).

Further reading

- Borland CD, *et al.* (1989). A simultaneous single breath measurement of pulmonary diffusing capacity with nitric oxide and carbon monoxide. *Eur Respir J*; 2: 56–63.
- Guenard H, *et al.* (1987). Determination of lung capillary blood volume and membrane diffusing capacity by measurement of NO and CO transfer. *Respir Physiol*; 70: 113–120.
- Hughes JMB, *et al.* (2012). Examination of the carbon monoxide diffusing capacity ($D_{L(CO)}$) in relation to its K_{CO} and V_A components. *Am J Respir Crit Care Med*; 186: 132–139.
- Hughes JMB, *et al.* (2013). The T_{LNO}/T_{LCO} ratio in pulmonary function test interpretation. *Eur Respir J*; 41: 453–461.
- Jones RS, *et al.* (1961). A theoretical and experimental analysis of anomalies in the estimation of pulmonary diffusing capacity by the single breath method. *Q J Exp Physiol*; 46: 131–143.
- Ogilvie CM, *et al.* (1957). A standardized breath holding technique for the clinical measurement of the diffusing capacity of the lung for carbon monoxide. *J Clin Invest*; 36: 1–17.
- Roberts CM, *et al.* (1990). Multi-breath and helium single breath dilution lung volumes as a test of airway obstruction. *Eur Respir J*; 3: 515–520.

Control of ventilation

Brian J. Whipp† and Susan A. Ward

The ventilatory control system is highly complex, involving:

- transmission of primary humoral stimuli from their sites of generation to the sensing elements;
- integration of chemoreceptor afferent activity within brainstem 'respiratory centres';
- generation of respiratory motor-discharge patterns;
- neuromuscular transmission at the respiratory muscles; and
- generation of appropriate pulmonary pressure gradients to produce the required airflow and ventilation.

Consequently, while inhalation of hypercapnic or hypoxic gas mixtures, either singly or in combination, is widely utilised to assess the normalcy of ventilatory 'chemoreflex' sensitivity, interpretation of responses should be made in the context of the entire 'input–output' relationship. Individuals with increased airway resistance or impaired respiratory muscle function, for example, may have an abnormally low overall ventilatory carbon dioxide or hypoxic response despite normal chemoreflex responsiveness.

Ventilatory response to inhaled carbon dioxide

The relationship between $V'E$ and arterial (a) or alveolar (A; typically end-tidal (ET)) carbon dioxide tension (PCO_2), with the subject sequentially inhaling a series of progressively greater hypercapnic inspirates (e.g. 3–6%), each for sufficiently long to establish a steady state, is used to estimate overall ventilatory carbon dioxide responsiveness. The resulting $V'E–PETCO_2$ relationship is

> **Key points**
>
> - Ventilatory carbon dioxide responsiveness is determined as the slope of the linear iso-oxic $V'E–PETCO_2$ relationship ($\Delta V'E/\Delta PETCO_2$), using steady-state, constant-concentration inspirates or hyperoxic rebreathing. $\Delta V'E/\Delta PETCO_2$ reflects central and, if PaO_2 is not excessive, also carotid chemoreceptor activity. Being appreciably shorter, the latter test is preferred, although $\Delta V'E/\Delta PETCO_2$ reflects only central chemoreflex activity.
>
> - Ventilatory hypoxic responsiveness is determined from the curvilinear isocapnic $V'E–PETO_2$ response, using steady-state, constant-concentration inspirates or rebreathing. It reflects solely carotid chemoreceptor activity. Expressing $V'E$ versus SaO_2 linearises the profile, with the slope ($\Delta V'E/\Delta SaO_2$) providing the hypoxic responsiveness index (however, PaO_2, not SaO_2, is the actual stimulus). This can also be estimated using the Dejours hypoxia-withdrawal test: abrupt oxygen administration from a prior hypoxic background acutely suppresses carotid-body activity to cause a transient, rapid $V'E$ decline; the maximum decrease as a fraction of the total hypoxic $V'E$ providing the hypoxic index.

typically linear in healthy, normoxic individuals, with a slope ($\Delta V'E/\Delta PETCO_2$) averaging ~2–3 $L \cdot min^{-1} \cdot mmHg^{-1}$. This slope reflects the carbon dioxide responsiveness of both the central 'chemoreceptors', located predominantly on the ventral medullary surfaces and also, if P_aO_2 is not excessive, the peripheral chemoreceptors (predominantly, if not exclusively, the carotid bodies in humans).

At P_aO_2 levels of ~90 mmHg, the central component accounts for 70–75% of the response, with the peripheral component accounting for the remainder. However, as the 'peripheral' component of carbon dioxide responsiveness increases with reductions of P_aO_2 below normal, $\Delta V'E/\Delta P_{ETCO_2}$ increases with greater, constant degrees of hypoxaemia and decreases with greater, constant degrees of hyperoxia. This results in a 'fan' of hypoxia-dependent carbon dioxide response slopes reflecting altered response 'sensitivity' (also termed 'potentiation'), with little or no change in the extrapolated $V'E$ intercept on the P_{CO_2} axis (fig. 1). By contrast, sustained metabolic acidaemia or alkalaemia results in a parallel shift by the carbon dioxide response relationship (*i.e.* no change in carbon dioxide 'sensitivity') with a reduced or increased $V'E$ intercept, respectively.

The increasing $\Delta V'E/\Delta P_{ETCO_2}$ with greater levels of simultaneous hypoxia reflects a progressively greater carotid-body response component; it is crucial, therefore, to maintain P_aO_2 constant (iso-oxic) during the test. Above a P_aO_2 of ~200 mmHg, the carotid-body component is effectively inactivated and hence the sufficiently hyperoxic carbon dioxide response entirely reflects that of the 'central' component. Interpretation depends on the relationships between the typically measured P_{ETCO_2} (or, less typically, P_aCO_2) and P_{CO_2} (and hydrogen ion concentration [H^+]) at each set of chemoreceptors; these relationships depend on factors such as the local-tissue perfusion, carbon dioxide production, carbon dioxide capacitance, H^+ buffering capacity and metabolic rate. The equilibrium process is rapid at the carotid body chemoreceptors, but is considerably delayed at the sites of central chemoreception.

It has been has proposed that three or more levels of inspired (I) P_{CO_2} should be used for $\Delta V'E/\Delta P_{ETCO_2}$ characterisation. Each level is maintained for ~8–10 min, with the average $V'E$ and P_{ETCO_2} over the final 2–3 min providing the steady-state values. Consequently, the test is time-consuming, although transiently overshooting P_{ICO_2} beyond the required level can reduce the time required to attain the new $V'E$ steady state.

This concern is obviated, to a considerable extent, by the rebreathing method of Read *et al.* (1967), which takes a small fraction of the time to perform while providing effectively the same $\Delta V'E/\Delta P_{ETCO_2}$ value as the steady-state method. The subject re-breathes from a 6–7-L bag initially containing ~7% carbon dioxide balance oxygen. The high initial P_{ICO_2} is designed to raise P_aCO_2 rapidly to, or close to, the mixed-venous level, such that the subsequent rebreathing provides an effectively linear increase in P_aCO_2; the high inspired oxygen tension (P_IO_2) maintains P_aO_2 above levels for which variations in carotid chemosensitivity would influence the response slope.

The rebreathing relationship is shifted to the right of the steady-state relationship, reflecting both the transit delay between the lungs and sites of chemoreception and the

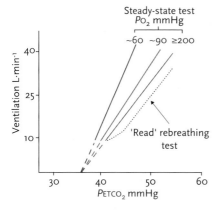

Figure 1. Steady-state ventilatory responses to inhaled P_{CO_2} at constant oxygen tension (P_{O_2}; solid lines). The dotted line depicts the response to progressively increasing P_{CO_2} (hyperoxic rebreathing test).

$V'E$ response kinetics. Consequently, as the test is designed to provide a constant rate of change of P_{CO_2} at the chemoreceptor sites, the rate of change of $V'E$ is compared with the rate of change of P_{ETCO_2} ($\Delta V'E/\Delta P_{ETCO_2}$). This is currently the more common means of assessing carbon dioxide responsiveness, although it is important to recognise that the carbon dioxide responsiveness obtained by this hyperoxic method reflects only central chemoreflex activity.

One must be careful, however, to assume that hypoxia does not influence central chemoreceptor responsiveness; it does indirectly by increasing cerebral blood flow. This tends to wash out CO_2 from the region, narrowing the difference between the local tissue P_{CO_2} and P_{aCO_2}.

Beginning at a value below the spontaneous control condition, carbon dioxide responsiveness is not characterised by the extrapolated dashed lines in figure 1. Rather, there is a region of virtual insensitivity to increasing P_{CO_2}, if previously lowered by, for example, acute hyperventilation or sufficient hypoxia. The transition from the insensitive to the sensitive region is considered to reflect a ventilatory recruitment threshold. The difference between this threshold and the lower P_{ETCO_2} at which apnoea ensues is thought to be important in conditions such as sleep apnoea. Also, as this threshold is lower in hypoxia than in hyperoxia, it can be used to further understand the interaction between peripheral and central chemoreceptor mediation. As a practical expedient, the difference in P_{ETCO_2} between these conditions at resting ventilation can be used as an index of the threshold change; Duffin (2011) has suggested P_{ETO_2} values of 150 and 50 mmHg for this assessment.

Estimation of ventilatory response to hypoxia

The $V'E$ response to hypoxia, if defined under isocapnic conditions, is considered solely to reflect carotid chemoreceptor activity. Both constant-concentration inspirate and rebreathing techniques have been successfully utilised for the characterisation.

The pattern of the $V'E$ response to a step decrease of P_{IO_2} is not monotonic, even with P_{ETCO_2} being maintained as constant by controlling the inspired level (i.e. isocapnic hypoxia). There is an initial increase to a peak, usually well within 5 min, followed by a slow reduction (termed 'hypoxic ventilatory decline') to a final steady state (fig. 2a). The initial increase is considered to be the carotid body component and the subsequent decline is thought to result from the hypoxia-mediated increase in cerebral blood flow. This reduces the degree of central chemoreceptor stimulation as a result of cerebral carbon dioxide wash-out, although an involvement of altered neurotransmission has also been proposed. If the hypoxic step is limited to the initial (or primary) response phase, then the resulting $V'E$–P_{aO_2} relationship over a range of increasingly hypoxic inspirates is curvilinear, with the $V'E$ rate of change approaching infinity at a P_{aO_2} of ~30 mmHg. Naturally, at higher isocapnic P_{CO_2} levels, the curvature constant of the response is increased as a result of greater hypoxic–hypercapnic interaction at the carotid bodies. It is recommended that the subject be switched to air or even a mildly hyperoxic mixture between successive hypoxic steady states to avoid possible depression of brainstem respiratory neurones. If, instead of isocapnia being maintained in this test, P_{aCO_2} is allowed to decrease spontaneously as $V'E$ increases (poikilocapnia), then both the peak initial $V'E$ response and the final level achieved after the hypoxic ventilatory decline are reduced.

A rebreathing test, notionally similar to the Read–Leigh test of CO_2 sensitivity, yields considerably greater data density in a significantly shorter period, although the requirement for isocapnia throughout the test does demand a degree of sophistication in avoiding, by means of a carbon dioxide-absorbing system, the otherwise progressive hypercapnia. The resulting curvilinear response to the progressive isocapnic hypoxia is shown in figure 2b for two subjects differing markedly in hypoxic sensitivity. There is little, from a physiological standpoint, to choose between an exponential and a hyperbolic

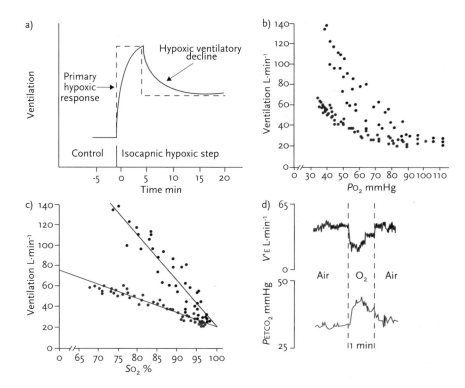

Figure 2. a) V'E time-course to prolonged isocapnic step-decrease in end-tidal oxygen tension (PO₂). b and c) Ventilatory response to progressive isocapnic hypoxia (in two subjects) as a function, respectively, of end-tidal PO₂, and oxygen saturation (SO₂). d) Ventilatory time-course to a hyperoxic step-increase in an exercising hypoxic subject with alveolar proteinosis. PETCO₂: end-tidal carbon dioxide tension. b and c) Reproduced from Rebuck et al. (1981) with permission from the publisher. d) Reproduced from Wasserman et al. (1989) with permission from the publisher.

characterisation of the response. The conflicting issues regarding the most appropriate index for hypoxic response characterisation appear to be obviated (on empirical grounds) by the demonstration that the curvilinear $V'E–PaO_2$ relationship can be transformed into a linear relationship by substituting SaO_2 for PaO_2 (fig. 2c):

$$V'E = G \cdot SaO_2 + V'E(o)$$

where $V'E(o)$ is the control $V'E$ and the slope parameter G is the hypoxic responsiveness quantifier. G has been shown to average ~1.5±1.0 (average±SD) L·min⁻¹·% decrease of SaO_2 in normal subjects. At higher isocapnic levels, G is increased as a result of the potentiating effect of carbon dioxide on carotid chemosensitivity, which sums with the further central carbon dioxide–H⁺ stimulation.

In addition to the ease of measuring SaO_2 noninvasively by pulse oximetry, and averting any assumption regarding the difference between $PETO_2$ and PaO_2, the linearity of the $V'E$ response makes this rebreathing method a very practical means of assessing hypoxic ventilatory responsiveness. It is important to recognise, however, that the ventilatory stimulus is PaO_2; SaO_2 is merely a practical expedient, with uncertainties regarding the influence of conditions altering haemoglobin affinity for oxygen.

The current degree of a subject's hypoxic ventilatory drive may be estimated by the hypoxia-withdrawal test of Dejours (1962).

If a particular level of P_{aO_2} is established by inhalation of a hypoxic gas mixture, or noting the spontaneous P_{aO_2} if the subject is already hypoxaemic (as in figure 2d for an exercising subject with alveolar proteinosis), then the abrupt administration of 100% oxygen will acutely suppress carotid-body hypoxic responsiveness and cause V'_E to fall transiently and rapidly. The maximum decrease in V'_E as a fraction of the total hypoxic V'_E provides the hypoxic index. In addition to the assumption (probably justified in humans) that the consequently high level of oxygen tension (P_{O_2}) actually silences the carotid bodies, the validity of the Dejours test (1962) depends upon the V'_E decrement reaching its nadir prior to the subsequently increased P_{aCO_2} (caused by the reduced V'_E) influencing central sites of carbon dioxide responsiveness. As the nadir of the response commonly occurs ~20–25 s after the hypoxic–hyperoxic transition, there is some uncertainty regarding this latter point. Although this test is quite easy to perform and provides a useful qualitative estimate of hypoxic responsiveness, it remains to be precisely standardised and quantified.

The peripheral-chemosensory potentiation of the carbon dioxide response by hypoxia may also be used to provide an index of hypoxic ventilatory responsiveness, as follows:

1) from the linear difference between the hyperoxic and the hypoxic carbon dioxide response, and

2) the increase in V'_E between the hyperoxic (peripheral chemoreceptors silenced) and the hypoxic (40 mmHg P_{aO_2}) carbon dioxide response relationship, measured at a standard target level of 40 mmHg P_{aCO_2} (ΔV_{40}).

Conclusions

While these approaches provide indices of acute ventilatory responsiveness, laboratory-based tests of more chronic blood–gas and acid–base regulatory challenges are less well standardised.

Further reading

- Cunningham DJC, et al. Integration of respiratory responses to changes in alveolar partial pressures of CO_2 and O_2 and in arterial pH. In: Widdicombe JG, et al., eds. Handbook of Physiology, Respiration. Vol II, Control of Breathing, Part 2. Washington DC, American Physiological Society, 1986; pp. 475–528.
- Dejours P (1962). Chemoreflexes in breathing. Physiol Rev; 42: 335–358.
- Dempsey JA, et al. (2004). The ventilatory responsiveness to CO_2 below eupnoea as a determinant of ventilatory stability in sleep. J Physiol; 560: 1–11.
- Duffin J (2011). Measuring the respiratory chemoreflexes in humans. Respir Physiol Neurobiol; 177: 71–79.
- Edelman NH, et al. Effects of CNS hypoxia on breathing. In: Crystal RG, et al., eds. The Lung: Scientific Foundations. 2nd Edn. New York, Raven Press, 1997; pp. 1757–1765.
- Read DJC, et al. (1967). Blood–brain tissue P_{CO_2} relationships and ventilation during rebreathing. J Appl Physiol; 23: 53–70.
- Rebuck AS, et al. Measurement of ventilatory responses to hypercapnia and hypoxia. In: Hornbein T, ed. The Regulation of Breathing. New York, Dekker, 1981; pp. 745–772.
- Severinghaus JW (1976). Proposed standard determination of ventilatory responses to hypoxia and hypercapnia in man. Chest; 70: Suppl. 1, 129–131.
- Wasserman K, et al. Respiratory control during exercise. In: Widdicombe JG, ed. International Review of Physiology, Respiratory Physiology III. Baltimore, Univ Park Press, 1981; pp. 149–211.

Arterial blood gas assessment

Paolo Palange, Alessandro Maria Ferrazza and Josep Roca

The fundamental function of the lung is to contribute to homeostasis by ensuring that pulmonary oxygen uptake ($V'O_2$) and carbon dioxide production ($V'CO_2$) match the body's bioenergetic requirements. We must look at pulmonary function as the first step of the oxygen transport chain from the atmosphere to mitochondria.

Arterial blood gas (ABG) analysis provides direct measurements of oxygen (PaO_2) and carbon dioxide tension ($PaCO_2$), and pH in arterial blood. In clinical practice, ABG analysis is needed to assess both severity and causes of pulmonary gas exchange impairment and acid–base (A–B) disequilibrium. ABG analysis is one of the most useful diagnostic tests, not only in the critical care setting but also in general clinical practice, to assess patients with respiratory diseases and those with other disorders with potential impact on pulmonary gas exchange and A–B disturbances (diabetes, heart failure (HF) and renal failure). Moreover, ABG analysis is mandatory to establish a diagnosis of respiratory failure.

Modern equipment for performing ABG assessment uses electrodes to measure PaO_2, $PaCO_2$ and pH. Other variables, such as bicarbonates (actual HCO_3^- and standard HCO_3^-), base excess (BE) and oxyhaemoglobin saturation (SaO_2), are computed using well-defined equations.

A simple and practical two-step approach for ABG interpretation in the clinical setting is illustrated in figure 1. The first step aims at the analysis of pulmonary gas exchange status based primarily on PaO_2 and $PaCO_2$, while the second step addresses the assessment of A–B status using $PaCO_2$, pH and, eventually, HCO_3^- (or BE). If serum electrolytes, and in

Key points

- ABG is mandatory for the diagnosis of respiratory failure and of A–B disorders.

- Pulmonary gas exchange status is best evaluated by the integrated reading of PaO_2 and $PaCO_2$.

- A–B status is best evaluated by the integrated reading of $PaCO_2$ and pH, with concomitant measurement of serum electrolytes.

- Mixed A–B disorders are very common in clinical practice.

- The correct interpolation of ABG represents a fundamental step for the diagnosis and treatment of A–B disorders.

- The study of serum chloride is fundamental to further investigate the causes of metabolic disorders affecting A–B equilibrium.

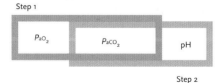

Step 1

Step 2

Figure 1. 'Two-step' approach for ABG interpretation.

particular chloride, are measured, a further insight into the differential diagnosis of metabolic A–B disorders can be obtained (third step).

Step 1: evaluation

Healthy subjects at sea level breathing room air (inspiratory oxygen fraction (FIO_2) 0.21) show PaO_2 values close to 90–95 mmHg. PaO_2 values <80 mmHg are considered arterial hypoxaemia and PaO_2 <60 mmHg indicates hypoxaemic respiratory failure. Because of the characteristics of the oxyhaemoglobin dissociation curve, a PaO_2 of 60 mmHg corresponds to a SaO_2 of ~90% and is located at the upper end of the steepest portion of the curve. PaO_2 values <60 mmHg will have a substantial impact, reducing arterial oxygen content and compromising tissue oxygenation. The accepted reference interval for $PaCO_2$ is 35–45 mmHg. By convention, hypercapnic respiratory failure is established at $PaCO_2$ >50 mmHg.

Abnormal respiratory gases in arterial blood are generally due to impaired pulmonary gas exchange. Intrapulmonary factors that may cause arterial hypoxemia are listed in table 1. Pulmonary alveolar ventilation ($V'A$)/perfusion (Q') mismatch is the most frequent determinant of hypoxaemia and hypercapnia in the clinical scenario. However, the identification of pulmonary shunt (perfusion of unventilated pulmonary units, $V'A/Q' = 0$) as the main cause of hypoxaemia in a patient with severe pneumonia has relevant therapeutic implications. It is of note, however, that alterations of extrapulmonary factors such as cardiac output, FIO_2, $V'O_2$ and $V'E$ are also determinants of PaO_2 and $PaCO_2$.

When $PaCO_2$ values are close to 40 mmHg, PaO_2 is an excellent indicator of the efficacy of the lung as an oxygen exchanger, but abnormal $PaCO_2$ values (hypercapnia or hypocapnia) may benefit from the integrated reading of PaO_2 and $PaCO_2$ values indicated in table 1. Such an integrated view can be numerically obtained by computing the alveolar–arterial oxygen tension difference ($PA-aO_2$) using the simplified formula

$$PA-aO_2 = ((PB-PH_2O) \cdot FIO_2 - PaCO_2/R) - PaO_2$$

where PB is barometric pressure, PH_2O is the partial pressure of water vapour in the airways and R is the respiratory quotient ($V'CO_2/V'O_2$, ~0.80 at rest).

At sea level, the normal expected $PA-aO_2$ value is <15 mmHg in young subjects and <20 mmHg in the elderly. Table 1 shows the contribution of the $PA-aO_2$ in the identification of the mechanisms of alteration of ABG.

To further understand the cause of arterial hypoxaemia, the effect of supplemental oxygen breathing on PaO_2 should be examined, keeping in mind that in the normal lung $PA-aO_2$ widens when breathing additional oxygen. While hypoxaemia due to pulmonary $V'A/Q'$ mismatch and diffusion defects is usually corrected by increasing inspired oxygen concentrations, this does not correct respiratory failure due to shunt.

A simple, but less accurate, way to compute $PA-aO_2$ is to use the rule of '130'. It is assumed that in a healthy subject, at sea level ($FIO_2 = 0.21$), the sum of PaO_2 and $PaCO_2$ should be ~130 mmHg. Consequently,

$$PA-aO_2 \approx 130 - (PaO_2 + PaCO_2)$$

The following examples illustrate the use of the rule. A patient with PaO_2 70 mmHg and

Table 1. $PA-aO_2$ in the evaluation of the causes of arterial hypoxaemia

Cause	PaO_2	$PaCO_2$	$PA-aO_2$
Hypoventilation	↓	↑	↔
$V'A/Q'$ mismatch	↓	↔ ↓ ↑	↑
Oxygen diffusion limitation	↓	↔ ↓	↑
Shunt	↓ ↓	↔ ↓ ↑	↑ ↑

PaCO$_2$ 60 mmHg (PA–aO$_2$ $\approx$130-(70+60)=0 mmHg) is hypoventilating a lung that is functionally 'normal', with a PA–aO$_2$ within the reference interval. However, a patient with hypoxaemic respiratory failure and hypocapnia (PaO$_2$ 50 mmHg, PaCO$_2$ 20 mmHg; PA–aO$_2$ $\approx$130-(50+20)=60 mmHg) shows worse pulmonary oxygen exchange (higher PA–aO$_2$) than a patient with respiratory failure and hypercapnia (PaO$_2$ 50 mmHg, PaCO$_2$ 50 mmHg; PA–aO$_2$ $\approx$130-(50+50)=30 mmHg). The computation of PA–aO$_2$ (and the use of the rule of 130) is not useful clinically when FIO$_2$ increases. Calculating the PaO$_2$/FIO$_2$ ratio is recommended to assess the efficacy of the lung as an oxygen exchanger in critical care when comparing ABG measurements taken at different values of FIO$_2$. Lung injury is defined as PaO$_2$/FIO$_2$ <300 mmHg while acute respiratory distress syndrome (ARDS) is associated with a PaO$_2$/FIO$_2$ <200 mmHg (table 2). Recently, three mutually exclusive categories of ARDS severity based on the degree of hypoxaemia have been proposed:

- mild (PaO$_2$/FIO$_2$ from 200 to ≤300 mmHg)
- moderate (PaO$_2$/FIO$_2$ from 100 to ≤200 mmHg)
- severe (PaO$_2$/FIO$_2$ ≤100 mmHg)

Step 2: diagnosis of A–B disorders

Arterial pH is highly regulated to be maintained between 7.38 and 7.42. In the clinical assessment of A–B equilibrium, two main determinants of arterial pH must be taken into account, namely

- the respiratory component (PaCO$_2$)
- the metabolic component

Hypercapnia (high PaCO$_2$) generates respiratory acidosis (low pH) whereas hypocapnia (low PaCO$_2$) is associated to respiratory alkalosis (high pH). In simple acute respiratory disorders, for each 10-mmHg variation in PaCO$_2$, the expected change in pH is 0.07 for acidosis and 0.08 for alkalosis, while in simple chronic respiratory disorders, it is 0.03 for both acidosis and alkalosis.

The metabolic component refers to the impact of nonvolatile molecules generating acidosis or alkalosis. The variable most often used to assess the metabolic component is bicarbonate concentration ([HCO$_3^-$]) computed through the Henderson–Hasselbalch equation:

$$pH = 6.1 + \log([HCO_3^-]/0.03 \cdot P\text{CO}_2)$$

where PCO$_2$ is carbon dioxide tension. In the past, the role of simple rules associating changes in PaCO$_2$ with changes in pH (and HCO$_3^-$) has been emphasised as useful for the diagnosis of simple and mixed A–B disorders. A graphical illustration of this approach in presented in figure 2.

Table 3 displays some examples of simple A–B disorders. The first two rows in table 3 indicate simple, uncompensated A–B disorders. The first row may correspond to a COPD patient with an episode of severe exacerbation showing acute hypercapnia leading to respiratory acidosis. The second

Table 2. Respiratory failure

Hypoxaemic respiratory failure
PaO$_2$ ≤60 mmHg, PaCO$_2$ normal or low, at sea-level (FIO$_2$ 0.21)
Hypoxaemia due to pulmonary V'A/Q' mismatching (PaO$_2$ rises with FIO$_2$)
Chronic respiratory diseases (only pulmonary fibrosis shows oxygen diffusion limitation with V'A/Q' mismatch)
Hypoxaemia due to intrapulmonary shunt (lung units with V'A/Q'=0) (PaO$_2$ responds to FIO$_2$) (PaO$_2$/FIO$_2$ ≤200)
Hypercapnic respiratory failure
PaCO$_2$ ≥50 mmHg and PaO$_2$ low, at sea-level (FIO$_2$ 0.21)
'Normal' lung (PA–aO$_2$ gradient preserved)
Reduced V'A due to extrapulmonary factors
Advanced chronic respiratory disease or severe exacerbation
Hypoxaemia due to pulmonary V'A/Q' mismatch

example fits any situation leading to hyperventilation and low $P\mathrm{aCO_2}$ that generates respiratory alkalosis (*e.g.* interstitial oedema in HF). The third row indicates an example of acidosis due to a metabolic disturbance (*e.g.* exercise-related increase in blood lactate, ketoacidosis, renal failure, *etc.*). Finally, the fourth example of A–B disequilibrium corresponds to a metabolic alkalosis that may be seen in patients with liquid depletion and low intracellular and serum potassium concentrations (*e.g.* excessive diuretic therapy).

Common causes of A–B disorders are illustrated in tables 4 and 5. It is of note that although they may begin as simple disorders (respiratory or metabolic), these often evolve to mixed A–B abnormalities.

Step 3: more on A–B disorders

To further investigate the causes of metabolic disorders, the measurement of serum electrolytes, and in particular chloride, is of great help. In fact, while respiratory disturbances directly affect pH by modifying $P\mathrm{aCO_2}$, metabolic disturbances can be derived from changes in the net difference between negative and positive charges dissolved in the serum (strong ions and weak acids). An increase in negative charges reduces pH, while a reduction increases pH (fig. 3). The negative charges that strongly influence the A–B equilibrium are chloride and the so-called non-measurable anions (see later). Several types of renal tubular acidosis impair renal chloride excretion, resulting in a net increase in serum chloride concentration and, thus,

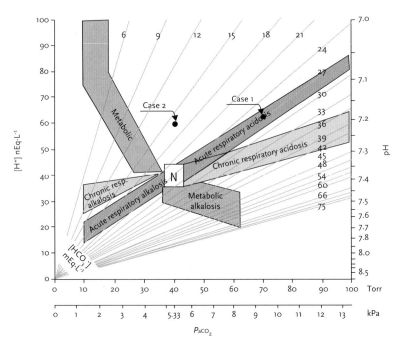

Figure 2. $P\mathrm{aCO_2}$–pH nomogram for the diagnosis of A–B disorders. $P\mathrm{aCO_2}$ and pH values that fall in the acute or chronic, respiratory or nonrespiratory (or metabolic) 'bands' should be considered 'simple' disorders (case 1: $P\mathrm{aCO_2}$ 70 mmHg, pH 7.19; acute respiratory acidosis). Values that fall between the respiratory and metabolic bands should be considered 'mixed' disorders (case 2: $P\mathrm{aCO_2}$ 40 mmHg, pH 7.20; acute respiratory and metabolic acidosis). N: normal. Reproduced and modified from Goldberg et al. (1973).

Table 3. *Examples of simple A–B disorders*

	pH	$P_{a}CO_2$	[HCO_3^-]
Respiratory acidosis	↓	↑	↔
Respiratory alkalosis	↑	↓	↔
Metabolic acidosis	↓	↓	↓
Metabolic alkalosis	↑	↑	↑

in metabolic acidosis. Lower gastrointestinal losses of sodium, potassium and water (diarrhoea) cause an increase in the serum concentration of chloride, thus resulting in hyperchloraemic acidosis. However, reduction of chloride (*e.g.* loop diuretics) causes metabolic alkalosis. The main mechanism that may cause metabolic alkalosis is the increase in renal ammoniagenesis that stimulates chloride excretion as ammonium chloride. Several factors can increase renal ammoniagenesis: primitive hyperaldosteronism, hypovolaemia (*e.g.* secondary hyperaldosteronism) and hypokalaemia. In the clinical setting, the causes of metabolic alkalosis can be classified as chloride-responsive or chloride-resistant based on the response to chloride salt administration (table 5). Negative charges other than chloride are usually calculated by the anion gap (AG) formula:

$$AG = [Na^+] - ([Cl^-] + [HCO_3^-])$$

The AG represents the amount of non-measurable anions (acids), and the normal value is around 12–14 mEq·L^{-1}. The most

common acids that cause high-AG metabolic acidosis are lactic acid (lactic acidosis), keto acids (diabetic or alcoholic acidosis) and inorganic acids (renal failure). The reduction in AG due to severe reduction in serum albumin can generate a mild metabolic alkalosis.

Conclusion

In clinical practice, the correct interpretation of ABG provides unique information on the characteristics and severity of lung gas exchange impairment and on A–B abnormalities. It represents a fundamental step towards an appropriate diagnosis of the patient and the adoption of the treatment strategy. Figure 3 summarises the interpretative 'integrative' approach to be used in the evaluation of the ABG. As a first step (step 1), the combined reading of $P_{a}O_2$ and $P_{a}CO_2$ values, on room air and during supplemental oxygen breathing, should be used to identify the causes and the severity of arterial hypoxaemia (blue squares and

Table 4. *Respiratory disorders*

Respiratory acidosis
Central nervous system depression, neuromuscular disorders
Chest wall abnormalities
Lung diseases
Respiratory alkalosis
Anxiety, central nervous system disorders
Hormones/drugs (catecholamine, progesterone, hyperthyroidism, salicylate)

Table 5. *Metabolic disorders*

Metabolic acidosis
Normochloraemic acidosis (or high anion gap acidosis)
Ketoacidosis
Lactic acidosis
Renal failure
Toxins
Hyperchloraemic acidosis (or normal anion gap acidosis)
Extra-renal loss of sodium
Renal tubular acidosis
Metabolic alkalosis
Chloride-responsive type
Gastric fluid loss
Volume contraction
Chloride-resistant type
Mineral corticoid disorders
Milk-alkali and Bartter syndromes
Hypoalbuminaemia

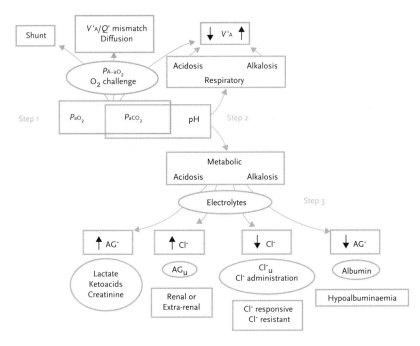

Figure 3. Comprehensive approach to ABG interpretation. AG: anion gap; U: urinary.

blue circles). As a second step (step 2), the combined reading of P_aCO_2 and pH is needed for the correct diagnosis of A–B disorders (red squares). Furthermore, the study of serum electrolytes, particularly serum chloride, may be of great help in the identification of the causes of metabolic disorders (red squares) (step 3).

Further reading

- ARDS Definition Task Force, *et al.* (2012). Acute respiratory distress syndrome: the Berlin Definition. *JAMA*; 307: 2526–2533.
- Astrup P (1956). A simple electrometric technique for the determination of carbon dioxide tension in blood and plasma, total content of carbon dioxide in plasma and bicarbonate content in 'separated' plasma at fixed carbon dioxide tension. *Scand J Clin Lab Invest*; 8: 33–43.
- Brackett NC Jr, *et al.* (1965). Carbon dioxide titration curve of normal man. Effect of increasing degrees of acute hypercapnia on acid–base equilibrium. *N Engl J Med*; 272: 6–12.
- Hughes JMB. Pulmonary gas exchange. *In:* Lung Function Tests: Physical Principles and Clinical Applications. Hughes JMB, *et al.*, eds. London, W.B. Saunders, 1999; pp. 75–79.
- Kassirer JP, *et al.* (1965). Rapid estimation of plasma carbon dioxide tension from pH and total carbon dioxide content. *N Engl J Med*; 272: 1067–1068.
- Kellum JA (2005). Clinical review: reunification of acid–base physiology. *Crit Care*; 9: 500–506.
- Kellum JA (2007). Disorders of acid–base balance. *Crit Care Med*; 35: 2630–2636.
- Narins RG, *et al.* (1980). Simple and mixed acid–base disorders: a practical approach. *Medicine*; 59: 161–187.

- Riley RL, *et al.* (1949). 'Ideal' alveolar air and the analysis of ventilation–perfusion relationships in the lungs. *J Appl Physiol*; 1: 825–847.
- Riley RL, *et al.* (1951). Analysis of factors affecting partial pressures of oxygen and carbon dioxide in gas and blood of lungs: theory. *J Appl Physiol*; 4: 77–101.
- Roca J, *et al.* (1994). Principles and information content of the multiple inert gas elimination technique. *Thorax*; 49: 815–824.
- Severinghaus JW, *et al.* (1958). Electrodes of blood P_{O_2} and P_{CO_2} determination. *J Appl Physiol*; 13: 515–520.
- Stewart PA (1983). Modern quantitative acid–base chemistry. *Can J Physiol Pharmacol*; 61: 1444–1461.
- Wagner PD (2003). The biology of oxygen. *Eur Respir J*; 31: 887–890.
- West JB (1971). Causes of carbon dioxide retention in lung disease. *N Engl J Med*; 284: 1232–1236.

Exercise testing

Paolo Palange and Paolo Onorati

The ability to exercise largely depends on the integrated physiological responses of the respiratory, cardiovascular and skeletal muscle systems. In healthy individuals, exercise tolerance is influenced by age, gender and level of fitness. In patients with lung diseases, exercise tolerance is typically reduced and limited by symptoms such as dyspnoea and leg fatigue.

Cardiopulmonary exercise testing (CPET), *i.e.* the study of ventilatory, cardiovascular and pulmonary gas exchange variables during symptom-limited incremental exercise, is considered the gold standard for evaluating the degree and causes of exercise intolerance in disease states (table 1). Moreover, CPET has been extensively used in patients with COPD, CF, interstitial lung diseases (ILDs), pulmonary vascular disorders (PVDs) and CHF.

- In COPD and CF, exercise tolerance is mainly limited by pulmonary mechanical

---

Key points

CPET is considered the gold standard for:

- an objective measure of exercise capacity,

- identifying the mechanisms limiting exercise intolerance,

- establishing indices of the patient's prognosis,

- evaluating the effects of therapeutic interventions.

---

abnormalities (*e.g.* reduction in ventilatory capacity, dynamic hyperinflation)
- In ILD, exercise tolerance is limited by ventilatory constraints and pulmonary gas exchange abnormalities (*e.g.* arterial oxygen desaturation).
- In PVD and CHF, both circulatory (*e.g.* reduced adaptation in cardiac output) and pulmonary gas exchange abnormalities contribute to exercise intolerance.

Exercise protocols

Maximal incremental test The symptom-limited maximal incremental exercise protocol is recommended as a first step in the evaluation of exercise tolerance. $V'E$, heart rate, oxygen uptake ($V'O_2$), carbon dioxide production ($V'CO_2$), and end-tidal oxygen and carbon dioxide tensions are the primary variables measured, typically on a breath-by-breath basis using computerised systems. Additional required measurements include ECG, blood pressure, dyspnoea, leg discomfort, exercise-related arterial oxygen desaturation and spirometry with flow–volume loop recording. Careful selection of patients minimises the likelihood of serious complications during maximal incremental exercise testing. Myocardial infarction (within 3–5 days), unstable angina, severe arrhythmias, pulmonary embolism, dissecting aneurism and severe aortic stenosis represent absolute contraindications to CPET. Resting lung function measurements and ECG are usually obtained before CPET. Cycle and treadmill exercise have been used interchangeably, although the former is largely used as the work rate for incremental and endurance tests is easier to quantify. As the exercise

Table 1. Some causes of exercise intolerance in lung diseases

Ventilatory limitation to exercise
Dynamic hyperinflation
Increased work of breathing
Pulmonary gas exchange abnormalities
Excessive perception of symptoms
Impaired cardiovascular response to exercise and reduced oxygen delivery
Peripheral muscle weakness/dysfunction

period should last 10–12 min, the work rate increment should be selected carefully. In patients with lung diseases, the usual rate of workload increase is 10 $W \cdot min^{-1}$, although slower or faster rates are possible in the very sick and in fitter patients, respectively. The maximal incremental exercise test is also used to determine the appropriate work rate for an endurance protocol.

Constant work rate (CWR) tests, on a cycle ergometer or on a treadmill, are used for the measurement of exercise 'endurance' tolerance and ventilatory and pulmonary gas exchange kinetics. CWR exercise results in steady-state responses when work rate is of moderate intensity (*i.e.* below the lactate threshold (θL); conversely, high-intensity CWR exercise (*i.e.* above θL) results in steady states either being delayed or not attained at all.

Walking tests, such as the 6-min walking test, have been increasingly used for the assessment of exercise tolerance in chronic lung diseases. The object of this test is to walk as far as possible in 6 min. The test should be performed indoors along a 30-m flat, straight corridor; encouragement significantly increases the distance walked. Measurements of S_{pO_2}, heart rate and exertional symptoms are recommended during this test.

Indications for CPET

In patients with lung diseases, exercise testing is mainly used for functional and prognostic purposes. Other indications include: detection of exercise-induced bronchocontriction; selection of candidates for surgery, including lung transplant; and evaluation of the effects of therapeutic intervention, including pulmonary rehabilitation.

Exercise variables and indexes

Maximal V'_{O_2} The classical criterion for defining exercise intolerance and classifying degrees of impairment is the maximal oxygen uptake (V'_{O_2}max). With good subject effort on an incremental test, V'_{O_2}max reflects a subject's maximal aerobic capacity. This index is taken to reflect the attainment of a limitation in the oxygen conductance pathway from the lungs to the mitochondria. Values <80% predicted are considered abnormal while values <40% predicted indicate severe impairment.

Lactate threshold θL is the highest V'_{O_2} at which the arterial lactate concentration is not systematically increased, and is estimated using an incremental test. It is considered an important functional demarcator of exercise intensity. Sub-θL work rates can normally be sustained for prolonged periods. θL is dependent on age, sex, body mass and fitness. Noninvasive estimation of θL requires the demonstration of an augmented V'_{CO_2} in excess of that produced by aerobic metabolism, and its associated ventilatory sequelae.

Oxygen pulse The oxygen pulse is the product of the stroke volume and the difference between the arterial oxygen content (C_{aO_2}) and the mixed venous oxygen content (C_{vO_2}). Given the Fick equation

$$V'_{O_2} = \text{cardiac output} \times (C_{aO_2}\text{-}C_{vO_2})$$

the oxygen pulse can be calculated as:

$$\text{Oxygen pulse} = V'_{O_2}/\text{heart rate}$$

In patients with ILD, the oxygen pulse at peak exercise is lower and its rate of increase with increasing work rate is usually reduced because of the reductions in stroke volume and C_{aO_2}. In PVD, the oxygen pulse is characteristically low at peak exercise and may not increase during incremental exercise, reflecting the abnormal cardiac output adaptation.

Heart rate reserve (HRR) The peak heart rate (HRpeak) achieved in a symptom-limited exercise test decreases with age. The most commonly used equation to predict HRpeak is

$$HR_{peak,pred} = 200\text{-age}$$

HRR is defined as the difference between HRpeak,pred and HRpeak. In healthy individuals, HHR is virtually zero; a high HRR is usually observed in patients with COPD, CF and ILD.

V'_E–V'_{CO_2} slope and ventilatory equivalent for carbon dioxide It is conventional to express the ventilatory response to exercise relative to V'_{CO_2}. It can be measured as the slope of the V'_E–V'_{CO_2} relationship ($\Delta V'_E/\Delta V'_{CO_2}$) over its linear region, i.e. typically extending from 'unloaded pedalling' to the respiratory compensation point. In normal individuals, $\Delta V'_E/\Delta V'_{CO_2}$ values of around 23–25 have been reported.

The adequacy of the ventilatory response to exercise is also expressed by the ratio V'_E/V'_{CO_2} that represents the litres of ventilation necessary to clear 1 L of carbon dioxide. Up to the respiratory compensation point, V'_E/V'_{CO_2} declines curvilinearly as work rate increases. It is common practice to record the value at θ_L ($V'_E/V'_{CO_2}@\theta_L$) or the minimum value. These have each been proposed to provide noninvasive indices of ventilatory inefficiency. In normal individuals, $V'_E/V'_{CO_2}@\theta_L$ values of 25–28 have been reported. Several factors may increase $\Delta V'_E/\Delta V'_{CO_2}$ and $V'_E/V'_{CO_2}@\theta_L$, such as hypoxaemia, acidosis, increased levels of wasted ventilation and pulmonary hypertension.

Breathing reserve (BR) provides an index of the proximity of the ventilation at the limit of tolerance (V'_{Emax}) to the maximal voluntary ventilation (MVV):

$$MVV = \text{resting } FEV_1 \times 40$$

BR can be defined as V'_{Emax} as a percentage of MVV:

$$BR = 1\text{-}V'_{Emax}/MVV$$

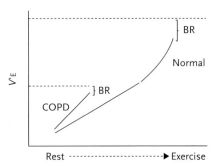

Figure 1. *Ventilatory response and limitation to exercise. Ventilatory limitation to exercise is typically observed in patients with COPD compared with normal subjects. In COPD, but also in CF and ILD, ventilatory reserve is reduced at peak exercise. See the main text for further comments.*

In COPD, CF and ILD, BR is usually reduced or absent at peak CPET exercise (fig. 1). Analysis of flow–volume loops is also emerging as an important tool to assess the degree of airflow and ventilatory limitation during exercise in patients with COPD.

Dynamic hyperinflation In normal subjects, end-expiratory lung volume (EELV) decreases with increasing work rate by as much as 0.5–1.0 L below functional residual capacity. Changes in EELV during exercise can be estimated by asking the subject to perform an inspiratory capacity manoeuvre at a selected point in the exercise test. In COPD, particularly in the advanced phases of the disease, EELV increases during exercise (i.e. dynamic hyperinflation) in spite of expiratory muscle activity.

Arterial oxygen desaturation During exercise, SpO_2 is normally maintained in the region of around 97–98%. However, arterial oxygen desaturation can be observed in patients with moderate–severe ILD and in patients with primary pulmonary hypertension.

Tolerable limit of exercise and 'isotime' measurements Tlim is the tolerable limit of exercise, expressed as function of time measured during CWR protocols. In clinical practice, high-intensity (around 70–80% of maximal work rate) CWR protocols are used for the evaluation of interventions. In addition to Tlim, measurement of pertinent physiological variables (*e.g.* $V'E$, inspiratory capacity and dyspnoea) at a standardised time (isotime) are obtained.

CPET response patterns

Ventilatory Response In normal individuals during incremental exercise, $V'E$ increases linearly relative to work rate or $V'O_2$. At some point, $V'E$ begins to increase more steeply in response to the development of lactic acidosis, to maintain acid–base homeostasis (normal individual in fig. 1). The ventilatory response to exercise in patients with lung disorders is increased (COPD patient in fig. 1). Conventionally, the ratio of $V'E$ at peak exercise to the estimated MVV represents the assessment of the ventilatory limitation or of the prevailing ventilatory constraints. Ventilatory limitation is commonly judged to occur when $V'E/MVV$ exceeds 85%. In lung diseases, the increase in $V'E/MVV$ may reflect a reduction in MVV or an increase in $V'E$. The ventilatory response during exercise is influenced by metabolic rate ($V'CO_2$), $PaCO_2$ and the physiological dead space fraction of the tidal volume (VD/VT). The relationship between these variables is described as:

$$V'E = (863 \times V'CO_2)/(PaCO_2 \times (1-VD/VT))$$

where $PaCO_2$ is expressed in Torr. In lung diseases, for a given $V'CO_2$ and $PaCO_2$, $V'E$ is usually increased because of a higher VD/VT. $\Delta V'E/\Delta V'CO_2$ or $V'E/V'CO_2@\theta L$ is often used in the functional assessment of patients with lung diseases (*e.g.* COPD, ILD and PVD) and cardiovascular disorders (*e.g.* CHF). $V'E/V'CO_2$ is usually increased, particularly in patients with PVD (fig. 2). Another particular behaviour of the $V'E$ response during exercise is the cyclic fluctuation of $V'E$ and expired gas kinetics, also defined as exertional oscillatory ventilation, which can occur in approximately one-third of patients with CHF. While the origin of such a ventilatory abnormality is still controversial, its clinical relevance in terms of a negative prognosis is well established.

Pulmonary gas exchange The efficiency of pulmonary gas exchange can be assessed by studying the magnitude of alveolar–arterial oxygen tension difference ($PA-aO_2$) at rest

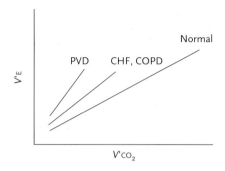

Figure 2. $\Delta V'E/\Delta V'CO_2$ during exercise. Different $\Delta V'E/\Delta V'CO_2$ slopes are seen in normal subjects and in patients with PVD, COPD and CHF.

and during exercise. Normally, PaO_2 does not decrease during exercise and $PA-aO_2$ at peak exercise usually remains below 20–30 Torr. In most patients with ILD and PVD, pulmonary gas exchange efficiency is impaired, as indicated by an abnormally large $PA-aO_2$ (>30 Torr) at peak exercise accompanied by arterial oxygen desaturation. These changes reflect regional ventilation–perfusion ratio dispersion and alterations in pulmonary capillary transit time resulting from the recruited pulmonary capillary volume becoming inadequate for the high levels of pulmonary blood flow.

Cardiovascular response CPET has proved very useful in the detection and quantification of cardiovascular abnormalities during exercise. The characteristic findings are a reduced $V'O_2max$, reduced θL, steeper heart rate–$V'O_2$ relationship (with a reduced heart rate reserve at peak exercise) and a shallower profile (or even flattening) of the oxygen pulse increase with increasing $V'O_2$. An abnormal cardiovascular response to exercise is observed in PVD and, in particular, in patients with idiopathic pulmonary arterial hypertension.

Exercise testing in prognostic evaluation

Exercise tolerance is well recognised as a valuable predictor of mortality in healthy subjects. This also appears to be the case in chronic pulmonary diseases. Exercise testing has become an essential component

Table 2. CPET prognostic indices

	COPD	ILD	CF	PVD	CHF
↓ $V'O_2max$	+	+	+	+	+
↑ $V'E/V'CO_2$		+			++
Arterial oxygen desaturation		++	+	+	
Exertional oscillatory ventilation					++

in the prognostic evaluation of patients with lung diseases (table 2).

Several studies have confirmed that $V'O_2max$ is superior to other indexes in the risk stratification of patients with end-stage lung diseases; many centres, however, use field tests for prognostic purposes.

Evaluating the effects of therapeutic interventions

High-intensity (75–80% of peak work rate) endurance CWR protocols performed on a cycle ergometer or treadmill to Tlim have been successfully used in COPD patients for the evaluation of the effects of therapeutic interventions (e.g. bronchodilators, oxygen, heliox and rehabilitation). These types of protocols have a greater power to discriminate therapy-induced changes in COPD patients, with a higher fractional improvement in exercise tolerance compared with incremental CPET. However, it should be recognised that the hyperbolic profile of the relationship between the power output and exercise duration (Tlim) (the 'power–duration curve') during CWR tests is responsible for a considerable proportion of variability in the improvement magnitude of Tlim. That is, Tlim is influenced by the pre-intervention work rate and exercise duration and their relative positioning on the power–duration profile. Without knowledge of these aspects, any change in Tlim to a single CWR bout must be cautiously interpreted in terms of realistic physiological benefits obtained from the intervention.

Further reading

- ATS Committee on Proficiency Standards for Clinical Pulmonary Function Laboratories. (2002). ATS statement: guidelines for the six-minute walking test. Am J Respir Crit Care Med; 166: 111–117.
- ERS Task Force on Standardization of Clinical Exercise Testing. (1997). Clinical exercise testing with reference to lung diseases: indications, standardization and interpretation strategies. Eur Respir J; 10: 2662–2689.
- Guazzi M, et al. (2012). Exercise oscillatory breathing and NT-proBNP levels in stable heart failure provide the strongest prediction of cardiac outcome when combining biomarkers with cardiopulmonary exercise testing. J Card Fail; 18: 313–320.
- Johnson B, et al. (2003). ATS/ACCP statement on cardiopulmonary exercise testing. IV. Conceptual and physiologic basis of cardiopulmonary exercise testing measurements. Am J Respir Crit Care Med; 167: 228–238.
- O'Donnell DE, et al. (2001). Dynamic hyperinflation and exercise intolerance in chronic obstructive pulmonary disease. Am J Respir Crit Care Med; 164: 770–777.
- Palange P, et al. (2007). Recommendations on the use of exercise testing in clinical practice. Eur Respir J; 29: 185–209.
- Ward SA, et al., eds. Clinical Exercise Testing. Sheffield, European Respiratory Society, 2007.
- Wasserman K, et al. Principles of Exercise Testing and Interpretation, 4th Edn. Philadelphia, Lippincott Williams & Wilkins. 2005.
- Whipp BJ, et al. (2009). Quantifying intervention-related improvements in exercise tolerance. Eur Respir J; 33: 1254–1260.

Bronchial provocation testing

Kai-Håkon Carlsen

As early as 1859, Sir Henry Hyde Salter described 'bronchial sensibility' in patients with asthma. Later, in 1945, Tiffenau suggested that measuring changes in expiratory flow after inhaling acetylcholine or isoproterenol could be helpful in assessing patients with airways disease. Ultimately, these observations led to the concept of bronchial hyperresponsiveness (BHR), which is defined as 'an increase in the ease and degree of airflow limitations in response to bronchoconstrictor stimuli *in vivo*' (Sterk, 1996).

BHR is assessed by bronchial provocation testing (BPT), which may be performed with several different aims in mind: it may be done as part of research or in the clinical setting, and with several different chemical substances; it may test specific bronchial responsiveness to an allergen (allergen BPT), or nonspecific bronchial responsiveness by BPT to histamine or methacholine, as well as several other different substances (table 1).

Methods of BPT

BPT can be divided into direct and indirect methods (Pauwels *et al.*, 1988). Methacholine and histamine BPT represent direct methods, using a transmitter (methacholine) or a mediator (histamine) substance as test agents. Indirect methods include exercise testing (which may also be regarded as BPT, but which otherwise is regarded to come outside the present topic), inhaled adenosine monophosphate (AMP), inhaled mannitol and eucapnic voluntary hyperpnoea (EVH) tests. The indirect tests have their effect through causing mediator or transmitter release from inflammatory cells and nerves.

Previously, BPT was performed qualitatively using a 10-fold increase in concentration of the test substance (Aas, 1970), whereas during the last 25 years, a doubling of the concentration/dose of the test substance has been used (Cockcroft *et al.*, 1977a).

Taking bronchial provocation with methacholine as an example, figure 1 shows the reduction in FEV1 caused by inhaling

> **Key points**
>
> - Bronchial challenge with methacholine/histamine is a sensitive measure of asthma but lacks specificity.
>
> - Indirect measures of bronchial responsiveness (exercise, inhaled AMP, hypertonic saline and mannitol, and EVH) are specific, but not sensitive, measures of asthma.
>
> - Indirect measures of bronchial responsiveness (exercise, *etc.*) respond rapidly (1–3 weeks) to inhaled steroids.
>
> - Direct measures of bronchial responsiveness (methacholine and histamine) respond slowly to inhaled steroids (>3 months).
>
> - Direct measures of bronchial responsiveness (methacholine and histamine) are presently the most exact monitoring tool for asthma.
>
> - BHR may predict later active asthma.

Table 1. *Different types of bronchial responsiveness assessed by different types of BPT*

Bronchial responsiveness	BPT substance
Specific	Allergen BPT
Nonspecific	
Direct	Methacholine
	Histamine
Indirect	Exercise test
	Exercise test while inhaling dry or cold air
	Inhaled AMP
	Inhaled mannitol
	EVH

doubling doses, with interpolation on the *x*-axis to determine the provocative concentration of methacholine causing a 20% decrease in FEV_1 (PC_{20}) (Cockcroft *et al.*, 1977a). Later, a simplification of the test was introduced by inhaling single doubling doses of methacholine, determining the provocative dose of the test agent causing a 20% decrease in FEV_1 (PD_{20}) (Yan *et al.*, 1983).

The test is performed under standardised conditions, with specified nebulisation rates for the tidal breathing method (PC_{20}), inhaling the test agent for 2 min, measuring FEV_1 and then inhaling the doubed concentration. The test is stopped when FEV_1 is reduced by $\geqslant 20\%$ and the PC_{20}/PD_{20} determined by interpolating the semilogarithmic dose–response curve (fig. 1).

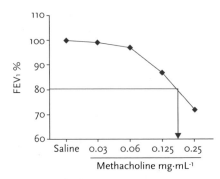

Figure 1. *Determination of PC_{20} by interpolation on the logarithmic x-axis.*

When determining bronchial responsiveness by measuring PD_{20}, the cumulated dose inhaled is determined. This is done by inhaling doubling doses of the test substance. The most often-used delivery device is an inspiration-triggered nebuliser enabling inhalation by controlled tidal ventilation, such as the Spira nebuliser (Spira Respiratory Care Centre, Hämeenlinna, Finland) (Nieminen *et al.*, 1988) or the Aerosol Provocation System (Jaeger, Würzburg, Germany). Alternatively, a handheld DeVilbiss nebuliser has been used (DeVilbiss Healthcare, Somerset, PA, USA) (Cockcroft *et al.*, 1977a). A joint Task Force of the European Respiratory Society and American Thoracic Society is presently revising the recommendations for bronchial challenges, including methacholine and histamine BPT. Recommendations given here may be superseded by new recommendations from that Task Force.

Determinations of PC_{20} or PD_{20} are used both for BPT with methacholine and histamine, as well as with AMP, and may be used for allergen BPT. BPT with mannitol was recently developed and launched commercially by inhaling cumulative doses through a powder inhaler. Here, a 15% reduction in FEV_1 (PD_{15}) is used as cut-off (Brannan *et al.*, 2005).

In EVH, the subject inhales dry air with 4.9% carbon dioxide for 6 min at a preferred ventilation rate of 85% of maximum voluntary ventilation (MMV), which is often calculated as $FEV_1 \times 30$, but a ventilation rate as low as

65% of MVV ($FEV_1 \times 22$) is acceptable (Rosenthal et al., 1984). A reduction in FEV_1 $\geqslant 10\%$ is taken as a positive test. EVH testing has been shown to be particularly sensitive for asthmatic athletes, particularly endurance athletes (Stadelmann et al., 2011; Cockcroft et al., 1977b).

Clinical relevance of BPT

Previously, allergen BPT was often used qualitatively to diagnose asthma and to demonstrate the reaction of the airways to the allergen. This has changed recently out of fear of worsening the asthma after such BPT. A long-lasting worsening of nonspecific BHR after performing an allergen BPT has been demonstrated (Cockcroft et al., 1977b). Thus, allergen BPT is now mostly a tool in research projects and not used in clinical practice.

However, different measures of nonspecific BHR are often used, both in a research context and a clinical setting. With the diagnosis asthma in mind, direct measures of BHR are seen as most sensitive for bronchial asthma, whereas indirect measures are considered to be more specific and less sensitive. In asthma patients from an outpatient clinic compared with healthy subjects, histamine bronchial responsiveness was found to be more sensitive, but less specific, for discriminating asthmatic from healthy subjects (Crockcroft et al., 1977a). Compared with exercise testing, methacholine BPT was more sensitive, but markedly less specific, for discriminating between asthma and other chronic lung diseases. When adding cold air inhalation to the exercise, sensitivity comparable to methacholine was reached, while maintaining the specificity (Carlsen et al., 1998).

In addition, other differences are found between direct and indirect BPT. Indirect bronchial responsiveness is rapidly influenced by treatment with inhaled steroids, with the first effects appearing after 1 week (Henriksen et al., 1983), whereas methacholine BPT needs several months of inhaled steroid treatment to show an effect (Essen-Zandvliet et al., 1992).

Results of BPT may be used to monitor the effect of treatment in asthma. It has been shown that methacholine BPT is superior to clinical assessment and lung function measurements in the follow-up of asthma patients. By monitoring the effect of treatment of asthma with inhaled steroids by follow-up using methacholine BPT, as compared with follow-up based upon clinical symptoms and lung function measurements, it was shown that follow-up by methacholine BPT improved asthma control and had a positive effect upon airway remodelling as assessed by bronchial biopsies (Sont et al., 1999). Thus, BPT with various substances and performed in a standardised measure is probably, at the present time, the best tool for monitoring asthma patients.

Methacholine BPT (PD_{20}) also has a role in predicting later active asthma, as shown by follow-up in a birth cohort study from 10 to 16 years of age (Riiser et al., 2012).

Further reading

- Aas K (1970). Bronchial provocation tests in asthma. *Arch Dis Child*; 45: 221–228.
- Brannan JD, et al. (2005). The safety and efficacy of inhaled dry powder mannitol as a bronchial provocation test for airway hyperresponsiveness: a phase 3 comparison study with hypertonic (4.5%) saline. *Respir Res*; 6: 144.
- Carlsen KH, et al. (1998). Cold air inhalation and exercise-induced broncho-constriction in relationship to metacholine bronchial responsiveness: different patterns in asthmatic children and children with other chronic lung diseases. *Respir Med*; 92: 308–315.
- Cockcroft DW, et al. (1977a). Bronchial reactivity to inhaled histamine: a method and clinical survey. *Clin Allergy*; 7: 235–243.
- Cockcroft DW, et al. (1977b). Allergen-induced increase in non-allergic bronchial reactivity. *Clin Allergy*; 7: 503–513.
- Dickinson JW, et al. (2006). Screening elite winter athletes for exercise induced asthma: a comparison of three challenge methods. *Br J Sports Med*; 40: 179–182.

- Essen-Zandvliet EE, *et al.* (1992). Effects of 22 months of treatment with inhaled corticosteroids and/or beta-2-agonists on lung function, airway responsiveness, and symptoms in children with asthma. *Am Rev Respir Dis*; 146: 547–554.
- Henriksen JM, *et al.* (1983). Effects of inhaled budesonide alone and in combination with low-dose terbutaline in children with exercise-induced asthma. *Am Rev Respir Dis*; 128: 993–997.
- Nieminen MM, *et al.* (1988). Methacholine bronchial challenge using a dosimeter with controlled tidal breathing. *Thorax*; 43: 896–900.
- Pauwels R, *et al.* (1988). Bronchial hyperresponsiveness is not bronchial hyperresponsiveness is not bronchial asthma. *Clin Allergy*; 18: 317–321.
- Riiser A, *et al.* (2012). Does bronchial hyperresponsiveness in childhood predict active asthma in adolescence? *Am J Respir Crit Care Med*; 186: 493–500.
- Rosenthal RR (1984). Simplified eucapnic voluntary hyperventilation challenge. *J Allergy Clin Immunol*; 73: 676–679.
- Salter HH. On Asthma: Its Pathology and Treatment. 1st Edn. London, J. Churchill, 1859.
- Sont JK, *et al.* (1999). Clinical control and histopathologic outcome of asthma when using airway hyperresponsiveness as an additional guide to long-term treatment. *Am J Respir Crit Care Med*; 159: 1043–1051.
- Stadelmann K, *et al.* (2011). Respiratory symptoms and bronchial responsiveness in competitive swimmers. *Med Sci Sports Exerc*; 43: 375–381.
- Sterk PJ (1996). Bronchial hyperresponsiveness: definition and terminology. *Pediatr Allergy Immunol*; 7: Suppl. 9, 7–9.
- Tiffeneau R, *et al.* (1945). Epreuve de bronchoconstriction et de bronchodilation par aérosols. *Bull Acad de Med*; 129: 165–168.
- Yan K, *et al.* (1983). Rapid method for measurement of bronchial responsiveness. *Thorax*; 38: 760–765.

Sputum and exhaled breath analysis

Patrizia Pignatti, Andrea Zanini, Sabrina Della Patrona, Federico Gumiero, Francesca Cherubino and Antonio Spanevello

Noninvasive techniques such as induced sputum and exhaled breath analysis have been successfully proven to reveal inflammatory status and to find indicators of airway oxidative stress involved in the pathogenesis of lung diseases. These techniques allow longitudinal sampling of inflammatory biomarkers in the lung of the same individual, providing a possibility to monitor the lung damage process and evaluate treatment strategies in patients with respiratory diseases, including children.

Induced sputum

Induced sputum is one of the most referenced methods used to determine airway inflammation in asthma, COPD and chronic cough, both in research and in clinical practice. The induced sputum technique is a relatively noninvasive method allowing sampling of low airway secretions from patients who are not able to produce sputum spontaneously.

Procedure Sputum induction consists of inhalation of ultrasonically nebulised saline solution (isotonic or hypertonic) over different time periods and subsequent expectoration of secretions. The subject is asked to inhale 200 mg salbutamol before induction, and FEV_1 is monitored before and after each inhalation to either prevent or detect possible bronchoconstriction.

After collection, the sputum sample is processed within 2 h according to a standardised method with mucolytic agents (dithiothreitol) and centrifugation is required to separate sputum cells from the fluid phase, which is stored at -80°C for soluble mediator evaluation. If the soluble

> **Key points**
>
> - Sputum and exhaled breath analysis are useful noninvasive tools to appraise airway inflammation, particularly in a longitudinal sense.
>
> - Eosinophils are the most significant sputum biomarkers for the evaluation of airway inflammation.
>
> - Many inflammatory mediators can be measured in the fluid phase of sputum but their usefulness remains at research level.
>
> - Nitric oxide is the most reliable exhaled biomarker to assess eosinophilic airway inflammation. Other exhaled biomarkers need further validation and a clear demonstration of their utility in the diagnosis and/or follow-up of airway diseases.

mediators are affected by mucolytic agents, sputum should be processed with phosphate buffer alone.

Safety issues Sputum induction is a simple, safe and well-tolerated procedure even in patients with severe lung diseases and exacerbations. It is recommended that experienced personnel apply standard operating procedures taking into consideration the degree of airway obstruction, use a modified protocol for subjects with severe airway obstruction, and assess lung function and symptoms during the procedure. Sputum induction is considered to be safe if the fall in FEV₁ is within 5% of baseline after waiting for 15 min. If a FEV₁ fall >20% occurs, the inhalation must be stopped. This adverse effect can affect 11% of asthmatics and patients with COPD.

Cell counts in different diseases A sputum sample from a healthy subject is rich in macrophages and neutrophils, and poor in eosinophils, lymphocytes and epithelial cells. The cut-off for sputum eosinophils varies from >2 or >3% according to different authors and European Respiratory Society (ERS) guidelines.

Asthma is characterised by sputum eosinophilia, which predicts a favourable response to corticosteroids. However, noneosinophilic asthma accounts for 25–55% of steroid-naïve asthmatics and is associated with a poor response to corticosteroids.

In up to 40% of subjects with chronic cough, a sputum eosinophil count >3% is seen. These subjects with cough, sputum eosinophilia and no lung function alterations receive the diagnosis of eosinophilic bronchitis, and have an objective response to corticosteroid treatment.

In COPD, neutrophils are usually increased and they are associated with reduced FEV₁, suggesting that neutrophilic airway inflammation is functionally relevant. A cut-off for sputum neutrophilia should take into account age, since neutrophils accumulate in the airways with ageing. Sputum eosinophilia could be present in subjects with COPD and usually predicts a response to corticosteroid therapy.

In figure 1, three representative examples of induced sputum are shown.

Many inflammatory mediators can be measured in the fluid phase of sputum. These mediators are granulocyte proteins, leakage markers, cytokines and chemokines, eicosanoids, and proteases. Unlike sputum cells, up to now, no determination of sputum soluble mediators has entered

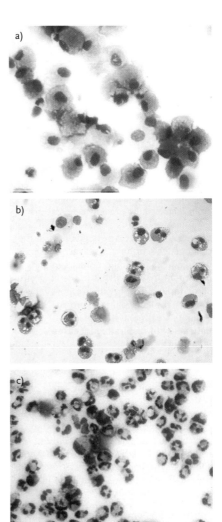

Figure 1. Three representative sputum samples. a) Sputum from a healthy subject containing mostly macrophages. b) Sputum from an asthmatic subject with eosinophilic inflammation. c) Sputum from a COPD subject with neutrophilic inflammation. Original magnification: 400×.

routine evaluation of airway inflammation. Recently, the application of new techniques, such as RT-PCR, *in situ* hybridisation, proteomics, *etc.*, has allowed a wider approach to the study of sputum soluble

Table 1. Biomarkers in induced sputum

Parameters	Asthma	COPD	CF	Sarcoidosis
Cellular phase				
TCC		↑	↑	
Eosinophils	↑			
Neutrophils		↑	↑	
Lymphocytes				↑
CD8$^+$		↑		
CD4$^+$				↑
Fluid phase	ECP	IL-8	IL-8	MMP-9
	MPO	IL-6	IL-17	
	Albumin	TNF-α	IL-23	
	Fibrinogen	IL-10	NE	
	Nonkinase plasminogen activator	IL-17		
	Plasminogen activator	Leptin		
	Neurokinin A	MPO		
	IL-5	HNL		
	IL-8	NE		
	IL-13	ECP		
	Cys-LTs	EPO		
	8-isoprostane	LTB$_4$		
	MMP-9/TIMP ratio	GRO-α		
	VEGF	MCP-1		
		GM-CSF		
		MMP-1		
		MMP-8		
		MMP-9		
		MMP-12		
		Hyaluronan		

↑: increased level; TCC: total cell count; ECP: eosinophil cationic protein; MPO: myeloperoxidase; IL: interleukin; Cys-LT: cysteinyl leukotriene; MMP: matrix metalloproteinase; TIMP: tissue inhibitor of metalloproteinases; VEGF: vascular endothelial growth factor; TNF: tumour necrosis factor; HNL: human neutrophil lipocalin; NE: neutrophil elastase; EPO: eosinophil peroxidise; LT: leukotriene; GRO: growth related oncogene; MCP: monocyte chemotactic protein; GM-CSF: granulocyte–macrophage colony-stimulating factor.

mediators in order to generate a disease associated pattern of mediators.

Table 1 summarises cellular and fluid phase markers of airway inflammation in different pulmonary diseases.

Reproducibility and validity Sputum induction is a reproducible, sensitive and valid method. A standardised methodology of sputum induction and processing was issued in 2002 by an ERS Task Force in order to provide guidance for the reproducibility of the results obtained.

Examination of samples obtained from patients with different respiratory diseases associated with distinct airway inflammatory patterns demonstrated significant differences in cell counts, confirming the validity of the technique. Reference values and the distribution of cell counts in induced sputum were established in a large number of samples from healthy subjects.

Exhaled breath

Measuring biomarkers in breath is useful for monitoring airway inflammation and oxidative stress. Exhaled breath analysis can be defined as analysis of exhaled gases and/ or exhaled breath condensate (EBC).

Variable-sized particles or droplets that are aerosolised from the airway lining fluid, distilled water that condenses from the gas phase out of the nearly water-saturated exhalate, and water-soluble volatiles that are exhaled and absorbed into the condensing breath are the main components of EBC.

Breath samples include:

- end-exhaled air, which represents the alveolar air
- mixed exhaled air, which represents the gas mixture coming from the dead space of the bronchial tree and the alveolar gas-exchange space

Sample collection and analysis Exhaled breath analysis is completely noninvasive, and is suitable for longitudinal studies and for monitoring the response to pharmacological therapy.

Breath analysis consists of direct (on-line) and indirect (off-line) reading methods. Breath analysis is immediately available in the on-line method. The use of indirect methods generally involves collecting and trapping the breath sample and subsequently transferring it to an analytical instrument.

The exhaled gases analysed include:

- exhaled nitric oxide fraction ($F_{e}NO$), which is a marker of airway inflammation
- carbon monoxide, a marker of inflammation and oxidative stress
- ethane, a marker of lipid peroxidation

For gas analysis, chemiluminescent or electrochemical methods and gas chromatography are the most sensitive methodologies used.

Figure 2 shows two commercially available portable $F_{e}NO$ analysers.

Furthermore, an increase in breath temperature can also be evaluated with a high-accuracy thermometer, which is associated with airway inflammation and remodelling.

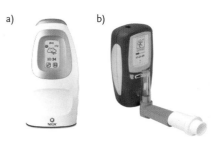

Figure 2. *Two commercially available portable $F_{e}NO$ analysers. a) Niox Mino (Aerocrine AB, Uppsala, Sweden). b) Quark NObreath (Cosmed, Rome, Italy). Images courtesy of the manufacturers.*

Exhaled breath can be condensed through cooling devices, resulting in 1–2 mL EBC over 10 min of tidal breathing. This procedure is noninvasive, simple and easy to perform in patients of any age. In-house and commercially manufactured condensers are available. For pH evaluation, argon deaeration of the EBC sample is needed.

The analysis of EBC is usually performed by immunoassays, mass spectrometry, high-performance liquid chromatography (HPLC), nuclear magnetic resonance, luminometry, spectrophotometry and pH measurement.

Biomarkers Several molecules can be detected in the exhaled air of healthy subjects and patients with inflammatory lung diseases (table 2).

Validity $F_{e}NO$ is the most reliable exhaled marker and is clinically used to assess eosinophilic airway inflammation. It is also useful for assessing adherence to inhaled steroid therapy and the need for further anti-inflammatory treatment in asthma, for differential diagnosis of cough, and for differentiating asthma from COPD. The role of $F_{e}NO$ in COPD is less clear. Smoking reduces $F_{e}NO$ levels, causing misleading results.

Immunoassays for many biomarkers still need to be validated by reference analytical techniques. Concentrations of markers are often close to the detection limit of the assays, making analytical data less reliable.

Table 2 Biomarkers in EBC

Biomarker	Clinical significance in asthma	Clinical significance in COPD
F2-isoprostanes	Increased, reflecting the severity of the disease and the degree of inflammation	Increased, reflecting the severity of the disease and the degree of inflammation
Leukotrienes	Elevated in both adults and children	
Prostanoids		Elevated in steroid-naïve and steroid-treated patients and correlated with the degree of airway inflammation
pH	Decreased and normalises with glucocorticoid therapy	
Hydrogen peroxide	Increased in both adults and children	Increased in patients with exacerbations
Nitrite/nitrate, nitrosothiol, nitrotyrosine	Increased and correlated with eosinophilic inflammation, reduced by corticosteroid therapy	Increased in early stages of exacerbations
FeNO	Increased and falls after treatment with corticosteroids	Increased during exacerbations and falls after inhaled steroids in stable COPD

Dilution of airway lining fluid may influence the results of biomarker analysis in EBC. A confident dilution marker for EBC has not been found yet. However, the use of dilution markers can be avoided by: 1) testing for multiple biomarkers and calculating ratios among them; and 2) identifying a substance that serves as an on–off indicator of an abnormality.

Standardisation and validation of exhaled breath analysis is important, and special attention should be given to:

- flow and time dependence
- influence of respiratory patterns
- origin of markers in EBC
- possible nasal, saliva and sputum contamination

New methodologies (HPLC/mass spectrometry, proteomics, metabolomics, etc.) able to define patterns of exhaled biomarkers specific for distinct airway diseases are under evaluation. Volatile organic compounds (VOCs) (carbon monoxide, ethane, pentane, etc.), in particular, are currently studied for their role in airway inflammation and oxidative stress.

The latest achievements in standardisation and validation of exhaled breath analysis have been presented in American Thoracic Society/ERS recommendations.

Conclusions

Noninvasive methods such as induced sputum and exhaled breath analysis have been successfully introduced in clinical practice and research to study airway inflammation involved in the pathogenesis of respiratory diseases.

Further reading

- American Thoracic Society, et al. (2005). ATS/ERS recommendations for FENO procedure. Am J Respir Crit Care Med; 171: 912–930.
- Barnes PJ, et al. (2006). Pulmonary biomarkers in chronic obstructive pulmonary disease. Am J Respir Crit Care Med; 174: 6–14.
- Brightling CE (2006). Clinical applications of induced sputum. Chest; 129: 1344–1348.

- European Respiratory Society Task Force. (2002). Standardised methodology of sputum induction and processing. *Eur Respir J*; 20: Suppl. 37, 1s–55s.
- Horváth I, *et al.* (2005). Exhaled breath condensate: methodological recommendations and unresolved questions. *Eur Respir J*; 26: 523–548.
- Hunt J (2007). Exhaled breath condensate: an overview. *Immunol Allergy Clin North Am*; 27: 587–596.
- Montuschi P (2007). Analysis of exhaled breath condensate in respiratory medicine: methodological aspects and potential clinical applications. *Ther Adv Respir Dis*; 1: 5–23.
- Pizzichini E, *et al.* (1996). Indices of airway inflammation in induced sputum: reproducibility and validity of cell and fluid-phase measurements. *Am J Respir Crit Care Med*; 154: 308–317.
- Spanevello A, *et al.* (1997). Induced sputum to assess airway inflammation: a study of reproducibility. *Clin Exp Allergy*; 27: 1138–1144.
- Spanevello A, *et al.* (2000). Induced sputum cellularity. Reference values and distribution in normal volunteers. *Am J Respir Crit Care Med*; 62: 1172–1174.

Bronchoscopy

Pallav L. Shah

Bronchoscopy is an essential tool for the pulmonologist that allows inspection and sampling of the airways. The procedure is usually performed with or without conscious sedation.

Equipment

The flexible bronchoscope has evolved from a fibreoptic instrument to videobronchoscopes, which are now almost universally used in most centres (fig. 1). The videobronchoscope consists of a video chip at the distal end, an instrument channel and optical fibres that illuminate the airways. The images obtained are then transmitted to a monitor. The distal end of the bronchoscope can be angled through to 180°. This, in combination with manual rotation movements, allows the bronchoscope to be manipulated in the airways.

Indications

Bronchoscopy provides diagnostic information in patients with suspected lung cancer or diffuse lung disease, and in patients with persistent infection or local pulmonary infiltrates (table 1).

Therapeutic bronchoscopy was traditionally performed for malignant disease. However, there are now a number of therapeutic procedures for emphysema and asthma:

- Clearance of airway secretions
- Removal of foreign bodies
- Palliation of endobronchial airway obstruction by tumour ablation or insertion of stents
- Bronchoscopic lung volume reduction for emphysema
- Bronchial thermoplasty for asthma:

Patient preparation

Patients should be given a full explanation of the procedure accompanied by written information. Below is a simple pre-procedure check list:

- Patient information – verbal and written
- Informed consent
- Full blood count and clotting – before transbronchial lung biopsy
- ECG if history of cardiac disease
- Ensure patients do not eat or drink for at least 4–6 h before the procedure
- Ensure patients have someone to take them home following the procedure if they receive sedation
- Patients are advised not to drive or operate machinery for at least 24 h after any sedation

Patients are monitored by continuous oximetry throughout the procedure. Those with pre-existing cardiac disease or hypoxia that is not fully corrected by oxygen therapy should undergo continuous ECG monitoring.

Key points

- Bronchoscopy provides diagnostic information in suspected lung cancer and diffuse lung disease, and in patients with persistent infection or local pulmonary infiltrates.

- Bronchoscopy also has therapeutic uses in tumour treatment, and more recently in asthma and emphysema.

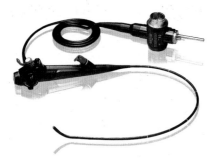

Figure 1. Flexible videobronchoscope (model BF-Q180; Olympus Europa, Hamburg, Germany).

Procedure

The oropharynx is anaesthetised with 4% lidocaine spray and the nasal passage with 2% lidocaine gel. Venous access should always be secured before the procedure and oxygen administered *via* a single nasal cannula. Bronchoscopy can be performed with or without sedation (fig. 2). The choice of sedative drugs varies with local practice. Midazolam at a dose of 2–5 mg administered intravenously is more commonly used and has the advantage of amnesic properties in addition to its sedative effect. Alternative agents are opiates, such as fentanyl or alfentanil, which also have antitussive properties. A number of institutions are now switching to nurse-administered sedation and using low-dose propofol infusions as a very short-acting general anaesthetic.

In the nasal approach, the bronchoscope is lubricated with 2% lidocaine gel and passed through the nares under direct vision. It is then inserted into the nasopharynx until the epiglottis is visualised.

In the oral approach, the patient is asked to bite gently onto a mouth-guard; the bronchoscope is then inserted through this mouth-guard into the posterior pharynx, to the level of the epiglottis.

The movement of the vocal cords is assessed and they are then anaesthetised using 2-mL aliquots of 2% lidocaine. When

Table 1. Indications for bronchoscopy

Investigation of symptoms
Haemoptysis
Persistent cough
Recurrent infection
Investigation of suspected neoplasia
Unexplained paralysis of vocal cords or hemidiaphragm
Stridor
Localised monophonic wheeze
Suspicious sputum cytology
Unexplained pleural effusions
Mediastinal tissue diagnosis and staging
Assess suitability for surgery
Staging of lung cancer
Assessment of persistent or recurrent infection
Identification of organisms
Evaluate airways
Assessment of diffuse lung disease

the coughing has subsided, the bronchoscope is advanced through the widest part of the glottis, taking care not to touch the vocal cords. The subglottic area of the trachea is very sensitive and patients initially feel as though they are choking. Further 2-mL aliquots of 2% lidocaine are administered in the trachea, carina, and right and left main bronchi. During bronchoscopy, the trachea, bronchi and airways down to the subsegmental level are carefully inspected for the presence of mucosal abnormalities, secretions, anatomical variants, malacia (degree of collapse of trachea and main bronchi in expiration) and endobronchial lesions (fig. 3). Narrowing of the bronchial tree as a result of external compression from large lymph nodes or masses is also noted.

Bronchoscopic sampling

Bronchoscopy also provides an opportunity to obtain a variety of samples which may aid diagnosis.

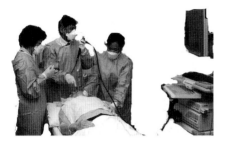

Figure 2. Performance of the bronchoscopy.

Bronchial washings The specimens are obtained by injection of 20 mL normal saline into the affected segment of the lung, followed by aspiration.

Bronchial brushings A fine cytology brush may be used to scrape cells from the surface of any visible lesion or from segments when the lesion is not visible at bronchoscopy. The bronchial brush specimen may be smeared onto a slide and fixed before cytological analysis, or shaken into saline or cytofix for cytospin preparations.

Bronchial biopsy Any endobronchial abnormalities should be biopsied. At least four samples should be obtained and placed in 10% formol saline solution. The diagnostic yield for polypoid lesions should be high (>90%) but is less for submucosal lesions.

Bronchoalveolar lavage (BAL) is used in the assessment of diffuse lung disease. The bronchoscope is wedged into the segment of interest and 50–60-mL aliquots of warm saline are injected into the segment. The fluid is then slowly aspirated using low-pressure suction or direct hand suction. A total of 150–250 mL is instilled and aspirated.

Transbronchial lung biopsy is used to obtain parenchymal lung tissue for the evaluation of diffuse lung diseases. It is particularly useful when a bronchocentric component is visible on CT scans. The closed biopsy forceps are advanced into a specific bronchial segment until they meet with resistance. The forceps are then withdrawn a short distance and the jaws opened. The

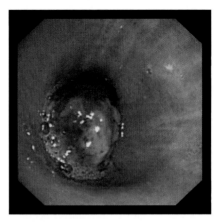

Figure 3. Image obtained through the videobronchoscope.

patient is asked to take a deep breath and the open forceps are advanced further. When there is further resistance, the patient is asked to breathe out and a biopsy sample is taken during expiration. Samples are obtained from the periphery of the lung.

Transbronchial fine-needle aspiration (TBNA) Mediastinal and hilar lymph nodes can be sampled by TBNA. The site of aspiration is planned on the basis of a cross-sectional CT. The needle is inserted at the desired point perpendicular to the airway wall. The needle is moved back and forth after penetration of the airway wall and suction applied with a 20-mL syringe. Samples collected can then be used to prepare slides, or be placed in cytofix or saline solution for cytological analysis. This is useful in the staging and diagnosis of suspected lung cancer. This should be performed prior to any other aspects of bronchoscopy so as not to carry over cells from endobronchial lesions into TBNA specimens and, hence, falsely up-stage the patient. Needle aspiration of submucosal lesions may also improve diagnostic yield. Overall, TBNA is a low-risk procedure with a good yield.

Complications

The adverse effects of flexible bronchoscopy may be due to the sedation, the local anaesthesia or the procedure. The overall incidence of complications is ~2%. Mortality from the procedure is <0.02%.

Sedative drugs may depress respiration and have cardiovascular effects (e.g. hypotension). Lidocaine may very rarely cause bradycardia, seizures, bronchospasm or laryngeal spasm.

The procedure may cause bronchospasm, laryngospasm, hypoxaemia or cardiac arrhythmias, particularly in patients with pre-existing cardiac disease or hypoxia not corrected by oxygen supplementation. Infection can be introduced by the bronchoscope. Therefore, it is essential to clean and disinfect all instruments before use. Haemorrhage and pneumothorax may follow transbronchial lung biopsy. The risk is 5–7%, and this is increased with paroxysmal coughing. Hypoxia and precipitation of respiratory failure are the main complications of BAL, particularly as the procedure is often performed in patients with diffuse lung disease.

Advanced diagnostic procedures

The airway is illuminated by blue light during fluorescence bronchoscopy. Normal tissue is visible as fluorescent green, whereas abnormal areas appear brown and red in colour. This absence of autofluorescence occurs in dysplasia, carcinoma in situ and invasive carcinoma, and may enable the earlier detection of endobronchial tumours. It is currently used as a research tool but may also be useful in routine practice. Narrow band imaging emphasises the blood vessels and increased capillary loops in the mucosa, which is associated with dysplasia and carcinoma in situ. Magnification of images and presentation at high definition further enhances the ability of the operator to detect subtle abnormalities.

Endobronchial ultrasound-guided (EBUS)-TBNA is performed with an integrated linear array ultrasound bronchoscope. It provides excellent ultrasound images of the mediastinum and tissue adjacent to the airways, and allows ultrasound-guided sampling of mediastinal lymph nodes or peribronchial tumour masses. The sensitivity of this technique is high. Its use is rapidly expanding and is establishing an important role in the diagnosis and staging of lung cancer. Its use for other disease, such as sarcoidosis and TB, is increasing.

A radial or mini-probe system can be used for localising peripheral pulmonary masses. These probes are passed through the instrument channel of a flexible bronchoscope into the desired segment with a guide sheath. The probe is manipulated in the airways with or without radiological guidance. Once the abnormal area is identified, the sheath is maintained in position, the radial ultrasound probe is removed, and washings, brushings and biopsies obtained via the guide sheath.

Cryoprobes may also utilised to obtain better tissue samples either endobronchially or for transbronchial lung biopsy. Patients need to be intubated with an endotracheal tube or laryngeal mask. The cryoprobe is passed through the instrument channel of the bronchoscope and applied to the tissue to be biopsied. The freezing effects cause the tissue to become adherent and gentle traction is applied to tear off a piece of the frozen tissue. The probe and bronchoscope need to be removed from the airway, and the piece of tissue thawed and placed in formalin. It is not possible to remove the probe through the instrument channel of the bronchoscope when there is tissue adherent to the tip, hence the need to intubate the patient. It is still possible to perform the procedure under sedation. If transbronchial lung biopsy is performed with cryoprobes, it is essential to use fluoroscopy in order to minimise the risk of a pneumothorax.

Therapeutic procedures

The therapeutic role of bronchoscopy is rapidly increasing. It is well established in the treatment of endobronchial tumour obstruction. A variety of techniques, such as cryotherapy, electrocautery or laser, can be utilised by flexible bronchoscopy to rapidly debulk tumours that are obstructing the main airways. Several clinical series have demonstrated that these techniques are very effective in palliating symptoms and improving the quality of life of patients with endobronchial tumour occlusion. They also reduce the risk of post-obstructive pneumonia. Where the airway wall structure has been extensively damaged or there is extrinsic compression from the tumour, endobronchial stents can be used to support the airways. Metal self-expanding stents can be inserted *via* a flexible bronchoscopy and are available in both uncovered and covered formats.

Brachytherapy is localised radiotherapy administered to an area of tumour infiltration. A blind-ending catheter is inserted through the instrument channel of the bronchoscope into the desired airway. The bronchoscope is then removed while maintaining the catheter in the appropriate position. The catheter can then subsequently be loaded with a remote device that is used to insert radiotherapy beads and, hence, deliver local radiotherapy. This technique can also be used to treat endobronchial obstruction. However, there is a risk of acute localised oedema following the procedure and treatment carries a significant risk of severe haemorrhage.

More recently, a number of innovations have been developed for the bronchoscopic treatment of patients with severe emphysema with significant hyperinflation. Endobronchial valves, such as zephyr valves and intrabronchial valves, can be used for bronchoscopic volume reduction. Other developments include airway stents, biological polymers, endobronchial coils and thermal vapour. Bronchial thermoplasty, a novel treatment for patients with moderate-to-severe asthma, is also delivered bronchoscopically. A special catheter is used to apply radiofrequency energy to the airways in order to destroy airway smooth muscle.

Further reading

- Shah PL. Atlas of Bronchoscopy. London, Hodder Arnold, 2011.
- Bronchoscopy International. www.bronchoscopy.org
- Interventional Bronchoscopy. www.interventionalbronchoscopy.co.uk

Bronchoalveolar lavage

Patricia L. Haslam

What it is and when to use it

Bronchoalveolar lavage (BAL) involves using a fibreoptic bronchoscope to wash a subsegment of the lungs with sterile physiological saline to sample components from the peripheral air spaces in health and disease. These include immune and inflammatory cells, other pathological cells or features, cytokines, enzymes, lipids or other secreted products, inhaled environmental or occupational agents, and infections. Since the 1960s, BAL has been used extensively in research and to assist in the diagnosis of peripheral lung diseases, notably diffuse interstitial lung diseases (ILDs), occupational lung diseases, rare lung diseases, thoracic malignancies and lower respiratory tract infections (table 1). Numerous publications, including guidelines from the European Respiratory Society (ERS) and American Thoracic Society (ATS), confirm that BAL cytological or microbiological findings can often increase diagnostic confidence. However, BAL itself is rarely specifically diagnostic and must be interpreted together with clinical, physiological, radiological and other multidisciplinary investigations.

Prior to 2000, BAL was routinely included in the diagnostic work-up of parenchymal lung diseases. Currently, for ILDs, specialists consider that HRCT patterns are often sufficiently diagnostic to avoid the need for BAL or lung biopsy. An ATS/ERS consensus terminology for the idiopathic interstitial pneumonias published in 2002 has also changed the way specialists diagnose and manage this subgroup of ILDs. However, BAL is still indicated whenever the preliminary clinical investigations plus HRCT fail to establish a confident diagnosis, or where additional information is needed to confirm, strengthen or exclude a diagnosis.

How to obtain a sample

This section will only describe the standardised BAL procedure recommended in Europe and BAL cytology methodology for investigation of adults with diffuse lung diseases where infection is not suspected. A modified BAL procedure is used for the specialist diagnosis of lower respiratory tract infections, designed to minimise contamination with irrelevant microorganisms and to target sites of maximal involvement.

For both research and routine applications, a standardised BAL procedure must be followed in order to minimise variability due to the unknown dilution factor during lavage

---

Key points

- BAL is used to sample immune and inflammatory cells and many other components from the peripheral air spaces of the lungs in health and disease.

- BAL is mainly used in research and to assist in the clinical diagnosis of ILDs or lower respiratory tract infections.

- BAL findings must be interpreted in conjunction with results from clinical, pathological and radiological investigations.

- A standardised procedure must be followed.

Table 1. *A guide to main types of BAL inflammatory cells and other cytological features in lower respiratory diseases*

	Predominant BAL inflammatory cell types increased compared with normal range[#]	Other characteristic cytological features
Lower respiratory tract infections		
Community-acquired; nosocomial pneumonia	Neutrophils very high in bacterial pneumonias	Intracellular bacteria in active pneumonia. Identify by special stains, cultures *etc.*
Opportunistic infections in AIDS; organ transplant recipients and patients on chemotherapy	Neutrophils often moderately increased	*Pneumocystis carinii* Cytomegalovirus Fungal infections Others by special stains, cultures *etc.*
Thoracic malignancies		
Adenocarcinoma or bronchoalveolar cell carcinoma	Not of diagnostic value	Tumour cells readily detectable
Metastatic or lymphangitic spread from nonpulmonary tumours	Not of diagnostic value	Tumour cells readily detectable
B-cell lymphomas	Lymphocytes often strikingly increased	Abnormal lymphocytes consistent with lymphoma can be demonstrated by special stains
Hodgkin's lymphoma		Reed–Sternberg cells
Rare lung diseases		
Alveolar lipoproteinosis	Not of diagnostic value	Globules of lipoprotein plus acellular debris Original BAL fluid 'milky'
Pulmonary haemosiderosis	Mainly macrophages containing particles similar to those in smoking but orange-brown	Majority of macrophages heavily laden with haemosiderin, Perl stain positive
Pulmonary Langerhans cell histiocytosis	Mainly macrophages containing smoking-related particles	>5% of the cells shown to be Langerhans cells by CD1a staining or electron microscopy
Fibrosing mineral dust diseases		
Asbestosis	Moderate increases in neutrophils with or without increased eosinophils or lymphocytes	Asbestos bodies indicating exposure
Talc pneumoconiosis	Insufficient information	Talc bodies indicating exposure

Table 1. Continued

Hard metal lung disease/giant cell interstitial pneumonia	Mild increases in neutrophils with or without increased eosinophils or lymphocytes	Refractile particles of hard metal in macrophages plus giant cells if also giant cell interstitial pneumonia
Drug-induced lung diseases		
Amiodarone-induced pneumonitis	Lymphocytes increased	Large phospholipid inclusions in macrophages
Acute alveolar haemorrhage	Not of diagnostic value	Numerous erythrocytes and 'bloody' fluid
Drug-induced eosinophilic pneumonia	Eosinophils very high	
Other pulmonary eosinophilias		
Idiopathic eosinophilic pneumonia	Eosinophils very high	
Allergic diseases: asthma; Churg–Strauss syndrome; bronchopulmonary aspergillosis	Mild to moderate increases in eosinophils plus lymphocytes	
Parasitic infections: schistosomiasis; Strongyloides	Eosinophils often high	
Acute respiratory distress syndrome	Neutrophils very high	
Idiopathic interstitial pneumonias		
Idiopathic pulmonary fibrosis	Moderate increases in neutrophils with or without increased eosinophils	
Nonspecific interstitial pneumonitis	Mild increases in lymphocytes plus neutrophils with or without increased eosinophils	
Cryptogenic organising pneumonia	Moderate increases in lymphocytes plus neutrophils	
Lymphoid interstitial pneumonia	Increases in lymphocytes	
Respiratory bronchiolitis-associated ILD	Mainly macrophages containing smoking particles plus a few neutrophils	
Desquamative interstitial pneumonia	Macrophages containing smoking particles plus moderate increases in neutrophils with or without increased eosinophils or lymphocytes	
Acute interstitial pneumonia	Neutrophils very high	

Table 1. Continued

Systemic connective tissue diseases		
Systemic sclerosis	Moderate increases in neutrophils with or without increased eosinophils or lymphocytes	
Sjögren's syndrome	Moderate increases in neutrophils with or without increased lymphocytes	
Granulomatous lung diseases¶		
Sarcoidosis	Moderate increases in lymphocytes with or without mild increases in neutrophils	CD4/CD8 ratios increased in about half of patients
Hypersensitivity pneumonitis/extrinsic allergic alveolitis	Lymphocytes very high Neutrophils and mast cells also increased after recent exposure	CD4/CD8 ratios frequently decreased
Chronic beryllium disease	Moderate to high increases in lymphocytes	CD4/CD8 ratios increased in nearly all Lymphocytes proliferate to beryllium salts

#: using differential percentage BAL cell counts (see main text for full explanation); ¶: excluding infections.

and many other potential sources of variability. There is still no globally agreed standard for the general conduct of BAL in adults for cytological and other purposes, but the ERS has long promoted BAL standardisation in a series of European guidelines. In 1999, the ERS published consensus guidelines recommending a standardised BAL procedure to use in adults based on the most comprehensive review of sources of variability for measurement of BAL components yet undertaken. The aim of using optimal BAL standardisation to minimise variability is to improve the reliability of quantitative measurements of all components. Minimising variability is an essential scientific requirement for research. However, a 2012 ATS clinical practice guideline on the clinical utility of BAL in ILD, recommends that 'the BAL target site be chosen on the basis of an HRCT performed before the procedure, rather than choosing a traditional BAL site.' This did not achieve full consensus because of the disadvantage that it would reduce BAL standardisation before it is known whether moving away from a standard BAL site would change diagnostic interpretation. To avoid compromising BAL standardisation, more research is needed into ILDs to compare lavages from both the standard BAL site and the site selected on the basis of HRCT, to conclude whether there is any clinical advantage to be gained. For now, the established standardised BAL procedure should also continue to be employed in patients with diffuse bilateral lung diseases. The standard site is also required to study healthy controls or patients with apparently 'normal' lungs, and to reduce variability for research. The site recommendation differs for patients with localised lung diseases such as some malignancies or infections, where BAL is targeted to the site of maximal involvement.

A protocol using the European recommended standard BAL procedure is as follows.

1) Perform BAL under local anaesthesia using fibreoptic bronchoscopy as part of pre-treatment assessment.

2) Proceed initially as for routine fibreoptic bronchoscopy:

- generally semisupine patient positioning;
- pre-medication with a sedating compound;
- local anaesthesia with lidocaine removing any excess prior to lavage.

3) For lavage, gently wedge the tip of the bronchoscope into an appropriate subsegmental bronchus. The recommended standard site is right middle lobe in diffuse lung diseases and healthy controls, but the area of greatest radiographic abnormality in localised lung diseases.

4) Sequentially introduce then aspirate standard aliquots (4×60 mL) of sterile physiological saline pre-warmed to body temperature through the application tube of the bronchoscope. Do not exceed total introduction volume of 240 mL.

5) Aspirate each aliquot, keeping dwell time to the minimum, using very low suction pressure (3.33–13.3 kPa/25–100 mmHg) to avoid airway collapse.

6) Collect the recovered fluid into a container to which cells are poorly adherent (e.g. siliconised glass or a non-cell adherent plastic designed for suspension tissue cultures).

7) Record the lavage site, total BAL fluid introduction volume and number of aliquots, and the total recovery volume.

8) Immediately send the BAL sample to the laboratory to enable processing to commence within 1 h because BAL cells deteriorate rapidly in saline.

9) Also send a patient protocol with age, sex, provisional diagnosis and other factors that influence BAL findings including smoking history (current, ex- or nonsmoker), current medications and associated diseases.

10) If biopsies are needed, perform these after BAL to avoid contamination of BAL with blood or bronchial tissue debris.

BAL is safe and side-effects are low, the same as for fibreoptic bronchoscopy alone, except for an increased risk of minor post-lavage pyrexia, which can be minimised by keeping total BAL introduction volumes to <300 mL.

Processing of samples for cytology

BAL cells deteriorate rapidly in saline and laboratory processing should commence a maximum of 1 h after BAL sample collection. To delay deterioration, BAL cells should be transferred into serum-free minimum essential medium containing 25 mM HEPES buffer (MEM-HEPES), which maintains pH 7.2–7.4 in an open system.

Non-cell adherent containers and pipettes must be used for all laboratory procedures. The processing procedure is as follows.

1) Measure the total volume of the BAL sample.

2) Record any abnormality in the gross appearance of the fluid, e.g. a milky appearance suggestive of alveolar lipoproteinosis or a very bloody appearance suggestive of acute haemorrhagic conditions.

3) Mix sample to ensure even suspension then divide into measured aliquots for different departments if required (e.g. ⩾20 mL for BAL cytology and flow cytometry, 10 mL for microbiology and 20 mL for electron microscopy).

4) For BAL cytology, the fluid aliquot should be mixed and a cell viability test conducted (e.g. trypan blue). Then, make a total count of nucleated cells (per mL) using an improved Neubauer counting chamber and white cell counting stain (e.g. Kimura stain). If the original BAL sample is too dilute for an accurate cell count, the count should be performed after separating the cells by centrifugation and resuspending them at a higher concentration.

5) Centrifuge the BAL sample at low speed ($300 \times g$ at $4°C$ for 10 min) to separate the cells and other insoluble components from the supernatant fluid. Aspirate the supernatant and aliquot it for storage at $-70°C$. Then, wash the BAL cell pellet in MEM-HEPES and resuspend it in a small

volume (1–2 mL) to achieve a more concentrated suspension. Perform a total cell count, and calculate the number of cells per mL and total in the original BAL fluid.

6) Adjust the volume of the cell suspension to a standard 1.5×10^6 cells·mL^{-1} to make cytocentrifuge slide preparations. Use 100-µL aliquots (1.5×10^5 cells) per slide (spin at $90 \times g$ for 4 min). Prepare at least six slides per patient. After air drying, fix two slides in methanol (not formalin, which impairs staining of mast cells). Stain with May–Grünwald–Giemsa for differential cell counting. Use other slides for special stains (e.g. Gomori–Grocott silver stain for fungi and *Pneumocystis carinii*, and Perl stain for haemosiderin-laden macrophages).

Mucus contamination of BAL samples, if very excessive, can cause serious technical problems in processing. When there is such heavy contamination from the upper airways, BAL results must be interpreted with caution. Mucus can be removed by filtering the lavage through cotton gauze or nylon mesh but this can cause loss of adherent cells, dust fibres and other components. An alternative to avoid such loss is to remove mucus by treating the BAL cell pellet with the mucolytic dithiothreitol.

Some workers consider that when BAL cells are in tissue culture medium, processing can be delayed for 24 h to enable long-distance transport to centralised processing centres. However, this is not advisable because granulocytes are short lived and apoptotic changes start within 9 h. Therefore, it is advisable to transfer BAL cells into tissue culture medium within 1 h and make cytocentrifuge preparations within 1–4 h. Staining of air-dried preparations can be delayed for $\geqslant 24$ h if necessary. It is essential that BAL is conducted by clinical and laboratory personnel who are highly trained in the procedure, applications and interpretation.

Differential cell counting and other cytological appearances

The standard approach to counting BAL cells in cytocentrifuge preparations is to express the count of each type as a percentage of the total BAL cells (differential percentage cell count). This proportionate approach is not affected by the unknown BAL dilution factor.

Differential cell counts are performed and other cytological features identified by examining May–Grünwald–Giemsa-stained cytocentrifuge slide preparations by light microscopy. First, low-power magnification ($\times 10$ and $\times 25$ objective lenses) is used to search the entire preparation and semi-quantitatively grade (on a scale from 0 to 5) any mucus and erythrocytes, and identify any unusual cytological features, such as inorganic dust particles or fibres, globules of lipoprotein, giant cells, malignant cells or microorganisms. Secondly, higher-power magnification ($\times 40$ or $\times 60$ objectives) is used to count all the immune and inflammatory cells and any other type of nucleated cells employing random-field counting methodology until a total of $\geqslant 400$ cells have been counted. The count for each cell type is then expressed as a percentage of the total cells counted (differential percentage BAL cell count). For diagnostic purposes, all nucleated cells, not only inflammatory cells, must be included in the count to ensure that important information is not omitted (e.g. malignant cells, giant cells and epithelial cells). The presence of >5% bronchial epithelial cells indicates excessive contamination from the upper airways and such samples are inadequate as a reliable indicator of alveolar events.

Abnormal cell appearances must also be reported, including proportions of foamy macrophages, multinucleate macrophages, giant cells, macrophages containing smoking-related particles, macrophages containing refractile or birefringent particles indicative of inorganic dusts, or macrophages heavily laden with haemosiderin confirmed by Perl staining, indicating possible pulmonary haemosiderosis.

When neutrophil counts are very high it is important to check for intracellular bacteria, which can indicate active bacterial pneumonia.

Table 2. Normal ranges for differential BAL cell counts

Cell type	Nonsmokers	Smokers
Macrophages	≥80	≥90
Lymphocytes	≤20	≤10
Neutrophils	≤3	≤4
Eosinophils	≤0.5	≤3
Mast cells	≤0.5	≤0.5
Plasma cells	0	0
Ciliated or squamous epithelial cells	≤5	≤5

Cata are presented as % total cells.

Fungal spores or hyphae may also be seen and their presence should be confirmed using Gomori–Grocott silver stain, which can also detect *P. carinii*.

Normal cell counts and the effect of smoking

BAL cells from healthy nonsmokers are mainly macrophages and a few lymphocytes but proportions of other cell types are very low. Smoking causes increases in BAL macrophages up to four-fold higher (total and per mL) in healthy smokers compared with nonsmokers; smokers also have slight increases in neutrophils. Thus, smoking must be taken into account when defining normal ranges and interpreting any BAL studies. Published normal ranges show considerable variability when cell counts are expressed per mL or absolute total numbers. However, results are very similar when expressed as differential percentage counts, consistent with these not being influenced by dilution.

The normal ranges that can be employed for differential BAL cell counts are shown in table 2. Smoking-related inclusions are frequent in macrophages from smokers.

Main applications in the diagnostic work-up of peripheral lung diseases

Although this section describes BAL procedures, it would be incomplete without a summary of how BAL is used in routine clinical investigation to increase confidence in the diagnosis of many parenchymal lung diseases. A quick guide showing the main types of increased BAL inflammatory cells

and other cytological features in a wide range of lower respiratory diseases is given in table 1.

Further reading

- American Thoracic Society, European Respiratory Society. (2002). International multidisciplinary consensus classification of idiopathic interstitial pneumonias. *Am J Respir Crit Care Med*; 165: 277–304.
- The BAL Cooperative Steering Group Committee. (1990). Bronchoalveolar lavage constituents in healthy individuals, idiopathic pulmonary fibrosis, and selected comparison groups. *Am Rev Respir Dis*; 141: Suppl. 5, S169–S202.
- Bradley B, et al. (2008). Interstitial lung disease guideline: the British Thoracic Society in collaboration with the Thoracic Society of Australia and New Zealand and the Irish Thoracic Society. *Thorax*; 63: Suppl. 5, v1–v58.
- Costabel U (2007). Ask the expert – diffuse interstitial lung disease. *Breathe*; 4: 165–172.
- Dombret MC, et al. (1998). The role of fibreoptic bronchoscopy in the diagnosis of bacterial infections. *Eur Respir Monogr*; 9: 153–170.
- Dhillon DP, et al. (1986). Bronchoalveolar lavage in patients with interstitial lung diseases: side effects and factors affecting fluid recovery. *Eur J Respir Dis*; 68: 342–350.
- Haslam PL, et al. (1999). Guidelines for measurement of acellular components and recommendations for standardization of bronchoalveolar lavage (BAL). Report of European Respiratory Society (ERS) Task Force. *Eur Respir Rev*; 9: 25–157.

- Haslam PL, et al. (1999). Report of ERS Task Force: guidelines for measurement of acellular components and standardization of BAL. Eur Respir J; 14: 245–248.
- Haslam PL. Bronchoalveolar lavage. In: Mitchell D, et al., eds. Sarcoidosis. London, Hodder Education, 2012; pp. 121–131.
- Klech H, et al. (1989). Technical recommendations and guidelines for bronchoalveolar lavage (BAL): report of the European Respiratory Society of Pneumology Task Group on BAL. Eur Respir J; 2: 561–585.
- Klech H, et al. (1990). Clinical guidelines and indications for bronchoalveolar lavage (BAL): report of the European Respiratory Society of Pneumology Task Group on BAL. Eur Respir J; 3: 937–974.
- Klech H, et al. (1992). Clinical guidelines and indications for bronchoalveolar lavage (BAL): report of the European Society of Pneumology Task Group on BAL. Eur Respir Rev; 2: 47–127.
- Luyt C-E, et al. (2010). Fibreoptic bronchoscopic techniques for diagnosing pneumonia. Eur Respir Monogr; 48: 297–306.
- Mayer KC, et al. (2012). An official American Thoracic Society Clinical practice guideline: The clinical utility of bronchoalveolar lavage cellular analysis in interstitial lung disease. Am J Respir Crit Care Med; 185: 1004–1014.
- Ohshimo S, et al. (2009). Significance of bronchoalveolar lavage for the diagnosis of idiopathic pulmonary fibrosis. Am J Respir Crit Care Med; 179: 1043–1047.
- Raghu G, et al. (2011). An official ATS/ERS/JRS/ALAT statement: idiopathic pulmonary fibrosis: evidence-based guidelines for diagnosis and management. Am J Respir Crit Care Med; 183: 788–824.
- Reynolds HY, et al. (1974). Analysis of proteins and respiratory cells obtained from human lungs by bronchial lavage. J Lab Clin Med; 84: 559–573.
- Woodhead M, et al. (2011). Guidelines for the management of adult lower respiratory tract infections – Summary: Joint Task Force of ERS and ESCMID. Clin Microbial Infect; 17: Suppl. 6, 1–24.

Fine-needle biopsy

Stefano Gasparini

Percutaneous (or transthoracic) fine-needle biopsy (PFNB) is a technique that allows cytohistological diagnosis of thoracic lesions. While the first reports on the use of transthoracic needle biopsy date back to the end of the 19th century, the modern era of PFNB did not begin until the mid-1960s when Nordenstrom (1965) introduced the use of fine needles (diameter <20 Gauge).

Indications

PFNB is indicated when a cytohistological diagnosis is required of peripheral lung lesions (nodules, mass or infiltrates) following a negative bronchoscopy. PFNB is also indicated for expansive lesions of the chest wall and pleura or for diagnosis of mediastinal masses, especially those located in the anterior mediastinum.

Key points

- PFNB is indicated when a cytohistological diagnosis of a peripheral lung lesion is required.

- PFNB may also be indicated for diagnosis of mediastinal mass and expansive lesions of the pleura and chest wall.

- The most common guidance system for PFNB is CT; biplane fluoroscopy and ultrasound can also be used.

- The sensitivity of PFNB for lung cancer is 85–95%.

- The most frequently reported complication is minor pneumothorax (25%).

Contraindications

Absolute contraindications are:

- contralateral pneumonectomy
- bleeding disorders
- an uncooperative patient
- uncontrollable cough
- suspected arteriovenous malformation or hydatid cyst

Relative contraindications that may increase the risk of complications are:

- respiratory failure
- severe COPD
- pulmonary arterial hypertension
- unstable ischaemic heart disease

Technique

Guidance systems Biplane fluoroscopy is the traditional guidance system for PFNB. Its main advantage is the real-time visualisation of the needle during the whole procedure. In recent years, CT has become the most common means of guidance. Although performing a CT scan is more time-consuming, it has several advantages:

- It helps determine the safest needle trajectory avoiding vascular structures, fissures, bullae and necrotic areas of the tumour;
- It allows an approach to lesions not visible on fluoroscopy, such as small lesions; and
- It avoids radiation exposure to the operators.

However, there are no studies that demonstrate a better sensitivity of CT compared with fluoroscopy. Ultrasound can also be used as a guidance system when the lesion is in contact with the thoracic wall.

Type of needle Commercially available needles are either:

1. aspiration needles that yield material satisfactory for cytological evaluation (Chiba, Franseen, Westcott or Nordenstrom); or

2. histology needles that yield a tissue core (Trucut, Menghini or Silverman).

Needle diameter should be <20 Gauge and generally 20–22 Gauge needles are utilised. The evidence is currently insufficient to support a difference between cytology needles and core-needle biopsy in identifying lung malignancies. Histology needles have a higher specificity to diagnose benign lesions and the use of a core-biopsy needle is recommended when either a benign lesion or a malignancy other than cancer (*i.e.* lymphoma) is suspected.

Results

The reported sensitivity of PFNB ranges from 60% to 97%. In patients with lung cancer, a diagnosis by PFNB is generally established in 85–95% of cases. Lower sensitivities are reported for benign lesions (4–14%). Sensitivity may be affected by the size and location of the lesion, number of needle passes, size of the needle, availability of immediate cytological assessment and experience of the operator. False-positive results are rare and the specificity of the technique is extremely high. However, it is important to emphasise that a non-diagnostic PFNB does not rule out the possibility of malignancy. Recent papers report the feasibility of PFNB for obtaining lung tumour samples suitable for gene mutation analysis (*i.e.* epidermal growth factor receptor).

Complications

The most frequently reported complication is minor pneumothorax, with an average incidence of ~25% (range 4–42%). Major pneumothorax, requiring chest tube drainage, occurs in ~6% of cases. Haemoptysis occurs in 5–10% of cases and is generally mild and self-limiting. Rare complications include air embolism (0.07%), haemothorax, empyema, tumour implantation along the needle tract and haemopericardium.

Further reading

- Gasparini S, *et al.* (1995). Integration of transbronchial and percutaneous approach in the diagnosis of peripheral pulmonary nodules or masses. Experience with 1,027 consecutive cases. *Chest*; 108: 131–137.
- Gould MK, *et al.* (2007). Evaluation of patients with pulmonary nodules: when is it lung cancer? ACCP evidence-based clinical practice guidelines (2nd edition). *Chest*; 132: Suppl. 3, 108s–130s.
- Nordenstrom B (1965). A new technique for transthoracic biopsy of lung changes. *Br J Radiol*; 38: 550–553.
- Shaham D (2000). Semi-invasive and invasive procedures for the diagnosis and staging of lung cancer. I. Percutaneous transthoracic needle biopsy. *Radiol Clin North Am*; 38: 525–534.
- Wiener RS, *et al.* (2011). Population-based risk for complications after transthoracic lung biopsy of a pulmonary nodule: an analysis of discharge records. *Ann Intern Med*; 155: 137–144.
- Yao X, *et al.* (2012). Fine-needle aspiration biopsy *versus* core-needle biopsy in diagnosing lung cancer: a systematic review. *Curr Oncol*; 19: e16–e27.
- Zhuang YP, *et al.* (2011). Use of CT-guided fine needle aspiration biopsy in epidermal growth factor receptor mutation analysis in patients with advanced lung cancer. *Acta Radiologica*; 52: 1083–1087.

Medical thoracoscopy/pleuroscopy

Robert Loddenkemper

Thoracoscopy was first used more than 100 years ago, primarily as a diagnostic procedure, but soon also as a therapeutic technique for lysis of pleural adhesions by means of thoracocautery (Jacobaeus operation) to facilitate pneumothorax treatment in TB. At the end of the last century, the addition of the term 'medical' was necessary in order to distinguish this procedure from 'surgical' thoracoscopy, which is much more invasive, using general anaesthesia, a double-lumen endotracheal tube and multiple points of entry. Other terms used are 'pleuroscopy', 'thoracoscopy for chest physicians' and 'local anaesthetic thoracoscopy'. Surgical thoracoscopy is better described as video-assisted thoracic surgery (VATS) which is performed in an operating room under general anaesthesia with selective intubation, whereas medical thoracoscopy can be performed under local anaesthetic or conscious sedation in an endoscopy suite using non-disposable rigid or semi-rigid (semi-flexible) instruments. It is therefore considerably less invasive, less cumbersome to the patient, and less expensive.

Nevertheless, medical thoracoscopy/pleuroscopy (MT/P) are invasive techniques that would be used only when other more simple methods fail. Today, it is considered to be one of the main areas of interventional pulmonology, and as such should be part of specialist pleural disease services. As with all technical procedures, there is certainly a learning curve before full competence is achieved. Therefore, appropriate training is mandatory. Actually, the technique is very similar to chest-tube insertion by means of a trocar, the difference being that, in addition,

the pleural cavity can be visualised (fig. 1) and biopsies can be taken from all areas of the pleural cavity including the chest wall, diaphragm, mediastinum and lung.

> **Key points**
>
> - MT/P has the advantage compared with VATS that it can be performed under local anaesthesia or conscious sedation, in an endoscopy suite using non-disposable rigid (or semi-rigid) instruments. Thus, it is considerably less expensive.
>
> - The leading indications for MT/P are pleural effusions, both for diagnosis – mainly in exudates of unknown aetiology – or for staging in diffuse malignant mesothelioma, lung cancer and for talc poudrage, the best conservative method today for pleurodesis.
>
> - MT/P can also be used efficiently in the management of early empyema and pneumothorax.
>
> - In the above indications, MT/P can replace most surgical interventions, which are more invasive and more expensive.
>
> - MT/P is a safe procedure, even easier to learn than flexible bronchoscopy, provided sufficient experience with chest-tube placement has been gained.
>
> - MT/P as part of the new field of interventional pulmonology should be included in the training programme of chest physicians.

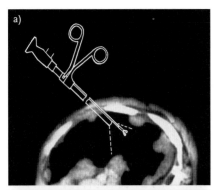

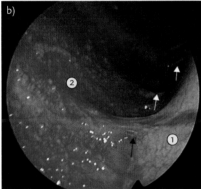

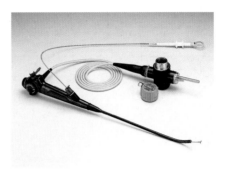

Figure 2. The semi-rigid (semi-flexible) pleuroscope. Reprinted with permission from Olympus Corporation, Tokyo, Japan. Reproduced from Loddenkemper et al. (2011).

Figure 1. a) Diagram of a CT scan showing several malignant lesions of the parietal pleura for which biopsies can be taken under visual control through the (rigid) thoracoscope. b) Tuberculous pleural effusion. After drainage of 800 mL of serous effusion, typical sago-like nodules on the reddened inflamed posterior chest wall, firm adhesions (arrows) between right lower lobe (1) and chest wall (2). Reproduced and modified from Loddenkemper et al. (2010).

There are two different techniques of diagnostic and therapeutic thoracoscopy, as performed by the pneumologist. One, very similar to the technique first described by Jacobaeus for diagnostic purposes, uses a single entry with a rigid, usually 9-mm, thoracoscope with a working channel for accessory instruments and an optical biopsy forceps under local anaesthesia. This single-entry technique has now been modified by the introduction of an autoclavable semi-flexible pleuroscope, which has the advantage that handling is very simple,

similar to a flexible bronchovideoscope (fig. 2).

The other technique uses two entries, one with a 7-mm trocar for the rigid examination telescope and the other with a 5-mm trocar for accessory instruments, including the biopsy forceps. For this technique, neuroleptic or general anaesthesia is preferred.

For cauterisation of adhesions and blebs, or in case of bleeding after biopsy, electrocoagulation should be available. For pleurodesis of effusions, 4–6 g of a sterile, dry, asbestos-free talc is insufflated through a rigid or flexible suction catheter with a pneumatic atomiser. In pneumothorax patients, 2–3 g of talc is sufficient. After thoracoscopy, a chest tube is introduced through which immediate suction is started carefully.

MT/P is a safe examination if the contraindications are observed and if certain standard criteria are fulfilled. An obliterated pleural space is an absolute contraindication. Relative contraindications include bleeding disorders, hypoxaemia and an unstable cardiovascular status, and persistent uncontrollable cough. The most serious, but fortunately least frequent, complication is severe haemorrhage due to blood-vessel injury during the procedure. However, this and pulmonary perforations, can be avoided by using safe points of entry

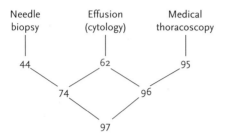

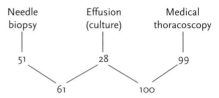

Figure 4. The different biopsy techniques used in the diagnosis of tuberculous pleural effusions and their sensitivity expressed in percentages (cytological and histological results combined). Prospective intra-patient comparison (n=100). Reproduced from Loddenkemper (1998).

Figure 3. The different biopsy techniques used in the diagnosis of malignant pleural effusions and their sensitivity expressed in percentages (cytological and histological results combined). Prospective intra-patient comparison (n=208). Reproduced from Loddenkemper (1998).

and a cautious biopsy technique. Reported mortality rates are very low (<0.001). The most frequent complication is nonspecific, transient fever.

Pleural effusions are by far the leading indication for MT/P, both for diagnosis, mainly in exudates of unknown aetiology, and for staging in diffuse malignant mesothelioma or lung cancer, and for treatment by talc pleurodesis in malignant or other recurrent effusions, or in cases of empyema. Spontaneous pneumothorax for staging and for local treatment is also an excellent indication. Malignant pleural effusions represent the leading diagnostic and therapeutic indication for MT/P. MT/P has a much higher diagnostic sensitivity and specificity in malignant pleural effusions than closed needle biopsy and pleural fluid cytology (fig. 3). Biopsies can be taken under direct visual control not only of the costal pleura, but also of the visceral and diaphragmatic pleura.

MT/P is helpful in the staging of lung cancer, diffuse malignant mesothelioma and metastatic cancers. In lung cancer patients, thoracoscopy can determine whether the tumour spread to the pleura is secondary to venous or lymphatic obstruction or is parapneumonic. As a result, it may be possible to avoid exploratory thoracotomy or to determine operability. In diffuse malignant mesothelioma, MT/P provides an earlier diagnosis and a better histological

classification due to larger and consequently more representative biopsies, including for hormone receptor determination in breast cancer, as well as a more precise staging.

An additional advantage is that the diagnostic procedure can easily be combined with the therapeutic procedure of talc poudrage which is, at present, the most successful conservative pleurodesis method.

In tuberculous pleural effusion, MT/P has a high diagnostic sensitivity of almost 100% (fig. 4). It provides a bacteriological confirmation of the diagnosis of TB much more often and, thus, the possibility to perform susceptibility tests, which may have a considerable impact on the correct treatment and final outcome in patients with drug resistances. In parapneumonic pleural effusion and empyema, MT/P offers the possibility to remove fibrinopurulent membranes and break up loculations, thus creating one single pleural cavity for successful local treatment.

In other pleural effusions, when the origin remains indeterminate, the main diagnostic value of MT/P lies in its ability to exclude, with high probability, malignant or tuberculous disease. In pneumothorax patients, MT/P allows talc poudrage for pleurodesis, which is highly effective in recurrence prevention.

For those who are familiar with the technique, other (mainly diagnostic) indications are biopsies from the diaphragm, the lung, *e.g.* in interstitial lung diseases, the mediastinum and the pericardium. In addition, MT/P offers a remarkable tool for research as a 'gold standard' in the study of pleural effusions.

Further reading

- Bridevaux PO, *et al.* (2011). Short-term safety of thoracoscopic talc pleurodesis for recurrent primary spontaneous pneumothorax: a prospective European multicentre study. *Eur Respir J*; 38: 770–773.
- Davies HE, *et al.* (2011). The diminishing role of surgery in pleural disease. *Curr Opin Pulm Med*; 17: 247–254.
- Grüning W, *et al.* Medical thoracoscopy/pleuroscopy. Procedure video; 2011. www.ers-education.org/pages/default.aspx?id=2375&dma=156667.
- Hooper CE, *et al.* (2010). Setting up a specialist pleural disease service. *Respirology*; 15: 1028–1036.
- Janssen JP (2010). Why you do or do not need thoracoscopy. *Eur Respir Rev*; 19: 213–216.
- Janssen JP, *et al.* (2007). Safety of pleurodesis with talc poudrage in malignant pleural effusion: a prospective cohort study. *Lancet*; 369: 1535–1539.
- Kern L, *et al.* (2011). Management of parapneumonic effusions and empyema: medical thoracoscopy and surgical approach. *Respiration*; 82: 193–196.
- Loddenkemper R (1998). Thoracoscopy: state of the art. *Eur Respir J*; 11: 213–221.
- Loddenkemper R, *et al.* (2004). Treatment of parapneumonic pleural effusion and empyema: conservative view. *Eur Respir Monogr*; 29: 199–207.
- Loddenkemper R, *et al.* Medical Thoracoscopy/Pleuroscopy: Manual and Atlas. New York, Thieme, 2011.
- Loddenkemper R, *et al.* (2011). History and clinical use of thoracoscopy/pleuroscopy in respiratory medicine. *Breathe*; 8: 145–155.
- Loddenkemper R, *et al.* (2011). Medical thoracoscopy/pleuroscopy: step by step. *Breathe*; 8: 157–167.
- Noppen M (2010). Pleural biopsy and thoracoscopy. *Eur Respir Monogr*; 48: 119–132.
- Rahman NM, *et al.* (2010). Local anaesthetic thoracoscopy: British Thoracic Society pleural disease guideline 2010. *Thorax*; 65: Suppl. 2, ii54–ii60.
- Rodriguez-Panadero F, *et al.* (2006). Thoracoscopy: general overview and place in the diagnosis and management of pleural effusion. *Eur Respir J*; 28: 409–422.
- Rodriguez-Panadero F, *et al.* (2012). Mechanisms of pleurodesis. *Respiration*; 83: 91–98.
- Tassi GF, *et al.* (2006). Advanced techniques in medical thoracoscopy. *Eur Respir J*; 28: 1051–1059.
- Tschopp JM, *et al.* (2011). Titrated sedation with propofol for medical thoracoscopy: a feasibility and safety study. *Respiration*; 82: 451–457.
- Tschopp JM, *et al.* (2006). Management of spontaneous pneumothorax: state of the art. *Eur Respir J*; 28: 637–650.
- Vansteenkiste J, *et al.* (1999). Medical thoracoscopic lung biopsy in interstitial lung disease: a prospective study of biopsy quality. *Eur Respir J*; 14: 585–590.

Thoracentesis

Emilio Canalis and Mari Carmen Gilavert

Thoracentesis (pleural tap; fig. 1) is a frequently performed procedure that is used to remove and analyse pleural fluid. Its goals may be diagnostic and/or therapeutic.

Diagnostic thoracentesis should be performed on almost all patients with a pleural effusion of unknown origin. Its main purpose is to differentiate between transudate and exudate. The number of diagnoses established by pleural fluid analysis varies with the population being evaluated. Careful history and physical examination, radiological evaluation, and ancillary blood tests are crucial in establishing a pre-test diagnosis.

The main purpose of therapeutic thoracentesis is to relieve dyspnoea and respiratory insufficiency caused by pleural effusion.

Patient position

A sitting position is preferred in conscious patients, as this will help the fluid to settle in the posterior and basal regions of the lung

---

Key points

- Thoracentesis may be diagnostic or therapeutic in patients with a pleural effusion.

- Ultrasound examination is valuable in guiding the procedure.

- There are no absolute contraindications, and complications are rare, but the possibility should be taken into account.

(usually the seventh to eighth intercostal spaces, although clinical examination may reveal different locations of the fluid).

Once a comfortable position for operating on the patient is achieved, the site for the puncture must be selected. This is decided according to the results of the physical examination and the radiological findings, which will indicate characteristics such as the size and localisation of the main effusion and whether it is free-organised, free-floating or encapsulated. Ultrasound examination is valuable to assess fluid presence accurately.

The puncture should be guided by ultrasound or attempted one intercostal space further down from where dullness on percussion starts. At least in pleural effusions of smaller size, ultrasound guidance is strongly recommended.

The thoracentesis set

The thoracentesis set is detailed in table 1.

Procedure

1. Under sterile conditions, the selected region of puncture is disinfected with povidone–iodine or alcohol, and a sterile draping, preferably with a centre hole, is taped to the patient's back.

2. Local anaesthesia is injected stepwise, at first with an intradermal injection producing a small wheal, then infiltrated subcutaneously and into the intercostal muscle down to the parietal pleura at the upper rim of the lower rib in order to avoid the intercostal nerve and vessels. During the injection, alternating aspiration is performed until the parietal pleura is penetrated and pleural fluid is aspirated. Then, 20–60 mL of

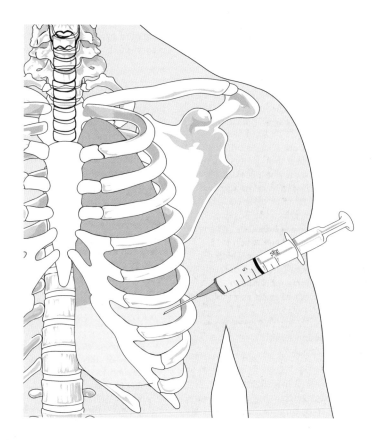

Figure 1. Thoracentesis needle through the intercostal space.

pleural fluid should be aspirated for fluid analysis.

Diagnostic thoracentesis can occasionally be carried out without local anaesthesia if the adult patient is calm, the puncture is anticipated to be easy, the subject is not obese and the operator is experienced.

3. For therapeutic thoracentesis, a catheter should be used, which is immediately connected to a closed three-way stop-cock. This allows aspiration syringes to be changed or facilitates connection to a suction device.

4. As soon as the procedure is finished, the needle or the catheter is removed and pressure is applied to the wound for a few minutes, followed by a sterile dressing.

5. Chest radiography should be carried out to exclude the development of a pneumothorax, unless the procedure has

Table 1. Thoracentesis set

Povidone–iodine solution or alcohol
Sterile drapes, gloves and gauzes
Abbocath-type needle catheters
Local anaesthesia
Syringes
Three-way stopcock
Aspiration set (if therapeutic)
Adhesive strips
Instrumentation table

been performed under ultrasound guidance without any problems.

Contraindications

Diagnostic thoracentesis has no absolute contraindications provided that it is done with caution by experienced persons. The following are relative contraindications.

- Altered coagulation. A decision must be taken as to whether thoracentesis is really needed. If so, it may be necessary to reverse anticoagulation or to administer fresh frozen plasma or platelets.
- Mechanical ventilation with positive pressure at the end of expiration. Whenever possible, mechanical ventilation is suspended briefly. If this is not possible, thoracentesis must be carried out with caution using ultrasound guidance.
- Local skin infections such as cellulitis or herpes zoster.
- Small effusions (this should be done under ultrasound control).

Complications

As with any invasive investigation, complications may occur, but these are rare. Patients have to be informed about possible complications when asked to give their informed consent. The most important are as follows.

Pneumothorax is usually only small if caused by entrance of air into the pleural cavity through the needle or the aspiration system. It can become larger if the lung is injured by the needle.

Hypotension may be induced by a vasovagal reaction when the parietal pleura is punctured. It can be avoided by careful local anaesthesia and prevented by administering atropine (not routinely necessary).

Bleeding can be prevented by avoiding the lower rim of the upper rib and by excluding coagulopathies.

Haemopneumothorax is rare when the aforementioned technique is observed and the patient has no bleeding disorder.

Re-expansion pulmonary oedema This can be prevented by removing less than 1–1.5 L of pleural fluid.

Additional recommendations

1. The region from the midclavicular line to the sternum should be avoided, as here the vessels are located in the centre of the intercostal space

2. Sterile conditions are mandatory during the whole procedure to prevent infection, which may lead to empyema.

3. For diagnostic purposes, 20 mL of pleural fluid is usually sufficient to assess the appearance of the fluid and for chemical, cytological and bacteriological analysis. Recent work recommends ~60 mL for cytology in case of suspected malignancy.

Further reading

- Abouzgheib W, et al. (2009). A prospective study of the volume of pleural fluid required for accurate diagnosis of malignant pleural effusion. Chest; 135: 999–1001.
- Alcaide MJ, et al. Toracocentesis y drenaje pleural [Thoracentesis and pleural drainage]. In: De Mendoza D, et al. Medicina Intensiva Respiratoria [Intensive Respiratory Medicine]. Tarragona, Silva ed., 2008.
- Chest Trauma. In: Advanced Trauma Life Support (ATLS) Course Manual. 7th Edn. Chicago, American College of Surgeons, 2004; pp. 107–121.
- Capizzi SA, et al. (1988). Chest roentgenography after outpatient thoracentesis. Mayo Clin Proc; 73: 948–950.
- Dev SP, et al. (2007). Videos in clinical medicine. N Engl J Med; 357: l5.
- Duncan DR, et al. (2009). Reducing iatrogenic risk in thoracentesis: establishing best practice via experiential training in a zero-risk environment. Chest; 135: 1315–1320.
- Feller-Kopman D, et al. (2009). Assessment of pleural pressure in the evaluation of pleural effusions. Chest; 135: 201–209.

Interventional pulmonology

Marc Noppen

Interventional pulmonology encompasses both diagnostic and therapeutic bronchoscopic, thoracoscopic and other techniques that go beyond everyday 'simple' procedures performed by pulmonary clinicians. In the context of pulmonary function testing and interventional pulmonology, the following discussion will be limited to the effects on interventional bronchoscopy of pulmonary function tests.

In addition, interventional bronchoscopy will be limited to all (rigid and flexible) bronchoscopic procedures designed to reopen obstructed central airways (including laser, electrocautery, cryotherapy, brachytherapy and photodynamic therapy) or to establish airway patency (airway stenting).

Over the past few decades, the literature on interventional bronchoscopy has mainly focused on the 'technicality' of the various procedures; data pertaining to functional assessment and evaluation are relatively scarce. Certainly, in the 'pioneer era' of interventional pulmonology, patients were referred in a (very) late stage of disease, with severe dyspnoea and/or stridor or signs of post-obstructive disease, requiring prompt intervention without additional testing. In stable and nonlife-threatened patients with or without symptoms, however, additional testing before proceeding with an intervention may be helpful in patient selection, and post-procedure testing may focus the usefulness and efficacy of an intervention. Thus, as more centres successfully perform various interventional bronchoscopic techniques, the need is increasing for a critical evaluation and selection of patients in order to understand the physiological effects of these interventions and gain an evidence-based, algorithmic integration of these techniques in the overall care of these patients. Alternatively, abnormalities observed during pulmonary function testing may prompt the clinician to suspect an upper (or central) airway stenosis (UAS).

In patients suffering from malignant airway stenosis, which is not candidate for, or is unresponsive to, 'classical' oncological treatments, the main interest of interventional pulmonological treatment should lie in the improvement of quality of life and the avoidance of death by suffocation.

Pulmonary function tests in UAS

Inspection of the maximal inspiratory and expiratory flow–volume loop is currently the most widely used method to detect/suspect

---

Key points

- Symptoms of central airway stenosis occur late, after ⩾50% (on exercise) or 80% (at rest) of the tracheal lumen is obstructed.

- The diagnostic accuracy of spirometric indices and visual flow–volume loop criteria in detecting central airway stenosis is relatively poor.

- Interventional bronchoscopic techniques have been shown to significantly improve objective pulmonary function and quality of life.

---

the presence of UAS (figs 1–3). However, significant changes in spirometry appear relatively late in the course of the stenosing process. The airway cross-sectional area has to be reduced by $\geqslant 50\%$ in order to cause breathing impairment, a clinical observation that recently has been corroborated by a fluid dynamic study of tracheal stenosis. There is also a very poor or even absent correlation between the severity of the UAS as determined by the flow loop analysis and its spirometrically derived indices, and breathing symptoms or radiological assessment of UAS. UAS becomes more easily symptomatic during exercise (from a tracheal diameter $\leqslant 8$ mm), whereas at rest the diameter has to be $\leqslant 5$ mm before symptoms occur. All of this may explain why the diagnostic accuracy of the various individual spirometric indices and visual flow–volume loop criteria in detecting UAS is relatively poor (area under the receiver operating curve <0.52).

Typical flow–volume appearances, however, may be helpful:

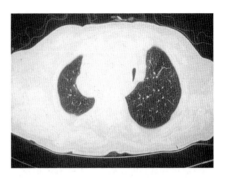

Figure 2. CT image of the patient in figure 1.

- a typical 'coffin' or 'box' appearance of the flow–volume curve is suspicious for a fixed UAS due to severe tracheal obstruction
- an isolated plateau during expiration is suspicious for an intrathoracic airway stenosis
- an isolated plateau of the inspiratory loop suggests extrathoracic obstruction

Obstructive lesions at multiple airway sites and associated abnormalities such as severe COPD may cause atypical flow–volume loop characteristics.

UAS may lead to typical flow–volume loop abnormalities and spirometric derived indices, but

- the diagnostic accuracy in detecting UAS of these tests is (very) low
- symptoms of UAS occur relatively late in the UAS process
- symptoms of UAS occur earlier during exercise

The most commonly used quantitative criteria to detect UAS include

- maximal expiratory flow at 50% FVC ($MEF_{50\%}$)/maximal inspiratory flow at 50% FVC ($MIF_{50\%}$) <0.30 for intrathoracic and >1 for extrathoracic stenosis
- FEV_1/MEF >10 mL·L^{-1}·min^{-1}
- $MIF_{50\%}$ <100 L·min^{-1}
- $FEV_1/FEV_{0.5}$ >1.5

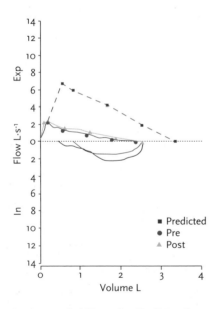

Figure 1. A typical flattened 'coffin' flow–volume loop curve in a patient with severe fixed tracheal obstruction due to an inoperable intrathoracic goitre. In: inspiration; Exp: expiration.

The visual criteria are the presence of a plateau, biphasic shape, or oscillations in

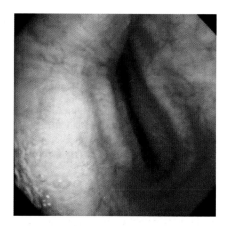

Figure 3. Bronchoscopic image of the patient in figure 1.

the inspiratory or expiratory curves. However, the absence of a good correlation between the severity of UAS as determined by flow–volume loop analysis and breathing symptoms or radiological assessment of UAS points to the need for a method that can detect and document UAS in patients at risk. Forced oscillation tests at different breathing flow rates provide an accurate and reproducible measure of UAS, namely flow dependence of resistance, as documented in a comparative prospective cohort analysis of 10 normal subjects, 10 COPD patients and 10 patients suffering from tracheal stenosis, before and after airway stenting (Verbanck *et al.*, 2010).

Impact of interventional bronchoscopy on pulmonary function

In most patients, but not all, pulmonary function significantly improves after restoration of central airway patency. Eisner *et al.* (1999) demonstrated mean improvements of 388 mL for FVC, 1288 mL for peak expiratory flow (PEF) and 550 mL for FEV_1 after stenting in nine patients. Gelb *et al.* (1992) showed increases in FVC from 64% to 73% predicted, and in FEV_1 from 49% to 72% predicted after stenting in 17 patients. Vergnon *et al.* (1995) showed mean improvements in FEV_1 (440 mL), PEF (920 mL·s⁻¹... $920\,mL·s^{-1}$), MEF_{25-75} (470 mL·s⁻¹... $470\,mL·s^{-1}$) and forced inspiratory volume in 1 s (310 mL)

after stenting in a total of 24 patients. Improvements were more pronounced in intra- and extrathoracic tracheal stenosis, as compared with bronchial stenosis. Noppen *et al.* (2004) showed improvements after tracheal stenting for inoperable benign thyroid disease (FEV_1 +470 mL, FVC +620 mL and PEF +79 $L·min^{-1}$) and after tracheal laser debulking and/or stenting for inoperable malignant thyroid disease (FEV_1 +540 mL, FVC +730 mL and PEF +96 $L·min^{-1}$) (figs 4 and 5). Oviatt *et al.* (2011) showed significant improvements in 6-min walk distance (99.7 m), FEV_1 (448 mL) and FVC (416 mL) 30 days after bronchoscopic treatment for malignant airway obstruction.

Ernst *et al.* (2007) showed improvements in some but not all patients stented for severe tracheomalacia, in terms of respiratory symptoms, quality of life, and functional status assessed by exercise testing and FEV_1. Overall, these retrospective and prospective observational case series, in selected patients, show significant but not homogeneous improvements in a number of functional parameters. Amjadi *et al.* (2008) and Oviatt *et al.* (2011) also documented significant and objective improvements in quality of life scores. Data on physiological effects of repermeabilisation techniques without additional stenting are even more scarce: objective improvements in pulmonary function were seen in 58% of patients after cryotherapeutic debulking of central airways,

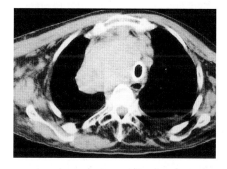

Figure 4. CT image of the patient in figure 1 after stenting.

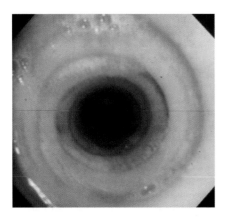

Figure 5. Patient in figure 1, 1 year after stent insertion.

and a trial of 19 patients with major airway obstruction due to lung cancer showed significant improvements in a variety of parameters including FEV1, FVC and ratio of forced expiratory/forced inspiratory flow rate at 50% of vital capacity, after endobronchial radiotherapy.

A breakthrough article by Miyazawa *et al.* (2004) shed more light on the underlying physiological phenomena occurring after airway stenting, including the heterogeneity of response. A total of 64 patients with extrinsic airway stenoses due to advanced malignancy were studied; patients were classified by location of the stenosis (tracheal, carinal, bronchial or multisite). Pulmonary function tests and CT were performed before and after stenting. Prior to stent insertion, patients underwent endobronchial ultrasound to evaluate the airway walls and ultrathin bronchoscopy to evaluate airway patency distal to the obstruction. Stents were placed at the visualised flow-limiting segments (choke points). Distinctive flow–volume loop patterns were found for each of the four types of stenosis. Most patients showed symptomatic improvement after stenting, and most flow–volume loops returned to normal. All 10 patients with multisite, extensive stenosis, however, showed persistent choke points, associated with

only minor improvements in symptoms and spirometry. Repeat endoscopy in these patients showed upstream displacement of choke points (distally from the inserted stents) and ultrasound showed destructed cartilage at these sites. Additional stenting at these sites then improved symptoms and pulmonary function to levels comparable with the other groups. This additional physiological and imaging information excluded all therapeutic failures.

Conclusions

When patients with UAS present with dyspnoea on exertion, and certainly with dyspnoea at rest, severe central airway stenosis is already present. In these patients, flow–volume loop analysis and spirometry will most probably show aberrations typical of UAS. However, as a screening tool in a general population, these aberrations show a poor accuracy in predicting UAS. Forced oscillation tests may prove to be more accurate in detecting and documenting UAS. In extremely symptomatic, almost suffocating patients, immediate intervention with repermeabilisation/stenting is warranted. In nonlife-threatening cases, pre-intervention pulmonary function testing may yield useful information on the type, site and extent of the stenosis, whereas post-procedure testing may be used to focus the response and can be used as a basis for post-procedure follow-up. In the case of a multisite, extensive stenosis, its relatively typical flow–volume loop pattern may be predictive of therapeutic failure of single-site stenting and may predict the necessity of additional stenting at upstream choke points. Interventional bronchoscopic procedures offer immediate (and often longstanding) palliation of respiratory symptoms, improvements in quality of life (and frequently length of life as well) and objective improvements in pulmonary function in the majority of patients. When used judiciously, they are an invaluable tool in the armamentarium of modern pulmonology.

Further reading

- Amjadi K, et al. (2008). Impact of interventional bronchoscopy on quality of life in malignant airway obstruction. Respiration; 76: 421–442.
- Brouns M, et al. (2007). Tracheal stenosis: a flow dynamics study. J Appl Physiol; 102: 1178–1184.
- Eisner MD, et al. (1999). Pulmonary function improves after expandable metal stent placement for benign airway obstruction. Chest; 115: 1006–1011.
- Empay DW (1972). Assessment of upper airways obstruction. BMJ; 3: 503–505.
- Ernst A, et al. (2004). Central airway obstruction. Am J Respir Crit Care Med; 169: 1278–1297.
- Ernst A, et al. (2007). Airway stabilization with silicone stents for treating adult tracheobronchomalacia: a prospective observational study. Chest; 132: 609–616.
- Gelb AF, et al. (1992). Physiologic studies of tracheobronchial stents in airway obstruction. Am Rev Respir Dis; 146: 1088–1090.
- Gittoes NJ, et al. (1996). Upper airways obstruction in 153 consecutive patients presenting with thyroid enlargement. BMJ; 312: 484.
- Goldman JM, et al. (1993). Physiological effect of endobronchial radiotherapy in patients with major airway occlusion by carcinoma. Thorax; 48: 110–114.
- Lund ME, et al. (2007). Airway stenting: applications and practice management considerations. Chest; 131: 579–587.
- Melissant CF, et al. (1994). Lung function, CT-scan and X-ray in upper airway obstruction due to thyroid goitre. Eur Respir J; 7: 1782–1787.
- Miller RD, et al. (1973). Evaluation of obstructing lesions of the trachea and larynx by flow–volume loops. Am Rev Respir Dis; 108: 475–481.
- Miyazawa T, et al. (2004). Stenting at the flow-limiting segment in tracheobronchial stenosis due to lung cancer. Am J Respir Crit Care Med; 169: 1096–1102.
- Modrykamien AM, et al. (2009). Detection of upper airway obstruction with spirometry results and the flow–volume loop: a comparison of quantitative and visual inspection criteria. Respir Care; 54: 474–479.
- Nishine H, et al. (2012). Assessing the site of maximal obstruction in the trachea using lateral pressure measurements during bronchoscopy. Am J Respir Crit Care Med; 185: 24–33.
- Noppen M, et al. (2004). Interventional bronchoscopy for treatment of tracheal obstruction secondary to benign or malignant thyroid disease. Chest; 125: 723–730.
- Oviatt PL, et al. (2011). Exercise capacity, lung function and quality of life after interventional bronchoscopy. J Thorac Oncol; 6: 38–42.
- Razi SS, et al. (2010). Timely airway stenting improves survival in patients with malignant central airway obstruction. Ann Thorac Surg; 90: 1088–1093.
- Rotman HH, et al. (1975). Diagnosis of upper airway obstruction by pulmonary function testing. Chest; 68: 796–799.
- Verbanck S, et al. (2010). Detecting upper airway obstruction in patients with tracheal stenosis. J Appl Physiol; 109: 47–52.
- Vergnon JF, et al. (1995). Efficacy of tracheal and bronchial stent placement on respiratory functional tests. Chest; 107: 741–746.
- Vincken W, et al. (1985). Flow oscillations on the flow–volume loop: a nonspecific indicator of upper airway dysfunction. Bull Eur Physiopathol Respir; 21: 559–567.
- Walsh DA, et al. (1990). Bronchoscopic cryotherapy for advanced bronchial carcinoma. Thorax; 45: 509–513.

Chest X-ray and fluoroscopy

Walter De Wever

Chest radiography is the most frequently used radiological chest imaging technique and also one of the most challenging. The technical aspects of this imaging modality are studied extensively. New approaches to image acquisition and display have been introduced in the past decade. As a general rule, establishing the presence of a lung disease process on the radiograph should constitute the first step in radiological diagnosis of chest disease. Its lower sensitivity demands greater accuracy in interpretation. This greater accuracy can be achieved by following a standardised and systemic approach to a complete review of a chest radiograph. Technical factors and the position of the patient should also be considered when a chest radiograph is reported. Comparing prior films with recent ones is mandatory for the evaluation of pulmonary diseases.

Basic radiographic techniques

Diagnostic accuracy in chest disease is partly related to the quality of the radiographic images themselves. Several variables, such as patient position, patient respiration and film exposure factors, must be taken into account to ensure image quality (table 1). Positioning of the patient must be such that:

- the X-ray beam is properly centred;
- the patient's body is not rotated; and
- the scapulae are rotated so that they are projected away from the lungs.

Patient respiration must be fully suspended, preferably at total lung capacity. Film exposure factors should be such that faint visualisation of the thoracic spine and the intervertebral disks on the posteroanterior

> **Key points**
>
> - Chest radiography is the first step in radiological diagnosis of chest diseases.
>
> - Although it is a common technique, achieving high image quality is challenging and depends on getting several factors right.
>
> - The move from film to digital imaging offers exciting opportunities to improve image consistency and data management.

(PA) radiograph is possible and that lung markings behind the heart are clearly visible. The exposure should be as short as possible, consistent with the production of adequate contrast. A high kilovoltage technique appropriate to the film speed should be used.

Projections

PA and lateral projection The most satisfactory routine radiographic views for evaluating the chest are the PA and lateral projections with the patient standing (fig. 1). The combination of these two projections provides very good three-dimensional information. In patients who are too ill to stand up, anteroposterior (AP) upright or supine projections offer alternative but considerably less satisfactory views. The AP projection is of inferior quality because of the shorter focal distance, the greater magnification of the heart and, often, the restricted ability of these patients to suspend respiration or achieve full

Radiographic appearance
Frontal view (PA view)
Area from the lower cervical spine to below the costophrenic angles
Sternoclavicular joints symmetrical about the midline
Shadows of the scapulae away from the lung field
Lateral view
Soft tissues of the axillae should be included
Respiration
End of normal inspiration
Positioning of the patient
Erect position
Very ill patients: horizontal or semierect
PA position
Film exposure factors
High kilovoltage
Focus: film distance
Must be kept constant for any particular department
150–180 cm

inspiration. Based on a review of the literature and the recommendations of the American College of Radiology and the American Thoracic Society, recommendations on the use of chest radiographs are summarised in table 2.

Lateral decubitus projection For the lateral decubitus projection, the patient lies on one side and the X-ray beam is oriented horizontally. This technique is particularly helpful for the identification of small pleural effusions. <100 mL of fluid may be identified on well-exposed radiographs in this position. Radiography in the lateral decubitus position is also useful to demonstrate a change in the position of an air–fluid level in a cavity or a freely moving intracavitary loose body (*e.g.* fungus ball in aspergilloma).

Lordotic projection The lordotic projection can be made in the AP or PA projection. For

this projection, the patient stands erect and the X-ray tube is angled 15° cephalad. The main advantage of this modification is its reproducibility. The lordotic projection can be used:

1) for improving the visibility of the lung apices, superior mediastinum and thoracic inlet; and

2) for identifying the minor fissure in suspected cases of atelectasis of the right middle lobe.

Oblique projection Oblique studies are sometimes useful in locating a pleural or chest wall disease process (*e.g.* pleural plaque); however, in most situations, CT is preferred.

Inspiratory–expiratory radiography

Comparison of radiographs exposed in full inspiration and maximal expiration may supply useful information in two specific situations.

- The first indication is the evaluation of air trapping, either focal or general. With air trapping, diaphragmatic excursion is reduced symmetrically and lung density changes little between expiratory and inspiratory radiographs.
- The second indication is when a pneumothorax is suspected and when the visceral pleural line is not visible on the standard inspiratory radiograph or the findings are equivocal. In these situations, a film taken in full expiration may show the line more clearly.

Bedside radiography

Chest radiography, performed at the bedside with portable apparatus, is one of the most frequently performed radiological examinations; however, this technique is also the examination with the most variation in image quality. The amount of diagnostic information provided by chest examinations performed with portable apparatus is high and many abnormalities are detected. These examinations are useful 76–94% of the time. However, poor image quality and day-to-day variations in film density interfere with the detection of interval changes in

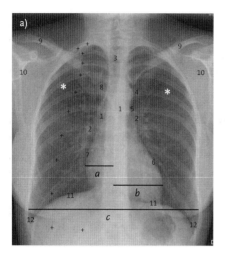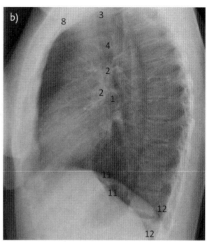

Figure 1. a) PA chest radiograph. Normal lungs are visible as black fields (air) (*) with superposition of multiple white linear structures (vessels and walls of airways). The lung hila consist of bronchi (main stem (1) and lobar bronchi) and vascular structures (pulmonary arteries (2) and pulmonary veins). A normal pleura is not visible on a chest radiograph. In the mediastinum, we can visualise the trachea (3) as a translucent tube on the midline, the aortic arch (4), the pulmonary trunk (5), the left border of the heart formed by the left ventricle (6) and the right border of the heart formed by right atrium (7). A normal heart has a normal cardiothoracic index: (a+b)/maximal diameter of the chest (c) must be <0.5. The bony components of the chest visible on the frontal view are: the ribs (+), the manubrium sternum (8), the clavicles (9), the scapulae (10) and the vertebral bodies on the midline. The diaphragm (11) is sharply delineated and the costophrenic angles (12) must be sharp and free. b) Lateral chest radiograph. The lateral chest film can be used to localise better the findings on the frontal view. Numbers and symbols are as for a).

patients with pulmonary diseases. The interpretation of a bedside radiograph requires extensive radiological experience to avoid misinterpretation of pleural and pulmonary disease. In addition, bedside radiography is an irreplaceable tool for detecting the malposition of tubes and lines and to identify associated complications. The need to improve the image quality of this examination has long been recognised but it is a difficult problem to solve.

Digital chest radiography

There have been many remarkable advances in conventional thoracic imaging over the past decade. Perhaps the most remarkable is the rapid conversion from film-based to digital radiographic systems. Digital radiography is the common name for different technologies that are characterised by a direct readout matrix that covers the whole exposure area. Conversion of X-ray intensity into electrical signals can either be direct (selenium-based systems) or indirect (scintillator/photodiode systems).

Advantages of digital radiography systems are:

- a high image quality; and
- the potential for dose reduction.

This technique is now the preferred imaging modality for bedside chest imaging because of its more consistent image quality. Digital radiography is rapidly replacing film-based chest units for in-department PA and lateral examinations. The final aim is to realise a completely integrated digital radiology department throughout the hospital connected to a large digital image archiving system. This concept, referred to as picture archiving and communication systems, represents the logical culmination of the

Table 2. Recommendations for the use of chest radiography

Indications

Signs and symptoms related to the respiratory and cardiovascular system

Follow-up of previously diagnosed thoracic disease for evaluation of improvement resolution, or progression

Staging of intrathoracic and extrathoracic tumours

Pre-operative assessment of patients scheduled for intrathoracic surgery

Pre-operative evaluation of patients who have cardiac or respiratory symptoms or patients who have a significant potential for thoracic pathology that may lead to increased peri-operative morbidity or mortality

Monitoring of patients who have life support devices and patients who have undergone cardiac or thoracic surgery or other interventional procedures

No indications

Routine screening of unselected populations

Routine pre-natal chest radiographs for the detection of unsuspected disease

Routine radiographs solely because of hospital admission

Mandated radiographs for employment

Repeated radiograph examinations after admission to a long-term facility

---

extensive research that is continuing in this area.

New developments in chest radiography

With the introduction of digital radiography, development of new techniques became possible. These techniques are dual energy, temporal subtraction, rib suppression technique and digital tomosynthesis.

Dual energy involves weighted subtraction of low- and high-energy images, and results in images representing bone structures or soft tissue. This technique can improve the detection of small, noncalcified pulmonary nodules and the detection of calcified chest lesions. Disadvantages of this technique are the higher radiation dose compared with standard digital radiography, the reduced signal to noise ratio and the need for additional hardware to perform this technique.

Temporal subtraction involves subtraction of a current image from a prior image of the same patient. With this technique, the detection of pathological changes over time becomes easier. Sophisticated algorithms are needed to eliminate detection errors

caused by differences in matching the projections of the two examinations.

Rib suppression technique This is a processing technique that suppress ribs in the image. Advantages of this technique over dual energy are:

- no need for an additional radiation dose or specialised equipment
- noise levels are not increased

Eliminating ribs has already shown to be effective in detection of lung lesions.

Digital tomosynthesis is a method of producing coronal cross section images using a digital detector and a chest X-ray system with a moving X-ray tube. This technique can improve the detection of pulmonary nodules by producing cross-section images without overprojection of the ribs or overlying vascular structures.

Chest fluoroscopy

Chest fluoroscopy was a popular procedure a generation ago. Patients were examined fluoroscopically in various projections and multiple spot radiographs were obtained with barium in the oesophagus. Examinations to evaluate pericardial effusion also were frequent. Overall diminution in cardiac pulsation and greater pulsation of the posterior cardiac wall in the lateral projection were thought to be signs of effusion. Other indications for fluoroscopy included the investigation of foreign bodies determined by air trapping and appropriate mediastinal shift, and the evaluation of diaphragmatic paralysis. This evaluation of diaphragmatic paralysis is still an indication for fluoroscopy today.

Dose and image quality in chest radiography

The radiation dose to the patient for chest radiography is relatively low but because of its frequent use, the collective dose can be considerable. The effective dose of a PA chest radiograph is about 0.02 mSv, which is about 0.5% that of a CT scan of the chest. The effective dose related to the lateral chest image is approximately two times higher compared with the dose of a PA projection. Studies indicate that dose reduction in PA chest images to at least 50% of commonly applied dose levels does not affect diagnosis in lung fields; however, dose reduction in the mediastinum, upper abdomen and retrocardiac areas appears to directly deteriorate diagnosis.

Further reading

- American College of Radiology. ACR Standard for the Performance of Pediatric and Adult Chest Radiography. Reston, American College of Radiology, 2001.
- American Thoracic Society (1984). Chest X-ray screening statements. *Am Thorac News*; 10: 14.
- Eisenhuber E, *et al.* (2012). Bedside chest radiography. *Respir Care*; 57: 427–443.
- MacMahon H, *et al.* (1991). Digital chest radiography. *Clin Chest Med*; 12: 19–32.
- Raoof S, *et al.* (2012). Interpretation of plain chest roentgenogram. *Chest*; 141: 545–558.
- Rigler LG (1931). Roentgen diagnosis of small pleural effusions: a new roentgenographic position. *JAMA*; 96: 104–108.
- Schaefer-Prokop C, *et al.* (2003). Digital radiography of the chest: detector techniques and performance parameters. *J Thorac Imaging*; 18: 124–137.
- Veldkamp WJ, *et al.* (2009). Dose and perceived image quality in chest radiography. *Eur J Radiol*; 72: 209–217.
- Wandtke JC (1994). Bedside chest radiography. *Radiology*; 190: 1–10.
- Zinn B, *et al.* (1956). The lordotic position in fluoroscopy and roentgenography of the chest. *Am J Roentgenol Radium Ther Nucl Med*; 75: 682–700.

Lung CT and MRI

Johny A. Verschakelen

CT is the second most important imaging modality of the chest and is, together with chest X-ray, one of the two basic imaging techniques used to visualise the lungs. Although there are indications to perform a CT of the chest in patients with a normal chest X-ray, this examination usually succeeds a chest X-ray on which a lesion is seen or suspected.

Except for visualisation of the heart and great vessels, MRI of the chest is less frequently used in daily clinical practice, but in selected cases, this imaging technique can sometimes add information to what is seen on CT.

Computed tomography

Since its introduction, CT has undergone several technical changes and improvements. The first scanners were 'incremental' CT scanners: in order to

complete one cross-sectional image, the patient needed to suspend respiration for a few seconds. After that, the table was moved and the next scan was performed. This was repeated about 25 times in order to image the entire thorax.

Spiral scanning (also known as helical or continuous volume scanning) has radically altered CT scanning protocols (table 1). In this technique, there is continuous patient movement with simultaneous scanning by a constantly rotating X-ray tube and detector system. While the first spiral CT scanners had only one row of detectors, todays scanners have multiple rows (multislice, multirow or multidetector row CT). This allows for a fast simultaneous acquisition of multiple images in the scan plane with one rotation of the X-ray tube around the patient. In this way, very good blood vessel opacification becomes possible using a limited amount of contrast (fig. 1). Spiral CT also offers flexible image reconstruction options, such as reconstructing images at various image thicknesses and two- and three-dimensional reconstructions.

Thin-section or high-resolution CT (HRCT) is a special type of acquisition technique that uses 0.5–1-mm slice thickness and high-frequency reconstruction algorithms to produce highly detailed images. It is used when detailed information on the lung parenchyma is needed. These thin slices can be obtained with the incremental acquisition technique in which 1-mm slices are produced with an image interval of 10–20 mm. However, with multislice spiral CT, it has become possible to produce a continuous set of thin slices of the entire chest. Although the quality of the individual

Key points

- CT is the second most important imaging modality of the chest.

- CT diagnosis of lung diseases is based on the study of their appearance and distribution patterns together with a careful analysis of patient data.

- CT interpretation of diffuse and interstitial lung diseases requires a formal multidisciplinary approach.

- MRI is second to CT when it comes to visualising pulmonary structure and pathology.

Table 1. *Advantages of spiral CT*

Sectional imaging without superposition of structures
Rapid acquisition within one breath hold
Very good blood vessel opacification in vascular studies using a limited amount of contrast
No respiratory misregistration between scans improving nodule detection
Fast and high-quality multiplanar and three-dimensional reconstructions

images may be somewhat reduced when multislice acquisition is used, the overall amount of information obtained is usually larger. Indeed, instead of a small number of axial slices with an image gap in between, a continuous dataset is obtained that allows the production of additional slices in different imaging planes. For this reason, this technique is currently replacing the incremental technique in most institutions, especially when it is the initial CT examination in a patient with a suspected lung problem. An important drawback may be the increased radiation dose. However, the lung parenchyma is very suitable for reduction of the radiation dose without important quality loss and first reports on the use of low-dose CT in demonstrating lung disease are indeed promising.

In addition, new reconstruction algorithms, such as iterative reconstruction, that allow further dose reduction without important loss in image quality are being developed.

Low-dose CT has been used in several lung cancer screening trials to examine whether any survival benefit can be found in patients with screen-detected cancers compared with the unscreened. The initial data from one trial showed a 20.3% reduction in lung cancer mortality among participants in the CT arm of the study. However, other articles have presented conflicting predictions of survival benefit and debate over the clinical utility of CT screening for lung cancer is ongoing. As mentioned earlier, a CT of the chest is usually performed when the chest X-ray is abnormal or suspicious for the presence of pathology,

although there are certainly indications for doing this examination even when the chest X-ray does not show any (obvious) abnormalities. Table 2 lists the most frequent indications for a CT of the chest.

Generally, the diagnosis of lung disease on a chest CT is based on three elements:

- Recognition of the appearance pattern of the disease *i.e.* classifying the abnormalities into a category that is based on their appearance
- Determination of location and distribution of the abnormalities in the lung: the distribution pattern
- Careful analysis of the patient data that are available at the time the CT scan is performed

Although in some cases, a diagnosis or a narrow differential diagnosis list can be proposed purely based on the study of the appearance and the distribution pattern of the disease on CT, the abnormalities seen in the lung should be carefully correlated with observations made on other radiological examinations and with all the clinical data that are available at the time of the CT examination. Particularly, diffuse and interstitial lung diseases are often very difficult to diagnose when the interpretation is only based on the CT presentation. Ideally, cooperation should be established between the clinician who is responsible for the patient, the radiologist and, when pathological information is present or probably required, the pathologist.

Continuous efforts are made to improve image quality and the diagnostic performance of CT imaging of the lung. Dual-energy CT scanning is helpful to study pulmonary perfusion in patients with pulmonary embolism (fig. 1). A further increase in the number of detector rows is feasible and may reduce acquisition time and, hence, image quality. Automated and semiautomated software packages will help to interpret the CT images.

Magnetic resonance imaging

Like CT, MRI produces multiplanar cross-sectional images, but allows for a greater

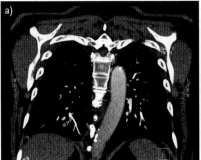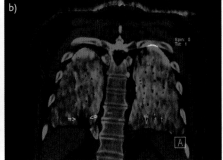

Figure 1. Dual-energy multislice spiral CT acquisition technique in a patient with pulmonary embolism. a) An enhancement defect is seen in a small branch of the right pulmonary artery (arrow). b) The perfusion scan shows a triangular area of decreased lung perfusion (arrows).

tissue characterisation because it has a better contrast resolution than CT (fig. 2). It also has the benefit of not using ionising radiation.

In MRI, tissue protons are exposed to a strong external magnetic field and realign along the plane of the magnetic gradient. From this position they are then deflected momentarily by applying a so-called radio frequency (RF) pulse. As they return to their original alignment, the protons emit a faint electromagnetic signal, which is detected by a receiving RF coil. When, in addition, a suitable gradient along the magnetic field is installed, signal detection can be confined to a pre-selected body plane. Processing of these data then yields a sectional image of the plane of interest.

Today, MRI has an established role in the imaging of the heart and the great thoracic vessels. For the chest wall, diaphragm, mediastinum and lung, MRI was, for many years, considered a useful 'problem-solving' technique in specific instances, in addition to CT. These instances included the identification of tumour invasion in the chest wall and mediastinal structures, the differentiation between solid and vascular hilar masses, the assessment of diaphragmatic abnormalities,

Table 2. Indications for CT of the chest

Abnormal chest X-ray
Further evaluations of a chest wall, pleural, mediastinal or lung abnormality seen on a chest X-ray
Rule out or confirm a lesion seen on a chest X-ray
Lung cancer staging and follow-up
Assessment of thoracic vascular lesions
Normal chest X-ray
Detection of diffuse lung disease
Detection of pulmonary metastases from a known extrathoracic tumour
Demonstration of pulmonary embolism
Investigation of a patient with haemoptysis
Investigation of patients with clinical evidence of a disease that might be related to the presence of chest abnormalities (e.g. pulmonary infection in an immunocompromised patient with fever)

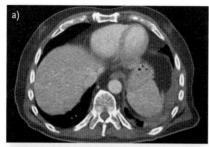

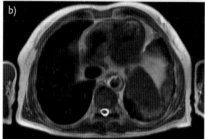

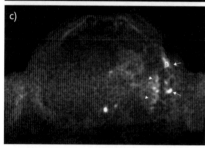

Figure 2. Patient with a left-sided malignant mesothelioma. Both a) CT and b) MRI show the irregular and nodular pleural thickening. There is suspicion of invasion in the diaphragm and spleen. c) Diffusion-weighted MRI shows increased signal in the spleen (arrowheads) indicating tumour invasion in this structure. In addition, increased signal is shown in the chest wall (arrows), suggesting chest wall invasion.

and the study and follow-up of mediastinal lymphoma during treatment. As mentioned earlier, nowadays most centres use multidetector spiral CT for thoracic imaging, including the areas thought previously to be the domain of problem-solving MRI.

Although it has become clear now that MRI will always be second to CT when it comes to the visualisation of pulmonary structure,

disease and patterns with high spatial resolution, the many research and development efforts that have been made during recent years have resulted in new and valuable applications that are very promising, and that could once be implemented in the clinical practice. There has been much interest in the role of MRI in the diagnosis of pulmonary embolism as a radiation-free alternative to CT. Some studies have shown that direct visualisation of the thrombus in the pulmonary artery is possible while others have concentrated on the study of lung perfusion, looking for decreased signal areas in the lung representing underperfused lung tissue on gadolinium-enhanced MRI. In addition, imaging of pulmonary ventilation by MRI has become possible. Hyperpolarised helium-3 gas has been used successfully to demonstrate perfusion changes in patients with asthma, COPD and CF, and hyperpolarised xenon-129, fluorine and oxygen-enhanced lung MRI are methods of gas imaging that have opened the field of imaging pulmonary ventilation by MRI. Diffusion-weighted magnetic resonance is another interesting application. This technique provides a measurement that reflects the random Brownian motion of water protons in biological tissue. This motion causes magnetic resonant signal loss that can be measured with the use of diffusion-sensitive sequences and that can be quantified by calculating the apparent diffusion coefficient. In the chest, it has been used successfully to differentiate between malignant and benign lesions.

Currently, most of these techniques remain in the experimental domain but it can be expected that some of them will reach daily clinical practice.

Further reading

- Aberle DR, *et al.* (2011). Reduced lung-cancer mortality with low-dose computed tomographic screening. *N Engl J Med*; 365: 395–409.

- Amundsen T, *et al.* (1997). Pulmonary embolism: detection with MR perfusion imaging of lung – a feasibility study. *Radiology*; 203: 181–185.
- Bach PB, *et al.* (2007). Computed tomography screening and lung cancer outcomes. *JAMA*; 297: 953–961.
- Bergin CJ, *et al.* (1990). MR evaluation of chest wall involvement in malignant lymphoma. *J Comput Assist Tomogr*; 14: 928–932.
- Bergin CJ, *et al.* (1993). Magnetic resonance imaging of lung parenchyma. *J Thorac Imaging*; 8: 12–17.
- Brown LR, *et al.* (1991). Masses of the anterior mediastinum: CT and MR imaging. *AJR Am J Roentgenol*; 157: 1171–1180.
- Coolen J, *et al.* (2012). Malignant pleural disease: diagnosis by using diffusion-weighted and dynamic contrast-enhanced MR imaging: initial experience. *Radiology*; 263: 884–892.
- Dawn SK, *et al.* (2001). Multidetector-row spiral computed tomography in the diagnosis of thoracic diseases. *Respir Care*; 46: 912–921.
- de Hoop B, *et al.* (2009). A comparison of six software packages for evaluation of solid lung nodules using semi-automated volumetry: what is the minimum increase in size to detect growth in repeated CT examinations? *Eur Radiol*; 19: 800–808.
- Gruden JF (2005). Thoracic CT performance and interpretation in the multidetector era. *J Thorac Imaging*; 20: 253–264.
- Gupta A, *et al.* (1999). Acute pulmonary embolism: diagnosis with MR angiography. *Radiology*; 210: 353–359.
- Heelan RT, *et al.* (1989). Superior sulcus tumors: CT and MR imaging. *Radiology*; 170: 637–641.
- Henschke CI, *et al.* (2006). Survival of patients with stage I lung cancer detected on CT screening. *N Engl J Med*; 355: 1763–1771.
- Kalender WA, *et al.* (1990). Spiral volumetric CT with single-breath-hold technique, continuous transport, and continuous scanner rotation. *Radiology*; 176: 181–183.
- Kauczor HU, *et al.* (1996). Normal and abnormal pulmonary ventilation: visualization at hyperpolarized He-3 MR imaging. *Radiology*; 201: 564–568.
- Klingenbeck-Regn K, *et al.* (1999). Subsecond multi-slice computed tomography: basics and applications. *Eur J Radiol*; 31: 110–124.
- MacFall JR, *et al.* (1996). Human lung air spaces: potential for MR imaging with hyperpolarized He-3. *Radiology*; 200: 553–558.
- Matoba M, *et al.* (2007). Lung carcinoma: diffusion-weighted MR imaging – preliminary evaluation with apparent diffusion coefficient. *Radiology*; 243: 570–577.
- Mirvis SE, *et al.* (1988). MR imaging of traumatic diaphragmatic rupture. *J Comput Assist Tomogr*; 12: 147–149.
- Muller NL (2002). Computed tomography and magnetic resonance imaging: past, present and future. *Eur Respir J*; 19: Suppl. 35, 3s–12s.
- Muller NL, *et al.* (1992). Value of MR imaging in the evaluation of chronic infiltrative lung diseases: comparison with CT. *AJR Am J Roentgenol*; 158: 1205–1209.
- Oudkerk M, *et al.* (2002). Comparison of contrast-enhanced magnetic resonance angiography and conventional pulmonary angiography for the diagnosis of pulmonary embolism: a prospective study. *Lancet*; 359: 1643–1647.
- Padhani AR (1998). Spiral CT: thoracic applications. *Eur J Radiol*; 28: 2–17.
- Padovani B, *et al.* (1993). Chest wall invasion by bronchogenic carcinoma: evaluation with MR imaging. *Radiology*; 187: 33–38.
- Silverman PM, *et al.* (2001). Common terminology for single and multislice helical CT. *AJR Am J Roentgenol*; 176: 1135–1136.
- Thieme SF, *et al.* (2008). Dual energy CT for the assessment of lung perfusion – correlation to scintigraphy. *Eur J Radiol*; 68: 369–374.
- Webb WR (1985). Magnetic resonance imaging of the mediastinum, hila, and lungs. *J Thorac Imaging*; 1: 65–73.

HRCT of the chest

Johny A. Verschakelen

High-resolution computed tomography (HRCT) is a CT acquisition and reconstruction technique that produces highly detailed images. It differs from 'classical' CT by the fact that thin slices (0.5–1 mm) are generated and that high-frequency reconstruction algorithms are used to improve image detail. As thin slices are necessary, the technique is also called thin-slice CT. Before the introduction of spiral CT, these thin slices were obtained by the 'incremental' acquisition technique in which 1-mm slices were produced with an image interval of 10 mm. Today, most institutions have spiral CT scanners and use multislice acquisition to obtain a continuous dataset of the entire chest that allows generation of a large number of adjacent thin slices. In this way, more information is obtained than with the incremental acquisition technique. In addition, images in other imaging planes and special reconstructions like maximal- and minimal-intensity projections (MIP and MinIP, respectively) can be made.

Because of the important image gap that existed when only incremental acquisition could be used – giving information about a small but well and equally distributed sample of the lung – the HRCT technique was (and still is) predominantly used to study diffuse and interstitial lung disease (DILD). It should be emphasised, however, that with the multislice spiral CT technique, thin and highly detailed images of the lung can be reconstructed from almost every CT examination.

HRCT and DILD

Since its introduction into clinical practice, the use of HRCT has constantly increased. This is related not only to the fact that this technique provides important morphological information on the lung parenchyma (it offers the highest image detail of the lung) but also because it helps to better understand the clinical and pathological course of some diseases, which has even resulted in the formulation CT classifications to categorise disease. HRCT is also partly responsible for the radical change in the diagnostic work-up of DILDs that has occurred the last 10 years. The historical gold standard of histologic diagnosis has been replaced by an integrative approach of clinical, radiological and, when necessary, pathologic data during multidisciplinary discussions. HRCT and

---

Key points

- HRCT is the imaging technique that offers the highest image detail of the lung parenchyma.

- HRCT is predominantly used to study DILDs but thin-slice CT can be useful in the study of focal lung abnormalities too.

- HRCT of the lungs is an essential element in the multidisciplinary discussion of patients with DILD.

- HRCT does not replace lung biopsy but helps to decide in which cases a lung biopsy will very likely give more (or important additional) information than CT and in which cases a biopsy is not needed.

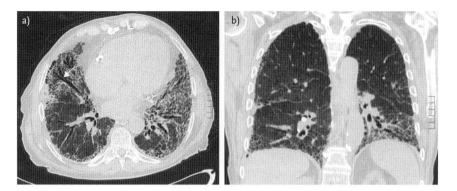

Figure 1. *Patient with IPF. CT shows the typical appearance and distribution pattern of IPF. Notice the traction bronchiectasis in the basal part of the middle lobe (arrow), a sign of pulmonary fibrosis. a) axial view; b) coronal view.*

histology are nowadays often considered as 'silver' standards. This does not mean that lung biopsy is less important but implicates that the multidisciplinary discussion defines in which cases a lung biopsy will very likely give more (or important additional) information than CT and in which cases a biopsy is not needed.

There are several reasons why HRCT plays an important role in this multidisciplinary discussion.

- Some DILDs can have a typical HRCT pattern and when this disease presents with such a pattern, HRCT may be very accurate in the diagnosis, *i.e.* HRCT may have a high positive predictive value (PPV). Idiopathic pulmonary fibrosis (IPF) is such a disease (fig. 1). The PPV of HRCT in IPF patients is >90% when a typical appearance pattern (predominant cystic, irregular linear pattern, traction bronchiectasis and no predominant ground-glass opacity) is combined with a typical distribution pattern (subpleural and basal lung). Unfortunately, a typical HRCT pattern of IPF is only seen in less than half of cases. In that situation, a part of the multidisciplinary discussion will be related to the question of whether the combination of HRCT with the clinical data is sufficient for diagnosis or whether an additional lung biopsy is necessary. Table 1 gives a list of diseases in which CT

can be diagnostic when a typical pattern is present.

- If it is decided that a lung biopsy is necessary, HRCT can help to determine the best location for taking the lung sample by suggesting the most likely areas of active disease and avoiding the areas of (nonspecific) terminal fibrosis.

- The information provided by HRCT and histology is very often complementary. While histology provides a microscopic view of a small part of the lung, HRCT gives a 'sub-macroscopic' or sub-millimetre view of the entire lung. Combination of this information can indeed result in a single diagnosis. It should be emphasised, however, that in some patients with DILD, multiple

Table 1. *Diseases that can present with a typical HRCT pattern*

IPF
Sarcoidosis
Langerhans' cell histiocytosis
Hypersensitivity pneumonitis
Lymphangitic spread of cancer
Silicosis and coalminers' pneumoconiosis
Alveolar proteinosis
Lymphangiomyomatosis
Cryptogenic organising pneumonia

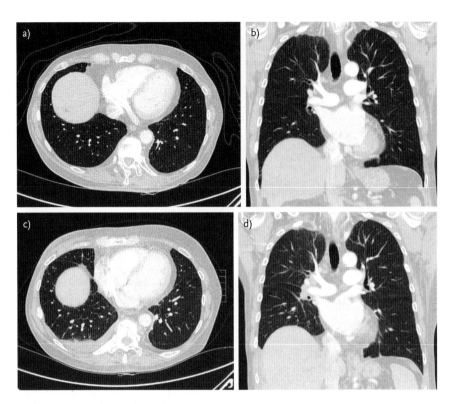

Figure 2. Patient with breast cancer developing lymphangitic spread of cancer. a, b) The first CT examination a) axial and b) coronal view shows a normal lung parenchyma. c, d) The second CT examination 6 months later shows a linear pattern in the right lower lobe caused by thickening of the interlobular septa together with the development of a pleural effusion. c) Axial view and d) coronal view.

pathologic and/or HRCT patterns can be seen simultaneously. In that situation, multidisciplinary discussion should determine the clinical significance of these individual patterns.

- HRCT can be helpful during follow-up of disease and in this way contribute to the diagnosis by providing information about speed of disease progression. HRCT also plays a role in patients with acute exacerbation of DILD and in the differential diagnosis with infection, left heart failure or other causes of acute lung disease.

HRCT and focal lung disease

As mentioned earlier, HRCT obtained by the incremental method was not suitable for the study of localised and focal lung abnormalities because of the image gap. The introduction of multislice spiral CT has made it possible to choose the slice thickness after the examination and highly detailed thin slices of the entire chest can be produced instead of, or in addition to, the thicker slices. In this way, it is possible to obtain not only additional detailed information of the focal lung lesion but also of the entire lung. Lymphangitic spread (fig. 2), lung perfusion defects in patients with pulmonary embolism, tumour extension into the surrounding lung, early pulmonary oedema and early small airway infection are examples of disorders that can be better appreciated on thin slices than on thick slices.

HRCT technique

The basic HRCT examination contains continuous axial 1-mm slices of the entire chest obtained with a multislice spiral CT scan at breath hold after deep inspiration. From these data, additional coronal reconstructions are usually made, as these are not only helpful to study the craniocaudal distribution of disease but often allow better visualisation of the presence and distribution of linear opacities. If desired, these CT data can also be used to calculate MIPs, which can be helpful to study small lesions and their relation to the pulmonary lobule, and MinIPs, which may be helpful to study low-attenuation lung disease. Expiratory HRCT (stopping breathing after deep expiration) should be performed when small airway narrowing is suspected. This expiratory HRCT can be obtained by the incremental method, in which 1-mm slices are produced with a larger image interval (20–30 mm), or by low-dose spiral CT. A lower radiation dose is used in this technique. Finally, it may be necessary to add a few slices in the prone body position. These are performed in patients suspected of having early DILD when supine CT shows minimal changes in the posterior and basal parts of the lung, areas that are often first involved in DILD but also often show a gravity-related perfusion increase. Prone CT scans are mostly able to differentiate between these entities as gravity-related changes will disappear in the prone body position. Administration of intravenous contrast is not necessary.

HRCT in the diagnosis of diffuse lung disease

As mentioned earlier, HRCT plays an important role in the process of making the diagnosis of diffuse lung disease. Interpreting a HRCT image of the lungs of a patient suspected of having DILD is a stepwise process. First, it is important to decide whether the lung changes are indeed resulting from a diffuse lung disease, i.e. a disease that is diffusely spread over an important part of the lung and shows CT changes that are composed in a repeating arrangement (pattern). If it very likely is a diffuse lung disease, the disease pattern should be determined: how does the disease appear, i.e. what is the appearance pattern (nodular or linear, increased or decreased attenuation), and where are the abnormalities located, i.e. what is the distribution pattern (which lung areas are involved and how does disease relate to the pulmonary lobule)? The disease pattern can be very typical (table 1) but is often atypical and a differential diagnosis list should be proposed. In both cases, it is important to have a multidisciplinary discussion in which the HRCT findings are correlated with the clinical findings. HRCT can then be helpful in the decision of whether a lung biopsy is necessary or not and, if so, of the best site to take the biopsy. Finally, the integration of the clinical, HRCT and pathological data may result in an assumed diagnosis or a differential diagnosis list, or the disease may be considered as unclassifiable.

Further reading

- American Thoracic Society/European Respiratory Society. (2002). International Multidisciplinary Consensus Classification of the Idiopathic Interstitial Pneumonias. *Am J Respir Crit Care Med*; 165: 277–304.
- Dodd JD, *et al.* (2008). Conventional high-resolution CT *versus* contiguous multidetector CT in the detection of bronchiolitis obliterans syndrome in lung transplant recipients. *J Thorac Imaging*; 23: 235–243.
- Flaherty KR, *et al.* (2004). Idiopathic interstitial pneumonia: what is the effect of a multidisciplinary approach to diagnosis? *Am J Respir Crit Care Med*; 170: 904–910.
- Hunninghake GW, *et al.* (2001). Utility of a lung biopsy for the diagnosis of idiopathic pulmonary fibrosis. *Am J Respir Crit Care Med*; 164: 193–196.
- Kawel N, *et al.* (2009). Effect of slab thickness on the CT detection of pulmonary nodules: use of sliding thin-slab maximum intensity projection and volume rendering. *Am J Roentgenol*; 192: 1324–1329.

- Mayo JR (2009). CT evaluation of diffuse infiltrative lung disease: dose considerations and optimal technique. *J Thorac Imaging*; 24: 252–259.
- Nishino M, *et al.* (2010). The spectrum of pulmonary sarcoidosis: variations of high-resolution CT findings and clues for specific diagnosis. *Eur J Radiol*; 73: 66–73.
- Nishino M, *et al.* (2010). Volumetric expiratory HRCT of the lung: clinical applications. *Radiol Clin North Am*; 48: 177–183.
- Quadrelli S, *et al.* (2010). Radiological *versus* histopathological diagnosis of usual interstitial pneumonia in the clinical practice: does it have any survival difference? *Respiration*; 79: 32–37.
- Raghu G, *et al.* (2011). An official ATS/ERS/JRS/ALAT statement: idiopathic pulmonary fibrosis: evidence-based guidelines for diagnosis and management. *Am J Respir Crit Care Med*; 183: 788–824.
- Schmidt SL, *et al.* (2009). Diagnosing fibrotic lung disease: when is high-resolution computed tomography sufficient to make a diagnosis of idiopathic pulmonary fibrosis? *Respirology*; 14: 934–939.
- Screaton NJ, *et al.* (2011). The clinical impact of high resolution computed tomography in patients with respiratory disease. *Eur Radiol*; 21: 225–231.
- Sverzellati N, *et al.* (2010). High-resolution computed tomography in the diagnosis and follow-up of idiopathic pulmonary fibrosis. *Radiol Med*; 115: 526–538.
- Wells AU (2003). High-resolution computed tomography in the diagnosis of diffuse lung disease: a clinical perspective. *Semin Respir Crit Care Med*; 24: 347–356.

Nuclear medicine of the lung

Antonio Palla and Duccio Volterrani

Nuclear medicine may contribute to the diagnosis of pulmonary embolism and inflammatory diseases, and the diagnosis and staging of lung cancer. Among several techniques available, perfusion and ventilation lung scintigraphy (PLS and VLS, respectively), gallium-67 scintigraphy, and positron emission tomography (PET) scintigraphy are of interest in clinical practice.

Diagnosis of pulmonary embolism

Thanks to its noninvasiveness, safety and low cost, PLS still remains the cornerstone of the diagnosis and follow-up of pulmonary embolism.

PLS has been proven to be useful for:

- diagnosis of pulmonary embolism
- detection of recurrences under treatment or after its discontinuation
- differential diagnosis between thromboembolic and nonthromboembolic pulmonary hypertension

Two main scintigraphic criteria must be considered for the diagnosis: 1) identification of perfusion defects corresponding to one or more pulmonary segments, and 2) diversion of pulmonary blood flow from lower and posterior lung regions. Perfusion defects are typically multiple, wedge-shaped and often bilateral. PLS has a sensitivity of 100%: it allows exclusion with certainty when the diagnosis is negative. The specificity varies in different reported series but, on average, does not reach acceptable values; to increase the specificity, VLS has been introduced, but it is cumbersome, time consuming and poorly

> **Key points**
>
> - Nuclear medicine of the lung has a role in the diagnosis of pulmonary embolism and inflammatory diseases, and in the diagnosis and staging of lung cancer.
> - Perfusion scintigraphy is key in the diagnosis and follow-up of pulmonary embolism as it is safe, cheap and noninvasive.
> - Gallium-67 scintigraphy is useful in identifying and localising intrathoracic inflammation and infection.
> - FDG-PET and PET/CT are used in diagnosis, treatment targeting and treatment in lung cancer.

available. Nowadays, VLS is only indicated in some individual patients with pulmonary embolism, since similar results can be obtained by using chest radiography. A few years ago, a new classification of perfusion defects was published in order to optimise its diagnostic usefulness in conjunction with chest radiography; this method has made it possible to obtain a diagnostic accuracy similar to that shown by angio-CT. PLS also plays a leading role in the follow-up of patients with pulmonary embolism, as it helps to monitor the efficacy of treatment in the first few days, it allows prompt detection of early and late recurrences and evolution towards pulmonary hypertension, and it may differentiate between thromboembolic pulmonary hypertension and other types of pulmonary hypertension.

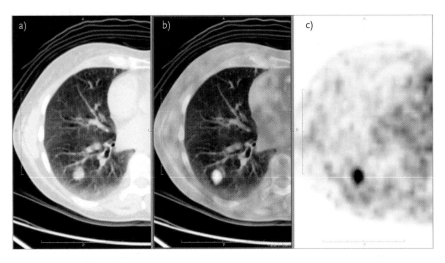

Figure 1. Solitary pulmonary nodule as it appears on a) chest CT, b) PET/CT and c) FDG-PET.

Diagnosis of inflammatory diseases

Gallium-67 citrate is the most widely employed positive tracer in order to identify and localise intrathoracic inflammations and infections. To acquire images, a scintillation gamma camera with a low-energy collimator is required. Gallium scintigraphy may help in evaluating the activity of granulomatous disorders and the efficacy of steroid treatment. In patients with sarcoidosis, it shows a high diagnostic sensitivity; in some cases, the presence of highly specific signs, such as 'panda' or 'lambda' signs, allows avoidance of invasive diagnostic tests. Moreover, this tracer may differentiate between sarcoidosis and non-Hodgkin's lymphoma, and detect multiple extrapulmonary sites of sarcoidosis. In addition, gallium scintigraphy is indicated in investigating metabolic activity in pulmonary infections and the efficacy of proper therapy. In the diagnosis of pulmonary TB, gallium scintigraphy may indicate the necessity of a bronchoalveolar lavage and the site where it should be performed. This occurs mostly in cases of suspected re-infection of areas of pleuroparenchymal fibrosis, in cases of suspicion where sputum is repeatedly negative and in immunocompromised patients. Finally, gallium scintigraphy may

be of value in the evaluation of the efficacy of chemotherapy in lymphomatous diseases and may help differentiate post-actinic fibrosis from residual tumour foci when a lung density persists after radiotherapy.

Lung cancer

PET is a nuclear medicine technique that produces a three-dimensional image of functional and biochemical processes within the body. Recently, PET has been combined with CT (PET/CT) (fig. 1); such fusion generally improves diagnostic accuracy by increasing specificity compared with PET alone. The most frequently used tracer is 2-[^{18}F]-fluoro-2-deoxy-D-glucose (FDG), a glucose analogue, the tissue concentration of which is directly related to glucose metabolism. The uptake of FDG may be evaluated by a semiquantitative measurement, the standardised uptake value (SUV), *i.e.* the ratio between the amount of tracer in a specific area and the amount potentially present if the tracer had been evenly distributed in the body.

FDG-PET has proven useful in:

- diagnosing and staging lung cancer
- monitoring the efficacy of treatment
- defining the biological target volume for radiation treatment planning

An indication of increasing clinical relevance of FDG-PET and PET/CT is the differentiation of benign from malignant solitary pulmonary nodules by replacing invasive modalities of investigation. A SUV of 2.5 has been reported as a guideline for the cut-off between benign (SUV <2.5) and malignant (SUV >2.5) lesions. A meta-analysis from 40 studies showed a sensitivity of 97% but a lower specificity (78%) due to FDG uptake within inflammatory/granulomatous lesions. However, a high rate of false-negative FDG results can occur when nodules are <1 cm (sensitivity of 69% for nodules of 5–8 mm). Moreover, some histotypes, such as bronchoalveolar carcinomas and well-differentiated neuroendocrine tumours, usually present a low glucose metabolic activity and cannot be correctly imaged by FDG-PET.

FDG PET is also a standard modality for staging nonsmall cell lung cancer. Several studies have demonstrated that PET is more accurate than CT in the staging of the mediastinum (N state). Due to its high negative predicted value, invasive staging procedures (mediastinoscopy) can be omitted in patients with a negative FDG-PET for mediastinal lymph node involvement. However, a positive finding should not preclude mediastinoscopy. Moreover, the addition of FDG-PET to the standard work-up can prevent unnecessary thoracotomies and change the therapeutic approach in a significant percentage of patients. PET is useful in disclosing distant metastases (M state) with a high sensitivity and specificity. However, PET cannot replace CT or MRI for detecting brain metastases. Moreover, the measurement of FDG SUV within the tumour correlates negatively with patient prognosis; early changes of FDG SUV during radiotherapy and chemotherapy can predict therapy efficacy; and PET is more accurate than contrast-enhanced CT for detecting residual tumour after radiotherapy and chemotherapy.

A recent indication of PET/CT is the definition of the biological target volume for radiation treatment planning. This approach has the goal of increasing the dose to the tumour and focusing the treatment planning to the biological target, which reveals an elevated glucose metabolism.

Further reading

- Bryant AS, *et al.* (2006). The maximum standardized uptake values on integrated FDG-PET/CT is useful in differentiating benign from malignant pulmonary nodules. *Ann Thorac Surg*; 82: 1016–1020.
- De Geus-Oei LF, *et al.* (2007). Predictive and prognostic value of FDG-PET in nonsmall-cell lung cancer: a systematic review. *Cancer*; 110: 1654–1664.
- Kita T, *et al.* (2007). Clinical significance of the serum IL-2R level and Ga-67 scan findings in making a differential diagnosis between sarcoidosis and non-Hodgkin's lymphoma. *Ann Nucl Med*; 21: 499–503.
- Liu SF, *et al.* (2007). Monitoring treatment responses in patients with pulmonary TB using serial lung gallium-67 scintigraphy. *Am J Roentgenol*; 188: 403–408.
- Miniati M, *et al.* (2008). Perfusion lung scintigraphy for the diagnosis of pulmonary embolism: a reappraisal and review of the prospective investigative study of pulmonary embolism diagnosis methods. *Semin Nucl Med*; 38: 450–461.
- Sostman HD, *et al.* (2008). Sensitivity and specificity of perfusion scintigraphy combined with chest radiography for acute pulmonary embolism in PIOPED II. *J Nucl Med*; 49: 1741–1748.
- Stein PD, *et al.* (2006). Multidetector computed tomography for acute pulmonary embolism. *N Engl J Med*; 354: 2317–2327.
- Van Tinteren H, *et al.* (2002). Effectiveness of positron emission tomography in the preoperative assessment of patients with suspected non-small-cell lung cancer: the PLUS multicentre randomised trial. *Lancet*; 359: 1388–1393.

Transthoracic ultrasound

Florian von Groote-Bidlingmaier, Coenraad F.N. Koegelenberg and
Chris T. Bolliger[†]

Key points

- Transthoracic ultrasound can be performed with the most basic ultrasound equipment and allows for immediate and mobile assessment of patients with a wide variety of respiratory diseases.

- The major indications for the use of transthoracic ultrasound are the description of pleural effusions, pleural thickening, diaphragmatic dysfunction, and chest wall and pleural tumours.

- Other applications of transthoracic ultrasound include the diagnosis of a pneumothorax, pulmonary consolidation, tumours, interstitial syndromes and pulmonary embolism.

- Furthermore, ultrasound is ideal to guide thoracentesis, drainage of effusions and other thoracic interventions, and is particularly useful in intensive care units where radiographic equipment is unavailable.

- Major advantages of the technique include its mobility, dynamic properties, lack of radiation and low cost.

- The ultrasonographic appearance of the normal thorax and the most common pathologies are reviewed in this section.

General technical aspects and appearance of the normal thorax

A low-frequency probe (*e.g.* 3.5 MHz) is routinely used for screening purposes, while detailed assessment of an abnormal chest wall or pleura can be performed with a high-frequency probe (*e.g.* 8 MHz).

Special attention must be paid to patient positioning. The posterior chest is ideally scanned in the sitting position whereas the anterior and lateral chest are best examined in the supine or lateral decubitus position.

Superficial muscles and fascia planes appear as a series of echogenic layers during the initial surveillance of a normal chest. Curvilinear structures on transverse scans, associated with posterior acoustic shadowing, represent the ribs.

The visceral and parietal pleura normally appear as one highly echogenic line. Movement of the lung with the respiratory cycle in relation to the chest wall on real-time ultrasound is called the 'lung sliding' sign.

Ultrasound cannot visualise normal aerated lung tissue. The large change in acoustic impedance at the pleura–lung interface, however, causes horizontal artefacts that are seen as a series of echogenic parallel lines equidistant from one another below the pleura. These bright but formless lines are known as reverberation artefacts or A-lines (fig. 1).

Chest wall pathology

Soft-tissue masses, such as abscesses, lipomas and a variety of other lesions, can be detected by ultrasound. These lesions are

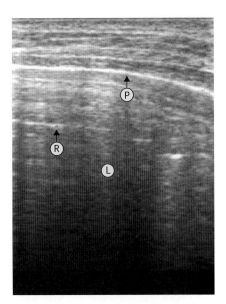

Figure 1. The typical appearance of a normal chest on ultrasound. A transverse view through the intercostal space is shown. The chest wall is visualised as multiple layers of echogenicity representing muscles and fascia. The visceral and parietal pleura appear as an echogenic bright line (two distinct lines sliding during respiration are visible on real-time ultrasound). Reverberation artefacts beneath the pleural lines imply an underlying air-filled lung. P: pleura; L: lung; R: reverberation artefact.

mostly benign, but variable echogenicity and nonspecific ultrasound findings make differentiation between various aetiologies difficult. Supraclavicular and axillary lymph nodes are usually accessible, and ultrasound may even help to distinguish benign from malignant lymph nodes. Hypoechoic masses disrupting the normal structure of a rib may represent bony metastases and can be seen on ultrasound.

Pleural pathology

Transthoracic ultrasound is most commonly used to investigate pleural effusions, and is more sensitive than decubitus radiographs at demonstrating minimal or loculated effusions. The ultrasound appearance of a pleural effusion depends on its nature and chronicity.

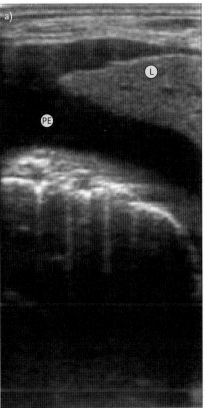

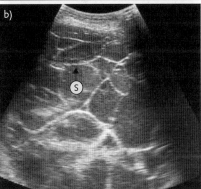

Figure 2. a) Example of an anechoic pleural effusion. It presents as an echo-free space between the visceral and parietal pleura. Compressive atelectasis of the lung may be seen as a tongue-like structure in a large effusion. Note the difference to the effusion in b), which is classified as complex septated. Multiple septa form many compartments in the same effusion. PE: pleural effusion; L: lung; S: septum.

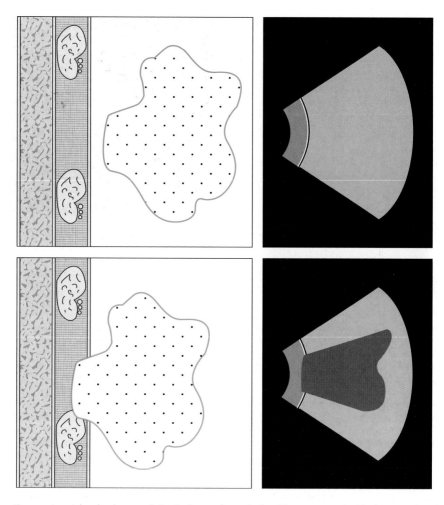

Figure 3. A peripheral pulmonary lesion is shown schematically without (top) and with (bottom) pleural contact. Only the lesion with pleural contact is visible on ultrasound. Reproduced from Diacon et al. (2005) with permission from the publisher.

Four appearances based on the internal echogenicity are recognised:

- anechoic
- complex but nonseptated
- complex and septated
- homogenously echogenic

Transudates are invariably anechoic, nonseptated and free flowing, whereas complex, septated or echogenic effusions are usually exudates. Malignant effusions are frequently anechoic. The atelectatic lung

inside a large effusion may appear as a tongue-like structure within the effusion. Inflammatory effusions are often associated with strands of echogenic material and septations that show more or less mobility with respiration and the cardiac cycle (fig. 2).

The volume of a pleural effusion can be estimated using the following classification:

- *minimal* if the echo-free space is confined to the costophrenic angle

- *small* if the space is greater than the costophrenic angle but still within the range of the area covered with a 3.5-MHz curvilinear probe
- *moderate* if the space is greater than a one-probe range but within a two-probe range
- *large* if the space is bigger than a two-probe range

Both small effusions and pleural thickening may appear as hypoechoic on ultrasound, so differentiation might be difficult. An important sign in favour of an effusion is mobility on real-time ultrasound.

Metastatic pleural tumours and malignant mesothelioma can be visualised as polypoid pleural nodules or irregular sheet-like pleural thickening. They are often associated with large pleural effusions. Benign pleural tumours are rare.

Qureshi *et al.* (2009) found that pleural thickening >1 cm, pleural nodularity and diaphragmatic thickening >7 mm were highly suggestive of malignant disease. In their study, ultrasound correctly identified 73% of malignant effusions.

The detection of a pneumothorax by means of ultrasound requires a greater deal of expertise than the detection of pleural fluid. A recent meta-analysis concluded that bedside ultrasonography had a higher sensitivity and similar specificity for the diagnosis of a pneumothorax when compared with chest radiography. The absence of normal lung sliding, the loss of comet-tail artefacts and exaggerated horizontal reverberation artefacts are reliable signs of the presence of a pneumothorax. Ultrasound is also the ideal tool to screen for a post-procedural pneumothorax after transthoracic procedures and transbronchial biopsy.

Pulmonary pathology

A lung tumour abutting the pleura will be detectable by ultrasound (fig. 3). In most cases, these tumours present as a hypoechoic mass with posterior acoustic enhancement (fig. 4). Visceral pleura or chest wall involvement is important for

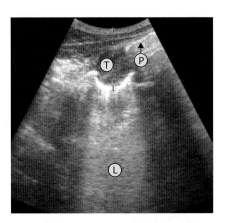

Figure 4. A sonographic image showing a solid lung lesion with posterior echo enhancement. Note that the tumour is abutting the pleura and is therefore visible on ultrasound. P: pleura; L: lung; T: tumour.

staging of malignant lung tumours. Loss of movement of a visualised tumour with respiration suggests infiltration beyond the parietal pleura.

Ultrasound can detect pneumonic consolidations provided they have contact with the pleura. Early pneumonic consolidation may appear very similar to the diffusely echogenic tissue-like texture of the liver. Both air and fluid bronchograms are usually seen within the consolidated lung. Noninfective causes of consolidations with similar appearance on ultrasound include pulmonary infarction, haemorrhage and bronchoalveolar carcinoma. Consolidation can be differentiated from an interstitial syndrome, for which long, laser-like vertical hyperechoic lines, called B-lines, are pathognomonic. Interstitial syndromes may include pulmonary oedema, interstitial pneumonia or diffuse parenchymal lung disease

A hypoechoic lesion with a well-defined or irregular wall abutting the pleura might represent a lung abscess. The centre of the abscess is most often anechoic but may reveal septations and internal echoes.

Another indication for the use of transthoracic ultrasound is the assessment of pulmonary and pleural-based cysts, which commonly appear as large, round anechoic lesions.

Conclusion

The value of ultrasound for chest physicians is firmly established. Basic thoracic ultrasonography is an elegant and inexpensive investigation that extends the physicians' diagnostic and interventional potential at the bedside in peripheral lung, pleural and chest wall disease.

Further reading

- Diacon AH, et al. (2005). Transthoracic ultrasound for the pulmonologist. Curr Opin Pulm Med; 11: 307–312.
- Ding W, et al. (2011). Diagnosis of pneumothorax by radiography and ultrasonography: a meta-analysis. Chest; 140: 859–866.
- Evans AL, et al. (2004). Radiology in pleural disease: state of the art. Respirology; 9: 300–312.
- Gorg C, et al. (1997). Sonography of malignant pleural effusion. Eur Radiol; 7: 1195–1198.
- Herth FJ, et al. (2004). Diagnosis of pneumothorax by means of transthoracic ultrasound: a prospective trial. Eur Respir J; 24: Suppl. 48, 491s–492s.
- Hirsch JH, et al. (1981). Real-time sonography of pleural opacities. Am J Roentgenol; 136: 297–301.
- Kocijancic I, et al. (2004). Imaging of pleural fluid in healthy individuals. Clin Radiol; 59: 826–829.
- Koegelenberg CF, et al. Pleural Ultrasound. In: Light RW, et al., eds. Textbook of Pleural Disease, 2nd Edn. London, Hodder & Stoughton, 2008; pp. 271–228.
- Koegelenberg CF, et al. (2011). Pleural controversy: closed needle pleural biopsy or thoracoscopy – which first? Respirology; 16: 738–746.
- Koegelenberg CF, et al. (2012). Transthoracic ultrasonography for the respiratory physician. Respiration; 84: 337–350.
- Koh DM, et al. (2002). Transthoracic US of the chest: clinical uses and applications. Radiographics; 22: e1.
- Kreuter M, et al. (2011). Diagnostische Wertigkeit der transthorakalen Sonografie vergleichend zur Thoraxubersicht beim Nachweis eines postinterventionellen Pneumothorax [Diagnostic value of transthoracic ultrasound compared to chest radiography in the detection of a post-interventional pneumothorax]. Ultraschall Med; 32: Suppl. 2, E20–E23.
- Lichtenstein DA, et al. (1995). A bedside ultrasound sign ruling out pneumothorax in the critically ill. Chest; 108: 1345–1348.
- Mathis G (1997). Thoraxsonography – part I: chest wall and pleura. J Ultrasound Med Biol; 23: 1131–1139.
- Mayo PH, et al. (2006). Pleural ultrasonography. Clin Chest Med; 27: 215–217.
- Qureshi NR, et al. (2009). Thoracic ultrasound in the diagnosis of malignant pleural effusion. Thorax; 64: 139–143.
- Tsai TH, et al. (2003). Ultrasound in the diagnosis and management of pleural disease. Curr Opin Pulm Med; 9: 282–290.
- Volpicelli G, et al. (2012). International evidence-based recommendations for point-of-care lung ultrasound. Intensive Care Med; 38: 577–591.
- Yang PC, et al. (1992). Value of sonography in determining the nature of pleural effusion: analysis of 320 cases. Am J Roentgenol; 159: 29–33.
- Yang PC (1997). Ultrasound-guided transthoracic biopsy of peripheral lung, pleural, and chest wall lesions. J Thorac Imaging; 12: 272–284.

Lung injury

Bernd Schönhofer and Christian Karagiannidis

Acute lung injury (ALI) and its most severe manifestation, acute respiratory distress syndrome (ARDS), are defined by physiological criteria (*i.e.* ratio of $P_{a}O_2$ to inspiratory oxygen fraction (FIO_2) $\leqslant$300 mmHg for ALI and $\leqslant$200 mmHg for ARDS, independent of positive end-expiratory pressure (PEEP)) and by bilateral pulmonary infiltrates as radiological criteria. Cardiac failure must be excluded based either on pulmonary artery wedge pressure (<18 mmHg) or on clinical evaluation of left ventricular function, if the invasive measurement is unavailable.

These criteria should be re-evaluated after 24 h, since their persistence is essential for the correct diagnosis of ALI/ARDS. Furthermore, timing may be of influence on the development of ALI/ARDS.

Lung oedema may evaluated by CT or other established methods.

ALI/ARDS may be caused by various aetiologies: direct lung injury, *e.g.* pneumonia, aspiration, toxic inhalation, near drowning or lung contusion; or indirect lung injury, *e.g.* sepsis, burn, pancreatitis or massive blood transfusion. The two aetiologies may coexist.

The exact incidence of ALI/ARDS is not known; its annual mortality rate has been estimated to be >30 000 patients per year in the USA. Despite recent advances in the understanding of the pathophysiology of ARDS, improvements in supportive care, and multiple therapeutic efforts directed at modifying the course of the condition, mortality rates are persistently 35–40%.

The pathophysiology of ALI/ARDS is related to altered pulmonary capillary permeability and increased intrapulmonary shunt, which is associated with impaired gas exchange. ARDS has been divided into three stages, in which an initial inflammatory phase (exudative) is followed by fibro-proliferation,

Key points

- ALI and its most severe manifestation, ARDS, are defined as $P_{a}O_2/FIO_2$ $\leqslant$300 mmHg and $\leqslant$200 mmHg, respectively, with bilateral infiltrates as radiological criteria. The ARDS Definition Task Force proposes a new classification according to the severity of ARDS, *i.e.* mild: $P_{a}O_2/FIO_2$ >200 mmHg and $\leqslant$300 mmHg; moderate: $P_{a}O_2/FIO_2$ >100 mmHg and $\leqslant$200 mmHg; and severe: $P_{a}O_2/FIO_2$ $\leqslant$100 mmHg, because of its better predictive value for mortality (fig. 1).

- Principles of protective ventilator settings for patients with ALI/ARDS are low tidal volume (*i.e.* V_T 6 mL per kg ideal body weight, plateau pressure <30 cmH_2O and peak pressure <35 cmH_2O).

- Permissive hypercapnia may be helpful to realise protective mechanical ventilation.

- Protection of the lungs may also be provided by the pump-driven veno-venous ECMO or pumpless ILA.

which can lead to established interstitial and intra-alveolar fibrosis, the final phase.

Mechanical ventilation itself can seriously damage lung parenchyma (ventilator-induced lung injury). ALI/ARDS often has systematic manifestations, triggering systemic inflammatory response syndrome, or in extremis multiple organ dysfunction syndrome.

In general, the spectrum of treatment ALI/ARDS includes supportive care, ventilator support and pharmacological treatment. The first principle of treatment is to identify potential underlying causes of ALI/ARDS. Furthermore, secondary lung injury, such as aspiration, barotraumas, nosocomial infections and oxygen toxicity, has to be avoided. The main aims of supportive care are maintaining oxygen delivery to end organs by avoiding anaemia and optimising cardiovascular function and body fluid balance; additionally, catabolism and nutritional support have to be balanced.

With regard to mechanical ventilation, the main goal is to improve oxygenation without increasing the iatrogenic effects caused by mechanical ventilation; there are different methods available. Among the methods related to the ventilatory setting, those found really effective are to reduce tidal volume and pressures and to apply PEEP to reduce the amount of nonaerated atelectatic lung.

Principles of protective ventilator settings for patients with ALI/ARDS are:

- Tidal volume 6 mL·kg^{-1} ideal body weight.
- Plateau pressure <30 cmH$_2$O, peak pressure <35 cmH$_2$O.
- This strategy of protective mechanical ventilation may be associated with permissive hypercapnia.

The 'optimal' setting of PEEP is not clear, since several methods have been proposed without any clear advantages over each other.

Higher PEEP (>15 cmH$_2$O) might be recommended in more severe ARDS patients. Prone position might be recommended in more severe ARDS patients, according to the expertise of the clinicians. Estimating the transpulmonary pressure by means of oesophageal pressure measurement might help to find the ideal PEEP level. Alternative methods of ventilation include high-frequency ventilation and airway pressure release ventilation.

Protection of the lungs may also be provided by pump-driven veno-venous extracorporeal membrane oxygenation (vv-ECMO), which improves both oxygenation and carbon dioxide removal, and allows a highly protective low tidal volume ventilation. Recently, the CESAR trial provides the first evidence that vv-ECMO is superior to conventional treatment in the most severe forms of ARDS. Moreover, a pumpless extracorporeal lung assist was developed using arterio-venous bypass, in which a gas exchange membrane is integrated (interventional lung assist). Interventional lung assist provides effective carbon dioxide elimination and a moderate improvement in oxygenation, and therefore allows a more protective mechanical ventilation.

Concerning pharmacological treatments of ALI/ARDS, inhaled nitric oxide has not been found to be particularly effective and there is no clear convincing data to support the

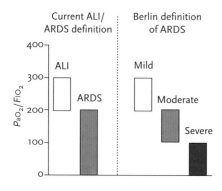

Figure 1. Current definition of ALI/ARDS and the Berlin definition of ARDS based on PaO$_2$/FIO$_2$ criteria.

widespread use of corticosteroids in both early and late phases of ALI/ARDS.

Finally, based on experimental models a series of molecular mechanisms offer innovative opportunities for cell or gene therapy. These need to be elaborated in human studies, however.

Further reading

- American Thoracic Society *et al.* (1999). International consensus conference in intensive care medicine: ventilator-associated lung injury in ARDS. *Am J Respir Crit Care Med*; 160: 2118–2124.
- The Acute Respiratory Distress Syndrome Network. (2000). Ventilation with lower tidal volumes as compared with traditional tidal volumes for acute lung injury and the acute respiratory distress sydrome. *N Engl J Med*; 342: 1301–1308.
- The ARDS Definition Task Force. (2012). Acute Respiratory Distress Syndrome. The Berlin Definition. *JAMA*; 307: 2526–2533.
- Dreyfuss D, *et al.* (1998). Ventilator-induced lung injury. Lessons from experimental studies. *Am J Respir Crit Care Med*; 157: 294–323.
- Gattinoni L, *et al.* (2005). The concept of 'baby lung'. *Intensive Care Med*; 31: 776–784.
- Marini JJ, *et al.* (2004). Ventilatory management of acute respiratory distress syndrome – a consensus of two. *Crit Care Med*; 32: 250–255.
- Matthay MA, *et al.* (2005). Acute lung injury and the acute respiratory distress syndrome: four decades of inquiry into pathogenesis and rational management. *Am J Respir Cell Mol Biol*; 33: 319–327.
- Peek GJ, *et al.* (2009). Efficacy and economic assessment of conventional ventilatory support *versus* extracorporeal membrane oxygenation for severe adult respiratory failure (CESAR): a multicentre randomised controlled trial. *Lancet*; 374: 1351–1363.
- Talmor D, *et al.* (2008). Mechanical ventilation guided by esophageal pressure in acute lung injury. *N Engl J Med*; 359: 2095–2104.

Respiratory failure

Nicolino Ambrosino and Fabio Guarracino

The respiratory system consists of two parts. The lung performs gas exchange and the pump ventilates the lung. The pump consists of the chest wall, including the respiratory muscles, and the respiratory controllers in the central nervous system (CNS) linked to respiratory muscles through spinal and peripheral nerves.

When respiratory failure ensues, the respiratory system fails in one or both of its gas exchange functions, i.e. oxygenation of mixed venous blood and/or elimination of carbon dioxide (fig. 1).

The diagnosis of respiratory failure is not clinical but based on arterial gas assessment: it is defined by a Pa_{O_2} <60 mmHg and/or Pa_{CO_2} >45 mmHg. These values are not rigid; they must serve as a general guide in combination with the patient's history and clinical evaluation. Respiratory failure may be acute, chronic or acute on chronic, with clinical presentation being quite different between these types.

Acute respiratory failure (ARF) may be life-threatening in clinical presentation, arterial blood gases and acid–base status; chronic respiratory failure is clinically indolent to unapparent, due to mechanisms of compensation for respiratory acidosis.

Respiratory failure due to lung diseases (e.g. pneumonia, acute lung injury, acute respiratory distress syndrome (ARDS), emphysema or interstitial lung disease) leads to hypoxaemia with normocapnia or even hypocapnia (type I respiratory failure).

Four pathophysiological mechanisms are responsible for hypoxaemic respiratory failure:

- ventilation/perfusion (V'/Q') ratio inequalities;
- shunt;
- diffusion impairment; and
- hypoventilation.

Hypoxaemia with hypoventilation is characterised by a normal alveolar–arterial oxygen difference, whereas disorders due to any of the other three mechanisms are

---

Key points

- Respiratory failure is failure of one or both of the respiratory system's gas exchange functions.

- It is diagnosed by arterial blood gas assessment.

- The clinical presentations of acute, chronic and acute-on-chronic respiratory failure can differ greatly.

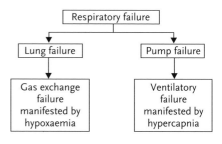

Figure 1. Types of respiratory failure. The respiratory system can be considered as consisting of two parts: the lung and the pump. Reproduced and modified from Roussos et al. (2003).

characterised by a widening of the alveolar–arterial gradient.

Abnormal desaturation of systemic venous blood in the face of extensive lung disease is an important mechanism of hypoxaemia.

Several non-COPD diseases may lead to hypoxaemic ARF, which is defined as a P_{aO_2}/inspiratory oxygen fraction (F_{IO_2}) ratio ⩽300 (table 1).

Hypoxaemia is treated with an increase in F_{IO_2} (the lower the V'/Q', the less the effect) and by recruiting airspaces with assisted ventilation. Airspace de-recruitment occurs when the transpulmonary pressure falls below the airspace collapsing or closing pressure, and when the transpulmonary pressure applied during inspiration fails to exceed the airspace opening pressure. Accordingly, airspace opening can be facilitated by increasing the transpulmonary pressure applied at the end of expiration (CPAP or positive end-expiratory pressure (PEEP)) and at the end of inspiration (inspiratory positive airway pressure).

Failure of the pump (e.g. neuromuscular diseases or opiate overdose) results in alveolar hypoventilation and hypercapnia with parallel hypoxaemia (type II respiratory failure).

In some diseases (e.g. COPD and cardiogenic pulmonary oedema), both conditions may coexist, hypoxaemia usually appearing first.

Hypercapnic respiratory failure may be the result of CNS depression, functional or mechanical defects of the chest wall, an imbalance of energy demands and supplies of the respiratory muscles, and/or adaptation of central controllers in order to prevent respiratory muscle injury and avoid or postpone fatigue (table 2). Hypercapnic respiratory failure may occur either acutely, insidiously or acutely upon a chronic carbon dioxide retention. In all of these conditions, the pathophysiological common mechanism

Table 1. The most common causes of hypoxaemic ARF

Cardiogenic pulmonary oedema
ARDS and ALI
Alveolar haemorrhage
Lobar pneumonia
Atelectasis
ALI: acute lung injury.

Table 2. Causes of acute hypercapnia

Decreased central drive
Drugs
CNS diseases
Altered neural and neuromuscular transmission
Spinal cord trauma
Myelitis
Tetanus
ALS
Poliomyelitis
Guillain–Barré syndrome
Myasthenia gravis
Organophosphate poisoning
Botulism
Muscle abnormalities
Muscular dystrophies
Disuse atrophy
Prematurity
Chest wall and pleural abnormalities
Acute hyperinflation
Chest wall trauma
Lung and airway diseases
Acute asthma
AECOPD
Cardiogenic and noncardiogenic oedema
Pneumonia
Upper airway obstruction
Bronchiectasis
Other causes
Sepsis
Circulatory shock
ALS: amyotrophic lateral sclerosis.

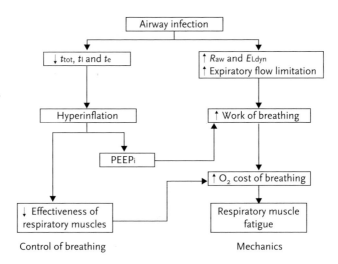

Figure 2. *Schematic representation of the sequence of responsible mechanisms that lead to acute-on-chronic respiratory failure in COPD patients.* t_{tot}: *total respiratory cycle time;* t_I: *inspiratory time;* t_E: *expiratory time;* R_{aw}: *airway resistance;* E_{Ldyn}: *dynamic elastance of the lung;* $PEEP_i$: *intrinsic PEEP. Reproduced and modified from Roussos et al. (2003).*

is reduced alveolar ventilation for a given value of carbon dioxide production.

Acute exacerbations of COPD (AECOPD) are periods of acute worsening that greatly affect the health status of patients, with an increase in hospital admission and mortality. Estimates of in-patient mortality range from 4% to 30% but patients admitted due to ARF experience a higher rate, in particular elderly patients with comorbidities (up to 50%) and those requiring intensive care unit admission (11–26%).

Many causes may potentially be involved in determining ARF during AECOPD, such as bronchial infections, bronchospasm, left ventricular failure, pneumonia, pneumothorax and thromboembolism. Acute-on-chronic respiratory failure due to AECOPD is characterised by the worsening of hypoxaemia, and a variable degree of hypercapnia and respiratory acidosis. The capacity of the patient to maintain acceptable indices of gas exchange during an AECOPD or the development of ARF depends both on the severity of the precipitating cause and on the degree of physiological dysfunction during the stable state, and the subsequent physiological reserve. Worsening of V'/Q' mismatching is probably the leading mechanism in the occurrence of the hypoxaemia by the enlargement of physiological dead space and the rise of wasted ventilation. The increase in airway resistance and the need for a higher V'_E may result in expiratory flow limitation, dynamic hyperinflation and related intrinsic PEEP with subsequent increased inspiratory threshold load and dysfunction of the respiratory muscles, which may lead to their fatigue. A rapid shallow breathing pattern may ensue in attempting to maintain adequate alveolar volume (V_A) when these additional resistive, elastic and inspiratory threshold loads are imposed on weakened respiratory muscles. Nevertheless, despite increased stimulation of the respiratory centres and large negative intrathoracic pressure swings, carbon dioxide retention and acidaemia may occur. Dyspnoea, right ventricular failure and encephalopathy characterise severe AECOPD complicated by ARF. Arterial pH reflects the acute worsening of V_A and, regardless of the chronic $P_{a}CO_2$ level, it represents the best marker of the ARF severity. Figure 2 shows a schematic representation of the sequence of responsible mechanisms that lead to acute-on-chronic respiratory failure in COPD patients.

Besides medical treatment of the underlying disease, oxygen supplementation and, eventually, ventilator assistance are appropriate therapy for acute-on-chronic respiratory failure. The goal of assisted ventilation (either invasive or noninvasive) during AECOPD is to unload the respiratory muscles and to reduce carbon dioxide by increasing V_A, thereby stabilising arterial pH until the underlying problem can be reversed.

Further reading

- Ambrosino N, *et al.* (1997). Advanced chronic obstructive pulmonary disease. *Monaldi Arch Chest Dis*; 52: 574–578.
- Ambrosino N, *et al.* (2008). Noninvasive positive pressure ventilation in the acute care setting: where are we? *Eur Respir J*; 31: 874–886.
- Calverley PMA (2003). Respiratory failure in chronic obstructive pulmonary disease. *Eur Respir J*; 22: Suppl. 47, 26s–30s.
- Donaldson GC, *et al.* (2006). COPD exacerbations – 1: epidemiology. *Thorax*; 61: 164–168.
- Koutsoukou A, *et al.* Acute and chronic respiratory failure: pathophysiology and mechanics. *In:* Fein AM, *et al.*, eds. Respiratory Emergencies. London, Hodder Arnold, 2006; pp.17–30.
- Patil SP, *et al.* (2003). In-hospital mortality following acute exacerbations of chronic obstructive pulmonary disease. *Arch Intern Med*; 163: 1180–1186.
- Plant PK, *et al.* (2003). Chronic obstructive pulmonary disease – 9: management of ventilatory failure in COPD. *Thorax*; 58: 537–542.
- Rossi A, *et al.* (1995). Intrinsic positive end-expiratory pressure (PEEPi). *Intensive Care Med*; 21: 522–536.
- Roussos C, *et al.* (2003). Respiratory failure. *Eur Respir J*; 22: Suppl. 47, 3s–14s.

NIV in acute respiratory failure

Anita K. Simonds

NIV is a key management tool in patients with acute hypercapnic respiratory failure, and meta-analyses confirm it markedly reduces mortality and morbidity in acidotic hypercapnic exacerbations of COPD (Lightowler *et al.*, 2003; Keenan *et al.*, 2003). NIV may also be used in other causes of acute ventilatory failure, such as neuro-muscular disease and bronchiectasis, but

these have not been subject to large randomised controlled trials (RCTs). A more limited role in hypoxaemic respiratory failure is described here. Levels of evidence to support NIV use in acute respiratory failure are shown in table 1.

NIV in acute exacerbations of COPD

NIV reduces endotracheal intubation rate, and decreases intensive care unit (ICU) and hospital duration of stay in acute acidotic exacerbations of COPD; therefore, it should be available in all respiratory centres that admit COPD patients with exacerbations. In a RCT (Plant *et al.*, 2000) carried out on a general respiratory ward NIV halved mortality from 20% to 10%, compared with standard COPD care. In patients already intubated, prompt extubation onto NIV reduces the duration of ventilation and ICU stay, and increases survival (tables 2 and 3). This is largely due to the fact that endotracheal tube-related nosocomial infections are reduced. Patients are also able to eat and drink normally and mobilise quicker. Most studies show improvements in arterial blood gases over the first hour of therapy and fall in carbon dioxide tension and respiratory rate have been shown to predict the success of therapy. Dyspnoea may decrease more rapidly with NIV than with conventional therapy (Bott *et al.*, 1993).

Indications NIV should be used in tachypnoeic, dyspnoeic acute COPD patients with a pH <7.35 and $PaCO_2$ >45 mmHg (6.0 kPa). In severe acidotic exacerbations (pH <7.30), the risk of NIV failure and need for intubation is higher but, providing patients are carefully monitored, NIV in a high-dependency unit or ICU may

Key points

- NIV is the gold standard therapy in acute dyspnoeic COPD patents with a pH <7.35 and $PaCO_2$ >45 mmHg (6.0 kPa) and has been shown to halve mortality in this situation.

- Patients with an acute exacerbation of COPD and pH <7.30 being treated with NIV should be managed in a high-dependency or ICU area as they are at risk of deterioration and requirement for invasive ventilation.

- In acute hypoxaemic respiratory failure, NIV and entrained oxygen therapy may be tried initially but if improvement in arterial blood gas tensions and dyspnoea do not occur rapidly, urgent consideration should be given to progression to invasive ventilation.

- A combination of NIV and cough assistance with insufflation–exsufflation may be helpful in neuromuscular patients with acute chest infection and reduced cough efficacy.

Table 1. *Levels of evidence for use of NIV in acute respiratory failure*

Strong evidence (level A)
Acute exacerbations of COPD
To facilitate weaning of COPD
Acute cardiogenic pulmonary oedema (*cf.* CPAP)
Immunocompromised patients
Reasonable evidence (level B)
Post-operative respiratory failure
'Do not intubate' patients
Upper airway obstruction, OSA, obesity, hypoventilation
CF, asthma
Case series/reports
Restrictive disorders
Acute respiratory distress syndrome

be tried first, as a failed trial of NIV leading to endotracheal intubation does not lead to higher mortality. Relative contraindications to NIV include mental obtundation due to severe hypercapnia, poor cough and bulbar function, upper airway obstruction, multiple comorbidities, and a very high severity score.

Practicalities of ventilator settings

Bilevel positive pressure devices are most commonly used together with full face mask to obviate leaks from the mouth. Inspiratory positive airway pressure (IPAP) is set to control $P_{a}CO_2$ and reduce the work of breathing; expiratory positive airway pressure (EPAP) is set to overcome episodes of upper airway obstruction and recruit alveoli. A back-up rate a few breaths below the patient's spontaneous breathing rate is usually chosen. Oxygen therapy should be entrained into the circuit as proximally as possible to the mask in order to titrate to the prescribed $S_{a}O_2$ (*e.g.* 88–92%). 'Intelligent' ventilators that add either an assured tidal volume or minute volume may be helpful in some patients but have not yet been shown to be superior to expert ventilator set-up. Careful attention to mask

fit is important as this helps encourage adherence to therapy. Before initiating NIV, advance planning should take place to clarify whether progression to endotracheal intubation is indicated and in accordance with the patient's wishes and best interests, in the event of NIV failure. An ERS Task Force survey (Nava *et al.*, 2007) showed that NIV was the ceiling of care in 31% of patients with acute exacerbations of COPD admitted to high-dependency units. As pointed out by Demoule *et al.* (2004), survival in patients with NIV as a ceiling of care is 50–60% for the episode, but one year after admission falls to 30%.

NIV in other causes of hypercapnic respiratory failure

NIV is used in acute hypercapnic exacerbations of CF and bronchiectasis. It may be helpful when combined with intensive physiotherapy and other airway clearance techniques (Demoule *et al.*, 2004) and, indeed, may allow physiotherapy sessions to be extended when these are carried out in patients simultaneously using NIV. In one study (Hodson *et al.*, 1991), NIV was used to bridge CF patients to transplantation.

NIV may also be used to reduce the work of breathing and improve arterial blood gas tensions in patients with respiratory muscle weakness due to neuromuscular conditions such as Duchenne muscular dystrophy, spinal muscular atrophy, myopathies and motor neurone disease. In these situations, if cough peak flow is $<160 \, L \cdot min^{-1}$, augmentation of secretion clearance with mechanical insufflation–exsufflation is likely to reduce the risk of intubation.

There are no RCTs of NIV in acute ventilatory failure in patients with obesity hypoventilation syndrome. However, nonrandomised comparisons suggest that NIV is more effective than CPAP in patients with significant hypercapnia and superior to endotracheal intubation in those without major comorbidity. EPAP should be titrated to control the OSA/hypopnoea component and IPAP to control $P_{a}CO_2$.

Table 2. Meta-analysis of NIV in acute COPD

Outcome	Patients n	Relative risk (95% CI)	Number needed to treat (95% CI)
Treatment failure	529	0.51 (0.38–0.67)	5 (4–7)
Mortality	523	0.41 (0.26–0.64)	8 (6–13)
Intubation	546	0.42 (0.31–0.59)	5 (4–7)
Complications	143	0.32 (0.18–0.56)	3 (2–4)

Reproduced and modified from Lightowler *et al.* (2003) with permission from the publisher.

NIV in acute hypoxaemic respiratory failure

Acute hypoxaemic respiratory failure (AHRF) occurs in a multiplicity of disorders including pneumonia, acute cardiogenic pulmonary oedema, acute lung injury, acute respiratory distress syndrome, and following immunosuppression, trauma and noxious gas inhalation. As the underlying pathophysiological mechanisms of ventilation–perfusion mismatch, shunt and diffusion difficulties differ from hypoventilation in acute ventilatory failure, one can predict that success rates with NIV will be lower. While ventilatory support is used to reduce the work of breathing, improve $PaCO_2$ control and recruit alveoli, it also buys time for other definitive therapies to take effect. Buying time may be more swiftly effective in, for example, acute pulmonary oedema, where diuretic and vasodilator therapy may be added, or pneumonia, where antibiotics can be introduced, compared with acute lung injury, where there is no specific therapy.

In several RCTs of patients with AHRF of mixed aetiology, NIV reduced the need for intubation, ICU stay and mortality (Wysocki *et al.*, 1995; Antonelli *et al.*, 1998). However, results are less clear-cut in pneumonia, where one study (Confalonieri *et al.*, 1999) showed a subgroup of patients with COPD and community-acquired pneumonia (CAP) experienced less intubation than the pneumonia group as a whole, and a further study (Jolliet *et al.*, 2001). suggests that those with severe CAP experienced a higher intubation rate and longer ICU stay. In highly infectious causes of pneumonia (*e.g.* severe acute respiratory syndrome and pandemic influenza), special measures are required when using NIV. Although NIV is categorised as an aerosol-generating procedure by some authorities, recent work (Simonds *et al.*, 2010) suggests it mainly generates large droplets (>10 μm in

Table 3. Meta-analysis of NIV in acute COPD

Outcome	Patients n	Weighted mean difference (95% CI)
Length of hospital stay days		
Trials in ICUs	138	-3.28 (-6.09– -0.67)
Trials in wards	408	-3.20 (-4.51– -1.89)
Total	546	-3.24 (-4.26– -2.06)
Respiratory rate at 1 h breaths·min^{-1}	380	-3.08 (-4.26– -1.89)
pH at 1 h	408	0.03 (0.02–0.04)
$PaCO_2$ at 1 h kPa	408	-0.40 (-0.78– -0.03)
PaO_2 at 1 h kPa	378	0.27 (-0.26–0.79)

Reproduced and modified from Lightowler *et al.* (2003) with permission from the publisher.

diameter). However, special precautions should be taken, including using personal protective equipment, a high-efficiency N95 microbial filter between the mask and exhalation valve, low pressures, and close attention to mask fit.

In acute cardiogenic pulmonary oedema, there have been several meta-analyses (Winck *et al.*, 2006; Masip *et al.*, 2005; Peter *et al.*, 2006) and a recent large RCT (Crane *et al.*, 2004). Results suggest that use of NIV and CPAP can reduce breathlessness and improve arterial blood gas tensions, and in the meta-analyses, NIV did reduce intubation; however, in the large RCT, which contained more patients than were included in the meta-analyses, there was no difference in mortality at 7 days between oxygen therapy, NIV and CPAP, and no differences in outcomes when NIV and CPAP were compared. A consensus is that medical therapy with nitrates is crucial first-line treatment, with the addition of CPAP in those with marked respiratory distress and NIV for those who are hypercapnic due to high work of breathing and/or concomitant COPD or neuromuscular disorder.

In all the causes of AHRF discussed here, NIV with entrained oxygen therapy may be tried initially but close monitoring is required and, if arterial blood gas tensions and dyspnoea are not relieved within the first hour of therapy or the patient's condition rapidly deteriorates, progression to use of invasive ventilation should be urgently considered.

Further reading

- Antonelli M, *et al.* (1998). A comparison of noninvasive positive-pressure ventilation and conventional mechanical ventilation in patients with acute respiratory failure. *N Engl J Med*; 339: 429–435.
- Bott J, *et al.* (1993). Randomised controlled trial of nasal ventilation in acute ventilatory failure due to chronic obstructive airways disease. *Lancet*; 341: 1555–1557.
- Confalonieri M, *et al.* (1999). Acute respiratory failure in patients with severe community-acquired pneumonia. A prospective randomized evaluation of non-invasive ventilation. *Am J Respir Crit Care Med*; 160: 1585–1591.
- Crane SD, *et al.* (2004). Randomised controlled comparison of continuous positive airways pressure, bilevel non-invasive ventilation, and standard treatment in emergency department patients with acute cardiogenic oedema. *Emerg Med J*; 21: 155–161.
- Demoule A, *et al.* (2006). Increased use of noninvasive ventilation in French intensive care units. *Intensive Care Med*; 32: 1747–1755.
- Fauroux B, *et al.* (2004). Setting of noninvasive pressure support in young patients with cystic fibrosis. *Eur Respir J*; 24: 624–630.
- Hodson ME, *et al.* (1991). Non-invasive mechanical ventilation for cystic fibrosis patients – a potential bridge to transplantation. *Eur Respir J*; 4: 524–527.
- Jolliet P, *et al.* (2001). Non-invasive pressure support ventilation in severe community-acquired pneumonia. *Intensive Care Med*; 27: 812–821.
- Keenan SP, *et al.* (2003). Which patients with an acute exacerbation of chronic obstructive pulmonary disease benefit from noninvasive positive pressure ventilation? A systematic review of the literature. *Ann Int Med*; 138: 861–870.
- Lightowler J, *et al.* (2003). Non-invasive positive pressure ventilation to treat respiratory failure resulting from exacerbations of chronic obstructive pulmonary disease: Cochrane systematic review and meta-analysis. *BMJ*; 326: 185.
- Masip J, *et al.* (2005). Noninvasive ventilation in acute cardiogenic pulmonary edema: systematic review and meta-analysis. *JAMA*; 294: 3124–3130.
- Nava S, *et al.* (2007). End of life decision-making in respiratory intermediate care units: a European survey. *Eur Respir J*; 30: 156–164.
- Peter JV, *et al.* (2006). Effect of non-invasive positive pressure ventilation (NIPPV) on mortality on patients with acute cardiogenic pulmonary oedema: a meta-analysis. *Lancet*; 367: 1155–1163.

- Plant PK, *et al.* (2000). Early use of noninvasive ventilation for acute exacerbations of chronic obstructive pulmonary disease on general respiratory wards: a multicentre randomised controlled trial. *Lancet*; 355: 1931–1935.
- Simonds AK, *et al.* (2010). Evaluation of droplet dispersion during non-invasive ventilation, oxygen therapy, nebuliser treatment and chest physiotherapy in clinical practice: implications for the management of pandemic influenza and other airborne infections. *Health Tech Assess*; 14: 131–172.
- Winck JC, *et al.* (2006). Efficacy and safety of non-invasive ventilation in the treatment of acute cardiogenic pulmonary oedema – a systematic review and meta-analysis. *Crit Care*; 10: R69.
- Wysocki M, *et al.* (1995). Noninvasive pressure support ventilation in patients with acute respiratory failure. A randomized comparison with conventional therapy. *Chest*; 107: 761–768.

Acute oxygen therapy

Anita K. Simonds

Acute oxygen therapy

Acute oxygen therapy is indicated to improve oxygen delivery in situations of cardiac and respiratory arrest, acute severe hypotension, low cardiac output states in the presence of metabolic acidosis and when SaO_2 is <90%. In respiratory conditions, oxygen therapy is prescribed to correct hypoxaemia, rather than to reduce breathlessness, and so should always be titrated to SaO_2 or blood gas measurements. In acutely ill patients, high-concentration oxygen therapy should be prescribed to correct SaO_2 to 94–98%. In those with hypercapnic respiratory failure or at risk of ventilatory decompensation (e.g. severe COPD, neuromuscular disease, obesity hypoventilation syndrome and chest wall disorders), a target SaO_2 of 88–92% should be the aim. If this cannot be achieved without progressive acidosis and hypercapnia, ventilatory support should be added. Indeed, in acute hypercapnic ventilatory failure, ventilatory support is usually the treatment of choice.

Key points

- Oxygen therapy is prescribed to correct hypoxaemia and should thus be titrated to SaO_2.

- In acutely hypoxaemic patients, oxygen should be delivered to correct SaO_2 to 94–98%.

- In those with hypercapnic respiratory failure or at risk of ventilatory decompensation, a target of SaO_2 of 88–92% should be the aim.

In emergency situations, oxygen therapy can be delivered by a high-concentration reservoir mask at a flow rate of 15 $L·min^{-1}$. In hypercapnic patients, 28% and 24% Venturi masks can be used. All acute patients require regular or continuous assessment by oximetry to ensure hypoxaemia has been corrected and the dose is still appropriate. Blood gas measurements are indicated if there is deterioration in SaO_2, features of carbon dioxide retention, such as drowsiness or flap, metabolic conditions, or low cardiac output state.

Long-term oxygen therapy

Chronic hypoxaemia occurs either due to ventilation–perfusion mismatch, alveolar hypoventilation or diffusion problems in chronic lung disease; in some conditions (e.g. COPD), all factors may be present. Long-term oxygen therapy (LTOT) is used to correct hypoxaemia diurnally and nocturnally in the majority of patients. In COPD, LTOT increases survival, reduces polycythaemia and, in some patients, may improve sleep quality and/or neuro-psychiatric symptoms. In individuals with chronic ventilatory failure due, for example,

Table 1. Assessment for LTOT

Consider assessment in
All patients with FEV_1 <30% predicted
Patients with cyanosis
Patients with polycythaemia
Patients with peripheral oedema
Patients with raised jugular venous pressure
Patients with SaO_2 on air ⩽92%

Table 2. Criteria for LTOT in steady-state patients

Chronic hypoxaemia (P_{aO_2} <7.3 kPa on air)
P_{aO_2} <8.0 kPa on air in addition to pulmonary hypertension, secondary polycythaemia, right heart failure or nocturnal desaturation

to chest wall disease, first-line treatment is assisted ventilation (*e.g.* NIV).

Patients should be assessed for LTOT in the presence of the features shown in table 1.

LTOT is prescribed for >15 h a day, *e.g. via* concentrator, to correct S_{aO_2} to ⩾90% in those patients listed in table 2.

Ambulatory oxygen therapy is added to correct hypoxaemia on exercise. In sedentary patients using LTOT, ambulatory oxygen is usually prescribed at the same flow rate as in daytime use. In active and mobile LTOT recipients and patients who desaturate on exertion but do not fulfil criteria for LTOT, optimum flow rates can be derived from a standard 6-min or shuttle walk, aiming to correct S_{aO_2} to >90%, reduce dyspnoea and increase exercise tolerance. There is no evidence to support the routine use of

short-burst oxygen therapy in COPD but it may be prescribed to palliate symptoms in end-stage disease. The evidence to support the use of short-burst oxygen in advanced cancer is minimal but it may be helpful in some individuals as part of a comprehensive supportive care plan.

Oxygen delivery systems

Oxygen can be delivered by oxygen cylinder, concentrator or liquid oxygen device. LTOT is more cost effectively delivered in the home by a concentrator. The advantages and disadvantages of the different systems are shown in table 3. LTOT patients should be regularly assessed (at least once a year) to check the suitability of flow rates, adherence to therapy and safety.

Table 3. Comparison of oxygen delivery devices

Delivery system	Advantages	Disadvantages
Compressed oxygen cylinder	Easily available No power required Economical in the short term	Frequent refills required High long-term cost Fire risk
Home concentrator	Permanent source No need for refills Economical in the long term	Power required Needs servicing and spare parts
Liquid oxygen	Small and portable No need for power	Refills required High cost Not widely available
Portable concentrator	Small and portable No need for refills Can be powered by car battery	High cost Limited battery life Cannot deliver high flow Pulsed or demand flow, so unsuitable for use during sleep F_{IO_2} during pulsed flow will vary according to pulse duration, trigger sensitivity and oxygen concentration delivered

Entrainment of oxygen therapy into NIV and CPAP circuits

In patients receiving acute or long-term therapy with NIV or CPAP, additional oxygen therapy may be required to correct SaO_2. Oxygen can be entrained into the circuit *via* a T-piece or through the mask. It is important to note that the more proximal the entrainment (*e.g.* ventilator side of exhalation port), the greater the inspiratory oxygen fraction (FIO_2) achieved. In addition, FIO_2 is likely to be lower than that achieved by delivering a similar oxygen flow rate without NIV/CPAP and difficult to predict accurately, as increases in inspiratory positive airway pressure may reduce FIO_2.

Further reading

- O'Driscoll BR, *et al.* (2008). British Thoracic Society Guideline for emergency oxygen use in adult patients. *Thorax*; 63: Suppl. 6, vi1–vi68.
- British Thoracic Society Working Group on Home Oxygen Services. Clinical component for home oxygen service in England and Wales. London, British Thoracic Society, 2006.
- Medical Research Council Working Party (1981). Long term domiciliary oxygen therapy in chronic hypoxic cor pulmonale complicating chronic bronchitis and emphysema. *Lancet*; 1: 681–685.
- Nocturnal Oxygen Therapy Trial Group (1980). Continuous or nocturnal oxygen therapy in hypoxaemic chronic obstructive lung disease, a clinical trial. *Ann Intern Med*; 93: 391–398.
- Thys F, *et al.* (2002). Determinant of FI,O_2 with oxygen supplementation during noninvasive two-level positive pressure ventilation. *Eur Respir J*; 19: 653–657.
- British Thoracic Society. Emergency Oxygen. www.brit-thoracic.org.uk/Clinical Information/EmergencyOxygen/tabid/219/ Default.aspx

Assessment for anaesthesia/surgery

Macé M. Schuurmans, Chris T. Bolliger[†] and Annette Boehler

Pre-operative assessment of pulmonary risk is important in order to identify patients at risk for peri-operative morbidity and mortality, to determine possible pre-operative interventions that are beneficial for outcome and to identify patients where surgery may be prohibitive.

Pre-operative evaluation for lung resection evaluates to what extent lung tissue can be resected without unacceptably increasing post-operative morbidity and mortality.

A careful history and physical examination are the most important tools for assessment of risk for post-operative pulmonary complications. Symptoms suggesting occult underlying lung disease (exercise intolerance, unexplained dyspnoea and cough) and the following risk factors for increased post-operative pulmonary complications need to be assessed.

Surgery-specific risk factors include:

- upper abdominal procedures
- aortic, thoracic, and head and neck surgery, including neurosurgery
- surgery lasting >3 h
- emergency procedures

Definite risk factors include:

- COPD
- CHF
- diminished general health status (American Society of Anesthesiologists (ASA) class $\geqslant 2$ (table 1))
- malnutrition (serum albumin $<35\,mg\cdot L^{-1}$)
- use of pancuronium as a neuromuscular blocker

> **Key points**
>
> - A careful history and physical examination is necessary to assess the risk of post-operative pulmonary complications
> - Pulmonary function testing is not routine except in the case of evaluation for lung resection
> - A number of strategies are available to reduce the risk of complications

Probable risk factors include:

- OSA
- general anaesthesia (when compared with spinal or epidural anaesthesia)
- pulmonary hypertension
- abnormal chest radiograph
- cigarette use within previous 8 weeks
- current upper respiratory tract infection

It is noteworthy that pulmonary function tests are not part of routine pre-operative assessment unless patients are being evaluated for lung resection (see later). Pulmonary function tests should also be performed in patients with unexplained dyspnoea or exercise intolerance, and when clinical evaluation cannot determine whether airflow obstruction has been optimally reduced in patients with previously diagnosed COPD or asthma. Well-controlled asthma (free of wheezing, and peak flows >80% of the predicted value or the patient's personal best) has been shown not to carry any added risk. Age and blood gases have no definitive role in the risk assessment when confounding issues such as comorbidities have been considered.

Table 1. ASA classification of pre-operative risk

ASA class	Systemic disturbance	PPC %	Mortality %
1	Healthy patient with no disease outside of the surgical process	1.2	<0.03
2	Mild-to-moderate systemic disease caused by the surgical condition or by other pathological processes, medically well controlled	5.4	0.2
3	Severe disease process that limits activity but is not incapacitating	11.4	1.2
4	Severe incapacitating disease process that is constant threat to life	10.9	8
5	Moribund patient not expected to survive 24 h with or without an operation	NA	34
E	Suffix to indicate emergency surgery for any class	Increased	Increased

PPC: post-operative pulmonary complications; NA: not applicable. Reproduced and modified from Koegelenberg *et al.* (2008) with permission from the publisher.

Patients with high risk (surgery-specific risk factor plus one or more definite risk factors) will benefit from the following strategies to reduce pulmonary complications.

Pre-operative interventions:

- smoking cessation for 8 weeks
- inhaled ipratropium or tiotropium for patients with clinically significant COPD
- inhaled β-agonists for symptomatic COPD and asthma patients
- pre-operative systemic glucocorticoids for COPD and asthma patients who are not optimised on inhalative treatment
- delay elective surgery if respiratory infection present
- antibiotics for patients with purulent sputum or change in sputum character
- inspiratory muscle training

Intraoperative interventions:

- choose alternative procedure lasting <3 h when possible (video-assisted thoracoscopic and laparoscopic procedures have ~1/10th the pulmonary complication rates of open procedures)
- minimise duration of anaesthesia
- regional anaesthesia (nerve block) in very high-risk patients
- avoid pancuronium

Post-operative interventions:

- deep-breathing exercises or incentive spirometry
- epidural analgesia instead of parenteral opioids, selective use of nasogastric tube if post-operative nausea or vomiting, inability to tolerate oral intake, or symptomatic abdominal distension

Cardiac evaluation:

- history, physical examination and resting ECG are frequently required for the initial estimate of the peri-operative cardiac risk
- the inability to climb two flights of stairs or run a short distance indicates poor functional capacity and is associated with an increased incidence of postoperative cardiac events
- the definitive assessment of cardiac risk should respect current guidelines for cardiologists

Pulmonary resection

Pulmonary resection is a high-risk procedure with a mortality of 2–3% for lobectomy and 4–6% for pneumonectomy in experienced centres. Clinical evaluation should focus on respiratory and cardiovascular pathology. Air flow limitation should be optimised before further evaluation, and cardiac disease identified and managed either medically or surgically. Initial pulmonary function evaluation should include at least FEV_1, FVC and $TLCO$. Values >80% predicted for FEV_1 and $TLCO$ are associated with an uncomplicated surgical course for resection up to a pneumonectomy. All other candidates should undergo a formal exercise test. Patients with a maximal oxygen uptake (V'_{O_2max}) >20 mL·kg^{-1}·min^{-1} (or >75% pred) tolerate pulmonary resection up to a pneumonectomy, and values >15 mL·kg^{-1}·min^{-1} are sufficient for lobectomy. Values <10 mL·kg^{-1}·min^{-1} are predictive of major post-operative complications and disability. Further evaluation according to a validated algorithm (fig. 1) necessitates the estimation of the relative contribution of the tissue earmarked for resection by means of the predicted post-operative (ppo) values of FEV_1, $TLCO$ and V'_{O_2max} ('split function'). The ppo values of these parameters are equal to their pre-operative values × (1-fractional contribution of the tissue earmarked for resection). There are three acceptable ways of estimating the relative functional contribution or split lung function:

1. anatomical calculation
2. quantitative CT
3. split perfusion scanning

Anatomical calculations are by far the simplest: the number of patent (or functional) segments that are due for resection is subtracted from the total number of segments (19) and this value is divided by 19 to give a fraction. The ppoFEV_1 is estimated to be equal to the pre-operative FEV_1 × ((19-patent segments removed)/19). Anatomical calculations have been shown to overestimate the functional loss so that patients who are deemed operable by anatomical calculations will generally not require radiological calculations.

Calculated ppo values based on lung perfusion scans (with technetium-99m-labelled macroaggregates) have been shown to correlate best with actual post-operative values. Densitometric calculations on the basis of CT are marginally less accurate than perfusion scans. The advantage of this method is the availability of the information,

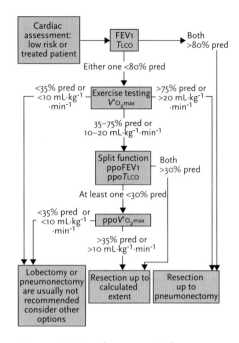

Figure 1. Algorithm for assessment of cardiopulmonary reserve before lung resection in lung cancer patients. Reproduced and modified from Brunelli et al. (2009).

as most lung resection candidates invariably have a pre-operative chest CT and modern software simplifies the three-dimensional reconstruction for the calculation of the relative volume of lung to be resected.

Simple stair climbing as a low-cost alternative to assess exercise capacity and operative risk is increasingly being used. A number of recent studies have shown that the ability to climb an elevation >22 m is correlated with a favourable surgical outcome for lung resection surgery. Patients unable to reach this elevation then require more sophisticated ergometric evaluation. Adding a time component to the evaluation of the stair climbing test appears to quantify the overall exercise performance more precisely: data from one recent study assessing additionally speed of ascent during stair climbing showed that patients reaching or passing the 20-m elevation mark within 80 s all had formal exercise tests permitting resection up to the extent of a pneumonectomy.

Lung volume reduction surgery for end-stage emphysema has partly redefined the limits of lung resection. Traditional cut-off limits are too prohibitive for these patients, as resection of largely nonfunctional emphysematous tissue leads to improved lung mechanics, improving the overall outcome. The latter is also partly true for moderate-to-severe COPD patients undergoing surgery for lung cancer. Patients with either ppoFEV1 or ppoTLCO <40% pred, or both parameters between 30% and 40% pred can undergo extensive resections such as lobectomy or even pneumonectomy with reasonable safety (mortality of 13.5%) if they have a ppo$V'O_2$max of >10 mL·kg^{-1}·min^{-1}. Survival following this strategy appears to be superior than for the nonsurgical strategy.

Further reading

- Bernasconi M, et al. (2012). Speed of ascent during stair climbing identifies operable lung resection candidates. Respiration; 84: 117–122.
- Bolliger CT, et al. (2002). Prediction of functional reserves after lung resection: comparison between quantitative computed tomography, scintigraphy, and anatomy. Respiration; 69: 482–489.
- Brunelli A, et al. (2009). ERS/ESTS clinical guidelines on fitness or radical therapy in lung cancer patients (surgery and chemoradiotherapy). Eur Respir J; 34: 17–41.
- Koegelenberg CFN, et al. Preoperative pulmonary evaluation. In: Abert RK et al., eds. Clinical Respiratory Medicine. 3rd Edn. Philadelphia, Elsevier, 2008.
- Puente-Maestú L, et al. (2011). Early and long-term validation of an algorithm assessing fitness for surgery in patients with postoperative FEV1 and diffusing capacity of the lung for carbon monoxide < 40%. Chest; 139: 1430–1438.
- Salati M, et al. (2012). Preoperative assessment of patients for lung cancer surgery. Curr Opin Pulm Med; 18: 289–294.
- Task Force for Preoperative Cardiac Risk Assessment and Perioperative Cardiac Management in Non-cardiac Surgery, et al. (2009). Guidelines for pre-operative cardiac risk assessment and perioperative cardiac management in non-cardiac surgery. Eur Heart J; 30: 2769–2812.
- von Groote-Bidlingmaier F, et al. (2011). Functional evaluation before lung resection. Clin Chest Med; 32: 773–782.

Long-term ventilation

Anita K. Simonds

Definition and prevalence

Long-term ventilation (LTV) is a term usually used to describe individuals using either NIV or tracheostomy-delivered ventilation for >3 months on a daily basis in the user's home or a long-term care facility. Lloyd-Owen *et al.* (2005) showed a prevalence rate of 6.6 per 100 000 of the population in Europe receiving LTV but there were widely varying practices ranging from a prevalence rate of 17 per 100 000 in France to <1 per 100 000 in Poland. Rates in Denmark, Germany, Spain, the UK and Italy were 9.6, 6.5, 4.1 and 3.9 per 100 000 respectively. Numbers will have grown since 2005, but these data exclude OSA patients using CPAP. There was also a north–south divide with more neuromuscular and chest wall patients receiving LTV in northern Europe and more chronic lung disease patients using LTV in southern Europe. As the prevalence of these conditions does not vary substantially, differences in the pattern of LTV are likely to be historical rather than evidence based.

Key points

- LTV is defined by the requirement for daily ventilatory support for >3 months.

- The majority of LTV recipients use NIV *via* pressure pre-set ventilators.

- NIV should be started for symptomatic nocturnal hypoventilation or daytime hypercapnia in restrictive disorders.

- NIV extends survival in MND/amyotrophic lateral sclerosis patients.

Pathophysiology

Chronic ventilatory decompensation occurs when the load placed on the respiratory system outstrips its capacity. This occurs in restrictive disorders, such as chest wall and neuromuscular disease, and in chronic lung diseases, such as COPD, CF and bronchiectasis. Disorders of ventilatory drive are less common but LTV is required in patients with congenital central hypoventilation syndrome (CCHS) or other acquired causes of failure of ventilatory drive, such as brain stem cerebrovascular or cervical spinal cord injury events. The clinical course in many patients is punctuated by episodes of acute-on-chronic ventilator failure precipitated by chest infections (*e.g.* COPD and CF). In others, there is a clear-cut vicious cycle of decline. For example, in chest wall or neuromuscular disease, small lung volumes lead to initially nocturnal hypoventilation and, ultimately, diurnal ventilatory failure if sleep-disordered breathing is not addressed.

Types of LTV

The greatest growth in LTV over the last two decades has been in the use of home NIV. This is virtually all mask ventilation or *via* oral/nasal interface, as very few patients receive domiciliary negative pressure ventilation (*e.g. via* cuirass or iron lung). The indications for tracheostomy ventilation are bulbar weakness leading to aspiration, near 24-h ventilator dependence, upper airway lesions, difficulties with NIV, neonatal age range and patient preference.

Ventilators

A survey of LTV in Europe (Lloyd-Owen *et al.*, 2005) showed nearly all patients were using positive pressure ventilators (mostly in pressure support mode) with <1% using volume ventilators. Dual-mode ventilators are obtainable but, perhaps not surprisingly, volume ventilators were most commonly used in neuromuscular and chest wall patients, and least frequently used in those with lung disease (COPD/ bronchiectasis). The choice of ventilatory mode and settings should match the underlying pathophysiology and be carefully titrated to the patient. Further considerations include the age and size of the patient, degree of ventilator dependency, and need for oxygen therapy. Humidification is required for nearly all tracheostomy patients and is indicated in some patients using long-term NIV (e.g. those with recurrent or viscid secretions).

The ventilator care plan should adapt to the patient, as patients with progressive disorders will become more ventilator dependent over time and require ventilatory support during the day, and/or progress from NIV to tracheostomy ventilation if bulbar function worsens; and in children, total ventilatory requirements will change with growth.

Tracheostomy

The choice of tracheostomy tube or cannula is dictated by:

- need for mechanical ventilation
- ability of the patient to defend the lower airway (adequate cough and bulbar function)
- temporary or permanent placement
- neck size and anatomy of the patient

The aim is to protect the airway and optimise ventilation while preserving speech and swallowing function, and minimising complications related to the tracheostomy tube such as sputum plugging, tracheal stenosis and pressure necrosis resulting in haemorrhage. Cuffed tracheostomy tubes may reduce aspiration risk in adults but cuff pressure should be monitored so that it does not exceed 25 mmHg. Fenestrated tubes have a window in the posterior curved region and a removable inner tube. The fenestration aids voice production and the

inner tube can be removed for cleaning, which can be helpful in weaning patients, but long-term use without the inner tube can be complicated by granuloma formation. In any patient with a long-term tracheostomy, correct size and placement, and regular inspection and bronchoscopy are recommended as follow-up.

Chest wall disorders

This group includes patients with scoliosis, old tuberculous lung disease, thoracoplasty and chest wall fibrosis. Patients with scoliosis at high risk of ventilatory decompensation are shown in table 1.

Neuromuscular disease

Neuromuscular disorders can be grouped into those in which the underlying condition is relatively static (e.g. previous poliomyelitis and phrenic nerve injury due to brachial neuralgia), those that are slowly progressive (e.g. Duchenne muscular dystrophy (DMD) and other myopathies) and those that are rapidly progressive (e.g. motor neurone disease and amyotrophic lateral sclerosis). Management plans should therefore take into account the natural history of the condition as well as current ventilator needs.

Most neuromuscular patients have normal lungs apart from occasional atelectasis, so they are relatively easy to ventilate with low pressures; back-up rates are usually required due to profound hypoventilation during REM (rapid eye movement) sleep. Careful consideration of the interface is required as individuals may not be able to affix a mask easily due to weak muscles of the upper

Table 1. Risk factors for ventilatory decompensation in scoliosis

Congenital or early-onset scoliosis
Thoracic curve >100°
Curve involves high thoracic and cervical vertebrae
Paralytic aetiology e.g. due to neuromuscular weakness
Vital capacity <50% predicted
Comorbidity e.g. COPD, morbid obesity

limb, and mid-facial hypoplasia may occur in children and young patients who start NIV before facial skeletal growth is complete. Near-100% 5-year survival has been reported in previous polio patients receiving NIV. In DMD patients, the use of NIV has extended median survival from 18 to 29 years (Eagle *et al.*, 2002; Simonds, 2006) and many young males with DMD are now surviving into their 30s and 40s.

In severe conditions such as Type 1 spinal muscular atrophy, where survival is poor, NIV may be used with the goal of palliating symptoms and allowing home discharge, rather than extending life expectancy.

Bourke *et al.* (2006) showed in a randomised trial of NIV in motor neurone disease (MND) (amyotrophic lateral sclerosis) that overall survival increased by ~7 months. This improvement was predominantly seen in patients with mild-to-moderate bulbar weakness and quality of life improvements were mainly seen in this group too. However, sleep-related symptoms improved, even in patients with severe bulbar disease. Although it is often reported that NIV cannot be used in MND patients with severe bulbar disease, this belief is overplayed, and a trial is recommended in all MND patients who wish to try NIV. Tracheostomy ventilation may be the only solution to aspiration pneumonia but in some bulbar patients, the combination of NIV, a cough assist device and percutaneous gastrostomy (PEG) feeding works as effectively.

Ventilatory support should be initiated in patients once daytime hypercapnia or symptomatic nocturnal hypoventilation is identified.

Spinal cord injury

Individuals with high spinal cord injury or bulbar lesions with no independent ventilatory capacity and an inability to clear secretions will usually require tracheostomy ventilation, but a proportion of quadriplegic patients with minimal ventilatory reserve may be managed by a combination of NIV and cough assist devices. As in other neuromuscular conditions, some patients may be able to augment spontaneous vital capacity by glossopharyngeal 'frog' breathing. Phrenic nerve pacing has a role in high spinal cord injury patients and central hypoventilation syndromes, but may need to be supplemented with other forms of ventilatory support and can only be effective if phrenic nerve integrity is maintained.

Central hypoventilation

CCHS affects ~1 in 200 000 and is due to mutations in the *PHOX2B* gene. More severe cases experience life-threatening episodes of apnoea or hypoventilation in the first months of life, complicated by other features of autonomic dysregulation such as cardiac arrhythmias or Hirschsprung's disease. In early infancy, use of ventilation *via* tracheostomy is recommended to optimise oxygenation and cognitive function. Transition to NIV may be possible later in childhood. Diaphragm pacing has been used in some CCHS children but often has to be combined with invasive ventilation or NIV. Other genetic syndromes associated with hypoventilation include Arnold–Chiari malformation and inborn errors of metabolism such as pyruvate dehydrogenase deficiency.

The obesity hypoventilation syndrome is a form of acquired hypoventilation and is defined by daytime PaCO$_2$ >45 mmHg (6.0 kPa) in the presence of a BMI >30 kg·m^{-2}. Obesity hypoventilation patients with mild hypercapnia (PaCO$_2$ <53 mmHg) with or without OSA may be successfully managed with CPAP therapy. More marked hypercapnia, acute acidotic ventilatory decompensation or failure to control sleep-disordered breathing with CPAP are indications for nocturnal NIV (Veale, 2008).

Chronic obstructive pulmonary disease

Although numerous selected series of hypercapnic COPD patients have shown physiological advantages of LTV, there is a dearth of adequately powered randomised controlled trials. Several are currently in progress. Meanwhile, McEvoy *et al.* (2009) randomised 144 COPD patients with FEV$_1$ <1.5 L or 50% predicted and stable PaCO$_2$

Table 2. *Discharge planning for home ventilator patients*

Stability and motivation of patient

Competency training of patient, family and carers

Arrangements for servicing and emergency back-up of ventilator equipment, including suction machines, cough assist devices and oxygen concentrator if required

Supply of disposables *e.g.* masks, suction catheters, ventilator circuits, filters

Liaison with all members of care team (home and hospital)

Follow-up assessments/appointments planned

Written guides to management of common problems *e.g.* chest infection

Suitable modifications to home environment

Risk management plan *e.g.* battery packs to cover power failure, smaller size tracheostomy tube if difficulties with tube replacement, low and high pressure and disconnection alarms

Anticipatory care plan detailing agreed actions in event of chest infection, hospital admission, and preferences regarding resuscitation status and intensive care unit admission

>45 mmHg to receive NIV plus long-term oxygen therapy (LTOT) or LTOT alone. The NIV group had an improvement in survival using an adjusted Cox model but there were no gains in quality of life. It may be that particular subgroups of COPD patients – those with less emphysema and a greater degree of nocturnal hypoventilation, and those with recurrent hypercapnic exacerbations or additional OSA – benefit most, but this remains to be seen. Pragmatically, current indications for LTV in COPD are chronic symptomatic hypercapnia, poor tolerance of LTOT leading to worsening carbon dioxide retention and recurrent admissions for acute-on-chronic hypercapnic respiratory failure responding to acute NIV.

There is a debate on the use of a high-intensity ventilatory approach in COPD patients (high pressure and controlled ventilation). This has been shown to reduce hypercapnia and improve exercise ability (Windisch *et al.*, 2005) but may be less easy to tolerate than lower pressures for some patients.

CF and bronchiectasis

Nocturnal NIV can reduce symptoms, including breathlessness, and improve nocturnal oxygenation, sleep quality, peak exercise level and quality of life in chronically hypercapnic adult patients with CF (Young

et al., 2008). Fauroux *et al.* (2008) has also shown stabilisation of lung function in younger CF patients treated for 1 year with nocturnal NIV. Use during physiotherapy can also prove beneficial. Effects on survival are less clear, other than in the situation where NIV is used to 'bridge' patients to transplantation.

Case–control studies of patients with bronchiectasis show improvements in oxygenation compared to LTOT alone and, in some groups, the frequency of infective exacerbations may be reduced. Both CF and idiopathic bronchiectasis patients experience ventilation/perfusion mismatch and diffusion problems, and so are likely to require a combination of NIV and LTOT, judged by overnight monitoring of Sa_{O_2} and Pa_{CO_2}.

Discharge planning and follow-up

Planning for discharge in patients receiving tracheostomy ventilation is necessarily more complex than in those using NIV. The key components of a successful discharge plan are listed in table 2.

Further reading

- Bourke SC, *et al.* (2006). Effects of non-invasive ventilation on survival and quality of life in patients with amyotrophic lateral sclerosis: a randomised controlled trial. *Lancet Neurol*; 5: 140–147.

- Eagle M, *et al.* (2002). Survival in Duchenne muscular dystrophy: improvements in life expectancy since 1967 and the impact of home nocturnal ventilation. *Neuromusc Disord*; 12: 926–969.
- Fauroux B, *et al.* (2008). Long-term non-invasive ventilation in patients with cystic fibrosis. *Respiration*; 72: 168–174.
- Lloyd-Owen SJ, *et al.* (2005). Patterns of home mechanical use in Europe: results from the Eurovent survey. *Eur Respir J*; 25: 1025–1031.
- McEvoy RD, *et al.* (2009). Nocturnal non-invasive ventilation in stable COPD: a randomised controlled trial. *Thorax*; 64: 561–566.
- Simonds AK (2006). Recent advances in respiratory care for neuromuscular disease. *Chest*; 130: 1879–1786.
- Veale D (2008). Respiratory complications of obesity. *Breathe*; 4: 210–223.
- Windisch W, *et al.* (2005). Outcome of patients with stable COPD receiving controlled non-invasive positive pressure ventilation aimed at maximal reduction of $Pa\text{CO}_2$. *Chest*; 128: 657–662.
- Young AC, *et al.* (2008). Randomised placebo controlled trial of non-invasive ventilation for hypercapnia in cystic fibrosis. *Thorax*; 63: 72–77.

Microbiology testing and interpretation

Magareta Ieven

In primary care, microbiological work-up in respiratory infections is primarily meant as an epidemiological investigation in order to guide future empiric antimicrobial policies. Hardly any study has shown that initial microbiological studies in primary care affect the outcome of respiratory infections. Therefore, recent guidelines confirm that microbiological tests such as Gram stains and cultures are not recommended as routine tests in the primary care setting. Nevertheless, an aetiological diagnosis, of both bacteria and viruses and mixtures of these in community-acquired pneumonia (CAP) or lower respiratory tract infections (LRTIs), may be helpful in guiding

---

Key points

For the aetiological diagnosis of LRTIs:

- Gram stain and culture of sputum are valuable in hospitalised patients, if of good quality, for the microbiological diagnosis of LRTI caused by *Streptococcus pneumoniae* or *Haemophilus influenzae*,

- Urinary antigen detection is a very helpful and rapid test for the diagnosis of pneumococcal or *Legionella* infections,

- Serology is rarely helpful in the management of the individual patient with LRTI,

- Molecular tests for the detection of respiratory viruses and atypical pathogens in specific patient populations are desirable.

---

treatment, particularly in the more severely ill or hospitalised patients. Diagnostic testing should not lead to delays in initiation of therapy, however. Even with extensive diagnostic testing, a specific aetiology is usually identified in only half of all patients, generally at least 1–2 days after the clinical diagnosis is made. With the advent of recently developed rapid techniques, such as immunochromatographic, urinary antigen and particularly nucleic acid amplification (NAA) tests, that produce results within 30 min or 4–5 h, microbiological information is becoming clinically useful (table 1).

Conventional culture techniques

Blood culture For the diagnosis of pneumonia, blood cultures have a very high specificity but are positive in only about 10–20% of untreated cases. In some studies, a direct correlation has been found between the severity of pneumonia (based on the Fine Severity Index) and blood culture positivity rate. Two sets of blood cultures should be performed in all patients with CAP who require hospitalisation; they should be obtained as early as possible in the disease and before any antibiotic treatment is started. If blood cultures are positive, *Streptococcus pneumoniae* is identified in ~60% and *Haemophilus influenzae* in 2–13%. Despite their low sensitivity, blood cultures in CAP are considered the gold standard for diagnosis of pneumonia because the organisms are recovered from a normally sterile source. Results may be available after 24–48 h.

Sputum Gram stain and culture The most frequently submitted specimen in cases of LRTI and, more specifically, in pneumonia is sputum.

183

Table 1. Diagnostic approach for the most common specific agents in LRTIs

Pathogen	Specimen	Rapid tests	Conventional tests	Comments
Streptococcus pneumoniae	Blood		Blood culture	Positive in 4–18% of cases when collected within 4 days
	Sputum	Gram stain	Culture	Only purulent samples acceptable; can be obtained in 35–40% of patients; informative if >90% Gram positive, diplococcic most relevant if Gram stain is informative
	BAL, PSB	Gram stain	Culture	Quantitative cultures
	Pleural exudates, TNA	Gram stain	Culture	Very specific; only considered if less invasive methods nondiagnostic
	Urine	Antigen test		Sensitivity 50–80% of bacteraemic cases; lacks specificity in children; more evaluation necessary
Haemophilus influenzae	Blood		Blood culture	Less frequently positive than for *S. pneumoniae*
	Respiratory specimens	Gram stain	Culture	
Legionella spp.	Urine	Antigen test		Sensitivity 66–95%
	Respiratory specimens	NAA	Culture	Culture on appropriate media; late results
	Serum		IgM and IgG serology	Acute and convalescent specimens; retrospective diagnosis
Chlamydophila pneumoniae, Mycoplasma pneumoniae	Respiratory specimens	NAA	Culture	Culture on appropriate medium; low sensitivity
	Serum		IgM and IgG serology	Acute and convalescent specimens; lack of sensitivity, specificity; not appropriate for individual patient management; retrospective results
Respiratory viruses	Respiratory specimens	Direct antigen tests, NAA	Virus isolation	Requirement for appropriate infrastructure; isolation less sensitive than NAA

NAA tests are not generally available yet and are not US Food and Drug Administration approved. BAL: bronchoalveolar lavage; PSB: protected specimen brush; TNA: transthoracic needle aspiration.

184

To be of value for microbial diagnosis and early guidance of therapy, sputum specimens must be representative of lower respiratory secretions and must be interpreted according to strict criteria by an experienced observer. The most widely used method to assess acceptability in this regard is based on cytological criteria. The specimen should therefore be screened by microscopic examination for the relative number of polymorphonuclear cells and squamous epithelial cells in a lower power (10×) field. Invalid specimens (⩾10 squamous epithelial cells and ⩽25 polymorphonuclear cells per field) should not be examined further. It may be difficult to obtain good-quality, purulent sputum. Many LRTI or pneumonia patients, particularly older ones, do not produce sputum. Satisfactory sputum specimens can be obtained in 32–55% of patients.

Large studies on the diagnostic value of Gram staining in primary care patients are lacking but some hospital-based studies show that in good-quality Gram-stained sputum, the presence of a single or a preponderant morphotype of bacteria (⩾90%) may be diagnostic. This is based on correspondence with the organisms recovered from blood cultures obtained in parallel, which are the gold standard. The study by Anevlavis *et al.* (2009) is the first reporting information concerning operating characteristics and the diagnostic value of sputum Gram staining in 1390 patients with bacteraemic CAP. The sensitivity of sputum Gram stain was 82% for pneumococcal pneumonia and 79% for *H. influenzae* pneumonia, with specificities ranging from 93% to 96%. Data from this study suggest that a properly collected and read Gram stain provides a simple, readily available, rapid and inexpensive test result, and can be a dependable test for the early aetiological diagnosis of bacterial pneumonia. Sputum with a mixed flora in the Gram stain has no diagnostic value. The sputum Gram stain is therefore valuable in guiding the processing and interpretation of sputum cultures.

The sensitivity and specificity of sputum cultures are reduced by contamination with flora colonising the upper respiratory tract.

The value of sputum cultures in establishing a bacterial cause of LRTI depends on how the specimens are collected and processed. The reported yield of sputum cultures has varied widely, from <20% for outpatients to >90% for hospitalised patients. The sputum Gram stain is valuable in guiding the processing and interpretation of sputum cultures. Sputum culture results are most convincing when the organism(s) isolated in culture are compatible with the morphology of the organisms present in the Gram stain. In the absence of an informative Gram stain, the predictive value of sputum culture is very low.

Rapid antigen tests

Urinary antigen tests The *S. pneumoniae* urinary antigen test has been shown to have a sensitivity of 65–100% and a specificity of >90% in adult CAP; however, weak positive results should be interpreted with caution. There is a relationship between the degree of *S. pneumoniae* urinary antigen test positivity and the pneumonia severity index. Therefore, the test could be reserved for high-risk patients for whom conclusive results of a sputum Gram stain are unavailable.

The urinary antigen test may also be applied to pleural fluid and serum samples with a sensitivity of 50% in bacteraemic patients and 40% in nonbacteraemic patients. In a retrospective study, a rapid immunochromatographic test (ICT) was performed on pleural fluid samples from 34 patients with pneumonia due to *S. pneumoniae*, and a number of control patients with effusions of non-pneumococcal origin or pneumonia of unknown aetiology. Data on blood cultures, pleural fluid cultures and urinary antigen tests were recorded. The ICT result was positive in 70.6% with pneumococcal pneumonia and negative in 93.3% of patients without pneumococcal pneumonia. The sensitivity of the pleural ICT is higher than that obtained for blood and pleural fluid cultures, but lower than the detection of pneumococcal antigen in urine samples. However, in some patients with pneumococcal pneumonia and a negative urinary antigen test result, a positive pleural fluid antigen test was detected. The ICT performed on pleural fluid samples therefore augments the standard diagnostic methods of blood and pleural fluid cultures, even in the case of prior antibiotic therapy, and enhances the urinary antigen assay. Vaccination does not result in a positive urinary antigen test. The immuno-chromatographic urinary antigen test for S. pneumoniae is therefore useful for the aetiological diagnosis of severe CAP, especially for patients without demon-strative results of a sputum Gram stain.

Urinary antigen detection is currently the most helpful rapid test for the diagnosis of a Legionella pneumophila serogroup 1 infection. Although >50 Legionella spp. have been identified, >90% of the isolates associated with legionnaires' disease are L. pneumophila and up to 84% of these are L. pneumophila serogroup 1. Several test formats have been developed, the enzyme immunoassay (EIA) format being more suited to test a larger number of specimens and taking a few hours to complete. The immunochromatographic format is better suited for single specimens and produces a result within minutes. These tests are particularly useful since culture of Legionella spp. is slow and takes 3–4 days. L. pneumophila serogroup 1 urinary antigen detection is frequently the first positive laboratory test in this infection. The sensitivity of the tests varies between 65% and 70% in unconcentrated urine and increases significantly after concentration of the specimen. In L. pneumophila infection, there is also a relationship between the degree of positivity of the urinary antigen test and the severity of disease: for patients with mild legionnaires' disease, test sensitivities range from only 40% to 50%, whereas for patients with severe legionnaires' disease who need immediate special medical care, sensitivities reach 88–100%.

Antigen tests on pharyngeal specimens A variety of antigen tests have been evaluated on respiratory specimens. During recent years, a considerable number of previously unknown respiratory viral agents have been discovered whose *in vitro* culture is very slow or even unrealised: human metapneumovirus, the novel coronaviruses NL63 and HKU1, and human bocavirus. Antigens of the many common respiratory viruses – influenza virus, respiratory syncytial virus (RSV), adenovirus and parainfluenza viruses – can be detected by direct immunofluorescence (DIF) or by commercially available EIAs. The sensitivities of these tests vary from 50% to >90% depending on the virus, the patient population studied and the sampling method used. For respiratory infections due to viruses, the optimal specimen is the nasopharyngeal aspirate. Alternatively, oro- or nasopharyngeal swabs can be obtained. A few studies comparing the respective efficacies of two structurally different swabs have been performed and conclude that nylon flocked swabs appear to be more efficient than rayon swabs, yielding significantly more total respiratory epithelial cells and more infected respiratory epithelial cells, which is likely to have a greater effect on diagnostic sensitivity both for antigen- and for PCR-based tests. For the detection of influenza virus infections, the sensitivity of immunofluorescence can be increased by inoculation of appropriate cells with clinical sample followed by immunofluorescence after 48 h. Several common respiratory viruses can be detected simultaneously by the use of pooled monoclonal antibodies. The sensitivity and positive predictive value of the DIF test is lower in adults and older people than in children. Rapid methods for the detection of influenza virus are of particular interest because of the availability of antiviral agents that must be given within 48 h after onset of symptoms.

Serology

Efforts have been made to diagnose infections caused by slowly growing or difficult-to-grow organisms by serology, particularly *Mycoplasma pneumoniae*, *Chlamydophila pneumoniae*, *Legionella* infections and respiratory viruses. It should be remembered that the most reliable serologic evidence of an ongoing infection is based on a four-fold increase in the titre of IgG (or IgG and IgM) antibodies during the evolution of the disease episode based on two serum samples collected at an interval of 14–21 days or longer, and/or the appearance of IgM antibodies during the evolution of the disease. IgM tests are usually less sensitive and specific than four-fold changes in antibody titres between paired specimens separated by several weeks. Solitary high IgG titres have no diagnostic meaning for an acute infection since the moment of the seroconversion is unknown and necessarily took place sometime before the illness under observation started.

The sensitivity and specificity of serological tests are related to the antigen used. For *M. pneumoniae* and *C. pneumoniae*, a great number of antigen preparations have been proposed: whole organisms, protein fractions, glycoprotein fractions and recombinant antigens. Several studies illustrate a lack of standardisation of antigens of *M. pneumoniae*.

For a number of respiratory agents, a variety of tests are available commercially. Some assays lack both sensitivity and specificity, emphasising the need for more validation and quality control.

IgM antibodies against *M. pneumoniae* require up to 1 week to reach diagnostic titres, and sometimes much longer. Anti-*M. pneumoniae* IgM antibodies can be detected in 7–25% (depending on the test applied) of acute sera and IgG antibodies in 41–63% of convalescent sera (depending on the timing of the second sample), illustrating the low incidence of IgM antibodies in the acute-phase serum specimens and importance of the delay between the two serum samples. Since IgM detection in the acute phase shows a moderate sensitivity, provided a specific test is used, further research is needed to better define the role of IgM serology: a combination of IgM antibody detection and PCR may be the most sensitive approach for early diagnosis of *M. pneumoniae* infections, especially in symptomatic children. It is critically important for current and future investigators to recognise the urgent need for the adoption of a more unified and consistent diagnostic approach. A common set of recommendations should be developed.

Legionella antibody tests also have a sensitivity of only 61–64%, depending on the assay applied, and do not substantially improve the diagnosis of legionellosis. The acute antibody test for *Legionella* in legionnaires' disease is usually negative or demonstrates very low titres. As for other aetiologies, high titres of IgG and/or IgM (above a certain threshold), present early during the disease, have been interpreted as diagnostic, but at least one study showed that this titre had a very low positive predictive value.

For respiratory viral infections, such as for influenza and RSV, a significant or four-fold IgG antibody increase is detected by EIA in approximately 80–90% of patients at only 20–30 days after the onset of disease.

The serological measurement of specific antibody responses mostly cannot offer an early diagnosis and, therefore, has limited application for an aetiological diagnosis and the routine management of the individual patient with LRTI. Consequently, it is an epidemiological, rather than a diagnostic, tool.

NAA tests

The newest approach in the diagnosis of respiratory tract infections is the detection of microbial nucleic acids by NAA tests. Culture procedures for viruses and fastidious bacteria, *M. pneumoniae*, *C. pneumoniae*, *L. pneumophila* and *Bordetella pertussis*, which do not normally colonise the human respiratory tract, are too insensitive and too slow to be therapeutically relevant, and these pathogens therefore should be detected using NAA tests, whose sensitivity is almost always superior to that of the traditional procedures.

A multitude of reports has appeared on the epidemiology of LRTIs but most are restricted to a few viruses (influenza, sometimes together with RSV, and rhino-, metapneumo- or coronaviruses) and/or to some population groups, *e.g.* children, adults or the elderly. Great variations occur as a function of time, place and the age-groups studied as well as in the diagnostic gold standard test used, varying between viral culture and serology. Although the role of some new viruses is becoming clearer in specific patient populations, more studies are needed to identify the clinical relevance of some others, such as the bocavirus. All these studies were performed with traditional NAA tests that require at least 1–2 days, producing *a posteriori* results that were unavailable to the clinician in time to have an impact on patient management. Real-time multiplex NAA tests offer a solution. To cover the wide spectrum of aetiological respiratory agents, a number of uni- and/or multiplex reactions are performed simultaneously. Both in-house and commercially available multiplex NAA tests for the simultaneous detection of two, three or up to 22 different respiratory pathogens, including the 'atypical' *M. pneumoniae, C. pneumoniae* and *L. pneumophila,* and respiratory viruses, with a mixture of primers, have been developed.

The combined use of single-target assays or of multiplex assays has increased the diagnostic yield in respiratory infections by 30–50%: combined with traditional bacteriological techniques to diagnose *S. pneumoniae* infections, >50% – and in some studies of CAP up to 70% – of aetiological agents can be detected.

The wider application of multiplex reactions during recent years has resulted in the detection of numerous simultaneous viral infections with widely varying incidences: from 3% to even 23% or 35%, depending on whether bacterial agents are also included. The divergent incidences may result from the variety of diagnostic panels applied. Combined viral and viral–bacterial infections are diagnosed but no preferential combinations have been found. The clinical significance of combined infections remains to be further clarified. Respiratory viruses have also been increasingly recognised as causes of severe LRTIs in immuno-compromised hosts. Respiratory infections are more common in solid organ recipients, particularly in lung transplant recipients. Infections are especially dangerous prior to engraftment and during the 3 months after

transplantation, in the setting of graft *versus* host disease. The origin of the infections is community-acquired as well as nosocomial.

As more epidemiological information on the role of a panel of respiratory viral pathogens becomes available, it is clear that screening for these viruses in specific patient populations, such as transplant patients, very young children or the elderly, is desirable, and preventive and therapeutic recommendations may take this information into account.

NAA tests are, however, not required for every purpose. For cohorting RSV-infected paediatric patients, the DIF tests can be as sensitive as an RT-PCR with results available within 60 min (and at lower cost than with NAA tests). Very rapid chromatographic tests are also available for RSV, which can be performed in the laboratory outside virology laboratory operating hours. These tests lack sensitivity, however, when applied to respiratory samples of adult patients.

Conclusion

In recent years, significant progress has been made in the microbiological diagnosis of respiratory infections. A straightforward interpretation of a good-quality, Gram-stained sputum sample has been established, and has been shown to be important for rapid diagnosis of pneumonia and the interpretation of culture results in severely ill patients.

The number of possible aetiological agents, viruses and fastidious bacteria has been extended, and their epidemiology has been clarified. Sensitive and rapid methods for their detection have been developed and are increasingly validated in clinical settings.

Amplification techniques are, at present, more expensive than conventional approaches. However, improvements in standardisation and automation for sample preparation and technical advances will lead to increased use of amplification methods and cost reductions to rates competitive with conventional methods. Several studies have tended to show cost efficiency of rapid diagnosis of acute respiratory infections resulting from reduced antibiotic use and complementary laboratory investigations, but most significantly from shorter hospitalisation and reduced isolation periods. Serological diagnosis of those cases that remain undetected by the NAA tests is of no clinical use, as it is available only after many days or even weeks.

Further reading

- Anevlavis S, et al. (2009). A prospective study of the diagnostic utility of sputum Gram stain in pneumonia. J Infect; 59: 83–89.
- Beersma MF, et al. (2005). Evaluation of 12 commercial tests and the complement fixation test for Mycoplasma pneumoniae-specific immunoglobulin G (IgG) and IgM antibodies, with PCR used as the 'gold standard'. J Clin Microbiol; 43: 2277–2285.
- Genne D, et al. (2006). Enhancing the etiologic diagnosis of community-acquired pneumonia in adults using the urinary antigen assay (Binax NOW). Int J Infect Dis; 10: 124–128.
- Ieven M, et al. (2012). Should serology be abolished in favour of PCR for the diagnosis of Mycoplasma pneumoniae infections? Curr Pediatr Rev 2012 [In press].
- Ieven M. (2007). Currently used nucleic acid amplification tests for the detection of viruses and atypicals in acute respiratory infections. J Clin Virol; 40: 259–276.
- Ieven M. Diagnosis of community acquired pneumonia. In: Torres A, ed. Community Acquired Pneumonia. Chichester, John Wiley and Sons Ltd, 2007; pp. 43–61.
- Loens K, et al. (2009). Optimal sampling sites and methods for detection of pathogens possibly causing community-acquired lower respiratory tract infections. J Clin Microbiol; 47: 21–31.
- Loens K, et al. (2003). Molecular diagnosis of Mycoplasma pneumoniae in respiratory tract infections. J Clin Microbiol; 41: 4915–4923.
- Loens K, et al. (2010). Acute respiratory infection due to Mycoplasma pneumoniae: current status of diagnostic methods. Eur J Clin Microbiol Infect Dis; 29: 1055–1069.
- Mahony JB. (2008). Detection of respiratory viruses by molecular methods. Clin Microbiol Rev; 21: 716–741.
- Templeton KE, et al. (2005). Improved diagnosis of the etiology of community-acquired pneumonia with real-time polymerase chain reaction. Clin Infect Dis; 41: 345–351.
- Woodhead M, et al. (2011). Guidelines for the management of adult lower respiratory tract infections. Clin Microbiol Infect; 17: Suppl. 6, E1–E59.

Upper respiratory tract infections

Gernot Rohde

Prevalence

Upper respiratory tract infections (URTIs) usually occur during the cold months,

---

Key points

- URTIs are the most common infectious illness in the general population, and are the leading cause of missed work and school.

- Most URTIs are viral in origin, and typical agents are rhinoviruses, coronaviruses, adenoviruses, coxsackieviruses, influenza and parainfluenza viruses, human metapneumovirus, and respiratory syncytial virus.

- URTIs rarely cause permanent sequelae or death but can progress to otitis media, bronchitis, bronchiolitis, pneumonia, sepsis, meningitis, intracranial abscess and other infections.

- Diagnosis is usually purely clinical; diagnostic investigations should only be performed in special circumstances, such as influenza, group A streptococcal pharyngitis, infectious mononucleosis and pneumonia.

- Infection will often be self-limiting, with no specific treatment necessary; the only indications for antibiotic treatment are group A streptococcal pharyngitis, bacterial sinusitis and pertussis.

---

mainly due to overcrowding inside buildings. The mean frequency is two to four episodes annually for adults. In children it is higher. Antigenic variation of hundreds of respiratory viruses allows repeated circulation in the community.

Spectrum

The upper respiratory tract comprises the airways above the vocal cords and consists of the nose, paranasal sinuses, pharynx and larynx. The most prevalent illness is the common cold (rhinosinusitis), followed by sinusitis, pharyngitis/tonsillitis and laryngitis (table 1).

The onset of symptoms usually begins 1–3 days after exposure to a microbial pathogen. The duration of the symptoms is typically 7–10 days but may be longer.

Transmission and predisposition

Transmission of pathogens is by aerosol, droplet or direct hand-to-hand contact. The pathogens invade the respiratory epithelium of the corresponding area. Sinusitis is often preceded by a common cold. There are predisposing conditions such as allergic rhinoconjunctivitis, nasal septum deviation, immunodeficiency or cocaine abuse. Smoking or exposure to second-hand smoke and travel are additional risk factors.

Pathogens

Most URTIs are viral in origin. More than 200 different viruses are known to cause the common cold. Typical viral agents that cause URTIs are rhinoviruses, corona-viruses, adenoviruses, coxsackieviruses, influenza and parainfluenza viruses, human

Table 1. *Signs and symptoms*

Upper respiratory tract infection	Symptoms	Signs
Common cold	Nasal congestion, mucopurulent nasal discharge, sneezing, sore throat, halitosis	Low-grade fever, nasal vocal tone, inflamed nasal mucosa
Sinusitis	Unilateral facial pain, maxillary toothache, headache, purulent nasal discharge	Swelling, redness, tenderness to palpation or percussion overlying the affected sinuses, abnormal transillumination
Pharyngitis	Sore throat, odynophagia or dysphagia, fever, absence of cough, halitosis	Pharyngeal erythema and exudate, palatal petechiae (doughnut lesions), tender anterior cervical lymphadenopathy, scarlatiniform rash, pharyngeal or palatal vesicles and ulcers (herpangina), tonsillar hypertrophy
Laryngitis	Hoarseness, voicelessness, dry cough, odynophagia or dysphagia, halitosis	Low-grade fever, cervical lymphadenopathy, inspiratory stridor, tachypnoea

metapneumovirus, respiratory syncytial virus and others.

Group A, but also group C and G, streptococci can cause pharyngitis (10–20% of cases), as well as other bacteria like *Neisseria gonorrhoeae*, *Corynebacterium diphtheriae* and atypical bacteria (*Chlamydia* and *Mycoplasma*). *Streptococcus pneumoniae*, *Haemophilus influenzae* and *Moraxella catarrhalis* can be the bacterial cause of rhinosinusitis. *Bordetella pertussis* or *Bordetella parapertussis* are the cause of whooping cough associated with laryngotracheitis.

Complications

URTIs usually are self-limiting and rarely cause permanent sequelae or death. However, they can progress to otitis media, bronchitis, bronchiolitis, pneumonia, sepsis, meningitis, intracranial abscess and other infections. Specific complications can occur with untreated group A streptococcal pharyngitis resulting in acute rheumatic fever (ARF), acute glomerulonephritis, peritonsillar abscess and toxic shock syndrome. Sinusitis can extend into surrounding deep tissue leading to orbital

cellulitis, subperiosteal abscess, orbital abscess, frontal and maxillary osteomyelitis, subdural abscess, meningitis and brain abscess. Epiglottitis, a presentation of laryngitis caused by *H. influenzae* type B (Hib), poses a risk of death due to sudden airway obstruction and other complications, including septic arthritis, meningitis, empyema and mediastinitis.

Diagnosis

In most cases, the diagnosis is purely clinical. History, inspection, palpation, percussion and auscultation (table 1) are sufficient. Additional diagnostic investigations should only be performed in special circumstances. These include suspicion of:

• influenza (perform pharyngeal swab for PCR)
• group A streptococcal pharyngitis (perform pharyngeal swab for rapid antigen detection test)
• infectious mononucleosis (there are usually additional symptoms such as hepatosplenomegaly and lymphocytosis; perform mononucleosis spot test in blood)

- Pertussis (perform serology or PCR on respiratory specimens, mostly nasopharyngeal swab)

Differential diagnosis

Influenza viruses can cause mild URTIs but also systemic disease. The definition of influenza-like illness is fever >38.5°C) and one of the following:

- cough
- sore throat
- headache
- muscle ache

Allergic rhinoconjunctivitis is characterised by oedema of the conjunctiva, itching and increased lacrimation additional to symptoms of rhinitis. It shows seasonal variation related to allergen exposure.

Acute thyroiditis can present as sore throat, a common symptom in URTIs. Investigation of thyroid hormones, thyroid-specific autoantibodies, ultrasound and radioactive iodine uptake can help with diagnosis.

Gastro-oesophageal reflux disease can clinically present as laryngopharyngitis and/or tracheobronchitis. History and oesophagogastroduodenoscopy in more severe cases should be performed.

Granulomatosis with polyangiitis (Wegener's) should be considered in patients with sinusitis not responding to therapy. Classic antineutrophil cytoplasmic antibodies and biopsy are key to diagnosis.

Asthma should be considered in patients with a nonresolving cough for >3 weeks.

Treatment

The vast majority of URTIs are viral in origin. In most cases, the infection will be self-limiting and no specific treatment is necessary. Sufficient fluid intake should be advocated. The effect of zinc and vitamin C is still debated. Echinacea seems to be effective in prevention and treatment of the common cold. Nonsteroidal anti-inflammatory drugs relieve fever, headache and malaise. In general, there is no role for antibiotic therapy in the management of common cold or any mild URTI. The only indications for antibiotic treatment are:

- group A streptococcal pharyngitis (oral penicillin or macrolide for 10 days)
- bacterial sinusitis, usually a sinusitis not resolving within 7 days (aminopenicillin with or without a β-lactamase inhibitor, second- or third-generation cephalosporins, macrolides, or trimethoprim-sulfamethoxazole for 7–10 days)
- pertussis (macrolides, alternatively trimethoprim-sulfamethoxazole or doxycycline for 7 days)

Nasal decongestants decrease symptoms in rhinitis and sinusitis, and topical nasal steroids improve sinusitis. Confirmed cases of influenza can be considered for therapy with neuraminidase inhibitors according to Centers for Disease Control and Prevention guidelines. New treatment options for the most prevalent respiratory pathogens, human rhinoviruses, are under development.

Prevention

Direct hand-to-hand contact is an important mechanism of pathogen transmission. Hence, frequent hand washing or disinfection in healthcare can limit spread of infection significantly. Influenza vaccination has been shown to be very beneficial and has to be advocated. In children, the routine administration of Hib vaccination has practically eradicated Hib as a cause of URTI; a herd effect can be demonstrated, as the introduction of the pneumococcal vaccine in children correlated with significant reduction in invasive pneumococcal disease in adults.

Further reading

- Arroll B, et al. (2005). Antibiotics for the common cold and acute purulent rhinitis. *Cochrane Database Syst Rev*; 3: CD000247.
- Centers for Disease Control and Prevention. Seasonal Influenza (Flu). www.cdc.gov/flu Date last updated: November 21, 2012.

- Choby BA (2009). Diagnosis and treatment of streptococcal pharyngitis. *Am Fam Physician*; 79: 383–390.
- Rosenfeld RM, *et al.* (2007). Clinical practice guideline: adult sinusitis. *Otolaryngol Head Neck Surg*; 137: 365–377.
- Meneghetti A, *et al.* Upper Respiratory Tract Infection. http://emedicine.medscape.com/article/302460-overview Date last updated: October 15, 2012.
- Mossad SB. Upper Respiratory Tract Infections. www.clevelandclinicmeded.com/medicalpubs/diseasemanagement/infectious-disease/upper-respiratory-tract-infection/ Date last updated: August 1, 2010.
- Musher DM (2003). How contagious are common respiratory tract infections? *N Engl J Med*; 348: 1256–1266.
- Poole MD, *et al.* (2005). Treatment of rhinosinusitis in the outpatient setting. *Am J Med*; 118: Suppl. 7A, 45S–50S.
- Rohde G (2007). Therapeutic targets in respiratory viral infections. *Curr Med Chem*; 14: 2776–2782.
- Shah SA, *et al.* (2007). Evaluation of echinacea for the prevention and treatment of the common cold: a meta-analysis. *Lancet Infect Dis*; 7: 473–480.
- Tiwari T, *et al.* (2005). Recommended antimicrobial agents for the treatment and postexposure prophylaxis of pertussis: 2005 CDC Guidelines. *MMWR Recomm Rep*; 54: 1–16.

Infective exacerbations of COPD

Marc Miravitlles

The American Thoracic Society/European Respiratory Society Task Force has defined the exacerbation of COPD as: 'an increase in respiratory symptoms over baseline that usually requires medical intervention'. In fact, the chronic and progressive course of COPD is often aggravated by short periods of increasing symptoms, particularly increasing cough, dyspnoea and production of sputum, which can become purulent. Patients with moderate-to-severe COPD present a mean of between one and two of these episodes or exacerbations per year. Patients with more advanced disease may suffer from an increasing number of exacerbations; however, some patients are more prone to suffer from exacerbations irrespective of the severity of airflow impairment – these are the frequent exacerbators, defined as those suffering from at least two exacerbations the previous year. It is estimated that ~30% of patients with moderate-to-severe COPD are frequent exacerbators.

Key points

- Up to 75% of COPD exacerbations are of infective aetiology.

- *Haemophilus influenzae* is the most frequent pathogen causing exacerbations.

- Relapse rate may be as high as 20%.

- Spectrum of antibacterial activity, risk factors for relapse and bacterial resistance to antibiotics are the criteria used for the selection of antibiotics.

Outcomes of exacerbations: risk factors for failure

The failure rate of ambulatory treatment of exacerbations of COPD ranges from 12% to 26%, and failure may lead to hospital admission. COPD severity is associated with a higher rate of severe exacerbation requiring hospitalisation. The mortality of patients admitted to hospital with COPD exacerbation is around 10–14% and the mortality of those admitted to an intensive care unit may be as high as 24%. Hospitalisation has an important impact on COPD patients; it is associated with a higher risk of short- and long-term all-cause mortality at any stage of severity of COPD. Frequent exacerbations have been demonstrated to have a negative impact on health-related quality of life in patients with COPD, and survival is significantly related to the frequency and severity of exacerbations. Identification of risk factors for failure of ambulatory treatment may allow the implementation of more aggressive broad-spectrum treatment and closer follow-up (table 1).

Aetiology of exacerbations

A variety of causes may deteriorate the clinical stability of patients with COPD: cold temperature, air pollution, lack of compliance with respiratory medication, worsening of comorbidities and pulmonary embolism, among others. However, up to three-quarters of exacerbations can be infectious in origin, with bacteria being responsible for three-quarters of these exacerbations. In addition, co-infection with respiratory viruses may be frequent in patients with severe COPD; this co-infection

Table 1. Risk factors for failure after ambulatory treatment of exacerbations of COPD

Coexisting cardiopulmonary disease
Increasing number of visits to the GP for respiratory problems (>3 per year)
Increasing number of previous exacerbations (>3 per year)
Increasing baseline dyspnoea
Severity of FEV$_1$ impairment (FEV$_1$ <35% predicted)
Use of home oxygen
Inadequate antibiotic therapy
GP: general practitioner.

has been identified in around 25% of admitted COPD patients with an exacerbation. Interestingly, the symptoms and signs of acute exacerbation in patients with COPD have been replicated experimentally *in vivo* by infecting subjects with respiratory viruses. This is a demonstration of the pathogenic role of viruses in exacerbations of COPD. Since no effective treatment exists for viral exacerbations, here we will focus on the management of bacterial exacerbations of COPD. The

most frequent microorganisms causing exacerbations are presented in table 2.

The role of bacteria in exacerbations has been a matter of controversy, as the respiratory secretions of some patients with stable COPD carry significant concentrations of bacteria. Therefore, the isolation of such microorganisms during exacerbations should not always be interpreted as a definite demonstration of their pathogenic role. However, studies performed with specific invasive techniques have shown that both the number of patients with pathogenic bacteria in respiratory secretions and their concentrations in bronchial secretions increase during exacerbations. The change in the colonising strain of bacteria is an important mechanism originating exacerbations. In this case, the host does not have protective specific antibodies against the new strain of bacteria, and the microorganism can thereby proliferate and cause the exacerbation.

Diagnosis of infective exacerbations

The combination of symptoms described by Anthonisen *et al.* (1987), *i.e.* increased

Table 2. Aetiology of exacerbations of COPD

Infectious exacerbations (~60–80% of all exacerbations)	
Frequent (70–85% of infectious exacerbations) *Haemophilus influenzae* *Streptococcus pneumoniae* *Moraxella catarrhalis* Viruses (influenza/parainfluenza, rhinoviruses, coronaviruses)	Infrequent (15–30% of infectious exacerbations) *Pseudomonas aeruginosa* Opportunistic Gram-negative bacteria *Staphylococcus aureus* *Chlamydia pneumoniae* *Mycoplasma pneumoniae*
Noninfectious exacerbations (20–40% of all exacerbations)	
Heart failure Pulmonary embolism Nonpulmonary infections Pneumothorax	

dyspnoea and increased production or purulence of sputum, have been widely used to identify exacerbations that require treatment with antibiotics. However, new studies have demonstrated that the presence of green (purulent) sputum as opposed to white (mucoid) is one of the best and easiest methods to predict the bacterial aetiology and the need for antibiotic therapy.

Unfortunately, no signs or symptoms can help the clinician to differentiate bacterial from viral exacerbations. Both viral and bacterial agents may co-infect a patient with COPD, and mixed infection is associated with higher inflammation, more severe symptoms and prolonged recovery time.

The degree of airflow impairment in COPD patients indicates the presence of different microorganisms during the course of exacerbations. Individuals with severe pulmonary function impairment, manifested by FEV_1 <50% predicted, are at a six-fold higher risk of developing acute exacerbations caused by *Haemophilus influenzae* or *Pseudomonas aeruginosa* than patients presenting FEV_1 >50% pred. Those with FEV_1 <30% pred have an even higher risk for *P. aeruginosa*. Other risk factors for infection with *Pseudomonas* include the presence of bronchiectasis, the previous isolation of *Pseudomonas* in a given patient and a recent previous courses of antibiotics.

However, the clinical presentation of exacerbation is not characteristic of any particular microorganism and no microbiological diagnostic test is available for differential diagnosis in primary care. To date, the best biomarker available for bacterial exacerbation of COPD is C-reactive protein (CRP), which can be quantified in capillary blood as a point-of-care test even in primary care.

Antibiotic treatment of exacerbations

Antibiotics have been shown to be superior to placebo in the treatment of exacerbations when all of the Anthonisen criteria are present; *i.e.* increased dyspnoea, increased production and purulence of sputum. The purulence of sputum has recently been

demonstrated to be very sensitive and specific for the diagnosis of bacterial exacerbation and indicates the need for antibiotic therapy. Therefore, most guidelines also recommend antibiotic therapy in patients with two of the three aforementioned criteria if one of them is increased in purulence of sputum.

On the other hand, placebo-controlled, randomised clinical trials and large observational studies have demonstrated the efficacy of antibiotics in the treatment of severe hospitalised exacerbation of COPD. Studies are ongoing to determine if patients with clear sputum can be safely treated without antibiotics in the hospital setting.

The antibiotic of choice may vary from country to country based on the prevalence of different bacteria and, more importantly, the differences in susceptibility of the causative bacteria to antibiotics. As an example, in 2000, the prevalence of macrolide-resistant *Streptococcus pneumoniae* in the UK was 12.2% but in France it was 58.1%, while the production of β-lactamase by *H. influenzae* was 13.9% in the UK and 33.1% in France.

Guidelines recommend the use of so-called first-line antibiotics, such as amoxicillin or tetracycline, in low-risk patients in countries with a low prevalence of antibiotic resist-ance, such as the Netherlands, UK and other northern European countries. However, in countries with a high percentage of resistant strains or in patients with risk factors for treatment failure, the choice of an antibiotic must consider amoxicillin–clavulanate, the respiratory fluoroquinolones (moxifloxacin and levofloxacin) or cephalosporins (cefditoren and cefuroxime). Table 3 describes the antibiotic alternatives according to the severity of COPD.

Nonantibiotic treatment of exacerbations

Acute exacerbations of COPD present with increasing dyspnoea in most cases. Both infectious and noninfectious exacerbations are the result of an ongoing inflammatory reaction in the bronchial mucosa, making anti-inflammatory and bronchodilator therapy mandatory.

Table 3. Risk classification and suggested antimicrobial therapy

	FEV₁ % pred	Most frequent microorganisms	Suggested treatment
Mild-to-moderate COPD without risk factors	>50	Haemophilus influenzae Moraxella catarrhalis Streptococcus pneumoniae Chlamydophila pneumoniae Mycoplasma pneumoniae	Amoxicillin Tetracycline In areas of high incidence of resistance: amoxicillin–clavulanate, cefditoren, cefuroxime
Mild-to-moderate COPD with risk factors[#]	>50	Haemophilus influenzae Moraxella catarrhalis PRSP	Amoxicillin–clavulanate Moxifloxacin/levofloxacin Cefditoren Cefuroxime
Severe COPD	30–50	Haemophilus influenzae Moraxella catarrhalis PRSP Enteric Gram-negative bacteria	Amoxicillin–clavulanate Moxifloxacin/levofloxacin
Very severe COPD	<30	Haemophilus influenzae PRSP Enteric Gram-negative bacteria Pseudomonas aeruginosa	Moxifloxacin/levofloxacin Ciprofloxacin if Pseudomonas is suspected Amoxicillin–clavulanate (if allergy to quinolones)[¶]

PRSP: penicillin-resistant S. pneumoniae. [#]: risk factors are explained in table 1; [¶]: in the case of intravenous therapy, other antibiotics can be used, such as piperacillin–tazobactam, imipenem or cefepime.

A short course of oral corticosteroids has been demonstrated to accelerate recovery from exacerbations and reduce the rate of relapse in patients with moderate-to-severe COPD. Patients can be treated with 0.5 mg·kg⁻¹ methylprednisolone or equivalent in a single morning dose for 7–14 days. Treatment for >14 days has not been demonstrated to be more beneficial and increases the likelihood of adverse side-effects. Inhaled bronchodilators, particularly short-acting inhaled β₂-agonists, must be given at increased doses during exacerbations. The short-acting bronchodilators may be prescribed with a chamber of inhalation or by nebulisation. In the acute phase, repeated doses every 30–60 min can be administered with close monitoring of clinical signs and arterial gas exchange with a pulse oximeter. If a prompt response to these drugs does not occur, the addition of an anticholinergic is recommended.

Oxygen therapy should be provided in cases of hypoxaemia. Adequate levels of oxygenation are PaO_2 >8.0 kPa or 60 mmHg, or SaO_2 >90%. These levels are easy to achieve in uncomplicated exacerbations. When oxygen is started, arterial blood gases should be checked 30–60 min later to ensure satisfactory oxygenation without carbon dioxide retention or acidosis.

The clinical and gasometric evolution of the patients will guide the decision to step down the treatment and discharge the patient from the emergency department or hospital. Family and home support is crucial in the first days after discharge.

In mild and moderate ambulatory exacerbations, clinical evaluation is required 48–72 h after initiation of therapy. In mild cases, this evaluation can be performed by telephone.

Further reading

- Anthonisen NR, *et al.* (1987). Antibiotic therapy in exacerbations of chronic obstructive pulmonary disease. *Ann Intern Med*; 106: 196–204.
- Daniels JMA, *et al.* (2010). Procalcitonin *versus* C-reactive protein as predictive markers of response to antibiotic therapy in acute exacerbations of COPD. *Chest*; 138: 1108–1115.
- García-Aymerich J, *et al.* (2011). Lung function impairment, COPD hospitalisations and subsequent mortality. *Thorax*; 66: 585–590.
- Hurst JR, *et al.* (2010). Susceptibility to exacerbation in chronic obstructive pulmonary disease. *N Engl J Med*; 363: 1128–1138.
- Llor C, *et al.* (2012). Efficacy of antibiotic therapy for acute exacerbations of mild to moderate COPD. *Am J Respir Crit Care Med*; 186: 716–723.
- Mallia P, *et al.* (2011). Experimental rhinovirus infection as a human model of chronic obstructive pulmonary disease exacerbation. *Am J Respir Crit Care Med*; 183: 734–742.
- Miravitlles M, *et al.* (2008). Antimicrobial treatment of exacerbation in chronic obstructive pulmonary disease: 2007 consensus statement. *Arch Bronconeumol*; 44: 100–108.
- Miravitlles M, *et al.* (2012). Sputum colour and bacteria in chronic bronchitis exacerbations: a pooled analysis. *Eur Respir J*; 39: 1354–1360.
- Niewoehner DE, *et al.* (1999). Effect of systemic glucocorticoids on exacerbations of chronic obstructive pulmonary disease. *N Engl J Med*; 340: 1941–1947.
- Papi A, *et al.* (2006). Infections and airway inflammation in chronic obstructive pulmonary disease severe exacerbations. *Am J Respir Crit Care Med*; 173: 1114–1121.
- Rothberg MB, *et al.* (2010). Antibiotic therapy and treatment failure in patients hospitalized for acute exacerbations of chronic obstructive pulmonary disease. *JAMA*; 303: 2035–2042.
- Seemungal T, *et al.* (2001). Respiratory viruses, symptoms, and inflammatory markers in acute exacerbations and stable chronic obstructive pulmonary disease. *Am J Respir Crit Care Med*; 164: 1618–1623.
- Sethi S, *et al.* (2002). New strains of bacteria and exacerbations of chronic obstructive pulmonary disease. *N Engl J Med*; 347: 465–471.
- Stockley RA, *et al.* (2000). Relationship of sputum color to nature and outpatient management of acute exacerbations of COPD. *Chest*; 117: 1638–1645.
- Woodhead M, *et al.* (2011). Guidelines for the management of adult lower respiratory tract infections. *Clin Microbiol Infect*; 17: Suppl. 6, E1–E59.

Pneumonia

Mark Woodhead

Background and definitions

Pneumonia is a condition caused by microbial infection within the lung parenchyma. This infection, together with the associated host inflammatory response, impairs normal alveolar function (*i.e.* gas exchange), which, together with the systemic effects of the infection, causes the clinical features of pneumonia. The gold standard for recognition of pneumonia is the presence of new lung shadowing on the chest radiograph in the setting of a compatible clinical illness.

Pneumonia is classified into groups that can be easily recognised and within which the causative pathogens, and hence the management, are different (table 1).

Community-acquired pneumonia (CAP) is that which occurs in the absence of immune compromise or prior hospital admission within the previous 30 days.

Key points

- Pneumonia is very common and has significant mortality.

- Severity assessment, aided by a severity assessment score, is a key management step.

- A variety of different pathogens can cause pneumonia.

- Antibiotic management is initially empirical, and based on guidelines and knowledge of local microbial patterns and resistance rates.

Epidemiology

CAP occurs in between one and 10 per 1000 of the adult population each year. It is more common in children aged <5 years and becomes progressively more common from age 40 years onwards, with a peak in the very elderly. It is more common in those with comorbidity, such as COPD, bronchiectasis, and chronic cardiac and renal disease. It occurs throughout the year with a peak during the winter months.

Nosocomial pneumonia can occur in anyone resident in hospital for ≥48 h. It is especially common in the intensive care unit >48 h after endotracheal intubation (ventilator-associated pneumonia (VAP)) with risk being proportional to the duration of intubation.

Two types of immune dysfunction predispose to pneumonia:

- humoral immune dysfunction, such as immunoglobulin deficiencies; and
- cell-mediated immune function in, for example, cancer chemotherapy, solid organ transplantation and bone marrow transplantation.

Aspiration pneumonia occurs especially in those with swallowing impairment and neurological impairment.

Most cases of CAP are managed in the community with a variable, but significant, proportion requiring hospital admission. Of those admitted, 5–10% may die and of those reaching the intensive care unit, 30–50% may die. Mortality is generally higher in nosocomial pneumonia and pneumonia in the immunocompromised.

Table 1. Pneumonia classification

Community-acquired pneumonia (CAP)
Hospital-acquired pneumonia (HAP) or nosocomial pneumonia
Ventilator-associated pneumonia (VAP)
Pneumonia in the immunocompromised
Aspiration pneumonia

Clinical features

The duration of illness before presentation is usually short. Classically, there is an abrupt onset with fever, shivers and pleuritic chest pain. A slower onset over a few days may also occur. Other common symptoms include cough, sputum production (which may be purulent or blood stained), breathlessness, muscle aches, headaches and anorexia. Nausea and diarrhoea are less common. In elderly patients, symptoms of cerebral dysfunction, such as confusion, incontinence or falls, may be the presenting feature.

Abnormalities on clinical examination include focal signs on chest examination, most commonly crackles. Only occasionally do the 'classical' features of lung consolidation occur: dullness to percussion, bronchial breathing and enhanced vocal resonance. Chest signs may, however, be absent, making the diagnosis difficult outside hospital. In addition, raised temperature, raised heart and respiratory rates, low blood pressure, and mental confusion may be found.

Clinical features are generally not helpful in predicting the causative organism. The Clinical Pulmonary Infection Score (CPIS) may be useful in nosocomial pneumonia.

Investigations including radiology

Investigations are unnecessary outside hospital but, in those admitted, are performed to aid precise diagnosis, assess illness severity and identify the microbial cause.

A chest radiograph is essential to confirm new lung shadowing in those admitted. Classically, such shadowing conforms to a lobar pattern and is associated with air bronchograms. More commonly, shadowing may occupy less than a whole lobe and may also be patchy, multilobar and bilateral. Additional features may include pleural effusion and, less commonly, cavitation and pneumothorax. The lower lobes are most commonly affected.

In routine blood tests, peripheral blood white cell count may be raised, especially in bacterial infection, but C-reactive protein and procalcitonin are probably more specific. Blood urea and creatinine are helpful in severity assessment and the assessment of renal impairment, and liver function tests may be abnormal. Measures of gas exchange, such as oxygen saturation and/or arterial blood gases, also aid assessment of illness severity and guide management.

In routine practice, tests to identify a microbial cause are positive in only about 15% of cases of CAP and hence seldom influence management. They are probably not indicated unless the patient is severely ill. In such cases blood culture, sputum Gram stain and culture, and urine tests for pneumococcal and *Legionella* antigens are indicated. Blood antibody levels or nose/throat secretion PCR-based tests for microbe-specific nucleic acids can be used for the detection of viruses and less common bacteria such as *Legionella, Mycoplasma* and *Coxiella*.

In nosocomial pneumonia, and especially in VAP, lower respiratory secretions should be sampled either by tracheal aspirate or from bronchoscopic specimens. The latter may also be of value in the immunocompromised.

Differential diagnosis

The differential diagnosis includes acute bronchitis, COPD exacerbation, left ventricular failure, pulmonary embolism, TB, exacerbation of pulmonary fibrosis and rare lung disorders (*e.g.* pulmonary eosinophilia).

Microbial aetiology and resistance

The same 10 pathogens commonly cause CAP worldwide, with *Streptococcus pneumoniae* being the most common overall and the most important cause of severe illness and death. *Mycoplasma pneumoniae* is also a common cause of mild illness, especially in young adults. Severe illness is most likely to be associated with *S. pneumoniae, Legionella*, staphylococcal or Gram-negative bacterial infection. *Legionella* infection may occur in outbreaks associated with a water aerosol source, such as showers or decorative fountains. Staphylococcal infection is especially common following influenza virus infection and in intravenous drug abusers. Influenza occurs in seasonal outbreaks during the winter months and occasional pandemics. It is the most common viral cause of CAP.

Bacterial antibiotic resistance varies in frequency between countries. Clinically significant resistance to penicillins in *S. pneumoniae* is rare but clinically significant macrolide resistance is more common, especially in Southern Europe (www.earss.rivm.nl).

Table 2. The CURB65 and CRB65 scores

Score 1 for each of
C: mental confusion
U: blood urea >7 mmol·L^{-1}
R: respiratory rate $\geqslant$30 breaths·min^{-1}
B: systolic blood pressure $<$90 mmHg or diastolic blood pressure $\leqslant$60 mmHg
65: age $\geqslant$65 years
Mild pneumonia: score of 0–1 (mortality 1.5%); moderate pneumonia: score of 2 (9%); severe pneumonia: score of 3–5 (22%).

Nosocomial pneumonia is most commonly caused by Gram-negative enterobacteria or *Staphylococcus aureus*. *Pseudomonas aeruginosa* and multiresistant bacteria (e.g. methicillin-resistant *S. aureus* (MRSA)) are important causes of VAP.

Humoral immune deficiency is associated with bacterial infection and cell-mediated

Table 3. European Respiratory Society/European Society for Clinical Microbiology and Infectious Diseases antibiotic guideline options for CAP

Outside hospital	Amoxicillin
	Tetracycline
Hospitalised	
Nonsevere	Aminopenicillin $\pm$ macrolide
	Aminopenicillin/β-lactamase inhibitor $\pm$ macrolide
	Non-antipseudomonal cephalosporin
	Cefotaxime or ceftriaxone $\pm$ macrolide
	Levofloxacin
	Moxifloxacin
	Penicillin G $\pm$ macrolide
Severe	
No *Pseudomonas* risk	Non-antipseudomonal cephalosporin III + macrolide
	Moxifloxacin or levofloxacin $\pm$ non-antipseudomonal cephalosporin III
Pseudomonas risk	Antipseudomonal cephalosporin + ciprofloxacin
	Antipseudomonal cephalosporin + macrolide + aminoglycoside[#]
	Acylureidopenicillin/β-lactamase inhibitor + ciprofloxacin
	Acylureidopenicillin/β-lactamase inhibitor + macrolide + aminoglycoside[#]
	Carbapenem[¶] + ciprofloxacin
	Carbapenem[¶] + macrolide + aminoglycoside[#]
Evidence does not clearly support one regime as better than another so a choice is provided. Decision will depend on local circumstances. [#]: gentamicin, tobramycin or amikacin; [¶]: meropenem is preferred.	

immune defects with viral and fungal infections such as *Pneumocystis jirovecii*.

Anaerobic bacteria may be important in aspiration pneumonia.

Severity assessment

Severity assessment is the key to deciding the place of care and should also guide diagnostic tests and antimicrobial therapy. This should be done through clinical judgement guided by objective severity scores. There are many of these, but the best validated for CAP are CURB65 (and its derivative CRB65) and the pneumonia severity index (PSI). The latter is based on a score from 20 variables and is often not practical in routine practice. The former is simpler and based on the number of severity variables present (table 2).

Management

Correction of gas exchange and fluid balance abnormalities, and the provision of appropriate antimicrobial therapy are the cornerstones of management. Outside hospital, rest, oral fluids and an oral antibiotic may be all that is required. In hospital, oxygen at a concentration to maintain S_aO_2 (92–95%) should be delivered. If this cannot be achieved, CPAP may be helpful. If there is an unacceptable rise in P_aCO_2, then assisted ventilation should be considered. A place for NIV in pneumonia management has yet to be proven.

Initial antibiotic therapy must be empirical and directed by illness severity according to national or international guidelines (table 3). Empirical antibiotics for CAP should always include pneumococcal coverage. Treatment for nosocomial pneumonia should be guided by knowledge of local microbial

causes and that for pneumonia in the immunocompromised by the type of immune suppression and likely pathogens. Duration of therapy is usually 7 days in uncomplicated cases but may need to be prolonged in severe illness. Failure to respond should prompt a re-evaluation of the correct diagnosis and a more detailed search for microbial cause, for example by bronchoscopy, as long as gas exchange function will allow.

Prevention

The main preventable risk for pneumonia is tobacco smoking. In those with comorbid disease and in the elderly, influenza and pneumococcal vaccination is indicated. Recent evidence suggests that conjugate pneumococcal vaccination in children not only reduces invasive pneumococcal infection in this group but also in adults.

Further reading

- Lim WS, et al. (2000). Severity prediction rules in community acquired pneumonia: a validation study. *Thorax*; 55: 219–223.
- Pugin J, et al. (1991). Diagnosis of ventilator-associated pneumonia by bacteriologic analysis of bronchoscopic and nonbronchoscopic 'blind' bronchoalveolar lavage fluid. *Am Rev Respir Dis*; 143: 1121–1129.
- Torres A, et al. Respiratory Infections. London, Hodder Arnold, 2006.
- Torres A, et al. (2009). Defining treating and preventing hospital acquired pneumonia: European perspective. *Intensive Care Med*; 35: 9–29.
- Woodhead M, et al. (2011). Guidelines for the management of adult lower respiratory tract infections – full version. *Clin Microbiol Infect*; 17: Suppl. 6, E1–E59.

Hospital-acquired pneumonia

Francesco Blasi

The currently proposed classification of hospital-acquired pneumonias includes hospital-acquired pneumonia (HAP), ventilator-associated pneumonia (VAP) and healthcare-associated pneumonia (HCAP) (table 1).

However, a statement issued by the European Respiratory Society/European Society of Clinical Microbiology and Infectious Diseases/European Society of Intensive Care Medicine calls for a redefinition of HCAP, particularly in terms of risk factors and microbial aetiology.

Epidemiology

The incidence of HAP is ~0.5–2.0% among all hospitalised patients and it is the second most common nosocomial infection, yet the first in terms of mortality (ranging from 30% to >70%). The incidence in different hospitals and different wards of the same hospital varies considerably. The main risk factors are: age, type of hospital and type of ward. Patients aged <35 years are less prone to developing HAP than elderly patients; the incidence of HAP may vary between five and 15 episodes per 1000 discharges. In large teaching hospitals, the incidence is higher than in district hospitals, possibly relating to differences in patient complexity. HAP is quite uncommon in paediatric and obstetric wards, and clearly most common in surgical wards and intensive care units (ICUs), particularly in ventilated patients, in whom the incidence may be >35 episodes per 1000 patient-days.

Pathogenesis and risk factors

The understanding of the pathogenesis of HAPs is a fundamental step for the comprehension of the risk factors involved. The main sources of HAP pathogens include:

- healthcare devices
- the environment
- the transfer of microorganisms between the patient and staff or other patients
- oropharyngeal and gastric colonisation, with subsequent aspiration of their contents into the lungs in patients with impaired mechanical, cellular and humoral defences.

Key points

- Incidence of hospital-acquired pneumonia is ~0.5–2%, with risk factors including age, type of hospital and type of ward.

- Mortality is high (30–70%).

- Diagnosis can be difficult, and requires a combined clinical and bacteriological approach.

- Antimicrobial therapy must be both prompt and appropriate, and should be modified as culture results become available.

Table 1. Definitions of HAP

HAP	Pneumonia that occurs ⩾48 h after admission, which was not incubating at the time of admission
VAP	Pneumonia that arises >48–72 h after endotracheal intubation

Table 2. Main recommendations for the management of modifiable risk factors for HAP and VAP

Host related	Adequate nutrition, enteral feeding *via* orogastric tubes Reduction/discontinuation of immunosuppressive treatments Prevent unplanned extubation (restraints, sedation) Kinetic beds Incentive spirometry, deep breathing and pain control
Device/treatment related	Minimise use of sedatives and paralytics Avoid gastric overdistention Avoid intubation and reintubation Expeditious removal of endotracheal and nasogastric tubes Semirecumbent positioning Drain condensate from ventilator circuits Endotracheal tube cuff pressure (>20 cmH$_2$O prevents leakage of bacterial pathogens around the cuff into lower respiratory tract) Continuous aspiration of subglottic secretions Use of heat–moisture exchangers (reduces ventilator circuit colonisation but not VAP incidence)
Environment related	Attention to infection-control procedures, *i.e.* staff education, hand washing, patient isolation Microbiological surveillance programme

Risk factors for the development of HAP can be differentiated into modifiable and non-modifiable conditions (table 2).

Microbiology

Gram-negative pathogens are the main cause of HAP. *Pseudomonas aeruginosa*, *Acinetobacter baumannii*, microorganisms belonging to the family Enterobacteriaceae (*Klebsiella* spp., *Enterobacter* spp., *Serratia* spp., *etc.*) and, under certain conditions, microorganisms such as *Haemophilus influenzae* are involved in HAP aetiology. Among Gram-positive pathogens, *Staphylococcus aureus, Streptococcus* spp. are the most common agents, accounting for 35–39% of all cases. Nonbacterial pathogens such as *Aspergillus* spp. and viruses (cytomegalovirus) have been described.

In general, there are significant geographical differences in the rates of resistance between some European areas and even within countries, from one hospital to another.

Taking into account the time course of pneumonia development, the expected pathogens in early-onset pneumonia (onset in ⩽4 days of hospital admission) include *S. aureus, S. pneumoniae* and *H. influenzae*, as well as nondrug-resistant Gram-negative enteric bacteria (GNEB), and in late-onset pneumonia (onset >4 days of hospital admission) include methicillin-resistant *S. aureus*, drug-resistant GNEB, *P. aeruginosa* and *A. baumannii* among other potentially drug-resistant microorganisms.

Diagnostic strategy

The clinical diagnosis of HAP is often difficult to establish. The American Thoracic Society/Infectious Diseases Society of America guidelines suggest the use of a

Table 3. Major points for HAP diagnosis

Medical history and physical examination Chest radiograph (posteroanterior and lateral) Blood gas analysis Blood cultures Thoracentesis if pleural effusion Endotracheal aspirate, bronchoalveolar lavage or protected brush sample for culture before antibiotic (negative results do not rule out viral or *Legionella* infections) Extrapulmonary site of infection should be investigated

Table 4. CPIS[#]

Criterion	0	1	2
Tracheal secretions	Absent	No purulent	Abundant and purulent
Chest radiograph infiltrates	No	Diffuse/patchy	Localised
Temperature °C	>36.5 and >38.4	<38.5 or >38.9	>39 or <36
Leukocytes cells·mL^{-1}	4000 and 11 000	<4000 or $>11\,000$	<4000 or $>11\,000$ + band forms $>50\%$ or >500
P_{aO_2}/F_{IO_2}	>240 or ARDS		<240, no ARDS
Microbiology[¶]	Negative	$\geqslant10^3$ and $\leqslant10^4$	Positive ($>10^4$)

F_{IO_2}: inspiratory oxygen fraction; ARDS: acute respiratory distress syndrome. [#]: CPIS is considered positive with a score $\geqslant6$; [¶]: tracheal aspirate.

combined clinical and bacteriological strategy. Table 3 summarises the major points and recommendations of the guidelines.

In case of doubt or relevant disagreement between the clinical presentation and the radiological findings, it is recommended to perform CT. The presence of new chest radiographic infiltrates plus one of the three clinical variables (fever $>38°C$, leukocytosis or leukopenia and purulent secretions) is sufficient to start antimicrobial treatment.

Concerning the diagnosis of VAP, the lack of accuracy of specific clinical signs of pneumonia led investigators to develop scores to identify respiratory infections. In particular, the Clinical Pulmonary Infection Score (CPIS) is based on six clinical assessments (temperature, blood leukocyte count, volume and purulence of tracheal

Table 5. Antimicrobial treatment of nosocomial pneumonia

	Recommended treatment options	Recommended dosages
Early-onset pneumonia without any additional risk factors[#]	Aminopenicillin plus β-lactamase inhibitor or second/third generation cephalosporin or respiratory fluoroquinolone	Amoxicillin-clavulanate 3×2.2 g Ampicillin sulbactam 3×3 g Cefuroxime 3×1.5 g Cefotaxime 3×2 g Ceftriaxone 1×2 g Levofloxacin 1×750 mg Moxifloxacin 1×400 mg
Late-onset or risk factors for multidrug-resistant pathogens	Anti-*Pseudomonas* β-lactams or carbapenems plus fluoroquinolone Addition of coverage for MRSA if suspected	Piperacillin/tazobactam 3×4.5 g Ceftazidime 3×2 g Imipenem 3×1 g Meropenem 3×1 g Ciprofloxacin 3×400 mg Levofloxacin 1×750 mg Vancomycin 2×1 g Linezolid 2×600 mg

MRSA: methicillin-resistant *Staphylococcus aureus*. [#]: ertapenem has been suggested; however, its use on a regular basis would lead to a considerable risk of overtreatment.

secretions, oxygenation, pulmonary radiographic findings, and semiquantitative culture of tracheal aspirate), each worth between 0 and 2 points (table 4). A CPIS value ≥ 6 is a threshold to accurately identify patients with pneumonia. However, the value of CPIS still needs to be validated in a large prospective study.

Treatment

Prompt administration of appropriate antimicrobial treatment is crucial in order to achieve an optimal outcome, and inappropriate antimicrobial treatment is associated with an excess mortality from pneumonia. Antibiotic selection for empirical therapy of HAP should be based primarily on the risk of multidrug-resistant pathogen infection. Table 5 shows the proposed empirical treatment approach.

Once the results of respiratory tract and blood cultures become available, therapy should be focused or narrowed, based on the identity of specific pathogens and their susceptibility to specific antimicrobials. An 8-day antibiotic course can be appropriate provided that the patient has a good clinical response and difficult-to-treat pathogens are not involved as an aetiological agent.

Further reading

- American Thoracic Society, et al. (2005). Guidelines for the management of adults with hospital-acquired, ventilator-associated, and healthcare-associated pneumonia. Am J Respir Crit Care Med; 171: 388–416.
- Ramirez P, et al. (2012). Measures to prevent nosocomial infections during mechanical ventilation. Curr Opin Crit Care; 18: 86–92.
- Torres A, et al. (2009). Defining, treating and preventing hospital acquired pneumonia: European perspective. Intensive Care Med; 35: 9–29.
- Torres A, et al. (2010). Treatment guidelines and outcomes of hospital-acquired and ventilator-associated pneumonia. Clin Infect Dis; 51: Suppl. 1, S48–S53.

Opportunistic infections in the immunocompromised host

Thomas Fuehner, Mark Greer, Jens Gottlieb and Tobias Welte

Pulmonary diseases remain prevalent among immunodeficient patients, manifesting as infections, malignancy, structural abnormalities such as bronchiectasis or primary ciliary dyskinesia (PCD), and inflammatory dysregulation. The causes of immunodeficiency are considered either primary (congenital) or acquired.

Primary immunodeficiency

Primary immunodeficiency results from either humoral or cellular immuno-deficiency, although clinical manifestations commonly result from a combination of both. Disorders of innate immunity

---

Key points

- Common causes of acquired immunodeficiency are immunosuppressive medication (corticosteroids, cytotoxic chemotherapy and biologicals), radiation, HIV infection and asplenia.

- The pathogen type depends on the nature of the underlying immune defects.

- Correct assessment of individual risk factors for pneumonia (community *versus* hospital acquired and immunosuppressed patient) helps to improve treatment.

- Diagnostic and treatment algorithms may help to reduce mortality and the use of antibiotics.

- These algorithms are solely defined for community- and hospital-acquired pneumonia in major guidelines.

---

commonly alter mononuclear phagocytic activity or the complement system. They have also been implicated in structural defects such as PCD and hereditary splenic deficiency. Cellular defects, typically involving either T-lymphocytes or both T- and B-lymphocytes are common causes of opportunistic infections, such as *Pneumocystis jiroveci* or cytomegalovirus (CMV) pneumonia. While particularly prevalent among newborns, isolated defects in humoral immunity may be compensated over subsequent months by persisting maternal antibodies. Impaired T-cell or phagocyte function increases the risk of opportunistic infections from particular opportunistic pathogens including *Pseudomonas*, *Burkholderia*, *P. jiroveci*, *Aspergillus* and CMV. However, the clinical course varies widely, with late presentation in older adults being a not uncommon feature in some syndromes, such as common variable immunodeficiency syndrome (CVID), in which patients are particularly susceptible to encapsulated microorganisms such as *Streptococcus pneumoniae* or *Haemophilus influenzae*.

Nontuberculous mycobacterial infections have been described in patients with genetic defects in the interleukin (IL)-12 and interferon (IFN)-γ pathways, as well as in patients with defective regulation of NF-κB (NF-κB essential modifier or NEMO defects).

Acquired immunodeficiency

Acquired immunodeficiencies remain much more prevalent than primary defects and result mainly from the use of cytotoxic medications in chemotherapy, biological treatments and steroids, and radiotherapy,

HIV infection and transplantation. In each of these patient groups, there is an increased susceptibility to specific groups of pathogens based primarily on the underlying immunological deficit. In comparison to other treatments, less is known about antibody-based treatments directed towards T- and B-cell function or tumour necrosis factor (TNF)-α, and these should be further evaluated when assessing individual patient risk.

Neutropenia Infection in neutropenic patients continues to pose major clinical challenges. Host defences are commonly impaired either by the underlying disease in primary deficiencies, or specific treatments or iatrogenic manipulation while hospitalised.

Due to a lack of neutrophil granulocytes, pulmonary infiltrations may be absent or difficult to identify. Current recommendations from the Infectious Disease Work Group of the German Society of Haematology and Oncology reflect this, recommending urgent thoracic CT in all patients with neutropenic fever failing to respond after 3 days of empirical antibiotic treatment (Maschmeyer et al., 2009). Pulmonary infiltrates, where present, require further investigation through bronchoalveolar lavage (BAL). Storage and transport of BAL samples is of critical importance, with 4°C considered the optimal temperature, and testing should ideally begin within 2–3 h of material recovery (Maschmeyer et al., 2009). Diagnostic work-up should include mycobacteria (microscopy, culture and PCR), P. jiroveci (immunofluorescence and PCR), Legionella spp. and galactomannan antigen testing for Aspergillus (Guo et al., 2010). Viral aetiologies should also be considered, particularly common respiratory pathogens, via immunofluorescence or PCR. CMV infections, including CMV pneumonia, may be detected via CMV antigen in blood, i.e. pp65, or CMV DNA, which is currently considered the gold standard (Hodinka, 2003).

The presence of Candida spp. on direct microscopy or even BAL culture requires careful interpretation and is not an automatic indication for treatment. Similar difficulties arise in diagnosing invasive pulmonary aspergillosis. In the absence of a confirmatory biopsy, diagnostic criteria including specific risk factors, CT criteria and corresponding microbiological findings (positive galactomannan antigen test, culture and PCR) are crucial in assisting with decision-making. Current guidelines recommend that all cases of 'probable' or 'proven' pulmonary aspergillosis be immediately treated (Ascioglu et al., 2002).

Bone marrow transplantation Patients undergoing allogenic stem-cell or bone marrow transplantation (BMT) are at understandably high risk of neutropenia, and impairment of barrier defences and both cell-mediated and humoral immunity. The degree of neutropenia reflects both the nature and duration of exposure to the precipitating factor. The resulting deficit facilitates even microorganisms with limited pathogenicity in causing serious infections. Patients undergoing allogenic stem-cell transplantation or BMT are subjected to sequential suppression of host defences, predisposing to variation in susceptibility to particular organisms at different phases following transplantation. The greatest infective risk, particularly of opportunistic pneumonias due to Staphylococcus aureus, Pseudomonas aeruginosa, Enterobacteriaceae, Aspergillus spp. or even CMV, occurs within the first few weeks following allogenic stem-cell transplantation.

Solid organ transplantation Due to their chronic immunocompromised state, infection represents a lifelong threat to patients after solid organ transplantation and remains a leading cause of early and late mortality. In addition to their direct impact, several studies have linked infection response processes with an increased predisposition to allograft rejection, especially in lung transplantation (LTx) (Fuehner et al., 2012).

While classical symptoms such as fever and cough may be masked in solid organ transplant recipients, this problem is of particular concern in LTx patients. In the early post-transplant phase, such infections are most commonly bacterial, followed by fungi and then viruses (Kotloff *et al.*, 2011). *P. aeruginosa* is the predominant pathogen, followed closely by *S. aureus*. Common gram-negative organisms causing post-transplant pneumonias include *Klebsiella* and *H. influenzae*.

CMV represents the commonest viral pathogen, occurring in approximately one-third of patients during the first year (Palmer *et al.*, 2010). CMV-naïve recipients (R⁻) receiving organs from seropositive donors (D⁺) are at the greatest risk of infection and are predisposed to particularly severe infection. Current guidelines recommend the use of ganciclovir/valganciclovir prophylaxis in D⁺/R⁻ for ⩾6 months following transplant (Kotton *et al.*, 2010).

Community-acquired respiratory viruses consisting mainly of adenovirus and influenza virus along with certain Paramyxoviridae – respiratory syncytial virus (RSV), parainfluenza virus and human metapneumovirus (hMPV) – have gained recognition as pathogens among LTx recipients (Kumar *et al.*, 2010; Gottlieb *et al.*, 2009). While treatment options remain limited, oral ribavirin may improve outcomes in paramyxoviral infections but may not be well tolerated in all patients (Fuehner *et al.*, 2011).

Fungal infections remain a constant, albeit less common, threat and are usually caused by *Aspergillus* or *Candida* species. However, pulmonary candidiasis is rare (Meersseman *et al.*, 2009), particularly among LTx recipients, and detection should be based on culture and histology of bronchial mucosa biopsies rather than BAL findings (Strassburg *et al.*, 2010). Conversely, the presence of *Candida* in blood cultures should, be considered significant, with immediate initiation of treatment. BAL analysis may be negative in up to 40% of patients with an invasive aspergillosis. Infections tend to be limited to the airways, with a preponderance towards bronchial anastomoses. Invasive disease at the anastomoses may result in erosion of the pulmonary artery precipitating catastrophic pulmonary haemorrhage. Voriconazole is the first-line treatment of invasive aspergillosis, with echinocandins and parenteral lipid formulations of amphotericin B used as second-line therapy. *Candida* infections generally respond well to fluconazole. In non-*albicans* species, however, fluconazole resistance is becoming increasingly prevalent (Schaberg *et al.*, 2010).

Due to a combination of lifelong co-trimoxazole prophylaxis and low-dose steroid treatment regimes, *P. jiroveci* pneumonia has become rare among adherent patients.

New immunosuppressive drugs In recent years, >40 monoclonal antibodies have been licensed for treatment of a wide variety of conditions. Inevitably, subsequent studies have alluded to an increased risk of severe infections in patients receiving antibody-associated immunosuppression (Keyser, 2011). Due to wide variations in immunological interactions, significant variability exists both in the pathogen spectrum and the severity of their effects (Curtis *et al.*, 2011). Their modes of action can be broadly classified into those affecting B-cell function such as rituximab (anti-CD20), those specifically binding T-cells such as alemtuzumab (anti-CD52), co-stimulatory T-cell antibodies such as abatacept, anti-TNF antibodies such as infliximab, adalimumab and certolizumab, and etanercept (anti-soluble TNF receptor) and tocilizumab (anti-IL-6)

HIV infection Reduced CD4⁺ cell counts, while not correlating directly, do appear to indicate an increased risk of opportunistic respiratory pathogens in HIV-infected patients. The common bacterial pathogens are *S. pneumoniae* and *Haemophilus* spp. (Benito *et al.*, 2012). Intravenous drug use and smoking appear to increase the pneumonia risk in these patients. Worldwide, *Mycobacterium tuberculosis* is the most important co-infection in HIV-infected patients and significantly influences AIDS-related mortality. *P. jiroveci* is the commonest nonbacterial pathogen. *Nocardia* spp., *Actinomyces* spp., *Rhodococcus* and *Cryptococcus* are rare opportunistic pulmonary pathogens occasionally diagnosed in European patients with poorly treated HIV.

Asplenia Antibody production and phagocytosis by splenic macrophages represent a fundamental aspect of defence against encapsulated bacteria. Following splenectomy, patients are at higher risk of infection with *S. pneumoniae*, *Haemophilus* spp. and *Neisseria meningitidis*. Mortality rates from overwhelming post-splenectomy infection (OPSI) are reported to be up to 600 times greater than in the general population. The overall incidence of septicaemia remains low, with an estimated lifetime risk for OPSI of ~5% (Lynch *et al.*, 1996).

Further reading

- Ascioglu S, *et al.* (2002). Defining opportunistic invasive fungal infections in immunocompromised patients with cancer and hematopoietic stem cell transplants: an international consensus. *Clin Infect Dis*; 34: 7–14.
- Benito N, *et al.* (2012). Pulmonary infections in HIV-infected patients: an update in the 21st century. *Eur Respir J*; 39: 730–745.
- Curtis JR, *et al.* (2011). The comparative risk of serious infections among rheumatoid arthritis patients starting or switching biological agents. *Ann Rheum Dis*; 70: 1401–1406.
- Fuehner T, *et al.* (2011). Single-centre experience with oral ribavirin in lung transplant recipients with paramyxovirus infections. *Antivir Ther*; 16: 733–740.
- Fuehner T, *et al.* (2012). The lung transplant patient in the ICU. *Curr Opin Crit Care*; 18: 472–478.
- Gottlieb J, *et al.* (2009). Community-acquired respiratory viral infections in lung transplant recipients: a single season cohort study. *Transplantation*; 87: 1530–1537.
- Guo YL, *et al.* (2010). Accuracy of BAL galactomannan in diagnosing invasive aspergillosis: a bivariate metaanalysis and systematic review. *Chest*; 138: 817–824.
- Hodinka RL. Human cytomegalovirus. *In*: Murray BE, ed. Manual of Clinical Microbiology. 8th Edn. Washington, ASM Press, 2003; pp. 1304–1318.

- Keyser FD (2011). Choice of biologic therapy for patients with rheumatoid arthritis: the infection perspective. *Curr Rheumatol Rev*; 7: 77–87.
- Kotloff RM, *et al.* (2011). Lung transplantation. *Am J Respir Crit Care Med*; 184: 159–171.
- Kotton CN, *et al.* (2010). International consensus guidelines on the management of cytomegalovirus in solid organ transplantation. *Transplantation*; 89: 779–795.
- Kumar D, *et al.* (2010). A prospective molecular surveillance study evaluating the clinical impact of community-acquired respiratory viruses in lung transplant recipients. *Transplantation*; 89: 1028–1033.
- Lynch AM, *et al.* (1996). Overwhelming postsplenectomy infection. *Infect Dis Clin North Am*; 10: 693–707.
- Maschmeyer G, *et al.* (2009). Diagnosis and antimicrobial therapy of lung infiltrates in febrile neutropenic patients: guidelines of the infectious diseases working party of the German Society of Haematology and Oncology. *Eur J Cancer*; 45: 2462–2472.
- Meersseman W, *et al.* (2009). Significance of the isolation of *Candida* species from airway samples in critically ill patients: a prospective, autopsy study. *Intensive Care Med*; 35: 1526–1531.
- Palmer SM, *et al.* (2010). Extended valganciclovir prophylaxis to prevent cytomegalovirus after lung transplantation: a randomized, controlled trial. *Ann Intern Med*; 152: 761–769.
- Schaberg T, *et al.* (2010). Management der Influenza A/H1N1 – Pandemie im Krankenhaus: Update Januar 2010. Eine Stellungnahme der Deutschen Gesellschaft fur Pneumologie und Beatmungsmedizin. [Management of a new influenza A/H1N1 virus pandemic within the hospital. Statement of the German Society of Pneumology.] *Pneumologie*; 64: 124–129.
- Strassburg A, *et al.* (2010). Infektionsdiagnostik in der Pneumologie. [Diagnosis of infections in pneumology.] *Pneumologie*; 64: 474–487.

Pneumonia in the immunocompromised host

Santiago Ewig

In contrast to community- and hospital-acquired pneumonia, pneumonia in the immunocompromised host is not defined by the setting of pneumonia acquisition but by the immune status of the host. In this context, immune suppression is best defined as a relevant risk for so-called opportunistic pathogens such as fungi, viruses, mycobacteria and parasites.

The expected pathogen patterns differ according to the type of immune suppression (table 1). Overall, there are five main types of immunosuppression:

- iatrogenic (through steroidal and nonsteroidal agents)
- neutropenia (usually through antineoplastic chemotherapy)
- haematopoietic stem-cell transplantation (HSCT)
- solid-organ transplantation
- HIV infection

Each immunosuppressive condition confers characteristic risk profiles for

pulmonary infections according to the type of immune failure. Some conditions additionally show time- or extent-dependent risk profiles.

Pulmonary infections in the immuno-compromised host usually constitute an emergency. Thus, immediate appropriate antimicrobial treatment is mandatory. Since the spectrum of potential pathogens is far more diverse than in immunocompetent hosts, a systematic approach to the management of these patients is required. This approach should include a comprehensive diagnostic evaluation, indications for empirical initial antimicrobial treatment and in the absence of definite pathogen identification, and for salvage management in case of treatment failure.

The basic diagnostic evaluation should include history, physical examination and chest radiography as well as a basic microbiological work-up (sputum and blood cultures). A CT scan of the lung (multi-slice scan and HRCT) is usually indicated in patients in whom a straightforward diagnosis cannot be made. It can be particularly valuable in patients at risk of fungi (Pneumocystis and Aspergillus). Bronchoscopy is usually indicated in patients with bilateral infiltrates, unusual clinical and radiographic presentations, or treatment failure. When performing bronchoscopy, particular care has to be taken to comply with the methodology of retrieving uncontaminated samples of the lower respiratory tract and a comprehensive evaluation of the samples retrieved. Bronchoalveolar lavage (BAL) is the most important sample, and stains and cultures should be investigated for all

Key points

- Different types of immuno-suppression confer vulnerability to different respiratory pathogens, which may be bacterial, viral, mycobacterial or fungal.
- The approach to treatment should include comprehensive diagnostic evaluation, indications for empirical antimicrobial treatment and a plan in case of treatment failure.

Table 1. Types of immunosuppression and typical infectious complications

Type of complication	Main immune disorder	Typical Infections
Iatrogenic (steroids)	Macrophages, T-cells	Bacteria, fungi (*Aspergillus* spp.), *Mycobacterium tuberculosis*
Iatrogenic (anti-TNF-α)	TNF-α	*Mycobacterium tuberculosis*
Neutropenia, HSCT	Neutrophils	
	Short duration (<10 days)	Bacteria
	Long duration (>10 days)	Additionally: fungi (*Aspergillus* spp.)
Solid-organ transplantation	Early (month 1): neutrophils	Bacteria
	Intermediate (months 2–6): macrophages, T-cells	Fungi, viruses, parasites
	Late (months >6): depends on extent of immune suppression	Variable
HIV infection	CD4$^+$ T-cell count >500 cells·μL^{-1}	No risk
	CD4$^+$ T-cell count 200–500 cells·μL^{-1}	Bacteria, *Mycobacterium tuberculosis*
	CD4$^+$ T-cell count <200 cells·μL^{-1}	Additionally: *Pneumocystis jirovecii*
	CD4$^+$ T-cell count <50 cells·μL^{-1}	Additionally: *Aspergillus* spp., atypical mycobacteria

TNF: tumour necrosis factor.

relevant pathogens. Occasionally, transbronchial biopsies and/or transbronchial needle aspiration may be rewarding.

Pneumocystis jirovecii pneumonia

P. jirovecii pneumonia in HIV-infected patients usually occurs in patients with <200 CD4$^+$ helper T-cells per microlitre. It presents with at least one of the following symptoms: fever, cough and dyspnoea on exertion; oral candidiasis is virtually always present. Chest radiography typically discloses bilateral interstitial infiltrates in a perihilar distribution but may also be normal in the early course. In the latter case, HRCT may reveal ground-glass opacities in a patchy or geographical distribution. Atypical cystic presentations may occur. Blood gas analysis shows wide alveolar–arterial gradients. The typical laboratory finding is an elevated lactate dehydrogenase level. Specific diagnosis is required and may be established by examination of induced sputum or BAL. The treatment of choice (also for prophylaxis) is trimethoprim-sulfamethoxazole. Second-line options include pentamidine and clindamycin/primaquine. Adjunctive steroids are indicated in patients with acute respiratory failure.

P. jirovecii pneumonia in non-HIV patients differs in that it presents more frequently as an acute-onset pneumonia and tends to be associated with higher mortality.

Cytomegalovirus pneumonia

Cytomegalovirus (CMV) pneumonia is defined as pulmonary signs and symptoms and the detection of CMV in pulmonary samples. Nevertheless, patients may shed CMV in the absence of CMV pneumonia. Co-infections with other opportunistic pathogens are frequently encountered. After introduction of CMV prophylaxis, the

Table 2. Diagnostic criteria for invasive aspergillosis

Definitive	Histological proof or positive culture from otherwise sterile site
Probable	Host factors + CT/tracheobronchitis + mycological criteria
Possible	Host factors + CT/tracheobronchitis

Host factors: several conditions associated with severe immunosuppression; CT: typical (albeit not specific) CT signs (*e.g.* the halo sign); tracheobronchitis: bronchoscopic visualisation of typical pseudomembranes on the tracheal mucosa (maybe subject to biopsy proof); mycological criteria: *e.g.* culture positive for *Aspergillus*, or positive galactomannan test in serum or BAL fluid. Information from the European Organization for Research and Treatment of Cancer/Invasive Fungal Infections Cooperative Group and the National Institute of Allergy and Infectious Diseases Mycoses Study Group (EORTC/MSG) Consensus Group.

incidence in allogeneic HSCT is 10–30%, with the highest risk in seropositive recipients, while it is rare in autologous HSCT (<10%). In addition, the onset is shifted to >100 days. Clinical presentation is unspecific. Radiologically, there is typically an interstitial pattern with tiny pulmonary nodules and patchy areas of consolidation. HRCT is more sensitive. Diagnosis is made by demonstration of inclusion bodies within epithelial cells of the lower respiratory tract (sensitivity 90%, specificity 98%). Culture of BAL fluid lacks specificity. The value of CMV pp65 antigen and PCR is controversial. The treatment of choice is ganciclovir and valganciclovir, combined with CMV immunoglobulin. Second-line agents are foscarnet and cidofivir. Antiviral prophylaxis and monitoring are the main preventive strategies.

Tuberculosis

Patients with reduced $CD4^+$ cell counts, and those on chronic steroid and anti-tumour necrosis factor (TNF)-α treatment are at increased risk of TB. Co-infection with TB and HIV alters the natural history of both diseases. TB in HIV-infected patients presents like primary infection (patchy infiltrates, mediastinal lymph node enlargement, pleural effusion and bacteraemia). Anti-TB treatment of pulmonary TB follows the rules of standard treatment (*i.e.* usually a 2-month regimen consisting of four first-line drugs (isoniazid, rifampicin, ethambutol and pyrazinamide) followed by a 4-month regimen consisting of two drugs (isoniazid and rifampicin)). Testing for drug

susceptibility is mandatory and treatment must usually be modified in the presence of resistance. Concurrent treatment of TB and HIV is challenging due to the many complex interactions of anti-TB drugs and antiretroviral agents. Patients who are candidates for chronic steroid or anti-TNF-α treatment should be evaluated for TB infection and, in the case of positive skin testing or interferon-γ release assay, receive prophylaxis.

Aspergillus pneumonia

Definite diagnosis of *Aspergillus* pneumonia in neutropenic patients requires tissue biopsy and can only rarely be established. Therefore, probable and possible diagnosis is based on a set of clinical, microbiological and radiographic criteria (table 2). HRCT is the method of choice to detect *Aspergillus* pneumonia early in its course. Typical, albeit not specific, signs of *Aspergillus* pneumonia include the 'halo' sign, as well as nodular and peripheral patchy densities near to vessels. The 'air crescent' sign, representing cavitation, is a late marker of *Aspergillus* pneumonia. The galactomannan antigen test in serum and BAL has a sensitivity of ~70% and a specificity of 90%. Bronchoscopy is usually indicated. Early initiation of treatment is crucial. The treatment of choice for definite *Aspergillus* pneumonia is voriconazole or, alternatively, liposomal amphotericin B. Second-line options include caspofungin and posaconazole. Mortality reaches 50–60%.

Further reading

- Agusti C, *et al*. Pulmonary Infection in the Immunocompromised Patient. Strategies for Management. Oxford, Wiley-Blackwell, 2009.
- Boersma WG, *et al*. (2007). Bronchoscopic diagnosis of pulmonary infiltrates in granulocytopenic patients with hematologic malignancies: BAL *versus* PSB and PBAL. *Respir Med*; 101: 317–325.
- Chan KM, *et al*. (2002). Infectious pulmonary complications in lung transplant recipients. *Semin Respir Infect*; 17: 291–302.
- D'Avignon LC, *et al*. (2008). *Pneumocystis* pneumonia. *Semin Respir Crit Care Med*; 29: 132–140.
- Davis JL, *et al*. (2008). Respiratory infection complicating HIV infection. *Curr Opin Infect Dis*; 21: 184–190.
- Duncan MD, *et al*. (2005). Transplant-related immunosuppression: a review of immunosuppression and pulmonary infections. *Proc Am Thorac Soc*; 2: 449–455.
- Feller-Kopman D, *et al*. (2003). The role of bronchoalveolar lavage in the immunocompromised host. *Semin Respir Infect*; 18: 87–94.
- Rañó A, *et al*. (2001). Pulmonary infiltrates in non-HIV immunocompromised patients: a diagnostic approach using non-invasive and bronchoscopic procedures. *Thorax*; 56: 379–387.
- Rosen MJ (2008). Pulmonary complications of HIV infection. *Respirology*; 13: 181–190.

Pleural infection and lung abscess

Amelia Clive, Clare Hooper and Nick Maskell

Pleural infection

Pleural infection occurs when micro-organisms, most commonly bacteria, enter the pleural space. This may be due to direct spread from an underlying pneumonia or may result from blood-borne spread of a systemic bacteraemia. It can be confirmed when pleural fluid has a positive Gram stain or culture, is frankly purulent or, in the context of sepsis, has an acidic pH (table 1). Pleural infection is a common and serious medical problem and the incidence is rising despite advances in medical management. It is associated with a mortality rate of 15–20%.

Epidemiology

- Pleural infection is most common in the elderly and children, but can occur at any age
- It is twice as common in males
- 20% of adults with pleural infection have diabetes mellitus
- Other important risk factors include aspiration, immunosuppression, poor dentition, pleural procedures, thoracic surgery and penetrating chest trauma

Pathophysiology Pleural infection most frequently follows community-acquired pneumonia (CAP) with bacterial migration from the lung parenchyma into a parapneumonic effusion. It may also follow hospital-acquired and aspiration pneumonia with effusion, traumatic or iatrogenic pleural penetration. Primary pleural infection is more common than previously thought, either as a result of translocation of bacteria from the oropharynx or as a consequence of bacteraemia from other sites.

> **Key points**
>
> - Pleural infection is common and serious, with a mortality rate of ~15%.
>
> - Blood, in addition to pleural fluid, should always be cultured. A higher microbiological yield is achieved if pleural fluid is sent in both a universal container and blood culture bottles.
>
> - Initial management is with broad-spectrum antibiotics and prompt chest drainage.
>
> - Lung abscess has a 10% mortality rate.
>
> - Invasive procedures are only required when a lung abscess does not respond to prolonged empirical antibiotics or an underlying neoplasm is suspected.

Bacteriology Bacteria are ultimately cultured from either pleural fluid or blood in 60–70% of cases of pleural infection. The microbiology of community-acquired pleural infection is different from that of hospital-acquired pleural infection and CAP, such that these should be considered three distinct diseases requiring different empirical antibiotic regimes. This is probably due in part to the differing environment within the pleural cavity, which is more hypoxic and has a lower pH than within the lung itself, making certain organisms (*e.g.* anaerobes) more pathogenic.

In community-acquired pleural infection, *Streptococcus* spp. (largely from the *Streptococcus anginosus* group (previously

Table 1. *Clinical classification of pleural infection*

	Simple parapneumonic effusion	Complex parapneumonic effusion	Empyema
Pleural fluid appearance	Straw coloured or bloody	Straw coloured, bloody or turbid	Frank pus
Pleural fluid pH	>7.2	Usually <7.2	Should not be measured
Pleural fluid Gram stain	Negative	May be positive	May be positive
Pleural fluid culture	Negative	May be positive	May be positive
Thoracic ultrasound appearance	Usually anechoic No pleural thickening	May show variable echogenicity, septations or loculations	Often homogenously echogenic Usually evidence of pleural thickening Loculations and septations may be present
Immediate management	Effusion will usually resolve with antibiotics for pneumonia alone Chest tube drainage can be performed if required for symptomatic relief of breathlessness	Intravenous antibiotics and chest tube drainage	Intravenous antibiotics and chest tube drainage

known as the *Streptococcus milleri* group) and *Streptococcus pneumoniae*) account for 50% of positive cultures. *Staphylococcus* spp., anaerobic and Gram-negative organisms make up the other half. Anaerobic organisms commonly co-exist with aerobes, particularly with the *S. anginosus* group. Atypical pneumonia organisms such as *Legionella* and *Mycoplasma* spp. are extremely unusual causes of pleural infection.

In nosocomial pleural infection, *Staphylococcus* spp. (including methicillin-resistant *Staphylococcus aureus* (MRSA)) and Gram-negative organisms are responsible for most positive culture results.

Investigations When a patient presents with sepsis and clinical and chest radiographic signs of a pleural effusion, a diagnostic pleural aspiration should always be performed to establish the presence of pleural infection.

Pleural fluid should always be sent for culture and cytological examination. The pH of nonpurulent pleural fluid should be measured, and fluid and blood should also be sent for protein and lactate dehydrogenase measurement.

In the correct clinical context, features suggesting that a parapneumonic effusion is complex and, hence, requires chest tube drainage include:

- a pleural fluid pH of <7.2 (or pleural fluid glucose of <2.2 mmol·L^{-1})
- positive pleural fluid culture or Gram stain
- purulent pleural fluid
- loculation or septation on thoracic ultrasound

A causative organism is not identified in up to 40% of patients with pleural infection, but if one is identified, it can be useful to guide antibiotic treatment. Culturing the fluid in blood culture bottles as well as a standard container has been shown to improve the microbiological yield and blood cultures may also help to achieve a microbiological diagnosis when there is no growth from pleural fluid.

Radiology Chest radiography often demonstrates a pleural effusion and consolidation. When pleural fluid has entered the organising phase there may be a lentiform pleural opacity (fig. 1).

Thoracic ultrasound is a useful bedside test in suspected pleural infection. It helps to differentiate simple parapneumonic effusions from empyema by the presence of septations and loculations, and should also be used to identify a safe site for fluid drainage. It also has a role in monitoring the degree of residual pleural fluid collection after a chest tube is placed, which may affect the subsequent management plan.

Contrast-enhanced CT demonstrates brightly enhancing pleural thickening in the organising phase of pleural infection. CT is only required when initial drainage of fluid is incomplete, for the planning of further

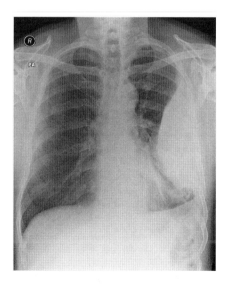

Figure 1. Chest radiograph of left empyema demonstrating a D-shaped, lentiform pleural opacity.

drains or thoracic surgical intervention or if other pathology such as pulmonary abscess, neoplastic lesions or oesophageal rupture is suspected.

Management The following steps should be implemented immediately:

- Broad-spectrum intravenous antibiotics
- Chest tube drainage
- Nutritional supplementation (oral or nasogastric)
- Thromboprophylaxis
- Vigilant monitoring for evidence of worsening sepsis indicating need for early thoracic surgery

Antibiotic choice is usually governed by local prescribing policies and should include antibiotics with broad-spectrum coverage and good penetration to the pleural space. Suitable combinations include penicillin–clavulanic acid in community-acquired infection and carbapenems with vancomycin in nosocomial infection. When cultures are available, antibiotics should be modified accordingly. As anaerobes can be difficult to culture, their presence should be assumed and cover continued, unless *S. pneumoniae* is isolated as this is not known to co-exist with anaerobes. Conventionally, $\geqslant 5$ days' intravenous antibiotics is followed by 2–4 weeks of oral treatment depending on clinical and radiological response.

In a clinically stable patient with a small empyema, chest tube drainage may be impractical and, hence, treatment with prolonged antibiotics and careful follow-up may suffice. However, in the majority of cases, drainage of the fluid is advocated. Small-bore (12–14 f) chest tubes are generally preferred to large-bore tubes as they can be placed *via* a Seldinger technique and are more comfortable for patients. There is no evidence that large-bore tubes achieve superior fluid drainage (although this is still the subject of some debate). Regular saline flushes (20 mL 6-hourly) may help to maintain tube patency and larger-volume 0.9% saline irrigation of the pleural space has been adopted by some European centres, with reports of improved primary treatment success rates, although this is not yet supported by published evidence.

The viscosity of the pleural fluid and degree of septation may impair tube drainage. Routine use of intrapleural fibrinolytics alone have not been shown to be of benefit. However, recent data suggests the combination of intrapleural tissue plasminogen activator (tPA) and DNase may result in improved radiological outcomes, and showed trends towards a reduction in need for surgery and duration of hospital stay. However, it has only been evaluated in a small number of patients and, therefore, its place in routine patient management is yet to be fully established.

Approximately 15–20% of patients will ultimately require surgical intervention for empyema, but selecting which patients are best suited to this approach can be challenging. The most compelling indication is failure of sepsis to improve despite appropriate antibiotics and tube drainage, but other reasons may include a significant residual pleural collection despite chest tube drainage. This assessment is usually made after 3–5 days of medical treatment. While surgical and anaesthetic complications are more common in the elderly and frail, the vast majority of deaths as a result of pleural infection occur in this group and, hence, early surgical referral for a limited surgical drainage procedure may be beneficial. Some European centres advocate early thoracoscopy for these patients.

Available approaches include:

- video-assisted thoracoscopic surgery (VATS)
- open thoracotomy and decortication
- rib resection and open drainage (often performed under local anaesthetic)
- mini-thoracotomy (usually VATS-assisted)
- thoracoscopy

Outcome It is not possible to reliably identify, by presenting radiological, pleural fluid or clinical feature,s which patients will go on to require thoracic surgery for empyema. However, a variety of risk factors for poor outcome have been identified,

including the elderly and hospital-acquired disease. Overall, mean mortality rates of 15% have been reported in a recent series, but vary depending on certain risk factors. In order to identify at presentation which patients are at the highest risk of a poor outcome, a validated clinical risk score is being developed, which may help guide early clinical management in those at highest risk. This has highlighted five particular risk factors for poor outcome, which include age, urea, albumin, hospital-acquired infection and nonpurulence.

Patients should be followed up for $\geqslant 3$ months to allow the early detection of recurrent sepsis or persistent breathlessness.

Lung abscess

Lung abscesses are caused when an area of infected lung becomes necrotic, which results in the development of a cavity within the lung itself. In contrast to pleural infection, the incidence and mortality rate of lung abscess have steadily declined since the advent of penicillin.

Risk factors include:

- male sex (2:1)
- immunocompromised states
- aspiration of any cause
- pneumonia (particularly *S. aureus* and *Klebsiella pneumoniae*).
- bronchial obstruction (*e.g.* endobronchial neoplasm is present in 10–20% cases)
- haematogenous spread of infection (*e.g.* tricuspid valve endocarditis and Lemierre's syndrome (whereby acute oropharyngeal infection caused by *Fusobacterium* spp., results in jugular vein thrombophlebitis and metastatic septic embolisation to the lung))

Diagnosis Symptoms may be acute or insidious in onset and commonly include cough, fever, chest pain, night sweats, weight loss and purulent or blood-stained sputum. There may be no specific examination findings or chest auscultation may mimic pneumonia. Anaemia is common in patients with a chronic lung abscess and inflammatory markers are likely to be raised.

Radiology Plain chest radiography classically demonstrates a well circumscribed opacity within the lung field, which is often thick walled and contains an air–fluid level. Right-sided abscesses are twice as common as left. Dependent segments are most commonly affected when the abscess is caused by aspiration of gastric contents.

CT is usually required to distinguish a parenchymal abscess from empyema and may assist in the detection of neoplastic lesions. Abscesses have an irregular wall and an indistinct outer margin that makes an acute angle with the chest wall. In contrast, an empyema is lenticular, well defined and causes compression of the underlying lung with vascular crowding (fig. 2).

The radiological appearances of a lung abscess may be mimicked by other pathologies, including:

- neoplastic lesions
- pulmonary vasculitis
- pulmonary infarction
- bullae and cysts
- rheumatoid nodules
- pneumoconiosis
- mycobacterial infection

Bacteriology and obtaining cultures The microbiology of lung abscesses has changed over recent decades, which is predominantly due to an increase in immunocompromise and immunosuppression. In >50% of

cases, lung abscesses are caused by more than one microorganism.

Anaerobes (*e.g. Fusobacterium*, *Prevotella* and *Peptostreptococcus* spp.), often originating from the oropharynx, are present in 30–50% and may be particularly important in the context of aspiration. However, aerobic bacteria now appear to be cultured more commonly than anaerobes (particularly *K. pneumoniae* and *S. aureus*).

Fungi, *Nocardia*, mycobacteria, *Amoeba*, actinomycosis and *Echinococcus* are more unusual causes of a parenchymal lung abscess, and immunocompromise may contribute to their development.

Most patients are treated effectively with broad-spectrum antibiotics in the absence of a microbiological diagnosis. Blood cultures should be sent and sputum cultured if available but, frequently, no organism is identified.

Bronchoscopy should be employed when there is particular suspicion of an underlying endobronchial neoplasm or inhaled foreign body. Culture of bronchial washings is of relatively low accuracy and often fails to focus antibiotic selection beyond empirical choices, but may help to investigate other potential causes of lung cavitation, such as malignancy or TB. Endobronchial drainage of large lung abscesses is not usually recommended due to the risk of sudden discharge of pus into the airway, which may result in asphyxiation and respiratory compromise.

Image-guided percutaneous aspiration using CT, ultrasound or fluoroscopy obtains a microbiological diagnosis in 80–90% of cases and changes antibiotic choice in up to 47%. Due to a relatively high risk of pneumothorax (~14%) as a complication of these techniques, it is usually reserved for cases that do not respond to empirical broad-spectrum antibiotics.

Management A prolonged course of antibiotics is the foundation of treatment and, often, up to 8 weeks of treatment is required depending on clinical and radiological response. β-lactam/β-

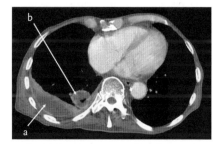

Figure 2. CT image of a) right pleural empyema and b) cavitating pulmonary abscess.

lactamase inhibitor combinations cover the majority of causative bacteria and are a good empirical choice. Local antibiotic policies differ and should be used to guide antibiotic choices.

Patients with very large abscesses should ideally be placed in the lateral decubitus position with the abscess side down. This may help to prevent spread of the infection to the contralateral lung and respiratory compromise should the abscess suddenly discharge the contents into the airway. Chest physiotherapy also plays an important role in management and postural drainage may help to clear secretions from the abscess itself. Preventative measures to avoid further aspiration of gastric contents are also important.

Fever and infective symptoms usually settle within a week of appropriate antibiotics. Failure to improve should raise the suspicion of drug-resistant organisms, such as MRSA (particularly in the case of hospital-acquired infection), or other pathologies, such as TB or malignancy. Sustained resolution of sepsis is the most important marker of successful conservative management as radiological resolution can take up to 3 months.

When appropriate antibiotic therapy fails, invasive intervention to drain the abscess itself may become necessary. This is more common in the elderly or immuno-compromised and for very large abscesses (>6 cm) and may be necessary in 11–21% of patients. This can either be performed using a percutaneous technique or surgery.

Image-guided percutaneous drainage is successful in 84% of cases and can be achieved with CT, ultrasound or fluoroscopic guidance. Complications such as bronchopleural fistulae, haemothorax and empyema are infrequent. As it is usually performed under local anaesthesia, this approach is preferred in patients with significant comorbidities.

The precise indications for surgical intervention are not well established, but it may be considered in the context of localised obstructing malignancy or life-threatening complications such as intractable haemoptysis, bronchopleural fistula or empyema. A VATS approach is less invasive than open surgical resection.

Perioperative mortality rates of up to 16% have been reported following surgery for lung abscess and, hence, an attempt at radiological drainage may be considered prior to undertaking a surgical procedure.

Lung abscesses are associated with a 10% mortality rate.

The elderly or immunocompromised and those with large abscesses (>6 cm), underlying malignancy, malnitrition or a delay in diagnosis and treatment have a particularly poor outcome.

Further reading

- Davies CW, et al. (1999). Predictors of outcome and long-term survival in patients with pleural infection. Am J Respir Crit Care Med; 160: 1682–1687.
- Davies CWH, et al. (2010). The British Thoracic Society Guidelines for the management of pleural infection. Thorax; 58: Suppl. 2, ii18–ii28.
- Grijalva CG, et al. (2011). Emergence of parapneumonic empyema in the USA. Thorax; 66: 663–668.
- Kioumis IP, et al. Lung abscess. http://bestpractice.bmj.com/best-practice/monograph/927/highlights/summary.html
- Maskell NA, et al. (2006). The bacteriology of pleural infection by genetic and standard methods and its mortality significance. Am J Respir Crit Care Med; 174: 817–823.
- Maskell NA, et al. (2012). Rapid Score – the first validated clinical score in pleural infection to identify those at risk of poor outcome at presentation. Am J Respir Crit Care Med; 185: A5341.
- Menzies SM, et al. (2011). Blood culture bottle culture of pleural fluid in pleural infection. Thorax; 66: 658–662.
- Mwandumba HC, et al. (2000). Pyogenic lung infections: factors for predicting clinical outcome of lung abscess and thoracic empyema. Curr Opin Pulm Med; 6: 234–239.

- Peña Griñan N, *et al.* (1990). Yield of percutaneous needle lung aspiration in lung abscess. *Chest*; 97: 67–94.
- Rahman NM, *et al.* (2011). Intrapleural use of tissue plasminogen activator and DNase in pleural infection. *N Engl J Med*; 365: 518–526.
- Van Sonnenberg E, *et al.* (1984). Lung abscess: CT guided drainage. *Radiology*; 151: 337–341.
- Yu H (2011). Management of pleural effusion, empyema and lung abscess. *Semin Interv Radiol*; 28: 75–86.

Influenza, pandemics and SARS

Wei Shen Lim

Seasonal and pandemic influenza

Virology Influenza viruses are RNA orthomyxoviruses with three main types, A, B and C. Viral surface proteins include haemagglutinin (H) and neuraminidase (N), which are involved in viral attachment and release respectively. There are 16 haemagglutinin (H1–H16) and nine neuraminidase types (N1–N9). Influenza viruses are described in a standardised manner according to their type/location of

Key Points

- Influenza is mostly a self-limiting viral upper respiratory tract infection that is managed in the community. Pneumonia is the most frequent serious complications of influenza.

- Neuraminidase inhibitors, such as oseltamivir and zanamivir, are effective in the prophylaxis and treatment of influenza A infection.

- The influenza A (H1N1) 2009 pandemic was of low severity compared to the other pandemics of the 20th century.

- The SARS outbreak of 2003 resulted in 8096 cases, of which 774 died.

- SARS-CoV is the causative agent of SARS. Bats are the natural reservoir for coronaviruses.

- The management of SARS is chiefly supportive. Basic infection control measures are the cornerstone of containment of any future outbreak.

first isolate/laboratory strain number/year of isolate/H and N subtypes, for example: influenza A/Hong Kong/1/68/H3N2 (the cause of the 1968 'Hong Kong' pandemic).

The natural reservoir hosts of all influenza A virus subtypes are water birds. The host specificity of the various influenza A virus subtypes is partially determined by the binding affinity of haemagglutinin to sialic acid residues on the host cell.

A notable feature of influenza A viruses is their propensity to undergo antigenic variation. The appearance of a novel antigenic type demonstrating efficient human-to-human transmission is a pre-requisite for a pandemic. Only influenza A viruses have been associated with pandemics.

Seasonal influenza Influenza is mostly a self-limiting upper respiratory tract infection that is managed in the community. In temperate climates, outbreaks of infections occur almost exclusively in winter. Attack rates are highest in young children and the elderly.

Influenza is highly transmissible. Human-to-human transmission occurs through large-droplet spread and direct contact with secretions (or fomites). There is also evidence supporting aerosol transmission although the extent and importance of this is debated.

The mean incubation period is 2–4 days with a range up to 7 days. An abrupt onset of high fever (up to 41°C) is the main presenting feature. The fever peaks within the first 24 h of illness and usually lasts for 3 days. Cough is the next commonest symptom (85%), which may be associated with sputum production in up to 40% of cases. Malaise (80%), chills (70%), headaches (65%) and myalgia (50%) may be prominent. Coryza and sore throat are reported in about half of patients. In addition, children may present with vomiting, diarrhoea and abdominal pain but these symptoms are uncommon in adults. The mean duration of symptoms is 4 days.

Complications of influenza Although influenza is mostly a self-limiting illness even without specific treatment, some patient groups experience significant morbidity and mortality. Persons at risk of complications from influenza include pregnant females, the frail elderly, those who are immunosuppressed, and those with chronic medical conditions such as heart disease, chronic respiratory disease (mostly asthma and COPD), cancer, diabetes, renal disease, rheumatologic disease, dementia and stroke. Rates of hospitalisation and death are increased in all these patient groups. Obesity (BMI >30 kg·m^{-2}) was also identified as being associated with adverse outcomes in patients hospitalised with influenza in the 2009 pandemic.

Pneumonia is the most frequent serious complication of influenza. Two main clinical patterns are described: primary viral pneumonia and secondary bacterial pneumonia.

Patients with primary viral pneumonia typically become breathless within the first few days of the onset of fever. This may be associated with tachypnoea, cyanosis and bilateral lung crackles on chest examination. The commonest chest radiographic abnormality is of diffuse bilateral interstitial infiltrates similar to pulmonary congestion. Progression to respiratory failure is well recognised. Mortality rates of 6–40% have been reported. In severe cases, pathological findings are similar to those seen in acute respiratory distress syndrome (ARDS).

Patients with secondary bacterial pneumonia complicating influenza typically experience an amelioration of the initial symptoms of viral infection. However, 4–10 days later, a recurrence of fever together with breathlessness and a productive cough ensues. Clinical features at this point are indistinguishable from community-acquired bacterial pneumonia. The commonest pathogens implicated are *Streptococcus pneumoniae*, *Staphylococcus aureus*, *Haemophilus influenzae* and *Streptococcus* spp.

In children, the commonest respiratory complication, though not the most serious, is otitis media.

In addition to the specific complications listed in table 1, patients with influenza may also experience a worsening of a pre-existing medical illness, such as COPD or cardiac failure.

Treatment There are two main classes of drug that are active against influenza. The M2 ion channel inhibitors, amantadine and rimantadine, are effective against influenza A.

Table 1. Complications of influenza in adults and children

Complication	Incidence	
	Adults	Children
Otitis media	Common	Very common
Secondary bacterial pneumonia	Common	Uncommon
Primary viral pneumonia	Common	Uncommon
Myositis	Uncommon	Rare
Myocarditis	Rare	Rare
Encephalitis/encephalopathy	Rare	Rare
Reye's syndrome		Rare
Febrile convulsions		Common

However, their use is hindered by the rapid emergence of resistance to these drugs together with a high incidence of side-effects. The neuraminidase inhibitors, oseltamivir and zanamivir, are effective against influenza A and B. Fortunately, although resistance to oseltamivir has been reported, this is not widespread in seasonal influenza A (H3N2). Oseltamivir is often generally preferred over zanamivir because of ease of administration (oral *versus* inhaled/intravenous). Newer neuraminidase inhibitors, such as peramivir and laninamivir, are also being clinically evaluated. A Cochrane meta-analysis of randomised controlled trials of neuraminidase inhibitors in the treatment of influenza reported that the efficacy of oral oseltamivir at 75 mg daily was 61% (risk ratio (RR) 0.39, 95% CI 0.18–0.85) and of inhaled zanamivir at 10 mg daily was 62% (RR 0.38, 95% CI 0.17–0.85). In clinical terms, this benefit translates to a shortening of the illness by 0.5–1 day. The review found the published evidence insufficient to answer the question of whether neuraminidase inhibitors are effective in reducing the complications of lower respiratory tract infection, antibiotic use or admissions to hospital. Oseltamivir use is associated with nausea (OR 1.79, 95% CI 1.10–2.93). A meta-analysis of observational cohort studies of patients with pandemic influenza A (H1N1) 2009 found that antiviral treatment was associated with reduced mortality, hospitalisation and otitis media. However, the quality of the evidence was graded as low or very low, reflecting the underlying risk of bias in these observational cohorts.

For critically ill patients with severe avian H5N1 influenza infection and for patients with severe H1N1 primary viral pneumonitis, an increased dose of antiviral treatment for an extended duration (*e.g.* oseltamivir 150 mg b.d. for 10 days in adults) has been used. This practice is not based on evidence from randomised controlled trials.

For selected critically ill patients with severe influenza-associated ARDS and in whom conventional ventilation is proving inadequate, extracorporeal membrane oxygenation (ECMO) should be considered based on experience from the 2009 H1N1 pandemic.

Management of influenza-associated exacerbations of underlying comorbid illnesses, such as COPD or heart failure, should follow the same principles for each specific condition regardless of influenza. Antibiotics are usually advised for patients with influenza-associated pneumonia or patients with severe influenza infection who are at high risk of developing secondary bacterial infections. The use of corticosteroids in severe influenza cannot be routinely advocated based on current data; observational cohort studies conducted during the 2009 H1N1 pandemic have reported mixed results including increased harm.

Chemoprophylaxis and vaccination Both oseltamivir and zanamivir, taken as prophylactic agents, reduce the chance of symptomatic, laboratory-confirmed influenza (RR 0.38, 95% CI 0.17–0.85 for zanamivir 10 mg daily; RR 0.39, 95% CI 0.18–0.85 for oseltamivir 75 mg daily). However, the effect of neuraminidase inhibitors on the prophylaxis of influenza-like illness (ILI), which includes infections other than influenza, is uncertain. Oseltamivir has also been demonstrated to be 58–84% efficacious as post-exposure prophylaxis.

Immunisation is the backbone of influenza prevention. The relative protective efficacy in children and young healthy adults is 70% to >90%. Efficacy is lower (~40%) in the elderly.

Oseltamivir resistance In 1977, influenza A (H1N1) re-emerged and co-circulated with influenza A (H3N2), with the latter remaining the dominant seasonal human influenza virus (fig. 1). During the 2007–2008 influenza season, oseltamivir-resistant seasonal influenza A (H1N1) viruses emerged suddenly and spread globally. These viruses carried a histidine-to-tyrosine mutation at residue 275 of the neuraminidase protein (H275Y). Laboratory and limited epidemiological data indicated that the viral fitness and virulence of these oseltamivir-resistant influenza A (H1N1) viruses were no different from those of oseltamivir-susceptible strains.

In the USA, the prevalence of oseltamivir resistance among seasonal influenza A (H1N1) viruses increased from <1% before the 2007–2008 influenza season to 12% during the 2007–2008 season and rose to >99% in the 2008–2009 season. This prompted the USA to issue guidelines at the time recommending the use of zanamivir or a combination of oseltamivir and rimantadine when oseltamivir-resistant seasonal influenza A (H1N1) virus infection was suspected.

H275Y mutations in pandemic influenza A (H1N1) 2009 viruses have also been identified. Fortunately, such oseltamivir-resistant isolates remain infrequent and sporadic, many occurring in immuno-suppressed patients who appear to be at risk of resistance developing during oseltamivir therapy.

Pandemic influenza In the 20th century, pandemics occurred in 1918 (H1N1), 1957 (H2N2), 1968 (H3N2) and 2009 (H1N1) (fig. 1). Each of these pandemics had a different impact and tempo. The 1918 pandemic was the deadliest, claiming the lives of an estimated 40–100 million people

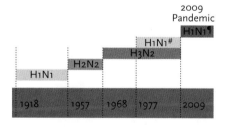

Figure 1. *Influenza pandemics and subtypes, 1918–2009. #: re-emergence of H1N1, possibly from accidental laboratory release – strain closely related to 1950 strain. ¶: new reassortment of six gene segments from triple-reassortant North American swine influenza virus lineages and two gene segments from Eurasian swine influenza virus lineages.*

globally. In contrast, the subsequent two pandemics were much less severe, accounting for an estimated 1–2 million deaths each.

The 2009 pandemic has been the best studied pandemic of the 20th century. The first cases were identified in Mexico in April 2009 and by June 2009, the World Health Organization had declared a pandemic. The pandemic influenza A (H1N1) 2009 virus was a triple-reassortant virus containing genes from human, swine and avian influenza viruses. It caused an infection that was clinically similar to seasonal influenza although gastrointestinal symptoms amongst adults were commoner than in seasonal influenza. Mainly children and young adults were affected and most illnesses were self-limiting. In persons >60 years old, pre-existing cross-reactive antibodies due to previous exposure to antigenically related influenza viruses provided protection against infection.

Compared to the other 20th century pandemics, overall hospitalisation and mortality rates were low. In the UK, the overall estimated case fatality rate was 26 per 100 000; lowest for children aged 5–14 years (11 per 100 000) and highest for those aged ≥65 years (980 per 100 000). Hospitalisation rates varied across countries. Of those hospitalised, 9–31% required intensive care support, predominantly because of diffuse viral pneumonitis or ARDS. The mortality of intensive care unit-admitted patients was 14–46%.

After 2009, some countries experienced a further wave of influenza A (H1N1) 2009 infections in the 2010–2011 influenza season. However, in the following 2011–2012 influenza season, influenza A (H3N2) predominated in most countries and overall influenza activity was much lower compared with previous years. Based on past events, the threat of a future pandemic remains but its timing and severity are not currently predictable.

Severe acute respiratory syndrome

Epidemiology The global outbreak of severe acute respiratory syndrome (SARS) in

2002–2003 affected 8096 individuals in 29 countries, 774 of whom died. The three most severely affected regions were mainland China, Hong Kong and Taiwan with 5327, 1755 and 674, cases respectively.

The first human case was identified in the city of Foshan in Guangdong Province, China on November 16, 2002 and the last known case of the initial outbreak experienced the onset of symptoms on June 15, 2003 in Taiwan.

A novel coronavirus, the SARS coronavirus (SARS-CoV), was identified as the causative agent of SARS in April 2003. Close human–animal contact associated with many of the early cases in China supported the concept of SARS as a zoonotic infection. While market animals such as the palm civet cat *Paguma larvata* have been identified as the likely animal sources of the 2003 outbreak, bats are now recognised as the natural reservoir for coronaviruses. Coronaviruses sharing 87–92% genome nucleotide identity with SARS-CoV have been found in horseshoe bats (*Rhinolophus* sp.). Accordingly, one hypothesis is that coronaviruses were transmitted from horseshoe bats to civet cats and then to humans (fig. 2).

Subsequent infections later in the course of the outbreak were due mainly to human-to-human transmission. Molecular evolutionary changes of SARS-CoV have been described that might explain the shift in mode of transmission. Nosocomial transmission was particularly high, with attack rates amongst healthcare workers in some centres ranging from 10% to 60%. In contrast, community transmission rates were much lower, with typically <10% of contacts infected.

The mean incubation period of SARS is estimated at 4–6 days with a maximum incubation period of 10 days. Overall, SARS may be considered to be low-to-moderately transmissible. A few remarkable super-spreading events (SSEs) were associated with SARS in which single individuals were responsible for infecting many more individuals than the average. In one SSE at the Prince of Wales Hospital, Hong Kong, a single patient infected 143 people.

Clinical features The clinical presenting features of SARS infection are nonspecific. Fever (93%), chills (61%), malaise (46%), cough (41%) and rigors (38%) were the predominant symptoms recorded in the Hong Kong-wide clinical database of SARS patients. High-volume, watery, nonbloody diarrhoea is present in a sizeable minority of patients (~20%) in the early stages of disease and increases in frequency (up to 70%) by the second week of illness. It is usually self-limiting. Similarly, respiratory symptoms of cough, breathlessness and sputum production are less frequently (<50%) encountered in the first 4 days of

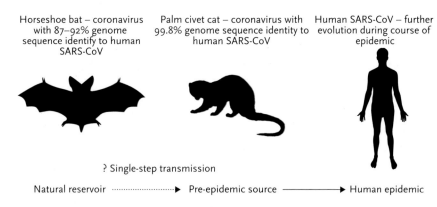

Horseshoe bat – coronavirus with 87–92% genome sequence identify to human SARS-CoV

Palm civet cat – coronavirus with 99.8% genome sequence identity to human SARS-CoV

Human SARS-CoV – further evolution during course of epidemic

? Single-step transmission

Natural reservoir ·····▶ Pre-epidemic source ──────▶ Human epidemic

Figure 2. Possible origin of SARS, based on phylogenetic studies.

illness, but increase to a peak (70%) by day 9 or 10 of illness. Typically, a dry cough is the first respiratory symptom. This is followed by breathlessness, which worsens at the start of the second week.

Radiological changes of airspace consolidation are usually unilateral and localised in the first week. The infiltrates are commoner in the lower lobes (70%) and the periphery (75%). Cavitation, lymphadenopathy and pleural effusions are not described in association with SARS infection. The extent of radiological abnormality correlates with severity of illness and prognosis.

Laboratory test abnormalities include lymphopenia, neutropenia, thrombocytopenia, and raised levels of lactate dehydrogenase (LDH), alanine aminotransferase (ALT), creatinine kinase and activated partial thromboplastin time.

Respiratory failure occurs in 20–25% of patients, mainly adults. Unusually, the incidence of barotrauma (manifesting as a pneumothorax or pneumomediastinum) was observed to be higher in severely ill patients with SARS than might be expected despite the use of low-volume, low-pressure mechanical ventilation strategies. The reason for this is unclear. Patients with SARS requiring critical care support have a mortality of ~25%. Features associated with a poor prognosis include advanced age, male sex, presence of comorbid illness, high serum LDH and neutrophilia at presentation, and an initial radiograph with more than one zone of involvement. Overall, adults suffer a more severe disease than children.

Virology SARS-CoV is detectable by RT-PCR and by culture from respiratory tract, faecal and urine samples. Virus RNA is also detectable in serum, plasma and cerebrospinal fluid, indicating multisystem infection. Diagnostic yields are better with nasopharyngeal aspirates and faeces compared with throat swabs. A retrospective diagnosis of SARS is possible using serological tests.

Clinical management The management of SARS is chiefly supportive.

Chemical compounds that have reported activity against SARS-CoV include glycyrrhizin, baicalin, reserpine, niclosamide, ribavirin, protease inhibitors (lopinavir and nelfinavir), interferon (IFN)-α and IFN-β. A comparative study using IFN alfacon-1 (n=22) and another using a lopinavir/ritonavir combination (n=41) suggested clinical benefit. However, there are no randomised controlled trials of treatment.

Corticosteroids were used during the SARS outbreak as an immunomodulatory agent with the intention of limiting the damage that might be caused by the host immune response. In reported series, there were large variations in type, dose, route and duration of corticosteroids used. Unsurprisingly, different conclusions about the efficacies of corticosteroids were drawn.

Basic infection control measures are the cornerstone of containment of any future outbreak. As subclinical infection with SARS has not been described and the peak in viral load occurs late (second week), effective infection control measures can often be instituted prior to widespread transmission.

Practice points regarding the clinical diagnosis of influenza or SARS

The early symptoms in both influenza and SARS are nonspecific, comprising primarily of a fever in association with respiratory symptoms, such as cough, and systemic symptoms, such as malaise or chills. A clinical diagnosis of influenza or SARS is, therefore, crucially dependent on epidemiological features. In the case of influenza, an ILI in the setting of local or community circulation of influenza viruses (*e.g.* during an influenza season or during a pandemic) greatly increases the likelihood that the illness is due to influenza virus infection: the positive predictive value of an ILI for laboratory-confirmed influenza can range from 20% to 70%. Alternative pathogens to consider in instances of an ILI include parainfluenza virus, adenovirus, rhinovirus, *Mycoplasma pneumoniae* and even *Streptococcus pneumoniae*. Similarly, a clinical diagnosis of SARS requires the establishment of an epidemiological link with another patient with SARS, or exposure to likely animal sources of SARS-CoV. Virological testing is necessary to make a definitive diagnosis in both influenza and SARS.

Further reading

- Cleri DJ, *et al.* (2010). Severe acute respiratory syndrome (SARS). *Infect Dis Clin North Am*; 24: 175–202.
- Hsu J, *et al.* (2012). Antivirals for treatment of influenza: a systematic review and meta-analysis of observational studies. *Ann Intern Med*; 156: 512–524.
- Jefferson T, *et al.* (2010). Neuraminidase inhibitors for preventing and treating influenza in healthy adults. *Cochrane Database Syst Rev*; 2: CD001265.
- Lew TW, *et al.* (2003). Acute respiratory distress syndrome in critically ill patients with severe acute respiratory syndrome. *JAMA*; 290: 374–380.
- Miller E, *et al.* (2010). Incidence of 2009 pandemic influenza A H1N1 infection in England: a cross-sectional serological study. *Lancet*; 375: 1100–1008.
- Monto AS *et al.* (2008). Seasonal and pandemic influenza: a 2007 update on challenges and solutions. *Clin Infect Dis*; 46: 1024–1031.
- Palese P (2004). Influenza: old and new threats. *Nat Med*; 10: S82–S87.
- Peiris JS, *et al.* (2003). The severe acute respiratory syndrome. *N Engl J Med*; 349: 2431–2341.
- Van Kerkhove MD, *et al.* (2011). Risk factors for severe outcomes following 2009 influenza A (H1N1) infection: a global pooled analysis. *PLoS Med*; 8: e1001053.
- Writing Committee of the WHO Consultation on Clinical Aspects of Pandemic (H1N1) 2009 Influenza, *et al.* (2010). Clinical Aspects of Pandemic 2009 Influenza A (H1N1) Virus Infection. *N Engl J Med*; 362: 1708–1719.
- Yip CW, *et al.* (2009). Phylogenetic perspectives on the epidemiology and origins of SARS and SARS-like coronaviruses. *Infect Genet Evol*; 9: 1185–1196.

Pulmonary tuberculosis

Giovanni Sotgiu and Giovanni Battista Migliori

The World Health Organization (WHO) has declared TB a global emergency due to its burden in terms of cases and deaths. Among the factors contributing to maintenance of the TB pandemic are:

- the large number of patients co-infected with HIV
- multidrug resistance to anti-TB drugs (*i.e.* strains resistant to at least isoniazid (H) and rifampicin (R))
- migration from high-incidence countries
- the social determinants of the disease (in particular, poverty, drug abuse and homelessness)

TB can affect virtually every organ, most importantly the lungs (pulmonary TB).

Key points

- With 8.8 million new cases (0.21 being MDR-TB) and 1.1 million deaths, TB is a first-class health priority.

- Diagnosis of pulmonary TB is simple, being primarily based on bacteriology (sputum smear microscopy and culture). Recently, a new molecular technique (Xpert MTB/RIF) for the rapid diagnosis of TB and rifampicin resistance has been recommended as the standard in Europe.

- Treatment of pan-susceptible cases of pulmonary TB is effective and cheap.

- Management of pulmonary TB in MDR-TB/HIV co-infected cases is particularly complicated.

Aetiology

TB is an infectious disease caused by aerobic, nonmotile, non-spore-forming bacteria belonging to the family *Mycobacteriaceae* in the order *Actinomycetales*. Among the species belonging to the *Mycobacterium tuberculosis* complex (*Mycobacterium africanum, Mycobacterium bovis, Mycobacterium canettii, Mycobacterium caprae, Mycobacterium microti* and *Mycobacterium pinnipedii*), the most frequent and important agent of human disease is *M. tuberculosis*. Mycobacteria are 2–4 μm long and 0.2–5 μm wide, with a bacterial generation time of 18–24 h. They are defined as acid-fast bacilli (AFB) by Ziehl–Neelsen staining, owing to their cell wall structure, which is crucial to their survival and characterised by a significant content of mycolic acid attached to the underlying peptidoglycan-bound polysaccharide arabinogalactan. An outermost structure, characterised by an elevated concentration of carbohydrates that function in cell–cell interactions, completes the mycobacterial envelope. The peptidoglycan network, located just outside the cell membrane, confers cell wall rigidity and protects a genome with ~4000 genes. Two groups of genes are crucial in the physiology of the mycobacteria: one encoding β-oxidation related-enzymes for energetic processes; and the other encoding PE and PEE families of proteins functioning in virulence and molecular mimicry processes. Furthermore, a relevant pathogenic role is attributed to the genes encoding glycolipids of the envelope, interplaying with the host innate and adaptive immune responses as well as with the metabolism of anti-TB drugs, due to their chemical characteristics.

Pathogenesis

Mycobacteria are spread through air droplets expelled by infectious pulmonary TB individuals coughing, sneezing or speaking. Close contacts (those with prolonged, frequent or intense contact with pulmonary TB cases) are at highest risk of becoming infected. Climate and human population density may affect the intensity and duration of human relationships and, consequently, the probability of close contact. The majority of mycobacteria, moved on droplet nuclei sized >5 µm, are trapped in the upper parts of the airways by the nasal vibrissae and by the mucus secreted by goblet cells, while the cilia of the epithelial cells constantly beat them upward for removal. Environmental factors like humidity, temperature and ventilation can modify the dimension and density of droplets containing mycobacteria. Bacteria in droplet nuclei sized 1–5 µm can bypass the mucociliary system and reach the alveoli, usually located in subpleural and in mid-lung zones, where they are rapidly engulfed by macrophages, which are part of the innate immune system and the most abundant phagocytic cells located in the alveolar spaces; they are readily active without requiring previous antigenic exposure. Macrophages engulfing mycobacteria transfer to draining lymph nodes in order to prime naïve lymphocytes, after having enrolled other mononuclear and nonmononuclear cells in the alveolar spaces. Mycobacteria significantly growing for the first 3 weeks are controlled by phagocytic cells, activated mainly by T-cells producing interferon (IFN)-γ. Infection could be crucially favoured by the slow pulmonary enrolment of T-cells. Numerous bacterial and host mechanisms are involved in the uptake of the mycobacteria, such as:

- mycobacterial lipoarabinomannans
- ligands for macrophage receptors
- complement proteins C2a and C3b, which bind to the cell wall and enhance recognition of the mycobacteria by effector macrophages

- Toll-like receptors
- nucleotide-binding oligomerisation domain-like receptors
- C-type lectins
- PE and PEE families of acidic, glycine-rich proteins
- induction of regulatory T-cells (delay of priming following the interaction with antigen-presenting cells and the production of interleukin-10)

Unfortunately, innate and adaptive immunity cannot eradicate mycobacterial strains and a latent TB infection (LTBI) follows in the majority of cases; rarely, infection progresses to active disease, called primary progressive pulmonary TB (common among children aged ⩽4 years). During the initial phase (2–12 weeks), the bacteria continue to multiply slowly but exponentially (a cell division every 25–35 h) and T-cells are attracted by cytokines released by macrophages. In the immunocompetent, the next defensive stage is formation of granulomata around mycobacteria, which limits bacterial replication and spread to other pulmonary sites, establishing latency of the infection (potential sustained T-cell responses). Granulomata, whose size range from 1 mm to 2 cm, are characterised by different macrophage populations that secrete pro- and anti-inflammatory cytokines, and by a chemical and physical microenvironment, which induces mycobacterial dormancy genes. $CD4^+$ T-cells, primed in the regional lymph nodes and migrating to the site of infection, produce cytokines that function in $CD8^+$ lymphocyte enrolment (e.g. interleukin-15), the activation of regulatory T-cells and the inhibition of mycobacterial replication (IFN-γ). Lesions in those with an adequate immune system undergo fibrosis and calcification, while in immunocompromised subjects, they progress to primary progressive pulmonary TB.

The majority of infected individuals developing pulmonary TB experience the disease within the first 2 years following infection. Dormant bacilli, however, may persist for years before being reactivated to produce secondary pulmonary TB. Overall, it is estimated that the lifetime risk of developing TB, given infection, is 5–10% in those who are immunocompetent and 5–10% per year in HIV-positive individuals. Age is an important determinant of the risk of disease after infection. Among infected subjects, the incidence is highest in childhood up to the age of 8 years (35–50% in children close contacts of contagious patients), with a second peak during adolescence and early adulthood. The risk may increase in the elderly, possibly because of waning immunity and comorbidities (*e.g.* diabetes mellitus, chronic renal failure, silicosis, gastrectomy, jejunoileal bypass, and solid and liquid neoplasias).

Epidemiology

WHO estimates that 8.8 (range 8.5–9.2) million new cases of TB occurred in 2010. India, China, South Africa, Indonesia and Pakistan recorded the highest incidence. Asia (South-East Asia and the Western Pacific region) accounts for 59% of global cases and Africa for 26%. TB/HIV co-infection was detected in 1.1 (range 1.0–1.2) million individuals, mainly living in the WHO African Region (82%). From 1990 to 1997, TB incidence decreased but the positive trend was reverted by the HIV/AIDS epidemic; however, the implementation and scale-up of several preventive measures, as well as the distribution of successful antiretroviral drugs, has favoured a positive declining trend since 2004 at an annual rate of -1.3%. However, the positive declining trend of TB prevalence since 1990 has not been affected by the HIV/AIDS epidemic. The estimated incidence in the WHO European region was 418 000 (range 335 000–496 000) in 2010, with four countries showing an elevated TB notification rate (*i.e.* Kazakhstan, Moldova, Georgia and Kyrgyzstan with 123, 115, 107 and 106 cases per 100 000 inhabitants, respectively). The global TB notification rate has declined since 2006, from 47.4 per 100 000 inhabitants to 43.2 per 100 000 inhabitants in 2010 (8.7% decrease).

Globally, 12 (range 11–14) million prevalent cases of TB were estimated to exist in 2010, equivalent to a prevalence of 178 cases per 100 000 population.

It was estimated that 210 000–380 000 (best estimate 290 000 individuals) cases of multidrug-resistant (MDR)-TB emerged worldwide in 2010, with an estimated prevalence of 650 000 cases. WHO identified 27 high MDR-TB burden countries, with almost half of them (13) located in the geographical area of the Former Soviet Union. Belarus and Moldova described the highest prevalence among new (26%) and previously treated (65%) patients. In 2006, a new drug-resistant form of TB was described and defined as extensively drug-resistant (XDR)-TB, characterised as MDR strains resistant to fluoroquinolones and to at least one second-line injectable drug (amikacin, capreomycin or kanamycin). The percentage of XDR-TB among MDR-TB cases was 12.2% in the WHO European Region. Globally, drug susceptibility testing (DST) to diagnose MDR/XDR-TB is performed only in <2% and 6% of new and previously treated TB cases, respectively; moreover, MDR-TB therapy was started in only 16% of the 290 000 MDR-TB cases in 2010. Those programmatic shortcomings in the diagnosis and treatment of drug-resistant cases will favour the emergence and spread of mycobacterial strains.

Approximately 1.1 (range 0.9–1.2) million TB patients died in 2010; an estimated 350 000 were HIV positive.

Clinical features

Before the HIV/AIDS epidemic, almost two-thirds of all TB cases were pulmonary; an increase in extra-pulmonary, and pulmonary and extra-pulmonary forms has been reported over recent decades.

Primary pulmonary TB frequently occurs without clinical signs and symptoms or takes a paucisymptomatic course resembling mild respiratory tract infection.

In the majority of cases, the primary infection is contained, largely resolves and a small calcified nodule (Ghon lesion) persists. Mostly in children and in individuals with impaired immunity, the primary infection can progress to pleural effusion; only in certain circumstances it may develop further to more acute infection, and induce fever, cough, pain and dyspnoea. In children aged <4 years, a systemic disease and/or meningoencephalitis can be diagnosed after primary regional lymphadenitis.

Secondary pulmonary or post-primary TB results from endogenous reactivation of a LTBI and is frequently located in pulmonary areas where the oxygen concentration is higher and favours mycobacterial replication (upper lobes).

Early clinical signs and symptoms consists of low-grade fever, asthenia, weight loss (inappetence and altered metabolism associated with systemic inflammatory response to mycobacteria) and night sweats. A mucopurulent cough develops in the majority of patients: a duration of at least 2–3 weeks has to be considered the main clinical symptom, whereas haemoptysis (*i.e.* coughing up of blood) in the late stages of the disease might be due to the rupture of a dilated vessel in a cavity (Rasmussen's aneurysm) or to an aspergilloma in an old cavity. A pleuritic process can cause chest pain. Rales and dullness can be detected in only a few individuals.

Diagnosis

At >100 years old, sputum smear microscopy (Ziehl–Neelsen staining) is still the most widely used technique for the diagnosis of pulmonary TB. Although highly specific, the lower limit of detection of microscopy is $0.5-1 \times 10^4$ organisms per mL sputum and only about half of all culture-positive cases have sputum smear-positive results. At least two sputum samples should be sent to the laboratory for a microscopic examination; at least one of them should be collected in the early morning. The first specimen is positive in 85.8% of the sputum smear positive individuals; the average incremental yield of the second specimen is 11.1%. However, sensitivity may be lower among HIV-infected subjects and in children. AFB microscopy is simple to perform but suboptimal results are described where adequate quality-assurance

programmes are absent. Over recent years, fluorescence microscopy was introduced in numerous laboratories, adding 10% sensitivity to that of conventional light microscopy. An increased sensitivity of 10–20% can be obtained after centrifugation and/or sedimentation. WHO has proposed a case definition for sputum smear-negative pulmonary TB based on three negative sputum smears, radiographic abnormalities consistent with active pulmonary TB and no response to a course of broad-spectrum antibiotics. Although sputum smear-negative pulmonary TB cases are not considered to be infectious, their high number is causing increasing concern in high HIV prevalence, low-income settings.

Sputum induction with hypertonic saline is a useful technique for diagnosing pulmonary TB in individuals who are either sputum smear negative or unable to produce sputum. Repeated sputum induction increases the yield of both smear and culture. It avoids invasive procedures and provides a means of diagnosis in resource-poor settings. It is worth noting that sputum induction should be carefully conducted in a well-ventilated setting, as it is a cough-inducing procedure with a high risk of mycobacterial exposure.

Mycobacterial culture is considered the gold standard; however, false-positive results do occur, primarily as a consequence of laboratory contamination. Moreover, several weeks are required for the performance of culture-based methods, although the use of liquid media has decreased pulmonary TB diagnosis time. DST for first- and second-line drugs is also useful in order to better define the phenotype of the isolated strain in culture-confirmed cases.

Molecular techniques (nucleic acid amplification (NAA)) based on gene amplification have shown an unpredictable sensitivity, particularly in sputum smear-positive cases and extra-pulmonary forms, and a low negative predictive value. The major limitation, mainly for low-income countries, is their current high cost and the risk of contamination (false-positive results). Recently, WHO endorsed a new molecular technique (Xpert MTB/RIF; Cepheid, Sunnyvale, CA, USA) for the rapid (~1 h 45 min) diagnosis of TB and rifampicin resistance, which is deemed a surrogate marker of MDR-TB. Rapid scale-up of this technique has started globally. In 2012, this technique was recommended in the European Union standards for TB care.

Chest radiology (fig. 1) and CT are useful tools that complement bacteriological examinations in the diagnosis of pulmonary TB. Although over- and under-reading have been described, these tools can offer important information to the clinician. Chest radiography is commonly used to screen individuals harbouring a significantly higher risk of pulmonary TB (e.g. prisoners, contacts of infectious cases, etc.).

Among the tools indirectly used to detect mycobacterial infection, the tuberculin skin test (TST) is widely used, even if several limitations, including poor specificity, difficult administration and the risk of anergy, are reported. It identifies adaptive immunity to mycobacterial antigens, injected intradermally as a protein precipitate (purified protein derivative (PPD)) in the volar part of the forearm (Mantoux test). PPD, constituted by different molecules, is derived by filtration of M. tuberculosis cultures.

False-negative reactions are common in immunocompromised patients and in those with overwhelming pulmonary TB. Positive

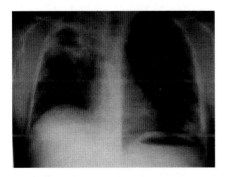

Figure 1. Improvement of pulmonary TB with a large cavity in the right upper lobe following adequate treatment.

results are obtained when patients have been infected with M. tuberculosis and when subjects have been sensitised by nontuberculous mycobacteria acquired environmentally or M. bovis bacille Calmette–Guérin (BCG) vaccination, because of the antigenic cross-reactivity of PPD.

Finally, IFN-γ release assays (IGRAs) have recently been introduced into clinical practice. They detect adaptive cellular immune reactivity towards M. tuberculosis-specific antigens encoded by genes located in the RD-1 genomic region. Their application in specimens collected from the infected organ (e.g. bronchoalveolar lavage) or tissue for the clinical diagnosis of TB is still under evaluation, but seems promising (specificity >80%). These techniques can increase the low specificity of TST based on the immune response (release of IFN-γ) to the 6-kDa early secreted antigenic target protein (ESAT-6), the 10-kDa culture filtrate protein (CFP-10) and TB7.7, which are antigens specific to M. tuberculosis and are not produced by M. bovis BCG or environmental mycobacteria. Although the diagnostic sensitivity of IGRAs performed using blood seems higher than that of TST, it is not sufficient to rule out TB. Their negative predictive value for progression from LTBI to active TB disease is 97.8–99.8% within 2 years.

Treatment

Individuals with active TB and positive sputum smear test results are the main source of TB transmission in the community owing to their high bacillary load. The most relevant priority in TB control programmes is the rapid identification of new cases of sputum smear-positive pulmonary TB and their effective treatment. It has been estimated that case-finding and effective treatment of sputum smear-positive individuals could halve the global number of TB cases within a decade.

Short-course regimens are divided into an initial or bactericidal phase and a continuation or sterilising phase.

WHO recommends treatment of new cases of pulmonary TB with a standardised regimen of four first-line anti-TB drugs, including isoniazid, rifampicin, pyrazinamide (Z) and ethambutol (E) for 2 months (intensive phase), followed by isoniazid and rifampicin for 4 months (continuation phase) (tables 1–3).

Fixed-dose combinations of two (isoniazid and rifampicin), three (isoniazid, rifampicin and pyrazinamide) and four (isoniazid, rifampicin, pyrazinamide and ethambutol) drugs are highly recommended.

Individuals with a previous TB diagnosis and treatment for >1 month are at higher risk of being infected with drug-resistant strains and, consequently, DST is necessary. In settings where rapid molecular-based DST is available, the results should guide the choice of the treatment regimen.

The standard re-treatment regimen containing first-line drugs (2HRZES/1HRZE/5HRE) is recommended by WHO for treatment of TB patients returning after default or relapsing from their first treatment course if country-specific data show low or medium levels of MDR in such patients.

If the setting-specific prevalence of MDR-TB is high, re-treatment cases should be managed as if they harbour MDR-TB strains. While rapid molecular-based methods allow a first orientation, DST for all second-line drugs should be promptly requested to allow the design of an adequate regimen.

Treatment duration is identical in HIV-positive and -negative patients. Antiretroviral therapy should be started within 2 months of the start of the anti-TB therapy in order to reduce the risk of death, irrespective of $CD4^+$ cell counts. However, drug–drug interactions, a relevant pill burden and the potential occurrence of immune reconstitution inflammatory syndrome (IRIS) can hinder an adequate management.

A regimen with at least four effective drugs is recommended for MDR-TB cases. At least four second-line drugs should be administered, with an injectable for the intensive phase of treatment (8 months).

Total duration should be ⩾20 months. Management of MDR/XDR-TB cases is more complicated from a clinical and public health perspective, being more expensive, more toxic and less efficacious (table 4).

Treatment of MDR- and XDR-TB cases should be managed in highly specialised reference centres by high skilled healthcare workers, identified by national authorities. Relevant clinical decisions (*e.g.* when to start and interrupt treatment, how to design the regimen, how to manage an adverse event, *etc.*) should ideally be taken within a team of experts with complementary competences (a consilium or similar body). Consilia, which are presently only available to cover internationally funded MDR-TB treatment projects, are considered by WHO to be important in ensuring the best possible management of these difficult-to-treat cases and to prevent development of super-resistance. The European Respiratory Society (ERS) and WHO are presently offering this service cost-free *via* an electronic platform through which clinicians will receive expert advice within 1 week (www.tbconsilium.org).

Scaling-up of culture and DST capacities, and the expanded use of high-technology assays for rapid determination of resistance (*e.g.* GeneXpert) are necessary if better control of MDR- and XDR-TB is to be achieved. The majority of resistant cases can be treated successfully if well-designed regimens are used and surgical options are carefully considered. Nevertheless, the development of new (more effective and less toxic) drugs to treat patients is urgently needed. Adherence to internationally agreed standards of care and control practices is imperative.

However, to reduce the emergence of new cases of TB, it is strategically crucial to identify and treat the infected subjects at higher risk of developing TB. National and international guidelines agree on the screening of HIV-positive patients, children and adults with close contact with an infectious case, individuals who are going to be treated with anti-tumour necrosis factor-α drugs. Isoniazid, administered for

Table 1. Anti-TB drugs, dosages and common adverse effects

Anti-TB drug	Recommended daily dosage	Common adverse effects (not exclusive)
Group 1: first-line oral agents		
Isoniazid	5 mg·kg^{-1} OD Should not exceed 300 mg per day Always consider co-administration of vitamin B6	Elevated transaminases Hepatitis Peripheral neuropathy GI intolerance CNS toxicity
Rifampicin	10 mg·kg^{-1} OD >50 kg: 600 mg <50 kg: 450 mg	Elevation of liver enzymes Hepatitis Hypersensitivity Fever GI disorders: anorexia, nausea, vomiting, abdominal pain Discoloration (orange or brown) of urine, tears and other body fluids Thrombopenia
Ethambutol	15–25 mg·kg^{-1} OD Maximum 2.0 g per day	Optic neuritis Hyperuricaemia Peripheral neuropathy (rare)
Pyrazinamide	30 mg·kg^{-1} OD Maximum 2.0 g per day	Arthralgia Hyperuricaemia Toxic hepatitis GI discomfort
Group 2: injectables		
Streptomycin[#]	0.75–1 g OD <50 kg: 0.75 g per day >50 kg: 1 g per day Maximum cumulative dose 50 g	Auditory and vestibular nerve damage (irreversible) Renal failure (usually reversible) Allergies Nausea Skin rash Neuromuscular blockade
Amikacin[¶]	0.75–1 g OD <50 kg: 0.75 g per day >50 kg: 1 g per day Maximum cumulative dose 50 g	Auditory and vestibular nerve damage (irreversible) Renal failure (usually reversible) Allergies Nausea Skin rash Neuromuscular blockade
Capreomycin[#]	0.75–1 g OD <50 kg: 0.75 g per day >50 kg: 1 g per day Maximum cumulative dose 50 g	Auditory and vestibular nerve damage (irreversible) Renal failure (usually reversible) Bartter-like syndrome Allergies Neuromuscular blockade

Table 1. Continued

Anti-TB drug	Recommended daily dosage	Common adverse effects (not exclusive)
Kanamycin¶	375–500 mg *b.i.d.* <50 kg: 0.75 g per day >50 kg: 1 g per day Maximum cumulative dose 50 g	Auditory and vestibular nerve damage (irreversible) Renal failure (usually reversible) Allergies Nausea Skin rash Neuromuscular blockade
Group 3: fluoroquinolones⁺		
Levofloxacin	500–1000 mg OD	GI discomfort CNS disorders Tendon rupture (rare) Hypersensitivity *Clostridium difficule* colitis
Ciprofloxacin	500–750 mg *b.i.d.*	GI discomfort CNS disorders Tendon rupture (rare) Hypersensitivity *Clostridium difficule* colitis
Moxifloxacin	400 mg OD	GI discomfort Headache Dizziness Hallucinations Increased transaminases QT prolongation *Clostridium difficile* colitis
Group 4: second-line oral agents		
Rifabutin	150–450 mg OD Consider monitoring drug levels	Anaemia GI discomfort Discoloration (orange or brown) of urine and other body fluids Uveitis Elevated liver enzymes
Ethionamide	0.75–1 g OD	Severe GI intolerance Nausea Vomiting Hepatitis CNS disorders
Prothionamide	0.75–1 g OD	Severe GI intolerance Nausea Vomiting Hepatitis CNS disorders

Table 1. Continued

Anti-TB drug	Recommended daily dosage	Common adverse effects (not exclusive)
Cycloserine	250 mg *t.i.d.* Maximum 1000 mg per day	CNS disorders Anxiety Confusion Dizziness Psychosis Seizures Headache
Terizidone	250 mg *t.i.d.* Maximum 1000 mg per day	CNS disorders Anxiety Confusion Dizziness Psychosis Seizures Headache
PAS	4 g *t.i.d.*	GI intolerance Nausea Diarrhoea Vomiting Hypersensitivity
Thioacetazone	50 mg *t.i.d.*	Hypersensitivity GI intolerance Vertigo Hepatitis
Group 5: oral reserve drugs with uncertain anti-TB activity		
Linezolid	600 mg OD (600 mg *b.i.d.* recommended for MRSA and VRE infections)	Thrombopenia Anaemia Neuropathy
Clofazimine	100 mg OD	Ichthiosis GI discomfort Nausea Vomiting Discoloration of the skin
Amoxicillin–clavulanate	875–125 mg *b.i.d.* or 500–250 mg *t.i.d.*	GI discomfort Diarrhoea Rash
Clarithromycin	500 mg *b.i.d.*	GI discomfort

PAS: para-aminosalicylic acid; OD: once daily; MRSA: methicillin-resistant *Staphylococcus aureus*; VRE: vancomycin-resistant *Enterococcus*; GI: gastrointestinal; CNS: central nervous system. [#]: intravenous/intramuscular administration only; [¶]: intravenous administration only; [+]: also available from intravenous administration.

6–12 months at a dosage of 5 mg·kg^{-1} per day, decreases the probability of developing active disease by 60% for a 2-year period. Longer duration is correlated with a higher probability of hepatic dysfunction, irrespective of efficacy. Other alternative regimens prescribed are: isoniazid and rifampicin for 3 months, or a weekly

Table 2. *Recommended treatment regimens for new TB cases*

TB treatment regimen		Notes
Intensive phase	**Continuation phase**	
2HRZE	4HR	Standard regimen
2HRZE	4HRE	Level of H resistance among new TB cases is high and H susceptibility testing result is not available before the continuation phase

Ethambutol (E) must be prescribed during the intensive phase in individuals with noncavitary, smear-negative pulmonary TB, or in HIV-negative patients with extrapulmonary TB. In TB meningitis, it should be replaced by streptomycin (S). Number preceding regimen indicates the length of treatment in months. H: isoniazid; R: rifampicin; Z: pyrazinamide.

administration of isoniazid and rifapentine for 3 months.

Prevention

In 1993, the United Nations stated that the global fight against TB must be a priority alongside with the fight against HIV/AIDS and malaria. On this basis, in 1996, WHO issued a public health strategy called DOTS (directly observed treatment, short course), aimed at diagnosing 70% of sputum smear-positive patients and successfully treating 85% of them by 2005. It was composed of five elements:

1. political commitment to TB control
2. bacteriological diagnosis through smear microscopy
3. supervised and standardised short-course therapy
4. supply of quality drugs without interruption
5. standardised recording and reporting system for treatment outcomes

In 1996, a new WHO strategy called STOP-TB was issued in order to address the new global epidemiological issues, such as MDR-TB and TB/HIV co-infection. It was aimed to meet the 2015 Millennium Development Goals (*i.e.* to halve TB prevalence and mortality compared to the data recorded in 1990) and showed a more comprehensive approach (for instance, involvement of the private sector, and engagement of the community and of all healthcare providers). WHO and partners are presently discussing the new post-2015 strategy, which will be centred around three main pillars:

1. intensified and innovative TB care
2. development and enforcement of bold health-system and social development policies
3. promotion and intensification of research and innovation

A relevant tool for the clinical and public health management of TB called the International Standards of Tuberculosis Care (ISTC) was developed by several stakeholders, coordinated by WHO, to give evidence-based standards. Recently, the ERS

Table 3. *Recommended treatment regimens for previously treated patients*

Probability of MDR-TB	
High (failure)	**Medium or low (relapse, default)**
Pending DST results: empirical MDR-TB regimen, modified once DST results are available	2HRZES/HRZE/5HRE, modified once DST results are available.

Number preceding regimen indicates the length of treatment in months. H: isoniazid; R: rifampicin; Z: pyrazinamide; E; ethambutol; S: streptomycin.

Table 4. General principles for designing an empiric regimen to treat MDR-TB

Basic principles	Comments
1. Use at least four drugs of know effectiveness or highly likely to be effective	Effectiveness is supported by a number of factors (the more of them that are present, the more likely it is the that drug will be effective). Susceptibility at DST No previous history of treatment failure with the drug No known close contacts with resistance to the drug DRS indicates resistance is rare in similar patients No common use of the drug in the area If at least four drugs are not certain to be effective, use five to seven drugs, depending on the specific drugs and level of uncertainty
2. Do not use drugs for which resistance crosses over	Rifamycins (rifampicin, rifabutin, rifapentine and rifalazil) have high level of cross-resistance Fluoroquinolones: variable cross-resistance; *in vitro* data show some later generation agents remain susceptible when earlier generation are resistant (clinical significance of the phenomenon still unknown) Aminoglycosides and polypeptides: not all are cross-resistant; in general, only kanamycin and amikacin are fully cross-resistant
3. Eliminate drugs likely to be unsafe for the patient	Known severe allergy or difficult-to-manage intolerance High risk of severe adverse effects including: renal failure, deafness, hepatitis, depression and/or psychosis Unknown or questionable drug quality
4. Include drugs from groups 1–5 in a hierarchical order, based on potency	Use any group 1 drugs that are likely to be effective (see principle 1 above) Use an effective injectable aminoglycoside or polypeptide (group 2 drugs) Use a later-generation fluoroquinolone (group 3) Use the remaining group 4 drugs starting from ethionamide (or prothionamide) to make a regimen consisting of at least four effective drugs plus pyrazinamide in the intensive phase of treatment Regimens should include at least pyrazinamide, a fluoroquinolone, a parenteral agent (kanamycin, amikacin or capreomycin), ethionamide (or prothionamide), and either cycloserine or PAS if cycloserine cannot be used An intensive phase of 8 months' duration is recommended; a total treatment duration of 20 months is recommended in patients without any previous MDR-TB treatment For regimens with up to four effective drugs, add second-line drugs most likely to be effective, to give five to seven drugs in total, with at least four of them highly likely to be effective The number of drugs will depend on the degree of uncertainty Use group 5 drugs as needed so that at least four drugs are likely to be effective
5. Be prepared to prevent, monitor and manage adverse effects for each of the drugs selected	Ensure laboratory services for haematology, biochemistry, serology and audiometry are available Establish a clinical and laboratory baseline before starting the regimen Initiate treatment gradually for a difficult-to-tolerate drug, splitting daily doses of ethionamide/prothionamide, cyclosporin and PAS Ensure ancillary drugs are available to manage adverse effects Organise intake supervision for all doses

DRS: drug resistance surveillance; PAS: para-aminosalicylic acid.

and the European Centre for Disease Prevention and Control adapted the ISTC to the European Union/European Economic Area scenario, focusing on the goal of TB elimination.

Only one vaccine is currently available for the primary prevention of TB: it consists of a live attenuated strain of *M. bovis* BCG, the efficacy of which has been proven in children for TB meningitis and miliary TB but not for pulmonary TB in endemic geographical areas. Safety concerns have been reported, particularly in HIV-positive patients.

The goal of the global elimination of TB, *i.e.* an incidence of new sputum smear-positive cases <1 per 1 million inhabitants, seems difficult to meet, but the epidemiological scenario could improve with a multi-sector approach oriented by the evidence-based WHO strategies.

Further reading

- Blasi F, *et al.* (2013). Supporting TB clinicians managing difficult cases: the ERS/WHO Consilium. *Eur Respir J*; 41: 491–494.
- Falzon D, *et al.* (2011). WHO guidelines for the programmatic management of drug-resistant tuberculosis: 2011 update. *Eur Respir J*; 38: 516–528.
- Fitzgerald D, *et al. Mycobacterium tuberculosis. In:* Mandell GL, *et al.*, eds. Principles and Practice of Infectious Diseases. 6th Edn. Philadelphia, Churchill Livingstone, 2005; pp. 2852–2886.
- Frieden TR, *et al.* (2003). Tuberculosis. *Lancet*; 362: 887–899.
- Getahun H, *et al.* (2010). HIV infection-associated tuberculosis: the epidemiology and the response. *Clin Infect Dis*; 50: Suppl. 3, S201–S207.
- Hopewell PC, *et al.* (2006). International standards for tuberculosis care. *Lancet Infect Dis*; 6: 710–725.
- Knechel NA (2009). Tuberculosis: pathophysiology, clinical features, and diagnosis. *Crit Care Nurse*; 29: 34–43.
- Mack U, *et al.* (2009). LTBI: latent tuberculosis infection or lasting immune responses to *M. tuberculosis*? A TBNET consensus statement. *Eur Respir J*; 33: 956–973.
- Migliori GB, *et al.* (2012). European Union standards for tuberculosis care. *Eur Respir J*; 39: 807–819.
- Orenstein EW, *et al.* (2009). Treatment outcomes among patients with multidrug-resistant tuberculosis: systematic review and meta-analysis. *Lancet Infect Dis*; 9: 153–161.
- Torrado E, *et al.* (2011). Cellular response to mycobacteria: balancing protection and pathology. *Trends Immunol*; 32: 66–72.
- Raviglione MC, *et al.* Tuberculosis. *In:* Fauci AS, *et al.*, eds. Harrison's Principles of Internal Medicine. 17th Edn. New York, McGraw-Hill Medical Publishing Division Inc., 2008; pp. 1006–1020.
- Sester M, *et al.* (2011). Interferon-γ release assays for the diagnosis of active tuberculosis: a systematic review and meta-analysis. *Eur Respir J*; 37: 100–111.
- World Health Organization. Multidrug and extensively drug-resistant TB (M/XDR-TB). Global report on surveillance and response. Geneva, WHO, 2010.
- World Health Organization. Global tuberculosis control 2011. Document WHO/HTM/TB/2011.16. Geneva, WHO, 2011.
- World Health Organization. Guidelines for the programmatic management of drug-resistant tuberculosis. Document WHO/HTM/TB/2008.402. Geneva, WHO, 2008.
- World Health Organization. Treatment of tuberculosis guidelines. Fourth Edition. Document WHO/HTM/TB/2009.420. Geneva, WHO, 2010.
- Yew WW, *et al.* (2011). Treatment of tuberculosis: update 2010. *Eur Respir J*; 37: 441–462.

Extrapulmonary tuberculosis

Aik Bossink

Definition

The World Health Organization(WHO) defines of extrapulmonary TB (EPTB) as 'A patient with tuberculosis of organs other than the lungs (e.g. pleura, lymph nodes, abdomen, genitourinary tract, skin, joints and bones, meninges). Diagnosis should be based on one culture-positive specimen, or histological or strong clinical evidence consistent with active extrapulmonary disease, followed by a decision by a clinician to treat with a full course of antituberculosis chemotherapy'.

A patient diagnosed with both pulmonary TB (PTB) and EPTB should be classified as a case of PTB.

The definition does not mention eyes or the ear–nose–throat region. However, these tissues are also, rarely, possible localisations.

General aspects of EPTB

Only a minority of TB cases (<30%) suffer from EPTB. However, this could be biased by the definition, because in countries with a differentiated registry (PTB, EPTB and EPTB+PTB), EPT localisations comprise nearly 50% of all cases. With the arrival of new, more sensitive detection methods, EPTB could well be even more common. EPTB has always been considered less important than PTB because of the low infectious potential and the difficulties involved in the diagnosis EPT.

In low-income countries, males appear to be affected by TB more often than females. However, in high-income countries, this difference is not so clear. This mechanism is not clearly understood. No evidence is available that EPTB affects one sex more often than the other.

Immunosuppression appears to be an important cause of EPTB and this is reflected by a sharp incline in reported cases of EPTB with the rise of the incidence of HIV infection. In high-income countries and countries with a lower incidence of HIV infection, biologicals like tumour necrosis factor-α inhibitors are relatively important causes of EPTB.

'The result of tuberculous bacillaemia must be the insemination in various parts of the body of foci most of which remain latent' (Wilkinson, 1940). Therefore, EPTB can be the result of a primary infection in severely immunocompromised hosts or can be the result of reactivation of dormant bacilli in previously infected subjects.

Sites of EPTB

The two most common localisations of EPT are the cervical lymph nodes and pulmonary pleura. Other sites are, in declining order, bones and joints, the meninges and central

---

Key points

- EPTB localisations appear in up to 50% of TB patients.

- Obtaining culture confirmation is essential in the treatment of both PTB and EPTB.

- Treatment of EPTB does not differ from PTB in the majority of EPTB localisations.

---

nervous system (CNS), abdominal lymph nodes, the peritoneum and gastrointestinal tract, the genitourinary tract, and the pericardium.

It should be noted that gastric aspirate from children with EPTB often contains mycobacteria. This is, however, not an indication of EPT but should be considered as local spread of mycobacteria by swallowing sputum.

In immunocompromised hosts, the presentation of EPTB is often different compared to immunocompetent hosts. Dissemination of the disease is more common and clinicians should be aware of other localisations. Dissemination is more likely because ill-formed granulomata are more common in immunocompromised hosts.

The term miliary TB is a radiological finding of chest radiography and should not be used in this context.

Diagnosis

In countries with all possible diagnostic resources, on average, 70% of all the TB cases are culture confirmed. One can imagine that in EPTB samples are more difficult to obtain compared with PTB samples. Furthermore, some of the EPTB localisations contain few mycobacteria. Culture or PCR confirmation will thus be lower in these cases. Using the Dutch TB registry, PTB is culture confirmed in nearly 80% and EPTB in about 60% of cases.

In low-income countries, specific staining is often the only available diagnostic tool and, because of its relative simplicity, should always be undertaken. A relatively novel method, the Xpert MTB/RIF assay (Cepheid, Sunnyvale, CA, USA), could well be promising in low-income countries with few laboratory facilities. This real-time automated nucleic acid amplification technique runs in a closed system and is suitable for use outside conventional laboratory settings. Most experience of the performance on this technique is based on sputum samples but a review (Lawn et al., 2012) mentions good performance in EPTB

samples. However, culture and drug susceptibility testing remain the cornerstone of adequate treatment.

Some promising reports of the use of interferon-γ release assays on materials other than blood in the diagnosis of EPTB (pleural, peritoneal, pericardial and meningitis TB) have been published. However, these tests are no proof of active infection, they will not provide culture results or drug susceptibility reports and can therefore only be supportive in the search for mycobacteria. However, it remains most important to obtain materials for culture and DST.

An increasing number of case and brief reports has been published on the use of 18-fluorodeoxyglucose (FDG) positron emission tomography (PET)/CT for the detection of both PTB and EPTB sites. Unfortunately, most prospective studies have been designed to differentiate between malignancies and TB. Nuclear medicine is, in general, not an appropriate tool to differentiate between these. However, FDG-PET/CT appears to have a high sensitivity in the detection of lymph-node TB and organ localisations. The performance on visceral TB localisations remains unclear. A recent review (Sathekge et al., 2012) concludes that 'Available data, reviewed above, suggest that SPECT [single-photon emission CT] and PET may prove to be valuable adjuncts for the differentiation of TB from malignant lung lesions, active from nonactive disease, and for treatment follow-up, and may thus play a major role in the work-up of TB patients'. It can be expected that with the use of more sensitive methods of detection, the proportion of EPTB localisations will increase.

Treatment

In general, treatment for EPTB does not differ from that for PTB. Depending on local or national guidelines, the treatment consists of a full course of at least four anti-TB drugs (isoniazid, rifampicin, ethambutol and pyrazinamide) in the first 2 months, and then another 4–7 months of isoniazid and rifampicin in culture-confirmed cases with normal drug susceptibility. In countries with a high prevalence of drug resistance for one or more of these drugs, a fifth or even sixth drug should be added awaiting culture and DST.

Specific localisations

Cervical lymph nodes Involvement of the lymph nodes or lymphadenitis is the most common localisation of EPTB. Concomitant pulmonary infection occurs in 5–10% of cases and, therefore, generalised symptoms are unusual. During medical treatment, the lymph nodes can rapidly increase in size (paradox reaction) and fine-needle aspiration of its content may prove beneficial in preventing fistula. In children, lymphadenitis is often caused by nontuberculous mycobacteria and this requires a different treatment approach. Confirmation of the causative organism is therefore crucial.

Other lymph nodes Other common sites of lymph node involvement are axillary, inguinal and abdominal. Culture results (*Mycobacterium tuberculosis versus* nontuberculous mycobacteria) for these localisations do not differ between children and adults.

TB of the pleura In general, TB pleurisy is one sided and the majority of cases have a tendency toward spontaneous resolution. Therefore, the diagnosis can be delayed for a prolonged period until a new effusion appears. Often, large amounts of pleural fluid are observed with relatively low numbers of mycobacteria. An accompanying hypersensitivity reaction is responsible for this phenomenon. Because of this low bacterial burden, the confirmation of TB can often be difficult. TB empyema is a rare condition compared with pleurisy, and often requires surgical drainage and decortication combined with medical treatment.

TB of the meninges and CNS Meningitis is the most common presentation of involvement of the nervous system. The infection can cause hydrocephalus and, through involvement of the cranial nerves,

paralysis of the abducens nerve. Classically, the patient is not able to look outward with one eye and this eye is rotated towards the nose. Neurological deterioration is classified in three grades based on the performance on the Glasgow Coma Scale. Apart from antibiotic treatment, it is recommended to add steroids (0.5 mg·kg^{-1}) in stage II and III. Survival is positively influenced by this regimen but neurological outcome is no better in the groups treated with steroids. Others recommend steroids independent of the stage. Antibiotic treatment should be for $\geqslant 9$ months. However, according to the British Infection Society guidelines, treatment should be continued for 1 year. WHO recommends replacing ethambutol with streptomycin in TB meningitis.

TB of the pericardium This condition is sometimes difficult to diagnose because, just like pleural effusion, the bacterial load is low. Pericardial effusion and, at a later stage, constrictive pericarditis can cause severe inflow limitation resulting in serious haemodynamic problems. To reduce the effusion and to prevent thickening of the pericardium, adjuvant steroids are recommended. No data are available on the amount and duration of steroid treatment. It seems reasonable to prescribe 0.5 mg·kg^{-1} for the first 2 months and then decrease the dose gradually to zero over a period of 4 months.

Bone and joint TB Any bone or joint can be affected but the classical lesion is a fracture of the vertebrae resulting in a kyphotic change of the spine (Pott's disease). In general, the larger bones and joints are more often affected compared with the smaller ones. Joint involvement presents as a monoarthritis. Diagnosis of both bone and joint involvement is generally made by biopsy. Aspiration of synovial fluid seldom yields the diagnosis. Medical treatment is the treatment of choice and should be prolonged to 9 months. Surgery is reserved for complicated cases such as neurological involvement or instability of the spine.

Further reading

- European Centre for Disease Prevention and Control, et al. Tuberculosis surveillance in Europe 2008. http://ecdc.europa.eu/en/publications/Publications/1003_SUR_tuberculosis_surveillance_in_europe_2008.pdf
- KNCV. Epidemiologie en surveillance [Epidemiology and surveillance]. www.kncvtbc.nl/nl/epidemiologie-en-surveillance
- Lawn SD, et al. (2012). Diagnosis of extrapulmonary tuberculosis using the Xpert® MTB/RIF assay. Expert Rev Anti Infect Ther; 10: 631–635.
- Sathekge M, et al. (2012). Nuclear medicine imaging in tuberculosis using commercially available radiopharmaceuticals. Nucl Med Commun; 33: 581–590.
- Thwaites GE, et al. (2004). Dexamethasone for the treatment of tuberculous meningitis in adolescents and adults. N Engl J Med; 351: 1741–1751.
- Thwaites G, et al. (2009). British Infection Society guidelines for the diagnosis and treatment of tuberculosis of the central nervous system in adults and children. J Infect; 59: 167–187.
- Wilkinson MC (1940). Pathogenesis of non-pulmonary tuberculosis. Br Med J; 2: 660–661.
- World Health Organization. Global Tuberculosis Control 2009: Epidemiology, strategy and financing. Geneva, WHO, 2009.
- World Health Organization. Global tuberculosis report 2012. www.who.int/tb/publications/global_report/en/
- World Health Organization. Treatment of tuberculosis: guidelines for national programmes. www.who.int/tb/features_archive/new_treatment_guidelines_may2010/en/index.html

Tuberculosis in the immunocompromised host

Martina Sester

The incidence of active TB and attendant mortality is increased in patients with impaired cellular immunity, such as HIV-infected patients, solid organ and stem cell transplant recipients, patients receiving tumour necrosis factor (TNF)-α antagonists, and patients with end-stage renal failure. The relative risk for TB varies with the type of immunodeficiency (table 1) and mortality rates may be as high as 75% (Sester et al., 2012). This emphasises the particular importance of the cellular arm of the adaptive immune response for efficient control of *Mycobacterium tuberculosis* (Sester et al., 2010, 2012; Bumbacea et al., 2012; Solovic et al., 2010). Moreover, the presence of *M. tuberculosis*-specific CD4[+] T-cell immunity is used as a surrogate marker for a previous contact (Mack et al., 2009). Consequently, a detailed knowledge of the pathomechanisms leading to increased incidence of TB in immunocompromised patients has also contributed to a better understanding of the principles of decreased test sensitivity in this vulnerable patient group.

Pathomechanisms of impaired TB control in immunocompromised patients

The general incidence of TB in immunocompromised patients may vary depending on the geographic location and may range from <1% to 15% in low- and high-prevalence countries, respectively. The relative risk of developing TB and its underlying pathomechanisms may differ widely among the various groups due to differences in the cause and extent of immunodeficiency (table 1). The dramatic reduction in CD4[+] T-cell numbers in HIV infected patients, in particular in those with AIDS, not only contributes to a severely impaired control of TB but also to a high percentage of false-negative diagnoses by immune-based tests (Sester et al., 2010). Similarly, immunosuppressive drug treatment after transplantation is associated with a decrease in T-cell function and may lead to a progressive decrease in *M. tuberculosis*-specific T-cell immunity over time (Sester et al., 2009). This not only facilitates reactivation but also contributes to a decreased sensitivity of immune-based testing (Bumbacea et al., 2012; Sester et al., 2009; Singh et al., 1998). The uraemia-associated immunodeficiency syndrome in patients with end-stage renal failure has been characterised by a defect in co-stimulatory signals to antigen-specific T-cells, thereby contributing to an impaired efficiency of vaccinations and increased risk of infectious complications including TB (Girndt et al., 2001). Finally, an increased incidence of active TB in patients receiving TNF-α antagonists is attributed to impaired T-cell function and failure to maintain the integrity of granulomata

Key points

- TB has a higher incidence among people with impaired cellular immunity.

- Diagnosis is often delayed owing to early lack of symptoms or unusual presentation.

- Screening for LTBI prior to immunosuppressive treatments can be a useful preventive measure.

Table 1. *Pathomechanisms and relative risk for TB in immunocompromised patients relative to persons without known risk factors (risk=1)*

Relative risk	Pathomechanism
100–170	Low $CD4^+$ T-cell counts
50–100	Low $CD4^+$ T-cell counts
20–74	Decreased T-cell function and numbers
10–25	Co-stimulation deficiency, chronic inflammation

in latently infected patients (Solovic *et al.*, 2010).

Clinical presentation of active TB in immunocompromised patients

Active TB in immunocompromised patients can pose a number of challenges. Due to the impaired immune response, patients may be clinically oligosymptomatic in the beginning of active disease, and its diagnosis is often delayed due to atypical presentations and more frequent extrapulmonary dissemination. Active TB is further aggravated by a significantly higher morbidity due to a more fatal course in the face of a weakened immune system (Sester *et al.*, 2012). In addition, treatment is frequently complicated due to complex drug interactions and altered pharmacokinetics (Bumbacea *et al.*, 2012). The treatment of TB is also more difficult to manage in HIV-infected patients, as immune restoration induced by antiretroviral therapy may be responsible for a paradoxical worsening of TB manifestations, a phenomenon defined as immune reconstitution inflammatory syndrome (IRIS) (Sester *et al.*, 2010).

Diagnosis and treatment of active TB

In active TB suspects, diagnosis should follow a clinical algorithm that includes acid-fast bacilli (AFB) staining from two sputum samples, and nucleic acid amplification (NAA) testing. In the case of negative results, bronchoalveolar lavage (BAL) should be obtained for microscopy, NAA and culture (Sester *et al.*, 2012; Lange *et al.*, 2010).

The first-choice treatment of immuno-compromised patients with active TB does not differ from immunocompetent

individuals, and should consist of a regimen including isoniazid, rifampicin, pyrazinamide and ethambutol for 2 months (2HRZE), followed by a continuation phase with isoniazid and rifampicin for 4 months (4HR). Treatment of active TB may be complicated by interactions between antibacterial and immunosuppressive or antiretroviral drugs. Evidence in favour of extending the continuation phase is limited. Longer duration is recommended in patients with cavitation on their initial chest radiograph and/or positive cultures after 2 months of treatment, or in patients with involvement of the central nervous system (Sester *et al.*, 2012).

Preventative approaches in immunocompromised patients

The increased risk of active TB in immunocompromised patients may result from an immunosuppression-induced reactivation of a previously acquired latent TB infection (LTBI) or new infections. While the extent of new infections is difficult to control as it largely depends on the overall prevalence of TB, the risk of progression from LTBI to active disease may be minimised by the early identification and treatment of latently infected patients (Sester *et al.* 2012). Although risk assessment in immunocompromised patients is often hampered by a low sensitivity of commonly used immune-based tests, current guidelines recommend regular screening for evidence of LTBI and – if possible – treatment prior to conditions of immunodeficiency, *i.e.* screening and treatment prior to transplantation or TNF-α antagonist therapy (Sester *et al.*, 2012; Bumbacea *et al.*, 2012; Solovic *et al.*, 2010; Singh *et al.*, 1998). Until recently, LTBI screening was exclusively carried out by the use of tuberculin skin testing (TST), where the cut-off of positivity is defined by the extent of immunodeficiency. At present, however, novel interferon-γ release assays (IGRAs) are more widely applied that are of higher specificity than TST. In addition, accumulating evidence suggests that IGRAs may be of higher sensitivity in immuno-compromised patients (Sester *et al.*, 2012).

Preventive chemotherapy should be given to patients with a positive immune-based test (TST ⩾5 or 10 mm depending on the type of immunodeficiency, or IGRA), signs of TB on chest radiograph in patients with no or insufficient previous TB treatment, or recent close contact with a patient with active TB in severely immunocompromised patients.

Among immune-based assays, IGRA testing is preferred over TST because of operational advantages, including internal positive controls. When using IGRAs as a predictive measure for development of active disease, a recent meta-analysis suggests that *in vitro* tests are superior for predicting development of TB (Diel *et al.*, 2011). Nevertheless, the actual risk of progression to active disease is still overestimated and may differ according to the local prevalence of TB (Rangaka *et al.*, 2012). The considerably low predictive value is due to the fact that a positive immune response towards *M. tuberculosis* does not necessarily reflect a true infection with viable bacilli that bears a higher risk of disease progression (Barry *et al.*, 2009). As decisions for chemoprophylaxis depend, to a great extent, on the results of immunodiagnostic testing, large studies are needed to determine more precisely the negative and positive predictive values of IGRAs in each specific population of immunocompromised patients and in regions of different TB prevalence.

Conclusions

TB in immunocompromised patients is more frequent than in the general population, and morbidity and mortality are high. This high mortality is primarily due to delayed diagnosis and increased incidence of disseminated disease. Risk assessment needs integrative

approaches that should consider clinical findings, the extent of immunodeficiency and the overall prevalence of TB.

Further reading

- Barry CE 3rd., *et al.* (2009). The spectrum of latent tuberculosis: rethinking the biology and intervention strategies. *Nat Rev Microbiol*; 7: 845–855.
- Bumbacea D, *et al.* (2012). The risk of tuberculosis in transplant candidates and recipients: a TBNET consensus statement. *Eur Respir J*; 40: 990–1013.
- Diel R, *et al.* (2011). Interferon-γ release assays for the diagnosis of latent *Mycobacterium tuberculosis* infection: a systematic review and meta-analysis. *Eur Respir J*; 37: 88–99.
- Girndt M, *et al.* (2001). Molecular aspects of T- and B-cell function in uremia. *Kidney Int Suppl*; 78: S206–S211.
- Lange C, *et al.* (2010). Advances in the diagnosis of tuberculosis. *Respirology*; 15: 220–240.
- Mack U, *et al.* (2009). LTBI: latent tuberculosis infection or lasting immune responses to *M. tuberculosis*? A TBNET consensus statement. *Eur Respir J*; 33: 956–973.
- Rangaka MX, *et al.* (2012). Predictive value of interferon-γ release assays for incident active tuberculosis: a systematic review and meta-analysis. *Lancet Infect Dis*; 12: 45–55.
- Sester M, *et al.* (2010). Challenges and perspectives for improved management of HIV/*Mycobacterium tuberculosis* co-infection. *Eur Respir J*; 36: 1242–1247.
- Sester M, *et al.* (2012). TB in the immunocompromised host. *Eur Respir Monogr*; 58: 230–241.
- Sester U, *et al.* (2009). Impaired detection of *Mycobacterium tuberculosis* immunity in patients using high levels of immunosuppressive drugs. *Eur Respir J*; 34: 702–710.
- Singh N, *et al.* (1998). *Mycobacterium tuberculosis* infection in solid-organ transplant recipients: impact and implications for management. *Clin Infect Dis*; 27: 1266–1277.
- Solovic I, *et al.* (2010). The risk of tuberculosis related to tumour necrosis factor antagonist therapies: a TBNET consensus statement. *Eur Respir J*; 36: 1185–1206.

Latent tuberculosis

Jean-Pierre Zellweger

Individuals who are in close contact with a patient with a transmissible form of TB, usually smear-positive pulmonary TB, may inhale droplets containing mycobacteria, which settle in the airways and give rise to a local inflammatory reaction. The risk of infection is related to the concentration of mycobacteria in the air and the duration of contact. Some exposed individuals develop active disease (TB) within a couple of weeks or months, others will control the incipient infection and stay, for a prolonged period (up to years), in a state of equilibrium called 'latent TB infection' (LTBI).

LTBI and risk of TB

Individuals with latent TB have no signs or symptoms of active disease, and only immunological markers of a prior contact with mycobacteria. It is therefore impossible to know whether individuals with LTBI still harbour living mycobacteria. The only gold standard for the infection is the development of the disease, which happens in a minority of exposed individuals. Why and how the infected individuals will develop TB is unknown. Estimates are that ~10% of infected individuals may develop TB, half of them within 2 years after infection, and 90% will never develop the disease. Some infected individuals have a higher risk of later reactivation than others (e.g. immunocompromised individuals, patients receiving immunosuppressive therapy and small children). As only a minority of contacts develop TB, there is a possibility that most contacts eradicate the mycobacteria but still retain an immunological marker of the infection, even in the absence of living mycobacteria.

Treatment of LTBI

As the persons in contact with a case of TB have a much higher risk of developing the disease in the future than the general population, particularly if they have a positive tuberculin reaction or a positive interferon-γ release assay (IGRA) test, the detection of LTBI among exposed contacts is important because a preventive treatment can reduce this risk. In countries or populations with a low incidence of TB, the search for latent infection among contacts

> **Key points**
>
> - The risk of LTBI depends on the intensity and duration of exposure to a source case with untreated pulmonary TB.
>
> - Some infected contacts will develop TB at a later time-point. Timely detection of infected contacts and preventive treatment of those at highest risk of reactivation is cost-effective and reduces the pool of future cases of active TB.
>
> - Before prescribing a preventive treatment, active TB should be excluded by a chest radiograph and, if abnormal, by a bacteriological examination of sputum.
>
> - The tests for the detection of latent infection are the tuberculin skin test and the IGRAs. The latter has the advantage of a greater specificity.

and the prescription of preventive treatment may contribute to the control of the disease by reducing the pool of potential future cases. The currently recommended preventive treatments are 9 months of isoniazid, 4 months of rifampicin, or 3 months of a combination of isoniazid and rifampicin. Recently, the use of rifapentine and isonazid once a week for 3 months has also been demonstrated to be very effective.

As the immunological reaction after the contact with mycobacteria needs several days or weeks to be complete, the proof of a recent sensitisation is usually not present before this time (the window period). Therefore, the search for latent infection is usually performed only 4–8 weeks after the last contact. In some cases, where the progression from infection to disease may be rapid (such as immunocompromised contacts or children aged <5 years), a first test with a clinical examination may be performed as soon as possible after the last contact and repeated several weeks later, if the results are negative. A test performed immediately after the last contact will usually indicate a prior sensitisation and may be observed among contacts born in a region with high prevalence of TB and in elderly people, independently of recent contacts.

Tests for detection of LTBI

The tests used for the detection of latent infection are all indirect and rely on the reaction between sensitised lymphocytes and antigens from *Mycobacterium tuberculosis*. The traditional test is the tuberculin skin test measuring the cutaneous reaction elicited by the intradermal injection of a mixture of antigens from *M. tuberculosis* cultures. New tests have recently been developed and introduced to the market, measuring *in vitro* the release of cytokines (interferon-γ) by lymphocytes incubated with two or three specific antigens present in *M. tuberculosis* but absent in *Mycobacterium bovis* bacille Calmette–Guérin (BCG) and in most nontuberculous mycobacteria (IGRAs). The *in vitro* tests are (at least) equally sensitive as the tuberculin test, but have the advantage of a greater specificity and,

therefore, avoid in practice the false-positive skin reactions elicited by prior BCG vaccination or contact with nontuberculous mycobacteria.

Detection in low-prevalence countries

In low-prevalence countries, the search for infected individuals is usually performed among persons who recently had contact with a patient with pulmonary TB (contact investigation), in healthcare workers potentially exposed to untreated cases of TB and in immunocompromised patients with a risk of reactivation that is higher than the general population if they are infected. Infected contacts considered at risk of developing TB in the future are either followed clinically or offered a preventive treatment. All contacts with immunological signs of infection (positive tuberculin skin test or IGRA) should have at least a chest radiograph for detecting signs of past or current TB. Before prescribing a preventive treatment in contacts with an abnormal chest radiograph, the presence of an active TB should be excluded by a bacteriological examination of sputum. The efficiency of the preventive treatment largely depends on the rate of treatment completion. Contacts of patients with multidrug-resistant TB have to be managed with special care.

Detection in high-prevalence countries

In high-prevalence countries, formal contact investigations are usually not performed, as most of the contacts may already have immunological signs of prior infection, but it is currently recommended to search for the presence of secondary cases of TB among the close relatives and to consider the protection of small children with a preventive treatment if one of the parents has a form of transmissible TB. The search for infection in HIV-positive contacts and prescription of preventive treatment is also recommended.

Controversies and open questions

There are still controversies about the definition of infectiousness (only smear-positive cases or all cases with pulmonary TB), the extent of the contact investigation (only close and prolonged contacts or all contacts) and the indications of preventive treatment (only infected contact with a high risk of reactivation or all contacts or individuals with a positive tuberculin or IGRA reaction). Prospective studies on the risk of reactivation among contacts with a positive immunological reaction will help to clarify these issues.

Further reading

- Abdool Karim SS, et al. (2009). HIV infection and tuberculosis in South Africa: an urgent need to escalate the public health response. *Lancet*; 374: 921–933.
- Andersen P, et al. (2007). The prognosis of latent tuberculosis: can disease be predicted? *Trends Mol Med*; 13: 175–182.
- Cardona PJ (2007). New insights on the nature of latent tuberculosis infection and its treatment. *Inflamm Allergy Drug Targets*; 6: 27–39.
- Diel R, et al. (2005). Cost-effectiveness of isoniazid chemoprevention in close contacts. *Eur Respir J*; 26: 465–473.
- Diel R, et al. (2011). Negative and positive predictive value of a whole-blood interferon-γ release assay for developing active tuberculosis: an update. *Am J Respir Crit Care Med*; 183: 88–95.
- Diel R, et al. (2011). Interferon-γ release assays for the diagnosis of latent *Mycobacterium tuberculosis* infection: a systematic review and meta-analysis. *Eur Respir J*; 37: 88–99.
- Erkens CG, et al. (2010). Tuberculosis contact investigation in low prevalence countries: a European consensus. *Eur Respir J*; 36: 925–949.
- European Centre for Disease Prevention and Control. Management of contacts of MDR TB and XDR TB patients. Stockholm, ECDC, 2012.
- Ferebee SH (1970). Controlled chemo-prophylaxis trials in tuberculosis: a general review. *Adv Tuberc Res*; 17: 28–106.
- Landry J, et al. (2008). Preventive chemotherapy. Where has it got us? Where to go next? *Int J Tuberc Lung Dis*; 12: 1352–1364.
- Mack U, et al. (2009). LTBI: latent tuberculosis infection or lasting immune responses to M. *tuberculosis*? A TBNET consensus statement. *Eur Respir J*; 33: 956–973.
- Mazurek GH, et al. (2010). Updated guidelines for using interferon gamma release assays to detect *Mycobacterium tuberculosis* infection – United States 2010. *MMWR Recomm Rep*; 59: 1–25.
- Moran-Mendoza O, et al. (2010). Risk factors for developing tuberculosis: a 12-year follow-up of contacts of tuberculosis cases. *Int J Tuberc Lung Dis*; 14: 1112–1119.
- National Tuberculosis Controllers Association. (2005). Guidelines for the investigation of contacts of persons with infections tuberculosis. Recommendations from the National Tuberculosis Controllers Association and CDC. *MMWR Recomm Rep*; 54: 1–47.
- Shapiro AE, et al. (2012). Community-based targeted case finding for tuberculosis and HIV in household contacts of patients with tuberculosis in South Africa. *Am J Respir Crit Care Med*; 185: 1110–1116.
- Sterling TR, et al. (2011). Three months of rifapentine and isoniazid for latent tuberculosis infection. *N Engl J Med*; 365: 2155–2166.

Nontuberculous mycobacterial diseases

Claudio Piersimoni

Nontuberculous mycobacteria (NTM) is the term indicating those *Mycobacterium* species that are different from *Mycobacterium tuberculosis* complex (MTC) and *Mycobacterium leprae*, whose detection in clinical samples is almost invariably associated with disease. The most important features distinguishing NTM from MTC include a lower pathogenicity and the lack of human-to-human transmission. In addition, *in vitro* resistance to first-line anti-TB drugs is an important distinctive issue. The majority of the >140 NTM species recognised has been associated with disease in man or animals.

Epidemiology and pathogenesis

NTM are widely distributed in both natural and man-made environments; organisms can be found in soil and water with high isolation rates. Human disease is suspected to be acquired by environmental exposure and pulmonary infection is likely to be *via* the aerosol route.

> **Key points**
>
> - Important features distinguishing NTM from MTC include lower pathogenicity and lack of human-to-human transmission.
>
> - Diagnosis of NTM disease requires both clinical and microbiological criteria to be met.
>
> - Treatment is disappointing and is characterised by long duration and side-effects, leading to poor compliance.

The epidemiology of NTM disease has been difficult to determine because reporting is not mandatory in most countries and differentiation between infection/colonisation and disease may be problematic. However, recent studies from North America and Europe have documented a steady increase of pulmonary disease over the past decade, reporting prevalence rates (range 1.08–8.6 cases per 100 000 persons) that may exceed those of TB.

Although much remains to be understood about the pathogenesis of NTM infections, the following is now well established.

- In HIV-infected patients, disseminated NTM infections occur only after the CD4$^+$ T-lymphocyte count has dropped below 50 cells·μL^{-1}.
- In HIV-uninfected patients, NTM infections may be associated with specific mutations in interferon-γ and interleukin-12 synthesis and response pathways.

The most common clinical manifestation of NTM infection is pulmonary disease, but lymphatic, skin/soft tissue, osteoarticular and disseminated disease are also important.

Pulmonary disease

In immunocompetent subjects, NTM lung disease presents as one of the following clinical forms.

Cavitary lung disease This pattern, which closely resembles pulmonary TB, involves the upper lobes of older males usually affected by a pre-existing destructive or obstructive lung condition such as pneumoconiosis, chronic bronchitis with emphysema (frequently associated with long-term, heavy smoking) and bronchiectasis. Thin-walled cavities with scarce parenchymal infiltrate and a marked pleural thickening are characteristic. Signs and symptoms include chronic cough with sputum production and weakness. With advanced disease, dyspnoea, fever, weight loss and haemoptysis can also occur.

Nodular bronchiectasis This pattern (also known as Lady Windermere syndrome) has been described in slender, elderly females with structural chest abnormalities (pectus excavatum, scoliosis and mitral valve prolapse) but no evidence of pre-existing lung disease. Indolent productive cough and purulent sputum are the most common presenting symptoms, while constitutional symptoms and haemoptysis are not common unless extensive disease is present. The radiographic findings include small nodular infiltrates and cylindrical bronchiectasis, predominately located within the middle lobe and lingula.

Hypersensitivity pneumonitis A syndrome indistinguishable from hypersensitivity pneumonitis has been reported in subjects exposed to household water laden with *Mycobacterium avium* complex (MAC) organisms (hot tubs and medicinal baths). Full recovery usually occurs without any specific therapy (simply by avoiding further contact with contaminated solutions) but

sometimes a combination therapy of steroids and antibiotics may be required.

In addition, NTM lung disease may be associated with the following conditions.

- HIV infection: although NTM are frequently recovered from respiratory specimens of HIV-infected subjects, extrapulmonary or disseminated disease are more likely to occur. The most relevant exception to this generalisation is *Mycobacterium kansasii*.
- Immune reconstitution disease: this clinical syndrome has been described in HIV-infected patients with poor immune function soon after the initiation of antiretroviral therapy (ART). ART-induced restoration of the immune response may cause subclinical mycobacterial disease to manifest suddenly or be 'unmasked'.
- Transplantation including both solid-organ and haematopoietic stem cell transplants: these infections generally occur late in the post-transplantation period, presenting as cutaneous lesions of the extremities, tenosynovitis, arthritis or pulmonary disease. Pleuropulmonary disease is the predominant manifestation among lung transplant recipients and also represents a significant proportion of NTM infections after heart transplant. The most common species reported to cause pulmonary disease include *M. kansasii*, *M. avium*, *Mycobacterium abscessus* and *Mycobacterium xenopi*.

Table 1. *American Thoracic Society criteria for diagnosis of pulmonary disease caused by NTM*

Clinical criteria (both required)
Pulmonary symptoms, cavitary or noncavitary lung disease
Appropriate exclusion of other causes for the disease
Microbiological criteria (only one required)
Positive culture results from at least two separate expectorated sputum samples
Positive culture results from at least one bronchial wash or lavage
A transbronchial or lung biopsy showing granulomata and/or AFB and positive culture for NTM
Biopsy showing granulomata and/or AFB and one or more sputa or bronchial washing that are culture-positive for NTM
AFB: acid-fast bacilli.

Table 2. Clinical and X-ray features of pulmonary infections caused by the most frequently encountered NTM

Species	Pathogenicity	Outcome	X-ray findings	Treatment (months)
MAC	Intermediate	Poor/fair	Upper lobe cavitations	Clarithromycin, ethambutol, rifampicin (18)
			Middle lobe bronchiectasis	Clarithromycin, ethambutol, rifampicin (18)
M. kansasii	High	Good	Upper lobe cavitations	Rifampicin, isoniazid, ethambutol (18)
M. malmoense	High	Fair	Upper lobe infiltrates	Rifampicin, ethambutol (24)
M. xenopi	Low	Poor	Upper lobe cavitations and nodules	Clarithromycin, rifampicin, ethambutol, moxifloxacin (18)
M. szulgai	High	Good	Upper lobe cavitations	Rifampicin, isoniazid, ethambutol, pyrazinamide (18)
M. simiae	Low	Poor	Upper lobe cavitations and nodules	Clarithromycin, moxifloxacin, co-trimoxazole (18)
M. abscessus	Intermediate	Poor	Multilobar interstitial and nodular lesions	Clarithromycin, amikacin, cefoxitin, tigecycline (6–12) Surgical resection

Reproduced and modified from Piersimoni *et al.* (2008) with permission from the publisher.

- Treatment with tumour necrosis factor-α antagonists
- CF

Laboratory diagnosis

Mycobacterial culture remains the cornerstone of definitive diagnosis. Therefore, appropriate, high-quality specimens properly collected from all patients with suspected NTM disease have to be sent to a certified laboratory. Due to the ubiquitous occurrence of NTM in the environment, the recognition of disease, as opposed to contamination of specimens or transient colonisation, may be difficult. While smear-positive samples strongly suggest an active disease, a single positive culture (especially with small numbers of organisms) does not suffice to set such a diagnosis. In this context, the American Thoracic Society has recently updated the criteria for the diagnosis of pulmonary disease caused by NTM (table 1).

It is necessary to fulfil all the above elements to establish a correct diagnosis. Although

these criteria are derived from experience with MAC, it is reasonable to believe they would work with other species provided that contamination of clinical specimens and medical devices with environmental NTM (pseudoinfection) has been excluded. Today, the combined use of automated liquid culture for detection and drug susceptibility testing (DST) plus the use of genetic probe technology for identification of mycobacteria is mandatory in all laboratories wishing to perform mycobacteriology.

Treatment

Treatment regimens for NTM disease are still largely undefined and outcome remains disappointing despite considerable upgrading in mycobacteriology and the availability of some new antimicrobials. Treatment success is impaired by the long duration of regimens, their side-effects and drug interactions, which prevent patients from full compliance (table 2). In addition, although many NTM species may be susceptible *in vitro* to one or more anti-TB drug, correlation between DST results and clinical outcome is poor.

Further reading

- Brown-Elliott BA, *et al.* (2012). Anti-microbial susceptibility testing, drug resistance mechanisms, and therapy of infections with nontuberculous mycobacteria. *Clin Microbiol Rev*; 25: 545–582.
- Clinical and Laboratory Standard Institute. Laboratory Detection and Identification of Mycobacteria. M48-A. Wayne, CLSI, 2008.
- Clinical and Laboratory Standard Institute. Susceptibility Testing of Mycobacteria, Nocardiae, and Other Aerobic Actinomycetes. M24-A2. Wayne, CLSI, 2011.
- Doucette K, *et al.* (2004). Nontuberculous mycobacterial infection in hematopoietic stem cell and solid organ transplant recipients. *Clin Infect Dis*; 38: 1428–1439.
- Field SK, *et al.* (2006). Lung disease due to the more common nontuberculous mycobacteria. *Chest*; 129: 1653–1672.
- Fujita G, *et al.* (2007). Radiological findings of mycobacterial diseases. *J Infect Chemother*; 13: 8–17.
- Glassroth J (2008). Pulmonary disease due to nontuberculous mycobacteria. *Chest*; 133: 243–251.
- Griffith DE, *et al.* (2007). An official ATS/IDSA statement: diagnosis, treatment, and prevention of nontuberculous mycobacterial diseases. *Am J Respir Crit Care Med*; 175: 367–416.
- Mangione E, *et al.* (2001). Nontuberculous mycobacterial disease following hot tub exposure. *Emerg Infect Dis*; 7: 1039–1042.
- Piersimoni C, *et al.* (2008). Pulmonary infections associated with non-tuberculous mycobacteria in immunocompetent patients. *Lancet Infect Dis*; 8: 323–334.
- Tortoli E (2007). Impact of genotypic studies on mycobacterial taxonomy: the new mycobacteria of the 1990s. *Clin Microbiol Rev*; 16: 319–354.
- Yew WW, *et al.* (2011). Update in tuberculosis and nontuberculous mycobacterial diseases 2010. *Am J Respir Crit Care Med*; 184: 180–185.

Laboratory diagnosis of mycobacterial infections

Claudio Piersimoni

Although the prevalence of TB in industrialised countries is low, one thing remains certain, TB, including multidrug-resistant (MDR) and extensively drug-resistant (XDR)-TB, is no longer restricted to developing regions of the globe. In addition, many species of nontuberculous mycobacteria (NTM) are now recognised as a cause of pulmonary disease in man with increasing frequency.

The rapid and accurate diagnosis of TB is of the utmost importance; it involves the isolation and identification of the aetiological agent, *Mycobacterium tuberculosis* complex (MTC), while design of an appropriate therapeutic regimen relies on the results of anti-TB drug susceptibility testing (DST).

Laboratory services are an essential component of effective TB control and elimination. Unfortunately, they are at the end of decision tree for the patient's health improvement; thus, they are unable to prevent delays in diagnosis related to both the patient and the physician.

Seven tests performed in clinical microbiological laboratories are recommended for TB control and elimination:

- microscopy for acid-fast bacilli (AFB)
- nucleic acid amplification (NAA)
- AFB detection by culture
- identification of cultured mycobacteria
- molecular detection of drug resistance
- DST for first-line drugs
- DST for second-line drugs

These tests should not only be available to every clinician involved in TB diagnosis and management but also be available in a timely manner according to well-defined turnaround times.

Specimen procurement, transport and processing

Success in detecting and isolating mycobacteria strongly depends on the following principles.

1. Select patients soundly suspected of having an active disease.
2. Submit appropriate specimens, collected from the body sites most likely to yield mycobacteria. Inappropriate or redundant specimens must be discouraged.
3. Ensure that adequate volumes of samples are properly collected, stored and delivered to the laboratory.

Most clinical specimens contain an abundance of nonmycobacterial organisms.

> **Key points**
>
> - Think of TB; if you do not, the laboratory cannot help you.
>
> - Do not use microbiological tests as screening tests.
>
> - Remember that the best way to improve testing sensitivity is to submit high-quality specimens.
>
> - Molecular tests cannot replace conventional culture.
>
> - If your laboratory does not meet current quality standards (testing and turnaround times), refer your specimens to a larger laboratory.

Unless an attempt is made to get rid of such contaminants, they will easily suppress the slow growth of mycobacteria. In addition, it is also necessary to liquefy respiratory samples so that mycobacteria can be easily harvested after centrifugation. This key procedure is referred to as 'decontamination', and is usually performed using a mixture of 1% N-acetyl-L-cysteine and 2% sodium hydroxide. As a rule of thumb, ideal decontamination should be mild enough to kill contaminants without damaging mycobacteria.

Microscopy

The first step in the laboratory diagnosis of TB is microscopic examination of sputum smears stained by an acid-fast procedure. Microscopy is rapid, easy and inexpensive, providing the physician with a presumptive diagnosis of TB and a simultaneous assessment of the patient's infectiousness.

Since the sensitivity of microscopy is relatively low, requiring 10^3–10^4 bacilli per mL of specimen to allow detection, smears should always be prepared from concentrated specimens. Centrifugation is a key step, and must be performed with sufficient g-force in appropriately refrigerated and enclosed biosafe centrifuges.

The acid-fast staining procedure depends on the ability of mycobacteria to retain dye when treated with acid or acid–alcohol solution. Two types of acid-fast stains are commonly used:

- the carbol fuchsin stain, which includes the Ziehl–Neelsen and Kinyoun methods
- a fluorochrome procedure using auramine O or auramine–rhodamine dyes

The latter provides a 10% more sensitive performance and also permits a faster screening of smears.

AFB seen on smear may represent either MTC or NTM. However, because of the infectious potential of MTC, sputum smear microscopy should be performed within one working day of specimen receipt and positive results should be reported immediately by telephone, fax or other electronic means, as soon as they are available.

Molecular detection of MTC

With the purpose of obtaining faster results and a more accurate diagnosis of TB than those achievable with microscopy and liquid culture, several molecular methods were introduced and have been evaluated worldwide.

These technologies allow for the amplification of specific target sequences that can be detected through the use of a complementary nucleic acid probe. Both RNA and DNA amplification systems have been developed.

Although many in-house amplification methods have been described in published studies, most amplification tests currently used in clinical laboratories are supplied commercially. While these assays have demonstrated an excellent specificity, their sensitivity cannot equal that of culture-based methods, especially for smear-negative samples. In a recent meta-analysis, pooled sensitivities and specificities of 85% and 97%, respectively, were reported.

NAA methods can be applied to decontaminated respiratory specimens within hours, producing a positive result with as few as 10^2 bacilli per mL of specimen. They should be performed within 48 h of specimen receipt. NAA tests are applied to smear-positive respiratory samples to provide rapid confirmation that the infecting mycobacteria belong to the MTC. In addition, it is recommended that NAA tests are used on the first sputum or other respiratory sample of all smear-negative TB suspects.

Since the clinical utility of NAA tests is for ruling in active TB, it is of utmost importance that they are employed on the basis of a sound clinical suspicion. Routine implementation of NAA testing without consideration of clinical data lacks cost-effectiveness and may be misleading.

Culture

All clinical specimens suspected of containing mycobacteria should be inoculated onto culture media for the following reasons.

- Culture is the most sensitive method, being able to detect as few as 10 mycobacteria per mL of specimen
- Growth of the organisms is necessary for proper species identification
- DST requires culture of the organism
- Genotyping of the cultured strain may be useful to study clusters of TB cases

Three different types of culture media are currently available: egg-based (Löwestein–Jensen), agar-based (Middlebrook 7H10 or 7H11 medium) and liquid (Middlebrook 7H9 and other 7H9-based commercial broths) whose selectivity may be greatly improved by adding antibiotics. A combination of liquid and solid culture gives the most rapid and optimal rates of mycobacterial recovery from clinical specimens.

Among liquid media, automated culture systems have been developed that are continuously monitored and also able to perform DST. Since none of the above liquid systems can distinguish between a pure and mixed mycobacterial culture, parallel culture on solid media will provide confirmation of a single colonial morphology. For these reasons, liquid culture systems should be available in all laboratories willing to perform mycobacteriology.

Identification

The genus *Mycobacterium* consists of >140 different species, all of which appear similar on acid-fast staining. More than two-thirds of them, both saprophytes and (potential) pathogens, may be recovered from human sources.

Causative agents of TB in humans (*M. tuberculosis, Mycobacterium bovis, M. bovis* bacille Calmette–Guérin (BCG), *Mycobacterium africanum, Mycobacterium caprae, Mycobacterium microti, Mycobacterium pinnipedii* and *Mycobacterium canettii*) are referred to as MTC and most clinical laboratories identify these organisms only to the level of the complex. This practice is supported by two rapid identification procedures that, based on distinctive molecular and antigenic characteristics of the MTC, have gained widespread use:

- nucleic acid hybridisation
- immunochromatographic assay

It is recommended that laboratories culture and identify MTC within 21 days of receiving the patient's specimen (table 1). This goal can be obtained only by combining liquid culture with the above rapid identification methods.

Drug susceptibility testing

DST should be performed on the initial isolate from all new TB cases. In addition, it should be repeated if the patient continues to be culture-positive after 2–3 months of treatment or exhibits positive culture after a period of negative cultures.

The source for DST may be either a smear-positive specimen (direct method) or, most often, growth is first isolated in pure culture from clinical specimens and then inoculated into a drug-containing medium (indirect method). Growth of mycobacteria in the presence of the drug(s) is then compared with a drug-free control.

Among different DST methods, the proportion method is the most widely used. It allows determining the proportion of MTC organisms that are resistant to a given drug at a single (critical) concentration. The susceptibility proportion was set at 1%, because higher proportions of drug-resistant bacilli were shown to be associated with treatment failure. The critical concentration of a drug is the level of drug that inhibits the growth of most organisms within the population of a wild-type strain without affecting the growth of strains recovered from clinically resistant patients (table 2).

Several studies have established that drug resistance in MTC isolates does not rely upon a 'on/off' mechanism, but, on the contrary, different mutations may lead to different levels of resistance. This means that

Table 1. Turnaround times for essential laboratory tests recommended by the American Thoracic Society to provide effective TB control and elimination

Test	Maximum turnaround time
Microscopy for AFB	≤24 h from receipt by laboratory
NAA assay	≤48 h from date of specimen collection
Mycobacterial growth detection by culture	≤14 days from date of specimen collection
Identification of cultured mycobacteria	≤21 days from date of specimen collection
DST	
First-line drugs	≤30 days from date of specimen collection
Second-line drugs	≤4 weeks from date of request

Reproduced and modified from American Thoracic Society et al. (2005) with permission from the publisher.

mutation(s) causing low-level resistance do not necessarily imply clinical resistance. Unfortunately, these data on different levels of resistance are not available when single critical concentrations are used. Moreover, the resistance level determined in vitro bears little relationship to the drug concentrations achievable in vivo.

Results of first-line drugs assay (isoniazid, rifampicin, ethambutol and pyrazinamide) should be reported within 4 weeks from specimen receipt. Although agar proportion is currently the reference method, two commercially available automated systems (BACTEC MGIT 960 (BD, Franklin Lakes, NUJ, USA) and ESP culture system (Thermo Scientific, East Grinstead, UK)) have been cleared for susceptibility testing of first-line drugs. The use of these liquid systems has not yet been approved for susceptibility testing of second-line drugs (amikacin, capreomycin, ethionamide, kanamycin, moxifloxacin, para-aminosalicylic acid, rifabutin, streptomycin and linezolid), which still relies on the agar proportion method.

Compared to other laboratory tests, accuracy is much more important than speed in the case of drug susceptibility. Thus, results should come from a small number of well-equipped, experienced laboratories enrolled in a national and/or supranational DST quality control scheme.

During the past 10 years, triggered by the increasing prevalence of MDR- and XDR-TB,

renewed efforts were spent to develop new drugs for the chemotherapy of TB. Several classes of drugs including diarylquinoline (bedaquiline), nitroimidazole (PA-824 and delamanid), and oxazolidine compounds have shown promise for the treatment of both fully susceptible as well as drug-resistant TB. These drugs have unique, new action mechanisms, and no cross-resistance between them and the existing TB drugs has been reported. To date, no information is available on DST for these new drugs.

Molecular detection of resistance

Although detection of drug resistance in MTC has traditionally been accomplished by culture-based assays, the emergence of MDR- and XDR-TB demands improved and faster detection methods. In this context, several molecular approaches have been developed aimed at detecting gene mutations known to be associated with phenotypic resistance to a particular drug.

As DNA sequencing (the reference method to look for specific mutations) would be almost impossible for most diagnostic laboratories, simpler procedures such as the line probe assay (LiPA) have recently been introduced. It relies on the reverse hybridisation of oligonucleotides on plastic strips to which specific probes have been immobilised. Amplified target sequences from the strain under evaluation are bound to probes and hybridisation is revealed by the development of a coloured line on the strip.

Table 2. Critical concentrations available for DST of MTC using commercial liquid media systems cleared for use by the US Food and Drug Administration and their equivalence in the agar proportion method

Antimicrobial agent	Concentration $\mu g \cdot mL^{-1}$		
	BACTEC MGIT 960	VersaTREK	7H10 Agar
Isoniazid	0.1	0.1	0.2
Isoniazid	0.4	0.4	1.0
Rifampicin	1.0	1.0	1.0
Ethambutol	5.0	5.0	5.0
Ethambutol	7.5	8.0	10.0
Pyrazinamide	100	300	NA
Streptomycin	1.0	NA	2.0
Streptomycin	4.0	NA	10.0

BACTEC MGIT 960 is manufactured by BD (Franklin Lakes, NJ, USA). VersaTREK is manufactured by Thermo Scientific (East Grinstead, UK). NA: not available. Reproduced from and modified from Clinical Laboratory Standards Institute (2011) with permission from the publisher.

There are currently three commercially available LiPAs for the rapid detection of drug resistance in MTC: the INNO-LiPA Rif TB (Innogenetics, Ghent, Belgium) for detecting resistance to rifampicin; the GenoType MTBDR*Plus* (Hain Lifesciences, Nehren, Germany) for the simultaneous detection of resistance to rifampin and isoniazid; and the newly released GenoType MTBDR*sl* (Hain Lifesciences), which detects the most frequent mutations associated with resistance to fluoroquinolones, aminoglycosides and ethambutol. These tests are validated for use in cultured strains as well as in smear-positive respiratory samples.

Real-time PCR technology has also been proposed for the rapid detection of drug resistance in MTC. Different assays have been developed, which include the XpertMTB/RIF (GeneXpert system; Cepheid, Maurens-Scopont, France), an automated molecular test for simultaneous detection of MTC and rifampicin resistance. This cartridge-based NAA assay employs a hemi-nested real-time PCR and requires just a single manual step with minimal sample manipulation. The remaining analysis is performed by the GeneXpert instrument, relatively rapidly ($\sim$2 h). Clinical validation trials performed in many different settings

showed a high diagnostic accuracy for rapid diagnosis of both smear-positive and -negative pulmonary TB. For diagnosis of rifampicin resistance, false-positive results were observed in settings characterised by a low prevalence of resistance. XpertMTB/RIF may have the potential to complement the current reference standard of TB diagnostics, and increase its overall sensitivity and speed. Further studies are required to determine the optimal level of the healthcare system where this system can be used cost-effectively.

Genotyping of MTC isolates

Genotyping or DNA fingerprinting of MTC refers to procedures developed to identify isolates that are identical in specific parts of the genome. The most extensively used method in the last two decades has been restriction fragment length polymorphism (RFLP) analysis of the distribution of the insertion sequence IS6110. The more recently developed spoligotyping and 24-locus variable number of tandem repeats (VNTR) techniques are similarly based on genetic polymorphism of additional mycobacterial repetitive sequences. The various DNA fingerprinting methods serve different purposes and have variable characteristics that enable their use in specific applications. They currently support routine contact tracing as well as investigations on person-to-person transmission, early disease outbreak identification and laboratory cross-contamination, and permit determination of whether new cases of TB are due to re-infection or re-activation. In addition, the recognition of different genotype families has facilitated studies on the population structure of MTC and its dynamic. Due to the fact that VNTR typing combines a more user-friendly technique with a significantly shorter turnaround time than RFLP typing, it is now considered the gold standard.

Organisation of laboratory services

Any TB laboratory-based diagnostic procedure should be performed by appropriately trained staff working to standardised operating procedures in appropriately equipped and safe laboratories, to well-defined national and international proficiency and quality standards. In this context, mycobacteriology laboratory consolidation at the regional level is strongly recommended.

Further reading

- American Thoracic Society, et al. (2005). Controlling tuberculosis in the United States. Am J Respir Crit Care Med; 172: 1169–1227.
- Centers for Disease Control and Prevention. (2009). Updated guidelines for the use of nucleic acid amplification tests in the diagnosis of tuberculosis. MMWR; 58: 7–10.
- Clinical and Laboratory Standard Institute. Laboratory Detection and Identification of Mycobacteria. M48-A. Wayne, CLSI, 2008.

- Clinical and Laboratory Standard Institute. Susceptibility testing of myco-bacteria, nocardiae, and other aerobic actinomycetes. M24-A2. Wayne, CLSI, 2011.
- Davies PDO, et al. (2008). The diagnosis and misdiagnosis of tuberculosis. Int J Tuberc Lung Dis; 12: 1226–1234.
- Drobniewski FA, et al. (2006). Recommended standards for modern tuberculosis laboratory services in Europe. Eur Respir J; 28: 903–909.
- Drobniewski FA (2003). Modern laboratory diagnosis of tuberculosis. Lancet Infect Dis; 3: 141–147.
- European Centre for Disease Prevention and Control. Mastering the basics of TB control: development of a handbook on TB diagnostic methods. Stockholm, ECDC, 2011.
- Ling DI, et al. (2008). Commercial nucleic-acid amplification tests for diagnosis of pulmonary tuberculosis in respiratory specimens: meta-analysis and meta-regression. PLoS One; 3: e1536.
- Palomino JC (2009). Molecular detection, identification and drug resistance detection in Mycobacterium tuberculosis. FEMS Immunol Med Microbiol; 56: 103–111.
- Parrish NM, et al. (2011). Role of the clinical mycobacteriology laboratory in the diagnosis and management of tuberculosis in low-prevalence settings. J Clin Microbiol; 49: 772–776.
- Tenover FC, et al. (1993). The resurgence of tuberculosis: is your laboratory ready? J Clin Microbiol; 31: 767–770.
- Weyer K, et al. (2013). Rapid molecular TB diagnosis: evidence, policy making and global implementation of Xpert MTB/RIF. Eur Respir J; 42: 252–271.

Chronic rhinitis

Arnaud Bourdin and Pascal Chanez

Rhinitis is one of the most common human diseases. Its most important features are inflammation and structural changes of the nasal mucosa. The causes are hetero-geneous and, if allergy and infections are dominant, it is often difficult to find a single common aetiology in chronic rhinitis. It is important to consider that rhinitis is often associated with sinusitis and lower airway diseases such as asthma. Rhinitis is a mild disease, but it interferes with sleep quality and daily life.

Epidemiology

Rhinitis is still increasing in prevalence in most countries. In some studies, 25–30% of the population suffers from rhinitis, which is often linked to IgE sensitisation. It may increase with age, as demonstrated in both children and adults, and there is growing evidence that emerging countries are affected by an increase in prevalence. Thus, rhinitis is an important health problem worldwide. It affects health-related quality of life in both adults and children. It is usually a mild disease, but its direct and indirect costs are substantial. Absenteeism from school or work is often reported by subjects suffering from rhinitis. Rhinitis is often associated with other IgE-related disease, and the continuum linking upper and lower airways is well represented by the association of rhinitis and asthma, which frequently coexist: asthma is present in 20–50% of patients with allergic rhinitis. Rhinitis is present in up to 80% of asthma patients. Whether allergic rhinitis precedes, triggers or precipitates asthma lacks supportive data. Atopic status plays a potentially prominent role in this relationship, although it is not a prerequisite. The risk factors for rhinitis need to be better known and understood in order for preventive measures to be implemented.

Definition and clinical aspects of rhinitis

Allergic rhinitis is defined as inflammation of the nasal mucosa characterised clinically by nasal discharge, blockage, sneezing and itch, with two or more symptoms occurring for >1 h on most days. It can be further classified as intermittent (symptoms occurring on <4 days out of 7 or for <4 weeks per year) or persistent (symptoms occurring on ≥4 days out of 7 or for ≥4 weeks per year). The impact of chronic rhinitis on sleep, daily activities, work or school is a major determinant of quality-of-life impairment in patients. The perception of nasal symptoms is highly variable, a fact illustrated in patients suffering from COPD, where a discrepancy between nasal inflammation and symptoms has been demonstrated. From a clinical point of view, it is thus difficult to rely on patients' reports of symptoms as the only way to assess rhinitis.

Key points

- The prevalence of rhinitis is increasing in most countries.

- Asthma is present in 20–50% of allergic rhinitis patients, while up to 80% of asthma patients have rhinitis.

- Treatment is anti-inflammatory and directed according to whether rhinitis is allergic or nonallergic.

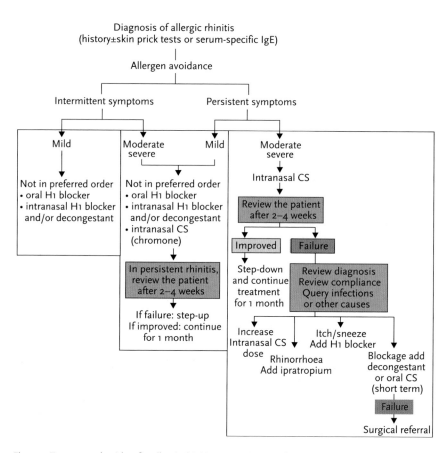

Figure 1. Treatment algorithm for allergic rhinitis. CS: corticosteroids. Reproduced and modified from the ARIA guidelines, with permission from the publisher.

Nonallergic rhinitis is difficult to differentiate clinically from allergic rhinitis. Exacerbations are usually associated with infections but several other triggers, including drugs, may cause recurrent symptoms.

Pathological and mechanistic aspects

Pseudostratified epithelium and a large, highly developed vasculature cover the nasal wall. Tight junctions, peptidases and a large antioxidant apparatus are key features of the anatomical barrier of the nasal epithelium. The mucosal-associated lymphoid tissue is developed in the nose. Structural abnormalities including changes of the basement membrane have been reported in

rhinitis. Inflammatory cells such as eosinophils, mast cells, T-cells and macrophages infiltrate the epithelium and submucosa. Mast cell-derived inflammatory mediators are overexpressed, such as histamine, chemokines and cytokines including interleukin (IL)-5, RANTES (regulated on activation, normal T-cell expressed and secreted), IL-4, IL-13 and granulocyte–macrophage colony-stimulating factor. Most of these molecules trigger a local eosinophilic inflammatory process. Allergens, microorganisms and pollutants are potential triggers that can generate acute and chronic inflammatory reactions through the epithelium. The release of various mediators is responsible for most of the clinical symptoms reported by patients. Nasal hypersecretion, sneezing and itching are related to the release of vasoactive and pro-inflammatory mediators such as histamine and sulfidoleukotrienes. Persistent nasal obstruction is linked to the perpetuation of inflammatory reactions mostly related, in allergic rhinitis, to eosinophilic infiltration.

Effects of anti-inflammatory treatment

Intranasal corticosteroids and intranasal or oral antihistamines have been shown to have effects on different aspects of inflammation in allergic rhinitis. Additionally, intranasal anticholinergic therapy provides relief for excessive rhinorrhoea, while leukotriene antagonists block the cysteinyl leukotriene receptor. Nasal obstruction improves significantly more with intranasal corticosteroids compared with most of the other pharmacological strategies. Specific immunotherapy using sublingual, oral or subcutaneous routes has been proven effective and safe in intermittent and persistent allergic rhinitis. Allergen avoidance is not effective in persistent allergic rhinitis. Several studies have demonstrated that the effective treatment of rhinitis decreases the burden of asthma as assessed by unscheduled visits to physicians and emergency rooms due to acute exacerbations.

Treatment should be directed according to the cause: nonallergic rhinitis should be treated by nasal decongestant and anticholinergic therapy; allergic rhinitis should be treated according to the Allergic Rhinitis and Its Impact on Asthma (ARIA) guidelines (fig. 1).

The term rhinitis covers a heterogeneous group of diseases. Allergic rhinitis and its associated diseases have been well defined and treatment is codified. Mucosal inflammation is the hallmark of rhinitis. Its natural history and its relationship with sinusitis and lower airway diseases need to be clarified. New treatments and management strategies are required, especially in the most chronic severe forms.

Further reading

- Allergic Rhinitis and its Impact on Asthma. www.whiar.org
- Bousquet PJ, et al. (2007). ARIA (Allergic Rhinitis and its Impact on Asthma) classification of allergic rhinitis severity in clinical practice in France. Int Arch Allergy Immunol; 143: 163–169.
- Carr WW, et al. (2008). Managing rhinitis: strategies for improved patient outcomes. Allergy Asthma Proc; 29: 349–357.
- Chanez P, et al. (1999). Comparison between nasal and bronchial inflammation in asthmatic and control subjects. Am J Respir Crit Care Med; 159: 588–595.
- Lipworth BJ, et al. (2000). Allergic inflammation in the unified airway: start with the nose. Thorax; 55: 878–881.
- Raherison C, et al. (2004). How should nasal symptoms be investigated in asthma? A comparison of radiologic and endoscopic findings. Allergy; 59: 821–826.
- Togias A (2003). Rhinitis and asthma: evidence for respiratory system integration. J Allergy Clin Immunol; 111: 1171–1183.

Asthma

Bianca Beghé, Leonardo M. Fabbri and Paul O'Byrne

Asthma is a chronic inflammatory disease of the airways characterised clinically by recurrent respiratory symptoms of dyspnoea, wheezing, chest tightness and/or cough, associated with reversible airflow limitation. Other characteristics of asthma are an exaggerated responsiveness of the airways to various stimuli, and, in most cases, a specific type of chronic inflammation of the airways characterised by an increased number of $CD4^+$ T-helper (Th) type 2 lymphocytes, eosinophils and metachromatic cells in the airway mucosa, increased thickness of the reticular layer of the epithelial basement membrane, and increased volume of airway smooth muscle (fig. 1).

Familial predisposition, atopy, and exposure to allergens and occupational sensitising agents are important risk factors for asthma, even though the causes of asthma – the factors responsible for the development of

asthma rather than its exacerbations – remain largely undetermined.

Asthma is a heterogeneous syndrome that, over the years, has been divided into many different clinical subtypes, *e.g.* allergic asthma, adult-onset asthma that is usually nonallergic, occupational asthma, asthma in smokers and asthma in the obese.

Minimum requirements for the diagnosis of asthma

The diagnosis of asthma is based on an appropriate clinical history, together with the demonstration of variable and/or reversible airflow limitation, using lung function tests, particularly peak expiratory flow (PEF) or spirometry. Allergy tests are also often performed during the initial assessment of a patient with suspected asthma, to identify possible triggers of asthma and to guide their avoidance.

Asthma clusters in families and its genetic determinants appear to be linked to those of other allergic IgE-mediated diseases. Thus, a personal or family history of asthma and/or allergic rhinitis, atopic dermatitis, or eczema increases the likelihood of a diagnosis of asthma.

Symptoms and medical history

Patients with asthma seek medical attention because of respiratory symptoms. A typical feature of asthma symptoms is their variability. One or more of the symptoms

- wheezing
- chest tightness
- episodic shortness of breath
- cough

Key points

- Asthma is diagnosed based on clinical history and lung function testing. Allergy testing may also have a role.

- The differential diagnosis is extensive. In particular, COPD may be difficult to distinguish from asthma.

- The goal of pharmacological asthma treatment is to achieve and maintain control of symptoms and prevention of exacerbations.

- Asthma is a chronic, lifelong disease and must therefore be managed in partnership with the patient.

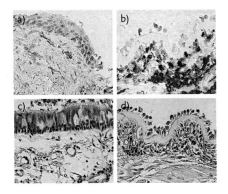

Figure 1. a, b) Photomicrographs showing bronchial biopsy specimens immunostained with anti-EG-2 (eosinophil cationic protein) a) from a patient with fixed airflow obstruction and a history of COPD and b) from a patient with fixed airflow obstruction and a history of asthma. The two patients had a similar degree of fixed airflow obstruction. In b), there is prominent eosinophilia beneath the destroyed epithelium that is not present in a). c, d) Photomicrographs showing bronchial biopsy specimens stained with haematoxylin and eosin c) from a patient with fixed airflow obstruction and a history of COPD and d) from a patient with fixed airflow obstruction and a history of asthma. The two patients had a similar degree of fixed airflow obstruction. In d), there is a thicker reticular layer of the epithelial basement membrane compared with c). Reproduced and modified from Fabbri et al. (2003) with permission from the publisher.

are reported by >90% of patients with asthma. However, the presence of these symptoms is not diagnostic because similar symptoms can be present with other respiratory or even cardiac diseases, or may be triggered by different stimuli in nonasthmatics, e.g. by acute viral infections. In some asthmatics, wheezing and chest tightness are absent, and the only symptom the patient complains of is chronic cough (cough-variant asthma).

Symptoms of asthma may be triggered or worsened by several factors, such as exercise, exposure to allergens, viral infections and emotions. Recurrent exacerbations of respiratory symptoms, worsening of lung function requiring change

of treatment, unscheduled requests for medical assistance and, sometimes, hospitalisation are also among the characteristic clinical features of asthma.

Physical activity is an important cause of symptoms for most asthma patients, particularly in children, and for some it is the only cause. Exercise-induced broncho-constriction usually develops not during exercise but 5–10 min afterward and resolves spontaneously within 30–45 min. Prompt relief of symptoms after the use of an inhaled β_2-agonist or their prevention by pre-treatment with an inhaled β_2-agonist before exercise supports a diagnosis of asthma.

Important aspects of personal history are exposure to agents known to worsen asthma in the home, such as dusty environments, forced air heating systems or exposure to allergens (e.g. pets, house dust mites or cockroaches) to which the patient is sensitised, workplace conditions, environmental tobacco smoke or even the general environment (e.g. diesel fumes in traffic).

Since respiratory symptoms of asthma are nonspecific, the differential diagnosis is quite extensive, and the main goal for the physician is to consider and exclude other possible diagnoses (table 1). This is even more important if the response to a trial of therapy has been negative.

When respiratory symptoms suggest asthma, the sine qua non condition for the objective diagnosis of asthma is the presence of reversible airflow obstruction. In patients who have persistent airway obstruction, reversibility may be demonstrated as response to treatment (e.g. 200–400 μg albuterol or after a period of regular treatment). In subject presenting without persistent airway obstruction, reversibility may be demonstrated either by measuring airway responsiveness or PEF variability.

Physical examination

In mild asthma, physical examination is usually normal under stable conditions, but becomes characteristically abnormal during

Table 1. *Differential diagnosis of asthma*

Localised pathology	Inhaled foreign body
	Endobronchial tumour
	Vocal cord dysfunction
Diffuse airway pathology	COPD
	Eosinophilic bronchitis
	Bronchiectasis
Other pathologies	Gastro-oesophageal reflux
	Left ventricular failure
	Pulmonary embolism
	Pulmonary eosinophilia

asthma attacks. Typical physical signs of asthma attacks are wheezing on auscultation, cough, expiratory rhonchi throughout the chest and signs of acute hyperinflation (*e.g.* poor diaphragmatic excursion on percussion or the use of accessory muscles of respiration). Some patients, particularly children, may present with a predominant nonproductive cough. In some asthmatics, wheezing, which usually reflects airflow limitation, may be absent or detectable only on forced expiration, even in the presence of significant airflow limitation; this may be due to hyperinflation or to very marked airflow obstruction. In these patients, however, the severity of asthma is mostly indicated by other signs, such as cyanosis, drowsiness, difficulty in speaking, tachycardia, hyperinflated chest, use of accessory muscles and intercostal recession.

Lung function tests

Spirometry Lung function tests play a crucial role in the diagnosis and follow-up of patients with asthma. Spirometric measurements – FEV_1 and slow vital capacity (VC) or FVC – are the standard means for assessing airflow limitation. Spirometry is recommended at the time of diagnosis and for the assessment of the severity of asthma. It should be repeated to monitor the disease and when there is a need for reassessment, such as during exacerbations.

Poorly or nonreversible airflow limitation is usually defined by the absolute reduction of

the post-bronchodilator FEV_1/FVC ratio to <0.7. However, because this parameter varies with ageing, it should be confirmed by post-bronchodilator FEV_1/VC values below the lower limit of normal, particularly in younger subjects. Measurements of residual volume and TLC may be useful in assessing the degree of hyperinflation and/or enlargement of airspaces. Lung volumes may help in the differential diagnosis with COPD but are not necessary for the diagnosis or for assessment of the severity of asthma. In asthma, airflow limitation is usually reversible, either spontaneously or after treatment, except for moderate/severe asthma with fixed airway obstruction (see later).

Peak expiratory flow An important tool for the diagnosis and subsequent treatment of asthma is the PEF meter. If spirometry does not reveal airflow limitation, then home monitoring of PEF for 2–4 weeks may help to detect an increased variability of airway calibre, and assist in making the diagnosis of asthma. Daily monitoring of PEF (at least in the morning at awakening and in the evening hours, preferably after broncho-dilator inhalation) is also useful to assess the severity of asthma and its response to treatment, and it can help patients to detect early signs of asthma deterioration. Diurnal variability is calculated as

$$\text{Diurnal variability} = \frac{PEF_{max} \text{-} PEF_{min} \times 100}{PEF_{max} + PEF_{min}/2}$$

where PEF_{max} and PEF_{min} are maximal and minimal PEF, respectively. A diurnal variability of PEF >20% is diagnostic of asthma and the magnitude of the variability

266

is broadly proportional to disease severity. PEF monitoring may be of use not only in establishing a diagnosis of asthma and assessing its severity but also in uncovering an occupational cause of asthma. When used in this way, PEF should be measured more frequently than twice daily and special attention should be paid to changes occurring in and out of the workplace.

Reversibility to bronchodilators Clinical and/or functional reversibility on repeated testing is required for the diagnosis of asthma. Thus, even a single reversibility test (defined as >12% reversibility and/or >200 mL in FEV$_1$ after bronchodilator) can establish the diagnosis. However, reversibility is often not present at the time of examination, particularly in patients on treatment, and thus the absence of reversibility does not exclude the diagnosis. Repeated testing of reversibility of both clinical features and functional abnormalities may be useful in obtaining the best level of asthma control achievable and/or the best lung function for individual patients achieving and maintaining lung function at the best possible level is one of the objectives of asthma management.

Airway hyperresponsiveness In patients who have symptoms consistent with asthma but have normal lung function, bronchial provocation tests with methacholine, histamine or exercise are helpful in measuring airway hyperresponsiveness and,

thereby, confirming or excluding the diagnosis of current asthma. These measurements are very sensitive, but poorly specific for a diagnosis of asthma. This means that while a negative test can be used to exclude a diagnosis of active asthma, a positive test does not always mean that a patient has asthma. While the measurement of airway hyperresponsiveness may be useful to confirm asthma in subjects with normal baseline lung function, it is not useful in the presence of irreversible airflow limitation and, thus, in the differential diagnosis between asthma and COPD.

Arterial blood gases

In severe asthma and, more importantly, during acute exacerbations of asthma, the measurement of arterial blood gases while the patient is breathing air and/or after oxygen administration is essential for the diagnosis of respiratory failure. This test should be performed in all patients with clinical signs of acute or chronic respiratory and/or heart failure, patients with an acute asthma exacerbation and PEF <50% predicted, patients who do not respond to treatment, and those with a $S_aO_2 \leqslant 92\%$.

Allergy tests

The presence of allergic disorders in a patient's family history should be investigated in all patients with symptoms of asthma. A history provides important

Table 2. History, symptoms and results of pulmonary function tests in the differential diagnosis between asthma and COPD

	Asthma	COPD
Onset	Mainly in childhood	In mid- to late adult life
Smoking	Often nonsmokers	Almost invariably smokers
Chronic cough and sputum	Often absent	Frequent (chronic bronchitis)
Dyspnoea on effort	Variable and reversible to treatment	Constant, poorly reversible and progressive
Nocturnal symptoms	Relatively common	Relatively uncommon
Airflow limitation	Increased diurnal variability	Normal diurnal variability
Response to bronchodilator	Good	Poor
Airway hyperresponsiveness	In most patients, with or without airflow limitation	In most patients, with airflow limitation

information about the patient's lifestyle and occupation, both of which influence exposure to allergens, and the time and factors possibly involved in onset and exacerbations of asthma. Skin tests with all relevant allergens present in the geographic area in which the patient lives are the primary diagnostic tool in determining allergic status. Measurement of specific IgE is not usually more informative than a skin test and is more expensive. Measurement of total IgE in serum has no value as a diagnostic test for atopy. The main limitation of methods to assess allergic status is that a positive test does not necessarily mean that the disease is allergic in nature or that it is causing asthma, as some individuals have specific IgE antibodies without any symptoms and these may not be causally involved. The relevant exposure and its relation to symptoms must be confirmed by patient history.

Additional tests

While the diagnosis and assessment of severity of asthma can be fully established on the basis of clinical history and lung function tests, additional tests are sometimes helpful to better characterise individual patients.

Imaging While chest radiography may be useful to exclude diseases that may mimic asthma, it is not required in the confirmation of the diagnosis and management of asthma. The utility of chest radiography is to exclude other conditions that may imitate or complicate asthma, particularly acute asthma. Examples include pneumonia, cardiogenic pulmonary oedema, pulmonary thromboembolism, tumours (especially those that result in airway obstruction with resulting peripheral atelectasis) and pneumothorax.

Assessment of airway inflammation While airway biopsies and bronchoalveolar lavage may provide useful information in research protocols, they are considered too invasive for the diagnosis or staging of asthma. In contrast, noninvasive markers of airway inflammation have been increasingly used in research protocols, particularly to differentiate asthma from COPD and measure response to treatment. These noninvasive measurements include induced sputum and exhaled nitric oxide fraction (*F*eNO) measurement. Induced sputum is not helpful in the diagnosis of asthma but can be very useful in the management of severe asthma. In particular, induced sputum helps identify the persistence of airway eosinophilia or airway neutrophilia in patients with difficult-to-treat asthma, which can be useful in deciding appropriate doses of inhaled corticosteroids and in reducing the risks of severe asthma exacerbations. *F*eNO is increased in atopic asthma but less so in nonatopic asthma. Again, it is not useful in diagnosis but can be helpful in

Table 3. Ancillary tests in the differential diagnosis between stable asthma and COPD

Ancillary test	Asthma	COPD
Reversibility to bronchodilator and/or glucocorticosteroids	Usually present	Usually absent
Lung volumes, residual volume, TLC	Usually normal or, if increased, reversible	Usually irreversibly increased
Diffusion capacity	Normal	Decreased
Airway hyperresponsiveness	Increased	Usually not measurable due to airflow limitation
Allergy tests	Often positive	Often negative
Imaging of the chest	Usually normal	Usually abnormal
Sputum	Eosinophilia	Neutrophilia
FeNO	Increased	Usually normal

monitoring adherence to inhaled corticosteroids, as it is effectively reduced by inhaled corticosteroids but not by bronchodilators.

Differentiating between asthma and COPD

Both asthma and COPD are characterised by chronic airway inflammation but with very different characteristics (fig. 1). In most patients, the clinical presentation and the history provide the strongest diagnostic criteria to distinguish asthma from COPD (table 2). Results of pulmonary function tests, particularly spirometric measurements that show a nearly complete reversibility of airflow limitation, will confirm a diagnosis of asthma, and measurements that show poorly reversible airflow limitation may help to confirm the diagnosis of COPD (table 2). Differential diagnosis between asthma and COPD becomes more difficult in elderly patients, in whom some features may overlap, such as smoking and atopy, and when the patient has airflow limitation that is poorly reversible after treatment. In these cases, symptoms, lung function, airway responsiveness, imaging and even pathological findings may overlap, and thus may not provide solid information to establish a diagnosis. Because an accurate diagnosis is needed to provide better treatment, it is important in these cases to undertake an individual approach and to perform additional tests. Reversibility to corticosteroids alone or in combination with long-acting bronchodilators, measurements of lung volumes and diffusion capacity, analysis of sputum and FeNO, and imaging of the chest may help to demonstrate whether asthma or COPD is the predominant cause of airflow limitation in these patients (table 3).

Table 4. Levels of asthma control

Assessment of current clinical control (preferably over 4 weeks)			
Characteristic	Controlled (all of the following)	Partly controlled (any measure present in any week)	Uncontrolled
Daytime symptoms	None (twice or less per week)	More than twice per week	Three or more features of partly controlled asthma present in any week[+,§]
Limitation of activities	None	Any	
Nocturnal symptoms/ awakening	None	Any	
Need for reliever/rescue treatment	None (twice or less per week)	More than twice per week	
Lung function (PEF or FEV_1)[#,¶]	Normal	<80% predicted or personal best (if known)	
Assessment of future risk (risk of exacerbations, instability, rapid decline in lung function, side-effects)			
Features that are associated with increased risk of adverse effects in the future include: poor clinical control, frequent exacerbations in the past year[+], admission to critical care for asthma, low FEV_1, exposure to cigarette smoke and high-dose medications			

[#]: not reliable for children aged ⩽5 years; [¶]: without administration of a bronchodilator; [+]: any exacerbation should prompt a review of maintenance treatment to ensure it is adequate; [§]: by definition, an exacerbation in any week makes that an uncontrolled week. Reproduced and modified from Global Initiative for Asthma (2012) with permission from the publisher.

Comorbidities of asthma

The coexistence of chronic rhinitis, nasal polyposis and sinusitis may contribute to the severity of asthma. There is evidence to show that adequate treatment of these upper airway diseases is beneficial to asthma by mechanisms that are not clearly understood. The 'one airway' concept has drawn attention to the importance of treating the whole respiratory tract when managing asthma. Gastro-oesophageal reflux is also occasionally associated with asthma, both in adults and in children, but treatment of reflux usually has little overall effect on mild-to-moderate asthma. A frequent and quite important comorbidity of asthma in adults is COPD, most likely due to smoking, which is as common in asthmatics as in the general population. Smoking modifies the airway pathology of asthmatics to a COPD-like pattern and reduces the response to treatment. Comorbidities may become important in severe asthmatics, whereas they play a much less important role overall in the clinical manifestations of mild-to-moderate asthma.

Management

Considering its chronic nature and life-long duration, asthma can be effectively managed only by developing a partnership between the patient and their doctor or health professional, who may provide the tools for guided self-management, and possibly a

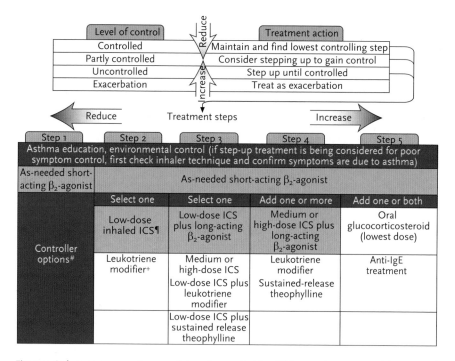

Figure 2. *Asthma management approach based on control for children aged >5 years, adolescents and adults. Alternative reliever treatments include inhaled anticholinergics, short-acting oral β_2-agonists, some long-acting β_2-agonists and theophylline. Regular dosing with short- and long-acting β_2-agonists is not advised unless accompanied by an inhaled glucocorticosteroid. ICS: inhaled corticosteroids. #: recommended treatment (shaded boxes) based on group mean data; individual patient needs, preferences and circumstances (including costs) should be considered. ¶: inhaled glucocorticosteroids. +: receptor antagonist or synthesis inhibitors. Reproduced and modified from Global Initiative for Asthma (2012) with permission from the publisher.*

written plan including self-monitoring, and periodically review of treatment and level of asthma control. Education plays a major role in this partnership.

Long-term pharmacological treatment The aim of pharmacological treatment of asthma is to achieve and maintain control of day-to-day symptoms, as well as preventing future severe asthma exacerbations (table 4), while using the safest treatment algorithm. While the initial treatment should be started according to the degree of asthma control at the first visit, subsequently treatment should be adjusted according to the level of asthma control achieved (fig. 2). Usually, regular treatment is lowered only after a significant period of acceptable asthma control (*e.g.* ⩾3 months). This means that monitoring of asthma is essential to maintain asthma control and establish the minimal treatment requirements. Step-up and -down of treatment are not standardised, and thus should be tailored to the individual patient to achieve and maintain control with the minimum amount of medication.

Medications to treat asthma can be classified as controllers or relievers. Medications are preferably administered by inhalation, as this approach is the most effective way to treat asthma and has the fewest side-effects. Controller medications (inhaled corticosteroids alone or in combination with long-acting β_2-agonists) are taken daily on a long-term basis to keep asthma under clinical control. In asthma, long-acting β_2-agonists should be used only in combination with inhaled corticosteroids when the latter are insufficient to achieve control, and should be discontinued only when control is maintained.

Only in patients not controlled by optimal doses of inhaled corticosteroids combined with long-acting β_2-agonists should other secondary agents may be considered. These include anti-leukotrienes, theophylline, systemic corticosteroids or anti-IgE monoclonal antibodies in very specific cases.

Reliever medications (predominantly short-acting β_2-agonists) are medications used on an as-needed basis that act quickly to reverse bronchoconstriction and relieve asthma symptoms. Ideally, if patients are adequately controlled, they should rarely need rescue medications. The use of a combination of an inhaled short-acting β_2-agonist and a corticosteroid both as controller and reliever is effective in maintaining high levels of asthma control.

Smoking asthmatics are resistant to anti-asthma medications and should be primarily treated for smoking addiction. Asthmatic smokers may develop features of COPD.

Specific immunotherapy in asthma is limited as:

1) it requires the identification of a single clinically relevant allergen

2) it can be used safely only in mild asthmatics who are usually well controlled by environmental interventions or pharmacotherapy

3) it may be associated with adverse events

Treatment of exacerbations

Shortness of breath, cough, wheezing and/or chest tightness may develop or worsen in a subject with asthma even when they are under regular treatment. Milder exacerbations are usually managed by the patients with an increased as-needed use of short-acting β_2-agonists alone or in combination in combination with inhaled steroids. More severe exacerbations or exacerbations that do not respond to the increased use of rescue medications require repetitive administration of rescue medication and systemic, preferably oral, corticosteroids, with oxygen supplementation in very severe cases (fig. 3). Severe exacerbations require medical attention and, in some instances, hospital admission.

Special considerations

Special considerations are required for patients with specific comorbidities, such as rhino/sinusitis and/or nasal polyps, aspirin-induced asthma (particularly if associated

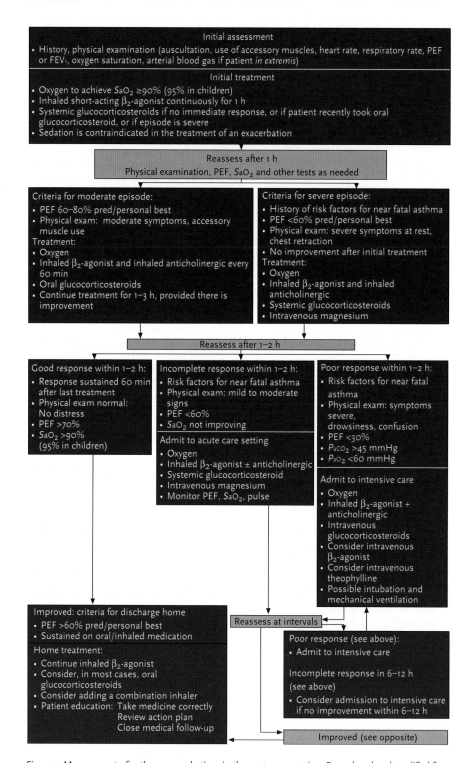

Figure 3. Management of asthma exacerbations in the acute care setting. Reproduced and modified from Global Initiative for Asthma (2012) with permission from the publisher.

with episodes of anaphylaxis), occupational asthma and obesity.

In addition, patients with asthma may require specific competent medical attention in case of smoking addiction, pregnancy, surgery, infections (*e.g.* influenza epidemics) and, more importantly, if asthma is severe.

Further reading

- Barnes PJ (2012).Severe asthma: advances in current management and future therapy. *J Allergy Clin Immunol*; 129: 48–59.
- Bateman ED, *et al.* (2011). Overall asthma control achieved with budesonide/formoterol maintenance and reliever therapy for patients on different treatment steps. *Respir Res*; 12: 38.
- Boulet LP, *et al.* (2011). Asthma-related comorbidities. *Expert Rev Respir Med*; 5: 377–393.
- Boulet LP, *et al.* (2012). A guide to the translation of the Global Initiative for Asthma (GINA) strategy into improved care. *Eur Respir J*; 39: 1220–1229.
- Brozek JL, *et al.* (2011). Grading quality of evidence and strength of recommendations in clinical practice guidelines part 3 of 3. The GRADE approach to developing recommendations. *Allergy*; 66: 588–595.
- Camargo CA Jr, *et al.* (2009). Managing asthma exacerbations in the emergency department: summary of the National Asthma Education and Prevention Program Expert Panel Report 3 guidelines for the management of asthma exacerbations. *J Allergy Clin Immunol*; 124: Suppl., S5–S14.
- Chung KF (2012). Inflammatory biomarkers in severe asthma. *Curr Opin Pulm Med*; 18: 35–41.
- de Groot EP, *et al.* (2010). Comorbidities of asthma during childhood: possibly important, yet poorly studied. *Eur Respir J*; 36: 671–678.
- Fabbri LM, *et al.* (2003). Differences in airway inflammation in patients with fixed airflow obstruction due to asthma or chronic obstructive pulmonary disease. *Am J Respir Crit Care Med*; 167: 418–424.
- Fattahi F, *et al.* (2011). Smoking and nonsmoking asthma: differences in clinical outcome and pathogenesis. *Expert Rev Respir Med*; 5: 93–105.
- Global Initiative for Asthma. Global Strategy for Asthma Management and Prevention 2012. www.ginasthma.org
- Global Initiative for Chronic Obstructive Lung Disease. Global Strategy for Diagnosis, Management, and Prevention of COPD 2012. www.goldcopd.org
- Hargreave FE, *et al.* (2009). The definition and diagnosis of asthma. *Clin Exp Allergy*; 39: 1652–1658.
- Holt PG, *et al.* (2012). Viral infections and atopy in asthma pathogenesis: new rationales for asthma prevention and treatment. *Nat Med*; 18: 726–735.
- Maestrelli P, *et al.* (2009). Mechanisms of occupational asthma. *J Allergy Clin Immunol*; 123: 531–542.
- Namazy JA, *et al.* (2011). Asthma and pregnancy. *J Allergy Clin Immunol*; 128: 1384–1385.
- O'Byrne PM (2011). Therapeutic strategies to reduce asthma exacerbations. *J Allergy Clin Immunol*; 128: 257–263.
- Parsons JP (2013). An official American Thoraeic Society clinical practice guideline. Exercise-induced bronchoconstriction. *Am Respir Crit Care Med*; 187: 1016–1027.
- Petsky HL, *et al.* (2012). A systematic review and meta-analysis: tailoring asthma treatment on eosinophilic markers (exhaled nitric oxide or sputum eosinophils). *Thorax*; 67: 199–208.
- Sin DD, *et al.* (2008). Obesity and the lung: 4. Obesity and asthma. *Thorax*; 63: 1018–1023.

Vocal cord dysfunction

Adel H. Mansur

Vocal cord dysfunction (VCD) is characterised by paradoxical vocal cord adduction during inspiration and/or expiration, leading to symptoms of breathlessness and wheeze. It is a poorly understood condition that often co-exists with asthma and chronic cough, and shares common triggers with them, such as psychological factors, gastro-oesophageal reflux and rhinosinus disease. The management of VCD focuses on establishing the correct diagnosis, identification and treatment of underlying triggers, and speech therapy. Further research is required to define VCD, establish its natural history and develop evidence-based therapies.

Terminology

Numerous terms have been used to describe VCD. These include hysteric croup, Munchausen's stridor, pseudo-asthma, factitious asthma, upper airway dysfunction, functional upper airway obstruction, irritable larynx syndrome, emotional laryngeal wheeze, laryngeal hyperresponsiveness and paradoxical vocal cord movement (PVCM). Indeed, there is disagreement over what

constitutes VCD, with some limiting it to an early description by Christopher et al. (1983) of a conversion disorder meeting a strict definition of inspiratory adduction and posterior chinking of vocal cords, to those who use an all-encompassing VCD definition of all cases demonstrating PVCM.

Epidemiology

While the true prevalence of VCD in the general population is unknown, it is more common in females, athletes, army recruits, asthmatics and patients with chronic cough (table 1). Using dynamic CT imaging, 50% of 46 difficult asthmatics demonstrated PVCM, which was severe in nine patients (Low et al., 2011).

Pathogenesis

VCD was seen largely as a conversion disorder of psychogenic origin. The larynx is innervated by a complex neurological network, and the association between stress and comorbid psychology and VCD attacks strengthened this view. More recently, it became apparent that PVCM 'VCD' exists outside the conversion disorder prototype. Laryngeal closure is a normal physiological reaction to exposure to irritants (e.g. aspiration), but this reaction normally only lasts for a few seconds. Acute (e.g. toxic fume inhalation) or recurrent irritation (e.g. repeated extreme cold air exposure) may lead to laryngeal hypersensitivity manifesting as vocal cord adduction and airflow limitation (Cukier-Blaj et al., 2008). Laryngeal hypersensitivity may form part of unified allergic airway syndrome with asthma and rhinitis. The association of laryngeal hypersensitivity with altered autonomic balance status maintained by

Key points

- VCD is not well understood, and there is as yet no consensus definition.

- Classically, symptoms appear abruptly, resolve quickly and do not respond well to asthma medication.

- Long-term treatment is based around speech therapy and psychotherapy.

Table 1. VCD prevalence in different patient groups.

Patient group	Prevalence %
Refractory asthma	5–10
Dyspnoea	2.8
Army recruits with stress-induced asthma	15
Olympic athletes	5
Childhood acute asthma[#]	14

The reported mean age at VCD diagnosis is 14.5 years in children and 33 years in adults. [#]: presenting to emergency department.

central brain activity have been postulated to underlie development of VCD (Ayers *et al.*, 2002).

Clinical presentation

VCD presentation varies from cases with predominant throat symptoms usually referred to ENT specialists, to asthma presenting to the respiratory clinic or angio-oedema presenting in an immunology clinic. Often, the diagnosis of VCD is made after treatment for asthma has not been successful.

Patients may report rapid-onset attacks of dyspnoea, which may be preceded by intense coughing, the sensation of strangulation or breathing through a straw, throat or upper chest tightness, dysphonia, or stridor. Classical VCD symptoms are of abrupt onset, resolve quickly and respond poorly to asthma medication.

Elucidation of triggers of VCD attacks is important for diagnostic and therapeutic purposes. Commonly associated triggers include exposure to cold air, exercise, inhalation of strong smells such as perfumes or chemical cleaning agents, smoke, cough, reflux, viral infections, allergens, and emotional stress. Psychological morbidity and sexual abuse are experienced in some VCD sufferers. The physical examination of patients with VCD is usually unremarkable outside symptomatic attacks. During symptoms, examination may reveal stridor or wheeze originating at laryngeal level with clear chest auscultation. The severity of respiratory distress varies from mild to severe with tachypnoea, but

oxygen saturation is often normal. Extreme forms of VCD can lead to collapse and loss of consciousness, usually leading to resolution of the attack or intubation. If intubated, the airway inflation pressure is characteristically normal.

Diagnosis

Flow–volume loops may show inspiratory loop truncation representing extrathoracic airflow obstruction. The maximum inspiratory/expiratory flow ratio at 50% FVC ($MIF_{50\%}/MEF_{50\%}$) can be reduced due to predominant inspiratory flow limitation. An abnormally high forced inspiratory flow at 25%/75% FVC ratio ($FIF_{25\%}/FIF_{75\%}$) would indicate an initially normal flow followed by rapid flow decline, reflecting PVCM during inspiration. However, various studies reported the insensitivity of spirometry for diagnosing VCD (Ruppel, 2009). Sensitivity of spirometry may be enhanced by histamine or other forms of airway challenge.

Impulse oscillometry (IOS) can discriminate between central and peripheral airway obstruction, and may be more sensitive than spirometry. Airway fluoroscopy and colour Doppler ultrasound imaging of vocal cord movement are other noninvasive tools that have not been standardised against laryngoscopy.

Integrated CT software programs have been used to obtain continuous dynamic axial, sagittal and coronal multiplanar images of the larynx, measuring airway diameters at the level of the vocal cords and the first tracheal ring. The ratio of vocal cord diameter to tracheal diameter was used as a marker of PVCM (Low *et al.*, 2011).

Laryngoscopy

VCD diagnosis is established by laryngoscopic demonstration of PVCM while the patient experiences spontaneous or induced symptoms. Bicycle ergometry combined with fibreoptic videolaryngoscopy has been developed as a diagnostic test for VCD in patients with exercise-induce dyspnoea. One study reported that if the symptom of dyspnoea appeared, the most frequent diagnosis was exercise-induced VCD (Tervonen *et al.*, 2009).

Agreed laryngoscopy standards have not been developed, with some advocating pre-procedure sedation and analgesia, while others recommend avoiding these measures. Following a short period of quiet breathing, specific manoeuvres such as repeating low- and high-pitched sounds, forceful inspiration and expiration are conducted to induce an attack (Wood *et al.*, 1996). Vocal cord movements are timed against respiratory cycle phases by putting a hand on the patient's chest. In VCD, the vocal cords adduct anteriorly, leaving an open posterior glottic chink (fig. 1). The adduction occurs during inspiration or throughout the respiratory cycle.

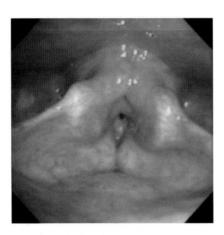

Figure 1. Laryngoscopy demonstrating inspiratory vocal cord adduction and posterior glottic chink.

False-negative PVCM can be secondary to gag reflex or coughing.

The larynx should also be inspected for signs of laryngopharyngeal reflux (Belafsky *et al.*, 2002). VCD should be distinguished from vocal cord immobility due to paralysis, amyotrophic lateral sclerosis, cricoarytenoid joint dysfunction and Reinke's oedema. Laryngeal electromyography (EMG) may help in differentiation. Normal laryngoscopy in the absence of symptoms does not exclude VCD. The presence of atypical features of asthma and/or VCD should prompt further investigations, such as CT of head, neck and thorax, and bronchoscopy.

Investigations directed at causes of VCD

A careful history is essential to guide investigations. The presence of concomitant rhinitis/asthma or allergic airway disease needs to be assessed by lung function, skin allergy testing, blood/sputum eosinophils and exhaled nitric oxide. Gastro-oesophageal reflux diseases symptoms or laryngeal refluxive changes on laryngoscopy should prompt further testing (*e.g.* oesophageal manometry and pH studies). Underlying psychological issues should be assessed.

Differential diagnosis

- Laryngeal oedema (angio-oedema)
- Allergic laryngitis
- Subglottic stenosis
- Laryngomalacia or tracheomalacia
- Vocal cord paralysis
- Systemic disease affecting the larynx/upper airways (*e.g.* relapsing chondritis or granulomatosis with polyangiitis (Wegener's))

Treatment

Diagnosis and treatment are best conducted in a multidisciplinary team setting comprised of a respiratory physician, speech therapist, ENT specialist and psychologist. The diagnosis is explained to the patient, preferably with the support of imaging or illustration. The patient's good understanding of VCD is prerequisite to effective treatment. A management plan should be formulated that bears in mind co-existing asthma. Due to VCD under-recognition, patients should carry an alert card listing medication and treatment strategy.

Treatment of acute attacks

The treating physician should adopt a calm, reassuring manner and ask the patient to focus on expiration with an 'S' sound that helps in diverting attention. A panting manoeuvre can abort acute attacks by inducing vocal cord abduction. Where hypoxaemia and hypercapnia have been excluded, sedation with benzodiazepines may help patient relaxation. Heliox gas mixture (e.g. 72% helium and 28% oxygen) can alleviate symptoms by enhancing upper airway laminar air flow. Intubation or tracheostomy should be avoided. In extreme cases presenting with an apparent life-threatening attack, the clinical decision will remain with the treating physician. If intubation is contemplated, prior inspection and documentation of the status of the vocal cords is recommended.

Long-term treatment

Speech therapy forms the mainstay of VCD treatment, with the primary aim of teaching patients to relax the upper airways and control the laryngeal area. It is conducted in four to six successive sessions to enable the patient to practice breathing techniques to abort or treat acute attacks (Wood et al., 1996). Patients are taught to exhale gently and avoid forceful inspiration in a rhythmic manner, followed by introduction of expiratory resistance by asking patient to produce sounds such as 'S'. The role of the speech therapist extends to making the diagnosis, identification and treatment of triggers, and relaxation therapy.

Psychotherapy should form an integral part of VCD management, given VCD's link to adverse psychology. Psychotherapy can include relaxation therapy, management of stress and anxiety, and development of coping strategies.

Other, unproven therapies for VCD include inhaled anticholinergic drugs to abort exercise-induced VCD attacks (O'Connell et al., 2006), enhancing inspiratory resistance by a face mask device, CPAP and vocal cord injection of botulinum toxin A (Botox). Tracheostomy has been used as a last resort in intractable cases.

Prognosis

The long-term outcome of VCD is unknown. VCD prognosis will probably depend on initial disease severity and associated morbidities. One study reported complete resolution of VCD within a 5-year time frame, with symptoms disappearing within 6 months in many who had a good response to speech therapy. However, intractable forms of disease did not seem to improve over a 10-year observation period (Doshi et al., 2006).

Conclusion

VCD is a relatively uncommon condition that mimics and co-exists with asthma, and presents episodically, thus making its diagnosis challenging and often delayed. Patients can become frequent healthcare users with substantial morbidity as result of erroneous diagnosis and toxic medication use. Establishing proper diagnosis and treatment can be effective and rewarding to both the patient and healthcare professionals.

Further reading

- Ayres JG, et al. (2002). Vocal cord dysfunction and laryngeal hyperrespon-siveness: a function of altered autonomic balance? Thorax; 57: 284–285.
- Belafsky PC, et al. (2002). Validity and reliability of the reflux symptom index (RSI). J Voice; 16: 274–277.
- Christopher KL, et al. (1983). Vocal-cord dysfunction presenting as asthma. N Engl J Med; 308: 1566–1570.
- Cukier-Blaj S, et al. (2008). Paradoxical vocal fold motion: a sensory-motor laryngeal disorder. Laryngoscope; 118: 367–370.
- Doshi DR, et al. (2006). Long-term outcome of vocal cord dysfunction. Ann All Asthma Imm; 96: 794–799.

- Low K, *et al.* (2011). Abnormal vocal cord function in difficult-to-treat asthma. *Am J Respir Crit Care Med*; 184: 50–56.
- Newman KB, *et al.* (1995). Clinical features of vocal cord dysfunction. *Am J Respir Crit Care Med*; 152: 1382–1386.
- O'Connell M, *et al.* (2006). Vocal cord dysfunction: ready for prime-time? *Ann All Asthma Imm*; 96: 762–763.
- Ruppel GL (2009). The inspiratory flow–volume curve: the neglected child of pulmonary diagnostics. *Respir Care*; 54: 448–449.
- Sullivan MD, *et al.* (2001). A treatment for vocal cord dysfunction in female athletes: an outcome study. *Laryngoscope*; 111: 1751–1755.
- Tervonen H, *et al.* (2009). Fiberoptic videolaryngoscopy during bicycle ergometry: a diagnostic tool for exercise-induced vocal cord dysfunction. *Laryngoscope*; 119: 1776–1780.
- Wood RP, *et al.* (1996). Vocal cord dysfunction. *J Allerg Clin Imm*; 98: 481–485.

Bronchitis

Gernot Rohde

Definition

Transient airway inflammation localised to the respiratory mucosa of the central airways and clinically characterised by cough and sputum production. Fever and dyspnoea can occur.

Symptoms

Cough is the cardinal symptom and is observed in 100% of cases. It usually persists for up to 2 weeks, but in 26% of cases it can stay for up to 8 weeks. Other symptoms include sputum production (90%), dyspnoea, wheezing (62%), rhonchi, chest pain, fever, hoarseness and malaise.

Epidemiology

Acute bronchitis is one of the most frequent human diseases worldwide, with children being most often affected. On average children contract bronchitis between two to six times per year, and adults two to three times per year. The prevalence in the UK is 44 cases per 1000 adults per year. 82% of episodes occur during the cold months.

Key points

- Respiratory viral infection is the most common cause of acute bronchitis.

- Acute bronchitis is usually a self-limiting disease.

- The diagnosis of acute bronchitis is purely clinical and in most cases symptomatic treatment is sufficient.

- Chronic bronchitis is defined clinically as productive cough for 3 months in each of two successive years.

Aetiology/risk factors

Respiratory infections are the main trigger of acute bronchitis. However, pathogens can only be detected in 55% of cases. Respiratory viruses are the most frequent pathogens. Rhinovirus, adenovirus, echovirus, influenza virus, parainfluenza virus, enterovirus, coronavirus, Coxsackie virus, human metapneumovirus and respiratory syncytial virus (RSV) represent the usual spectrum. Parainfluenza viruses, enteroviruses and rhinoviruses mainly infect in the autumn, while the influenza viruses, RSV and coronaviruses mainly infect in the winter and early spring. Typical bacteria are *Streptococcus pneumoniae*, *Haemophilus influenzae* and *Moraxella catarrhalis*. Atypical bacteria, *e.g. Mycoplasma pneumoniae* or *Chlamydia pneumoniae*, and *Bordetella pertussis* also play a role.

Specific risk factors have not been dentified and it is currently not clear whether cigarette smoking increases the risk of acute bronchitis. There are epidemiological data showing that the frequency of bronchitis is increased after school holidays, which indicates that crowding facilitates the dissemination of respiratory infections.

Prognosis

Acute bronchitis is usually a self-limiting disease. However there are only sparse data on prognosis and rate of complications. In a study investigating 653 previously healthy adults with lower respiratory tract symptoms, 20% of patients had persistent symptoms. In 40% of these patients, there was reversible airway obstruction. In another study, a third of patients developed asthma or chronic bronchitis symptoms.

Diagnosis

Diagnosis is purely clinical. Cough, sputum production and optionally accompanied by dyspnoea and/or wheezing, are suggestive. Tachycardia and tachypnoea are usually absent, and vital signs are normal. Complicated cases show fever; however, in these cases differential diagnosis like pneumonia or systemic influenza should be considered. Clinical signs of pneumonia, *e.g.* rales, egophony, dullness on percussion, should be absent. Acute bronchitis should be differentiated from asthma, which typically presents as progressive cough accompanied by wheezing, tachypnoea, respiratory distress and hypoxaemia. It should also be distinguished from bronchiectasis, a distinct phenomenon associated with permanent dilatation of bronchi and a chronic cough. Laboratory investigations are not necessary. In more severe cases, sputum culture can be considered to guide antibiotic therapy.

Therapy

Therapeutic goals are the reduction of symptoms and the prevention of complications, with as few side-effects as possible. Antibiotic therapy cannot be recommended generally, but in patients with fever and/or comorbidities, aminopenicillins or cephalosporins (second generation) can be administered. Dextromethorphan has been shown to reduce cough efficiently. In patients with dyspnoea and/or wheezing, short-acting bronchodilators can be beneficial.

Chronic bronchitis

Chronic bronchitis is defined clinically as chronic productive cough for 3 months in each of two successive years in a patient in whom other causes of productive chronic cough have been excluded. Cigarette smoking is by far the most important and preventable risk factor. Chronic bronchitis is a major component of chronic obstructive pulmonary disease.

Further reading

- American Thoracic Society (1962). Chronic bronchitis, asthma, pulmonary emphysema: a statement by the committee on diagnostic standards for non-tuberculous disease. *Am Rev Respir Dis*; 85: 762–768.
- Antó JM, *et al.* (2001). Epidemiology of chronic obstructive pulmonary disease. *Eur Respir J*; 17: 982–994.
- Boldy DA, *et al.* (1990). Acute bronchitis in the community: clinical features, infective factors, changes in pulmonary function and bronchial reactivity to histamine. *Respir Med*; 84: 377–385.
- Chesnutt MS, *et al.* Lung. *In*: Tierney LM, ed. Current Medical Diagnosis and Treatment, 41st Edn. New York, Lange Medical/McGraw-Hill, 2002; pp. 269–362.
- Jonsson JS, *et al.* (1998). Acute bronchitis and clinical outcome three years later: prospective cohort study. *BMJ*; 317: 1433.
- Macfarlane JW, *et al.* (2001). Prospective study of the incidence, aetiology and outcome of adult lower respiratory tract illness in the community. *Thorax*; 56: 109–114.
- Wenzel RP, *et al.* (2006). Acute bronchitis. *N Engl J Med*; 355: 2125–2130.
- Williamson HA Jr (1987). Pulmonary function tests in acute bronchitis: evidence for reversible airway obstruction. *J Fam Pract*; 25: 251–256.

Gastro-oesophageal reflux

Lieven Dupont

Gastro-oesophageal reflux (GOR), defined as the retrograde flow of gastric contents into the oesophagus, is a normal physiological phenomenon that occurs to some extent in most people. Brief exposure of the oesophagus to gastric contents does not necessarily result in injury or disease. When reflux is prolonged and/or when there is a breakdown of the defence mechanisms that act to protect mucosal integrity, symptoms and/or lesions in the oesophagus occur. This is then referred to as gastro-oesophageal reflux disease (GORD). GORD is an increasingly prevalent condition that affects >20% of the Western population. Although GORD often causes typical symptoms such as heartburn or regurgitation, 32% of the patients with reflux disease have extraoesophageal symptoms, including respiratory and ENT symptoms and disorders. The relationship between reflux and respiratory symptoms is frequently difficult to establish with a high degree of certainty and diagnostic, as well as therapeutic, management remains largely empirical. In contrast to oesophageal GORD manifestations, efficacy of acid-suppressive therapy in extraoesophageal GORD symptoms has not been equally well established.

Key points

- GORD is a common disorder caused by the reflux of gastric contents into the oesophagus because of impaired function of the LOS and may result in oesophageal and extraoesophageal symptoms.

- The relationship between reflux and respiratory symptoms or disorders is frequently difficult to establish with a high degree of certainty.

- Diagnostic, as well as therapeutic, management remains largely empirical.

- Treatment with PPIs has been shown to improve cough in patients with acid GOR-induced cough but the effect of PPIs remains disappointing when treating GOR in other respiratory diseases.

- Antireflux surgery is associated with improved allograft function after lung transplantation.

Mechanisms of increased reflux

The oesophagogastric junction (OGJ) is the first line of defence against reflux. It comprises two important components: the lower oesophageal sphincter (LOS) and the crural diaphragm that regulate the exchange of contents between the oesophagus and the stomach. Transient lower oesophageal sphincter relaxations (TLOSRs), defined as relaxations of the LOS not triggered by swallowing, account for the majority of reflux episodes, both in healthy subjects and in GORD patients. Not all TLOSRs are associated with reflux. In healthy subjects, almost half of the TLOSRs are followed by a reflux episode, which is significantly higher in GORD patients, where ~70% of the TLOSRs lead to reflux. A hiatal hernia, which is the separation of the LOS from the crural diaphragm, further diminishes the capacity of the OGJ to prevent reflux. GORD patients have a higher gastro-oesophageal pressure gradient during a TLOSR than healthy subjects. The higher pressure gradient is due to a higher intra-abdominal pressure and correlates with BMI. Although a delay in gastric emptying has been shown in ~30% of GORD patients, a clear causal relationship between rate of gastric emptying and reflux parameters remains controversial.

Pathophysiology

There are a number of potential mechanisms of interaction between the oesophagus and the lung that explain the complex interplay between GOR(D) and respiratory symptoms and disease:

- aspiration of gastric contents into the airways
- stimulation of a vagally mediated reflex pathway
- hypersensitivity

Direct microaspiration of (duodeno)gastric refluxate into the airway occurs as a consequence of failure of the normal protective mechanisms against foreign material, *i.e.* reflex contraction of the upper oesophageal sphincter and closure of the glottis and vocal cords. Aspiration can be demonstrated by the presence of pepsin and bile acids in saliva, sputum or bronchoalveolar lavage (BAL) fluid. While pepsin and bile acids are clearly increased in patients with CF and idiopathic pulmonary fibrosis (IPF), and after lung transplantation, there was no difference between chronic cough, patients with asthma and healthy controls.

Aspiration of (duodeno)gastric contents into the lungs can lead to chemical injury, which may be followed by an inflammatory response, characterised by the recruitment of neutrophils to the airways. It has been widely accepted that acid causes damage to bronchial epithelial cells, but recent data demonstrated that nonacidic gastric contents are also important in the pathogenesis of reflux-induced airway inflammation. Pepsin and bile acids may even cause cell damage at normal pH, which may explain why some patients have refractory symptoms on maximal proton pump inhibitor (PPI) therapy.

The oesophagus is innervated by sensory-type nociceptors that express the TRPV1 channel. These afferents of the vagus nerve converge centrally with capsaicin-sensitive C-fibres and capsaicin-insensitive, acid-sensitive mechanoreceptors from the respiratory tract. The convergence of these vagal afferent neurons in the brainstem may allow sensitisation of vagally mediated reflexes from the (distal) oesophagus to be triggered by chemical or mechanical stimuli. A vagally mediated oesophageal–bronchial reflex has been postulated to account for the association between acid reflux and cough or asthma.

Oesophageal sensory stimulation can release tachykinins into the airways and may increase the bronchomotor responsiveness to airway stimuli, resulting in bronchospasms. It has also been postulated that chronic exposure of the oesophageal mucosa to gastric juices can produce long-lasting hypersensitivity to a variety of stimuli that cause cough symptoms even in the absence of increased oesophageal acid exposure or esophagitis.

GOR in asthma and COPD

GORD is a common condition among patients with obstructive pulmonary diseases. At least one-third of asthmatics present with GORD (prevalence 34–89%) and 50–60% of COPD patients have abnormally high oesophageal acid exposure times. Often, COPD or asthmatic patients with GORD do not have typical symptoms of GORD. The relationship between GOR and the clinical course of asthma and COPD needs to be better understood but it has been shown that that abnormal GOR may worsen asthma symptoms and has been associated with increased risk of asthma and COPD exacerbations. Oxygen desaturation coincides with episodes of increased oesophageal acidity in 40% of patients with severe COPD and GORD.

Several mechanisms may be involved (vagus nerve mediated mechanisms, chronic microaspiration and bronchial hyperreactivity). β_2-agonists and theophylline decrease LOS tone and may consequently promote oesophageal reflux. Airway obstruction resulting in increased thoracic pressure changes, hyperinflation and exaggerated diaphragmatic flattening may also contribute to the occurrence of GOR.

Multiple trials have examined the treatment of GORD with histamine antagonists or PPIs in asthma. A Cochrane systematic review concluded that acid-suppressive therapy did not result in a consistent benefit in patients with asthma. Similarly, there was no effect on lung function, airway responsiveness or asthma symptom control. Even though nine out of 12 trials included in the meta-analysis reported at least one significant outcome, there was no consistency in these effects. The Study of Acid Reflux in Asthma (SARA), a large randomised control trial evaluated high-dose PPI (esomeprazole 40 mg *b.i.d.*) in patients with uncontrolled asthma that did not have typical GOR symptoms. PPI therapy did not improve asthma control, quality of life or lung function and, although 40% of these patients had abnormal asymptomatic acid GOR upon oesophageal pH monitoring, there was also no improvement with PPIs in this subgroup. A recent study in children yielded similar results. However, these studies did not test for nonacid reflux and did not evaluate the effect of treating nonacid reflux on asthma control. A retrospective study showed improvement of FEV1 with antireflux surgery in patients with adult-onset asthma, typical reflux symptoms and proximal extent of the reflux.

No large-scale studies have evaluated therapeutic options for GOR in patients with COPD. Uncontrolled data suggest that PPI treatment may decrease the number of COPD exacerbations. Future randomised controlled trials are needed.

For patients with asthma or COPD and who have typical reflux symptoms, empirical prescription of acid suppression therapy is appropriate but the effect on respiratory end-points may be limited. Current evidence does not support the initiation of empirical acid suppression therapy in asthma patients who lack symptoms that suggest the presence of GORD. Additional testing by means of endoscopy and ambulatory pH/impedance is indicated in asthma or COPD

patients with a suspected GORD syndrome who do not respond to an empirical trial of PPI therapy, in elderly patients with asthma or COPD, or in patients with severe refractory asthma.

GOR-induced cough

Studies have determined GOR to be a cause of chronic cough in >40% of patients referred for specialist evaluation. GOR-induced cough is currently thought to occur predominantly *via* an oesophageal–bronchial reflex. Studies using combined pH/impedance and cough monitoring have shown that both acid and nonacid reflux events can be associated with cough. The acidity of the refluxate may thus be unimportant if the oesophageal–bronchial reflex is already sensitised. Findings of an equal number of cough events preceding as well as following reflux also suggest the possibility that cough may precipitate TLOSRs. Reflux should not be considered as a single independent cause but rather as a contributing factor as well as a consequence of chronic cough.

Only a minority of patients with chronic cough and GORD have typical digestive symptoms and/or clear evidence of oesophagitis. As a result and in accordance with published guidelines, objective evaluation of GOR is indicated in patients with chronic cough. Detection of both acid and nonacid reflux events with simultaneous cough detection allows for an objective assessment of the relationship between the two.

Treating GOR with the therapeutic strategies currently available may result in only a partial symptomatic improvement, as chronic cough is often a multifactorial process. The treatment of cough-associated reflux with acid-suppressive therapy has been evaluated in many uncontrolled and a few controlled trials. A Cochrane review concluded that PPI administration was not efficacious for cough associated with GORD symptoms in children. There was insufficient evidence to conclude that treating GOR with PPI in adults with cough was beneficial, although a slight improvement in cough scores was found in those receiving PPIs. Further randomised, parallel-design, placebo-controlled, double-blind trials are needed. Based on these data, an empirical course of PPIs for 8 weeks could be advocated in all patients with possible reflux-induced cough, especially in patients who also have typical reflux symptoms. Prokinetic drugs have no efficacy in GORD-related cough and gastric emptying has not been shown to be delayed in patients with GOR-related cough. In patients who failed to respond to empirical therapy with PPIs, reflux-induced cough is not necessarily excluded, as nonacid reflux may also be implicated. Fundoplication provides an alternative method to treat GORD, which similarly controls acid and nonacid reflux. Uncontrolled studies with surgical treatment in patients with possible reflux-induced cough showed a positive response in 56–100% of surgically treated patients. A positive symptom association between acid or nonacid reflux was a good predictor of successful surgical outcome. In selected patients with refractory acidic or nonacidic reflux and a documented correlation between reflux episodes and cough, antireflux surgery may be indicated for long-term control.

GOR in advanced lung disease

GOR is an important comorbidity in patients with bronchiectasis. The prevalence of abnormal GOR in CF is estimated to be between 35% and 81%, and a somewhat smaller increase in GORD prevalence has also been reported in patients with non-CF bronchiectasis. Acid GOR is most predominant in CF, but weakly acidic GOR may also occur. CF patients with increased GOR often have a high proximal extent of the reflux into the oesophagus. Many CF patients have oesophageal hypomotility and low basal LOS pressure. The number of TLOSRs is similar to controls but TLOSRs in CF patients are more often associated with reflux, due to an more pronounced reduction in thoracic pressure during inspiration. Patients with CF have a high risk of gastric aspiration, as demonstrated by increased bile acids in saliva, sputum or in BAL fluid. Half of the CF patients with

increased GOR or gastric aspiration do not present oesophageal symptoms like heartburn or regurgitation. The characteristics of GOR and the material aspirated depend on the genotype, with bile acid aspiration being more important in $CFTR^{\Delta F508}$ homozygotes.

The available evidence suggest a possible relationship between GOR, aspiration and the severity of CF lung disease, generation of cough symptoms, airway inflammation, and the progression of the lung disease. CF patients with increased oesophageal acid exposure have more cough and a positive association between GOR and cough is associated with poorer lung function. Bile acid levels in sputum correlate with elastase levels in sputum and FEV_1; raised pepsin levels in BAL fluid are associated with higher levels of interleukin (IL)-8 in the BAL fluid. GOR might also be involved in earlier onset of first acquisition of Pseudomonas aeruginosa and the pathogenesis of CF exacerbations.

Retrospective data suggested that CF patients on acid suppression therapy had a smaller yearly decline of FEV_1. However, a Cochrane review failed to show any relationship between reflux treatment and improvement of pulmonary damage in CF. Antireflux surgery may be considered as a more efficacious treatment of GOR in CF patients and uncontrolled studies showed an improvement in FEV_1 decline and cough symptoms and a reduction in CF exacerbation rate.

GOR may play a role in the pathogenesis and/or progression of IPF as a recurrent inflammatory stimulus. Studies have found a high prevalence of reflux (36–87%) among patients with interstitial lung diseases (ILDs), especially those with IPF or connective tissue disease (CTD)-associated ILD. Hypopharyngeal multichannel intraluminal impedance measurement in patients with IPF demonstrated frequent occurrence of abnormal proximal reflux events despite the absence of typical GOR symptoms and a frequently negative DeMeester score. Aspiration, assessed by means of increased BAL fluid pepsin levels, was associated with an increased odds ratio for an acute exacerbation in IPF patients. Pre-transplant patients with IPF undergoing antireflux surgery had reduced supplementary oxygen dependence compared with other pre-transplant patients with IPF. There are anecdotal cases of IPF disease stability and less radiological fibrosis on HRCT following treatment for reflux. In addition, a recent cohort analysis found that the use of medications to suppress reflux was an independent predictor of longer survival time.

GOR and microaspiration have also been implicated as a potential nonalloimmune cause of lung allograft rejection (bronchiolitis obliterans syndrome (BOS)) after lung transplantation. Standard oesophageal pH recordings indicated an increased oesophageal acid exposure in >70% of lung transplant patients. Luminal gastric components such as pepsin and bile acids have been demonstrated in the bronchial material of lung transplant recipients and were more prevalent in the lungs of patients with BOS. Aspiration of bile acids was related to weakly acidic reflux events, especially during the night, and was associated with a reduced concentration of pulmonary surfactant collectin proteins, reduced freedom from BOS and reduced survival. Aspiration, even in the absence of an increased number of GOR events, might therefore be a risk factor for the development of BOS after lung transplantation. Retrospective studies have linked prophylactic antireflux surgery to improved allograft function and decreased incidence and/or severity of BOS.

While it cannot be absolutely proven that disease stability is related to the control of reflux, the aforementioned study data suggest that a subset of patients with advanced lung disease may benefit from antireflux therapy. Proximal gastrointestinal tract motility studies, pH/impedance testing and markers of microaspiration appear to be important in management decisions. Future studies should seek to identify the most effective tool to determine the timing and efficacy of antireflux treatment.

Sleep and GOR

Sleep-related reflux is common, affecting between 47% and 79% of GORD patients. Between 54% and 57% of GORD patients and 25% of the general adult population report heartburn during the night. Sleep-related reflux is more commonly associated with oesophageal mucosal injury, malignant transformation and extraoesophageal manifestations of GORD. Poor quality of sleep and sleep disturbances have also been recently documented in a significant number of GORD patients with night-time reflux.

Sleep-related GOR occurs primarily during arousals or conscious awakenings in the first few hours of the sleep period and is primarily caused by TLOSR. Most conscious awakenings during sleep that also demonstrated reflux were not associated with typical GORD-related symptoms. Testing for reflux may thus be helpful in patients without typical GOR symptoms who have disrupted sleep without an identifiable cause found despite having undergone polysomnography sleep testing.

Up to 62% of OSA patients have sleep-related GOR symptoms and CPAP improves GOR symptoms and reduces oesophageal contact times. Treatment of sleep-related GOR includes behavioural treatment (weight loss, not eating prior to bedtime and avoiding foods known to worsen GOR) and PPI therapy given an hour before the last meal. Fundoplication can be helpful in selected patients with GOR and OSA.

Management of GORD

In general practice, most cases of GORD are diagnosed on the basis of typical symptoms and the response to inhibition of gastric acid secretion. Endoscopy, oesophageal manometry or acid instillation in the oesophagus (Bernstein test) have limited sensitivity and specificity for the diagnosis of GORD. 24-h oesophageal pH monitoring can provide useful information, in particular through the assessment of the temporal association between symptoms and reflux events. The addition of impedance monitoring to pH monitoring further improves GOR diagnosis as it also detects nonacid reflux events and allows testing while the patient is taking a PPI. The detection of biomarkers of aspiration (*e.g.* pepsin and bile acid concentrations in saliva, sputum or BAL fluid) has increasingly been recognised as a tool to identify patients at risk of disease worsening due to GORD but, currently, there is no consensus on how best to detect aspiration.

Medications interfering with acid production, especially the PPIs, are the cornerstone of GORD treatment. Acid-suppressive therapy is highly effective in the healing and maintenance of oesophagitis, but seems to be poorly effective when GORD is presumed to underlie extraoesophageal symptoms. Symptoms that persist during standard acid suppressive therapy regimens have also been related to nonacid reflux. There is little evidence that further intensification of acid suppression beyond high-dose PPIs twice daily is of any benefit for these patients. Dopaminergic antagonists with prokinetic activity (metoclopramide and domperidone) enhance gastric emptying and gastroduodenal coordination, but they do not appear to improve LOS pressure or reduce reflux events. Serotonin receptor prokinetic agents (cisapride and tegaserod) might be useful in the treatment of GOR but these drugs are no longer available due to concerns over possible adverse cardiovascular side-effects. A number of selective $5\text{-}HT_4$ agonists/antagonists (prucalopride and mosapride) show some promise and are undergoing investigation for reflux treatment. Baclofen is a γ-aminobutyric acid (GABA) receptor blocking agent that diminishes acid and nonacid reflux through GABA receptor inhibition of TLOSRs and is now being used off label in the treatment of GOR. Baclofen may also reduce the exposure to duodenogastric reflux but its use has been limited by side-effects. Other GABA agonists (arbaclofen and lesogaberan) are currently under evaluation for their ability to reduce TLOSRs and improve reflux and symptoms that are refractory to PPI therapy. Other pathways that are under investigation include mucosal protective agents, inhibitors of

acid-sensitive ion channels, metabotropic glutamate receptor-5 antagonists and endoscopic antireflux procedures.

At present, the only alternative is a surgical fundoplication. Laparoscopic antireflux surgery creates a mechanically competent cardia, and is more effective in preventing microaspiration and in eliminating proximal reflux. However, not all patients are eligible for surgery, the intervention is not without complications and poor responders to PPI therapy are also less certain to experience symptom relief from surgery. The key is thus the identification of patients who, with certainty, have GOR as an important cause of their pulmonary symptoms.

Further reading

- Asano K, *et al.* (2009). Silent acid reflux and asthma control. *N Engl J Med*; 360: 1551–1553.
- Blondeau K, *et al.* (2008). Gastro-oesophageal reflux and aspiration of gastric contents in adult patients with cystic fibrosis. *Gut*; 57: 1049–1055.
- Dettmar PW, *et al.* (2011). Reflux and its consequences – the laryngeal, pulmonary and oesophageal manifestations. *Aliment Pharmacol Ther*; 33: Suppl. 1, 1–71.
- Dupont LJ, *et al.* (2009). Emerging risk factors for bronchiolitis obliterans syndrome: gastro-oesophageal reflux and infections. *Eur Respir Monogr*; 45: 212–225.
- Galmiche JP, *et al.* (2008). Respiratory manifestations of gastro-oesophageal reflux disease. *Aliment Pharmacol Ther*; 27: 449–464.
- Meyer KC, *et al.*, eds. Gastroesophageal Reflux and the Lung. New York, Springer, 2013.
- Pashinsky YY, *et al.* (2009). Gastroesophageal reflux disease and idiopathic pulmonary fibrosis. *Mt Sinai J Med*; 76: 24–29.
- Sweet MP, *et al.* (2009). Gastro-oesophageal reflux and aspiration in patients with advanced lung disease. *Thorax*; 64: 167–173.

COPD and emphysema

Eleni G. Tzortzaki and Nikolaos M. Siafakas

Chronic obstructive pulmonary disease (COPD) is a major cause of morbidity and mortality worldwide. It affects ~10% of the general population but its prevalence among smokers may reach as much as 50%; COPD is projected to rank as the fifth largest worldwide burden of disease by 2020. According to the Global Initiative for Chronic Obstructive Lung Disease (GOLD) 2013 report, COPD is a preventable and treatable disease characterised by airow limitation that is not fully reversible. The airow limitation is usually progressive and is associated with an enhanced inammatory response of the lungs to noxious particles or gases, primarily caused by cigarette smoking. Exacerbations and comorbidities contribute to the overall severity in individual patients. The cardinal symptoms of COPD – dyspnoea, cough and sputum production – are chronic and progressive.

Key points

- COPD is a heterogeneous disease, with two main phenotypes: chronic bronchitis and emphysema.

- A strong genetic component, in conjunction with environmental insult, probably accounts for the development of COPD.

- Smoking cessation is the single most effective intervention in COPD prevention and treatment.

- Bronchodilators are central to symptomatic treatment, backed up if necessary by other interventions.

COPD comprises pathological changes in four different compartments of the lungs (central airways, peripheral airways, lung parenchyma and pulmonary vasculature), which are variably present in individuals with the disease. Airflow limitation in COPD is caused by the presence of an inflammatory cellular infiltrate in the small airways, remodelling and thickening of the airway wall. The destruction of alveoli and enlargement of airspaces, which are anatomical hallmarks of emphysema, contribute to the loss of elastic recoil and the loss of outward traction on the small airways, leading to their collapse on expiration. These result in airflow obstruction, air trapping and hyperinflation. In general, the inflammatory and structural changes in the airways increase with disease severity and persist even after smoking cessation.

Chronic obstructive bronchitis and/or emphysema

COPD is a heterogeneous disease; two main phenotypes of the disease are recognized: chronic bronchitis and emphysema.

Chronic bronchitis is characterised by cough and sputum production for ⩾3 months in each of two consecutive years. The symptoms may precede the development of airflow limitation by many years. Inflammation and secretions provide the obstructive component of the disease. In contrast to emphysema, chronic bronchitis is associated with a relatively undamaged pulmonary capillary bed. Emphysema is present to a variable degree but is usually centrilobular rather than panlobular. The body responds by decreasing ventilation and increasing cardiac output (ventilation/perfusion (V'/Q') mismatch), leading to hypoxaemia, polycythaemia and increased carbon dioxide retention, and eventually these patients develop signs of right heart failure.

Emphysema The second major COPD phenotype is the emphysematous patient. Emphysema is defined by destruction of airways distal to the terminal bronchiole, and gradual destruction of alveolar septa and the pulmonary capillary bed, leading to a decreased ability to oxygenate blood. The body compensates with lowered cardiac output and hyperventilation. This V'/Q' mismatch results in relatively limited blood flow through a quite well oxygenated lung with normal blood gases and pressures. Eventually, due to low cardiac output, the rest of the body suffers from tissue hypoxia, pulmonary cachexia, muscle wasting and weight loss.

Diagnosis and assessment

A clinical diagnosis of COPD should be considered in any patient who has dyspnoea, chronic cough and/or sputum production, a history of exposure to risk factors for the disease (tobacco smoke, occupational dusts and chemicals) and a family history of COPD (table 1). Overall COPD assessment should include the evaluation of current symptoms, the degree of airflow limitation, the risk of exacerbations and comorbidity. Combined COPD assessment including symptoms, spirometric classification and risk of exacerbation is presented in table 2, categorising COPD patients in four groups (A, B, C and D).

First, assess symptoms using either the modified Medical Research Council (mMRC) questionnaire or the COPD Assessment Test (CAT). Although the mMRC questionnaire is a validated tool to assess disability due to dyspnoea and CAT has a broader coverage of patients' health status, the proposed classification cut-offs are relatively arbitrary. Thus, further real-life studies are needed to better assess COPD patients.

Table 1. Risk factors for COPD

Genes
Exposure to particles
Tobacco smoke
Occupational dusts, organic and inorganic
Indoor air pollution (heating and cooking with biomass fuel)
Outdoor air pollution
Lung growth
Oxidative stress
Sex
Age
Respiratory infections
Socioeconomic status
Nutrition

Secondly, assess disease severity by spirometry and by the frequency of exacerbations. Spirometry is required to assess the degree of airflow limitation as it is the most widely available and reproducible lung function test. The presence of a post-bronchodilator FEV_1/FVC ratio <0.70 confirms the presence of airflow obstruction, and thus of COPD. The classification of severity of airflow obstruction in COPD into four stages it is presented in table 3. Where possible, values should be compared to age-related normal values (a cut-off based on the lower limit of normal (LLN) values for FEV_1/FVC) to avoid overdiagnosis of COPD in the elderly and less frequent diagnosis in adults younger than 45 years.

COPD exacerbations deteriorate health status, and enhance lung function decline and mortality. Thus, the assessment of exacerbation risk can reflect the risk of poor outcome and prognosis. The best predictor of having frequent exacerbations (two or more exacerbations per year) is a history of previous episodes, especially hospital admissions, as the exacerbation rate varies greatly between patients.

Comorbidities such as cardiovascular disease, skeletal muscle dysfunction, metabolic syndrome, osteoporosis,

Table 2. COPD severity assessment

	Group A: low risk, fewer symptoms	Group B: low risk, more symptoms	Group C: high risk, fewer symptoms	Group D: high risk, more symptoms
Spirometric stage	FEV_1 ⩾50% pred	FEV_1 ⩾50% pred	FEV_1 <50% pred	FEV_1 <50% pred
Symptoms	mMRC grade 0–1 or CAT score <10	mMRC grade ⩾2 or CAT score ⩾10	mMRC grade 0–1 or CAT score <10	mMRC grade ⩾2 or CAT score ⩾10
Exacerbations per year	0–1	0–1	⩾2	⩾2

% pred: % predicted.

depression and lung cancer can occur frequently in patients with COPD. Comorbidities influence mortality and hospitalisations independently, and should thus be recognised and treated properly in all COPD patients.

Risk factors

Although smoking is the best-studied COPD risk factor, it is not the only one and there is consistent evidence from epidemiological studies that nonsmokers may develop chronic airflow obstruction (table 1). Other factors, such as indoor air pollution from burning biomass fuels for cooking and heating, are important causes of COPD in many developing countries, especially among females. Nevertheless, not all subjects exposed to noxious agents develop COPD. Thus, a strong genetic component in relation with an environmental insult

(gene–environment interaction) most probably accounts for the development of the disease (table 1). Familial clustering of COPD has been observed and twin studies have supported the concept of a genetic predisposition to COPD. Among the candidate genes that have been studied in COPD are genes that regulate the production of proteases and antiproteases, genes that modulate the metabolism of toxic substances in cigarette smoke, genes involved with mucociliary clearance, and genes that influence inflammatory mediators.

Although rare, hereditary α_1-antitrypsin (AAT) deficiency is the best documented genetic risk factor for emphysema. The AAT gene is located on chromosome 14q23.1–3 and is a serum protein made in the liver that is capable of inhibiting the activity of serine proteases. Neutrophil elastase is the main target of AAT; if not inactivated by AAT,

Table 3. Spirometric classification of airflow obstruction in COPD based on post-bronchodilator FEV_1

All stages	FEV_1/FVC <0.70
Stage I: mild	FEV_1 ⩾80% pred
Stage II: moderate	FEV_1 ⩾50– <80% pred
Stage III: severe	FEV_1 ⩾30– <50% pred
Stage IV: very severe	FEV_1 <30% pred or <50% pred plus chronic respiratory failure[#]

% pred: % predicted. [#]: respiratory failure is defined as P_aO_2 <60 mmHg with or without P_aCO_2 >50 mmHg while breathing air at sea level. Respiratory failure may also lead to effects on the heart such as cor pulmonale (right heart failure). Clinical signs of cor pulmonale include elevation of the jugular venous pressure and pitting ankle oedema. Patients may have stage IV COPD even if their FEV_1 is >30% pred whenever these complications are present. At this stage, quality of life is significantly impaired and exacerbations may be life threatening. Reproduced and modified from GOLD (2013) with permission from the publisher.

neutrophil elastase destroys lung connective tissue, particularly elastin, and this leads to the development of emphysema. Over 90 different phenotypes of AAT have been described. The common gene variants are M, S and Z. Emphysema associated with AAT deficiency is typically panlobular, characterised by uniform destruction of the pulmonary lobule. Cigarette smoking is the biggest risk factor for the development of emphysema and airflow obstruction in AAT deficiency, and current smokers have an accelerated decline in FEV_1 compared with ex-smokers and never-smokers with AAT deficiency. Homozygous Z patients have a very low AAT levels and generally show a rapid decline in FEV_1 even without smoking. However, this homozygous state is rare in the general population (one in 5000 live births) and, thus, as genetic risk factor, it can explain <1% of COPD.

Recently, epigenetic mechanisms, such as acquired somatic mutations, have been explored in COPD. Somatic mutations are not heritable, although the susceptibility to acquiring such mutations might be controlled by inherited genes. Under normal conditions, cells are equipped with a number of repair pathways that remove damage and restore DNA. However, increased and persistent oxidative stress (e.g. due to cigarette smoking) may inactivate the human DNA mismatch repair system, leading to acquired mutations. Smoking-induced acquired somatic alterations have been detected in COPD patients.

Management

The overall approach to managing stable COPD is based on an individualised assessment of disease severity and response to various therapies. Patients who still smoke should be encouraged to quit. Smoking cessation is the single most effective intervention to reduce the risk of developing COPD and stop its progression, and can have a substantial effect on subsequent mortality.

The goals of therapy are to prevent and control symptoms, reduce the frequency and severity of exacerbations, and improve

Table 4. The recommended therapeutic management per severity group

	Group A: low risk, fewer symptoms	Group B: low risk, more symptoms	Group C: high risk, fewer symptoms	Group D: high risk, more symptoms
First-choice treatment	SABA p.r.n. or SAMA p.r.n.	LABA or LAMA	ICS+LABA or LAMA	ICS+LABA and/or LAMA
Second-choice treatment	LABA or LAMA or SABA and SAMA	LABA and LAMA	LABA and LAMA LAMA and PDE4i or LABA and PDE4i	ICS+LABA and LAMA or ICS+LABA and PDE4i or LAMA and LABA or LAMA and PDE4i
Alternative choice	Theophylline	SABA and/or SAMA Theophylline	SABA and/or SAMA Theophylline	Carbocisteine SABA and/or SAMA Theophylline

Treatments are presented in alphabetical order not in order of preference. SABA: short-acting β₂-agonist; SAMA: short-acting muscarinic antagonist; LABA: long-acting β₂-agonist; LAMA: long-acting muscarinic antagonist; ICS: inhaled corticosteroid; PDE4i: phosphodiesterase-4 inhibitor. Reproduced and modified from GOLD (2013) with permission from the publisher.

exercise tolerance, thus improving overall the quality of life. A summary of the proposed pharmacological management across COPD groups is presented in table 4. Bronchodilator medications are central to the symptomatic management of COPD. These drugs improve emptying of the lungs, tend to reduce static and dynamic hyperinflation, and improve exercise performance. Inhaled therapy is preferred and bronchodilators are prescribed either on an as-needed basis or on a regular basis, although it is evident that regular treatment with long-acting bronchodilators is more effective and convenient than treatment with short-acting ones. Treatment with a long-acting inhaled anticholinergic drug reduces the rate of COPD exacerbations and improves the effectiveness of pulmonary rehabilitation. A combination of β_2-agonist and an anticholinergic produces better and more sustained improvements in FEV_1 than either drug alone. The addition of inhaled glucocorticosteroids is appropriate for symptomatic COPD patients in groups C and D and repeated exacerbations according to the guidelines (table 4). This treatment does not modify the long-term decline of FEV_1 but it has been shown to reduce the frequency of exacerbations and improve the health status of COPD patients. Recent data, however, based on a single large study of patients with FEV_1 <60% predicted, indicate that regular treatment with inhaled glucocorticosteroids can decrease the rate of decline of lung function. Long-term treatment with oral glucocorticosteroids should be avoided in COPD because side-effects such as steroid myopathy may contribute to muscle weakness, decreased functionality and respiratory failure in patients with advanced COPD. The regular use of mucolytic and antioxidant agents has been evaluated in COPD patients without significant overall benefit, although there has been a study reporting reduced frequency of exacerbations. The regular use of antibiotics, other than for treating infectious exacerbations of COPD, is not recommended. The regular use of antitussive medications is also not recommended as cough, although a troublesome symptom, has a significant

protective role. There has been some recent evidence regarding the use of statins and long-term macrolide treatment in decreasing COPD exacerbations but these are not standard recommendations.

Influenza vaccination and pneumococcal polysaccharide vaccine are strongly recommended for all COPD patients, as they decrease serious illness and death rates by ~50%.

Pulmonary rehabilitation aims to improve exercise capacity, reduce symptoms and improve overall quality of life. It is a multidisciplinary programme ideally involving several types of health professionals. COPD patients at all stages of disease appear to benefit from exercise training programmes although benefit decreases after a rehabilitation programme ends. Pulmonary rehabilitation improves dyspnoea, improves quality of life scores, reduces the number of hospitalisations and days in the hospital, reduces anxiety and depression related to COPD and improves survival. A comprehensive rehabilitation programme includes exercise training, education and nutrition counselling.

Nutritional status is an important factor in determining symptoms, respiratory function and prognosis in COPD. Both extremes (overweight and underweight) are detrimental. A reduction in BMI, seen in ~25% of stage III and IV COPD patients, is an independent risk factor for mortality. The present evidence suggests a combination of nutritional support and exercise regimes should be used to induce anabolic action.

Further reading

- Blamoun AI, et al. (2008). Statins may reduce episodes of exacerbations and the requirement for intubation in patients with COPD: evidence from a retrospective cohort study. *Int J Clin Pract*; 62: 1373–1378.
- Castaldi PJ, et al. (2011). The association of genome-wide significant spirometric loci with chronic obstructive pulmonary disease susceptibility. *Am J Respir Cell Mol Biol*; 45: 1147–1153.

- Celli BR, *et al.* (2004). Standards for the diagnosis and treatment of patients with COPD: a summary of the ATS/ERS position paper. *Eur Respir J*; 23: 932–946.
- Celli BR, *et al.* (2005). Airway obstruction in never smokers: results from the Third National Health and Nutrition Examination Survey. *Am J Med*; 118: 1364–1372.
- Celli B, *et al.* (2008). Effect of pharmacotherapy on rate of decline of lung function in chronic obstructive pulmonary disease: results from the TORCH study. *Am J Respir Crit Care Med*; 178: 332–338.
- Coventry PA (2009). Does pulmonary rehabilitation reduce anxiety and depression in chronic obstructive pulmonary disease? *Curr Opin Pulm Med*; 15: 143–149.
- DeMeo DL, *et al.* (2004). α_1-Antitrypsin deficiency. 2: Genetic aspects of α_1-antitrypsin deficiency: phenotypes and genetic modifiers of emphysema risk. *Thorax*; 59: 259–264.
- Global Initiative for Chronic Obstructive Lung Disease. Global Strategy for the Diagnosis, Management and Prevention of COPD. www.goldcopd.org/uploads/users/files/GOLD_Report_2013_Feb20.pdf
- Hersh CP, *et al.* (2005). Attempted replication of reported chronic obstructive pulmonary disease candidate gene associations. *Am J Respir Cell Mol Biol*; 33: 71–78.
- Hogg JC (2004). Pathophysiology of airflow limitation in chronic obstructive pulmonary disease. *Lancet*; 364: 709–721.
- Nici L, *et al.* (2009). Pulmonary rehabilitation: what we know and what we need to know. *J Cardiopulm Rehabil Prev*; 29: 141–151.
- Qiu W, *et al.* (2011). Genetics of sputum gene expression in chronic obstructive pulmonary disease. *PLoS One*; 6: e24395.
- Seemungal TAR, *et al.* (2008). Long term erythromycin therapy is associated with decreased COPD exacerbations. *Am J Respir Crit Care Med*; 178: 1139–1147.
- Silverman EK, *et al.* (1996). Risk factors for the development of chronic obstructive pulmonary disease. *Med Clin North Am*; 80: 501–522.
- Stoller JK, *et al.* (2005). α_1-antitrypsin deficiency. *Lancet*; 365: 2225–2236.
- Tager IB, *et al.* (1976). Household aggregation of pulmonary function and chronic bronchitis. *Am Rev Respir Dis*; 114: 485–492.
- Tzortzaki E, *et al.* (2012). Oxidative DNA damage and somatic mutations: a link to the molecular pathogenesis of chronic inflammatory airway diseases. *Chest*; 141: 1243–1250.
- Tzortzaki EG, *et al.* (2009). A hypothesis for the initiation of COPD. *Eur Respir J*; 34: 310–315.
- Zheng JP, *et al.* (2008). Effect of carbocisteine on acute exacerbation of chronic obstructive pulmonary disease (PEACE study): a randomized placebo-controlled study. *Lancet*; 371: 2013–2018.

Exacerbations of COPD

Alexander J. Mackay and Jadwiga A. Wedzicha

Definition

COPD is a chronic inflammatory airway condition associated with episodes of acute deterioration termed exacerbations. An exacerbation of COPD is defined in the 2011 revision of the Global Strategy for the Diagnosis, Management and Prevention of COPD as an acute event characterised by a worsening of the patient's respiratory symptoms that is beyond normal day-to-day variations and leads to a change in medication. However, around half of all COPD exacerbations identified by symptom worsening are not reported, hence may not be treated, and thus could remain unidentified if a strict healthcare utilisation definition for exacerbations is used. For this reason, considerable interest exists in the potential of patient reported outcomes, such as the Exacerbations of Chronic Pulmonary Disease Tool (EXACT) to detect and quantify the severity of exacerbations.

Burden

Exacerbations are important events in the natural history of COPD; they have been shown to drive lung function decline and are responsible for much of the morbidity and mortality associated with this highly prevalent condition. Unreported exacerbations are also important events, significantly impairing quality of life. Exacerbations are also among the most common causes of medical admission and are costly to health services.

Patients hospitalised with exacerbations of COPD are a particularly vulnerable group. Every new, severe exacerbation that requires hospitalisation increases the risk of a subsequent exacerbation, and every new severe exacerbation increases the risk of death, up to five times after the tenth hospitalisation when compared with after the first COPD hospitalisation. Mortality peaks in the first week after admission, stabilising after 3 months and long-term prognosis is poor, with all-cause mortality approaching 50% at 3 years post discharge. Advanced age and severe lung function impairment, in addition to diabetes and poor health status, are particular risk factors for mortality. Inpatient mortality of patients admitted with COPD exacerbations in the UK is 7.4%, and rises to 25% for those patients with

---

Key points

- Exacerbations are important events; they drive lung function decline and are responsible for much of the morbidity and mortality associated with COPD.

- The majority of COPD exacerbations are triggered by respiratory viral infections and/or bacterial infections.

- The 'frequent exacerbator' phenotype is stable over time and exists across all GOLD stages.

- Frequent exacerbators exhibit faster decline in lung function, have worse quality of life, increased risk of hospitalisation and greater mortality.

- Both pharmacological and nonpharmacological therapies exist that can help prevent COPD exacerbations.

---

hypercapnic respiratory failure treated with NIV. Thus prevention, early diagnosis and prompt, effective management is vital to improve exacerbation recovery, ameliorate the effects on quality of life and reduce the risk of hospitalisation.

Causes

Exacerbations are associated with increased systemic and airway inflammation, and may be precipitated by environmental factors. However, the majority of COPD exacerbations are triggered by bacterial and/ or respiratory viral infections (fig. 1).

Infection Bacteria are isolated from sputum in 40–60% of acute exacerbations of COPD, and respiratory viruses are identified in 40– 60% of exacerbations with rhinovirus being the most prevalent species identified. Experimental infection models provide direct evidence that the symptomatic and physiological changes seen in acute exacerbations of COPD can be precipitated by rhinovirus infection. Furthermore, viral and bacterial infections demonstrate a synergistic effect at exacerbation; exacerbation symptoms, decline in FEV_1, and inflammation all being more severe in the presence of bacteria and viruses. These subjects are discussed further in the section on Infective exacerbations of COPD.

Air pollution Extensive data exists to support a role for air pollution in the aetiology of some COPD exacerbations. The Air Pollution and Health, a European Approach (APHEA) collaboration examined short-term effects of air pollution on mortality and morbidity of COPD in six European cities and found that increased levels of environmental pollutants (sulfur dioxide, nitrogen dioxide, ozone and particles) were associated with elevated relative risks of daily admissions for COPD.

Low temperature COPD exacerbations are more common and may be more severe in the winter months when there are colder temperatures; small but significant falls in lung function occur with a reduction in outdoor temperature during the winter in COPD patients. The mechanisms behind these observations are not clearly understood but may relate to increasing prevalence of respiratory viruses in the low temperature winter months and/or increased susceptibility to upper respiratory tract viral infections in cold weather.

Cardiovascular disease, comorbidities and exacerbations

Comorbid ischaemic heart disease is associated with longer exacerbations characterised by increased dyspnoea and wheeze. The presence of cardiac complications is increasingly being recognised as a predictor for COPD outcome. Data from The Health Improvement Network (THIN) database demonstrated a 2.27-fold increased risk of myocardial infarction 1– 5 days after outpatient exacerbations (defined by the prescription of both steroids and antibiotics). And in hospitalised exacerbations, raised troponin, chest pain and serial ECG changes are common, with one in 12 patients meeting the criteria for myocardial infarction. Furthermore, elevated troponin levels predict 30-day mortality in hospitalised COPD exacerbations, and so these studies challenge the way that exacerbations are conventionally treated. Patients receiving β-blockers appear to have a reduced risk of COPD exacerbations and a lower mortality from exacerbations. Therefore, COPD patients in the future, especially those with elevated cardiac biomarkers, may be considered for increased cardiac treatment at exacerbation.

Diabetes is also an important influence on COPD exacerbations. Comorbid diabetes mellitus prolongs the length of stay in hospital and increases the risk of death in patients hospitalised with acute exacerbations of COPD.

Frequent exacerbator phenotype

Patients with a history of frequent exacerbations have a worse quality of life, increased risk of hospitalisation and greater mortality (fig. 2). Frequent exacerbators also exhibit a faster decline in lung function and may have worse functional status, as measured by time outdoors. Thus, it is vital to identify patients at risk of frequent exacerbations.

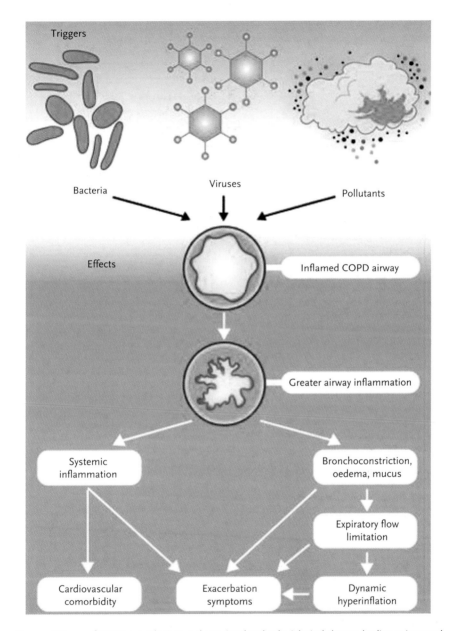

Figure 1. *Triggers of COPD exacerbations and associated pathophysiological changes leading to increased exacerbation symptoms. Reproduced from Wedzicha* et al. *(2007) with permission from the publisher.*

Exacerbations become more frequent and severe as COPD severity increases. However, one distinct group of patients appear to be susceptible to exacerbations, irrespective of disease severity. This phenotype of susceptibility to exacerbations is stable over time and the major determinant of frequent exacerbations is a

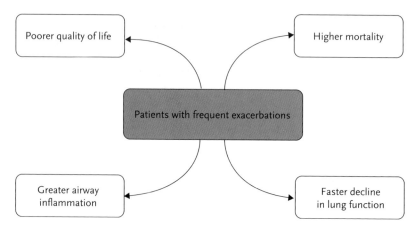

Figure 2. Effect of COPD exacerbations in the group with frequent exacerbations. Reproduced from Wedzicha et al. (2007) with permission from the publisher.

history of prior exacerbations. This phenomenon is seen across all GOLD stages (Global Initiative for Chronic Obstructive Lung Disease), including patients with stage II disease, of whom 22% had frequent exacerbations in the first year of the ECLIPSE study (the Evaluation of COPD Longitudinally to Identify Predictive Surrogate Endpoints). Therefore, suggesting patients with frequent exacerbator phenotypes are prone to exacerbations as a result of intrinsic susceptibility, and develop exacerbations when exposed to particular triggers, like respiratory viruses.

Susceptibility to exacerbations Respiratory viruses are more likely to be detected in patients with a history of frequent COPD exacerbations, suggesting that frequent exacerbators may be more susceptible to respiratory viral infections. Cells from patients with COPD manifest increased viral titre and copy number following rhinovirus infection compared to controls and intercellular adhesion molecule (ICAM)-1, the rhinovirus major group receptor, is upregulated on the bronchial epithelium of patients with COPD.

Frequent exacerbators also have elevated airway inflammation when stable, as measured by sputum interleukin (IL)-6 and IL-8 levels, in addition to a higher incidence of lower-airway bacterial colonisation.

Haemophilus influenzae enhances rhinovirus serotype 39-induced protein expression of IL-8 and epithelial-derived neutrophil attractant-7 chemokines, which are increased in the sputum and airways of patients with COPD exacerbations. *H. influenzae* also increases the expression of ICAM-1 and Toll-like receptor-3 and augments binding of rhinovirus to cultured cells. Through such mechanisms, patients colonised with bacteria may be more susceptible to the development of virally triggered exacerbations.

Exacerbation prevention

Vaccines In retrospective cohort studies of community-dwelling elderly patients, influenza vaccination is associated with a 27% reduction in the risk of hospitalisation for pneumonia or influenza and a 48% reduction in the risk of death. A pneumococcal polysaccharide vaccine has been shown to reduce the incidence of community-acquired pneumonia in COPD patients under the age of 65 years and those with severe airflow obstruction, although no mortality benefit was demonstrated. As a result, influenza and pneumococcal vaccines are recommended in the majority of patients with COPD.

Inhaled corticosteroids and long-acting bronchodilators The ISOLDE study (Inhaled

Table 1. Strategies to prevent COPD exacerbations

Pharmacological therapies	Nonpharmacological therapies
Vaccines	Pulmonary rehabilitation
Inhaled corticosteroids	Home oxygen therapy
Long-acting bronchodilators (LABA and LAMA)	Home ventilatory support
Combinations of LABA and inhaled corticosteroids	
Phosphodiesterase-4 inhibitors	
Mucolytics	
Long-term antibiotics	

Steroid in Obstructive Lung Disease in Europe) showed a 25% reduction in exacerbation frequency with inhaled corticosteroids (ICS). Long-acting β-agonists (LABA) also reduce exacerbation frequency, and in the TORCH study (Towards a Revolution in COPD Health), in which 6112 patients were followed for over 3 years, both inhaled fluticasone and salmeterol reduced exacerbation frequency when administered separately in comparison to placebo. The combination of fluticasone and salmeterol reduced exacerbation frequency further, in addition to improving health status and lung function in comparison to placebo. The combination of ICS and LABA also resulted in fewer hospital admissions over the study period and trended towards a mortality benefit, although this did not reach statistical significance. Reduction in exacerbation frequency has also been found with other LABA/ICS combinations, such as formoterol and budesonide.

Long-acting antimuscarinics (LAMA) also reduce exacerbation frequency. In the UPLIFT trial (Understanding Potential Long-Term Impacts on Function with Tiotropium), 5993 patients were randomised to tiotropium or placebo for a 4-year duration, with concomitant therapy being allowed. Although the primary end-point of the trial (reduction in the rate of decline in FEV_1) was negative, tiotropium was associated with a reduction in exacerbation risk, related hospitalisations and respiratory

failure. The POET-COPD trial (Prevention of Exacerbations with Tiotropium in COPD) showed that in patients with moderate-to-very-severe COPD, tiotropium is more effective than salmeterol in preventing exacerbations.

Newer bronchodilators, such as indacaterol, may also play a role in future maintenance regimens to reduce COPD exacerbations. To date, indacaterol has shown comparable exacerbation reduction rates in comparison with tiotropium in short clinical trials; however, whilst indacaterol in combination with tiotropium has recently been shown to provide enhanced bronchodilation compared to tiotropium alone, further research is required to assess if this combination provides synergistic benefits to reduce exacerbation frequency.

Phosphodiesterase-4 inhibitors Inhibit the airway inflammatory processes associated with COPD. Evidence from a pooled analysis of two large placebo-controlled, double-blind multicentre trials revealed a significant reduction of 17% in the frequency of moderate (glucocorticoid treated) or severe (hospitalisation/death) exacerbations. However, only patients with an $FEV_1 < 50\%$ (GOLD stage III and IV), presence of bronchitic symptoms and a history of exacerbations were enrolled. There are no comparator studies with ICS. Weight loss was also noted in the roflumilast group, with a mean reduction of 2.1 Kg after 1 year, and was highest in obese patients. Therefore, following treatment with roflumilast, weight needs to be carefully monitored.

Mucolytics The routine use of these agents is not recommended as only a few patients with viscous sputum appear to derive some small benefit from mucolytics.

Long-term antibiotics At present there is insufficient evidence to recommend routine prophylactic antibiotic therapy in the management of stable COPD, but some studies have shown promise. Erythromycin reduced the frequency of moderate and/or severe exacerbations (treated with systemic steroids, treated with antibiotics, or hospitalised) and shortened exacerbation length when taken twice daily over 12 months by patients with moderate-to-severe COPD. The macrolide azithromycin has been used as a prophylaxis in patients with CF and, when added to usual treatment, azithromycin has also been shown to decrease exacerbation frequency and improve quality of life in COPD patients. However the benefits were most significant in the treatment-naïve patients with mild disease (GOLD stage II), and significant rates of hearing decrement (as measured by audiometry) and antibiotic resistance were found. In addition, a recent large epidemiological study has suggested a small increase in cardiovascular deaths in patients receiving azithromycin, particularly in those with a high baseline risk of cardiovascular disease.

Furthermore, intermittent pulsed moxifloxacin, when given to stable patients, has been shown to significantly reduce exacerbation frequency in a per-protocol population, and in a *post hoc* subgroup of patients with bronchitis at baseline. However, this reduction did not meet statistical significance in the intention-to-treat analysis and further work is required in this area.

Hence, before prescription of long-term antibiotics in COPD, patients should be:

- Treated with an optimum combination of inhaled therapy
- Show evidence of ongoing frequent exacerbations

- Be carefully assessed for risk of potential cardiovascular and auditory side effects.

Pulmonary rehabilitation with home oxygen and ventilatory support There is some evidence from clinical trials that pulmonary rehabilitation programmes reduce hospital stay. There is evidence from epidemiological studies that home oxygen and ventilator support may reduce hospital admission, but controlled trials have not yet addressed these issues. These subjects are discussed in detail in the sections on Pulmonary rehabilitation, Acute oxygen therapy and Long-term ventilation.

A summary of the different therapies used to prevent COPD exacerbations is given in table 1.

Further reading

- Albert RK, et al. (2011). Azithromycin for prevention of exacerbations of COPD. N Engl J Med; 365: 689–698.
- Anderson HR, et al. (1997). Air pollution and daily admissions for chronic obstructive pulmonary disease in 6 European cities: results from the APHEA project. Eur Respir J; 10: 1064–1071.
- Calverley PM, et al. (2009). Roflumilast in symptomatic chronic obstructive pulmonary disease: two randomised clinical trials. Lancet; 374: 685–694.
- Calverley PM, et al. (2007). Salmeterol and fluticasone propionate and survival in chronic obstructive pulmonary disease. N Engl J Med; 356: 775–789.
- Donaldson GC, et al. (2002). Relationship between exacerbation frequency and lung function decline in chronic obstructive pulmonary disease. Thorax; 57: 847–852.
- Donaldson GC, et al. (2009). Increased risk of myocardial infarction and stroke following exacerbation of COPD. Chest; 137: 1091–1097.
- Global Initiative for Chronic Obstructive Lung Disease. Global Strategy for the Diagnosis, Management and Prevention of COPD. www.goldcopd.org/guidelines-global-strategy-for-diagnosis-management.html

- Hurst JR, *et al.* (2010). Susceptibility to exacerbation in chronic obstructive pulmonary disease. *N Engl J Med*; 363: 1128–1138.
- Mahler DA, *et al.* (2012). Concurrent use of indacaterol plus tiotropium in patients with COPD provides superior bronchodilation compared with tiotropium alone: a randomised, double-blind comparison. *Thorax*; 67: 781–788.
- Mallia P, *et al.* (2011). Experimental rhinovirus infection as a human model of chronic obstructive pulmonary disease exacerbation. *Am J Respir Crit Care Med*; 183: 734–742.
- McAllister DA, *et al.* (2012). Diagnosis of myocardial infarction following hospitalisation for exacerbation of COPD. *Eur Respir J*; 39: 1097–1103.
- Nichol KL, *et al.* (2007). Effectiveness of influenza vaccine in the community-dwelling elderly. *N Engl J Med*; 357: 1373–1381.
- Patel AR, *et al.* (2012). The impact of ischemic heart disease on symptoms, health status, and exacerbations in patients with COPD. *Chest*; 141: 851–857.
- Ray WA, *et al.* (2012). Azithromycin and the risk of cardiovascular death. *N Engl J Med*; 362: 1881–1890.
- Roberts CM, *et al.* (2011). Acidosis, non-invasive ventilation and mortality in hospitalised COPD exacerbations. *Thorax*; 66: 43–48.
- Sajjan US, *et al.* (2006). *H. influenzae* potentiates airway epithelial cell responses to rhinovirus by increasing ICAM-1 and TLR3 expression. *FASEB J*; 20: 2121–2123.
- Schneider D, *et al.* (2010). Increased cytokine response of rhinovirus-infected airway epithelial cells in chronic obstructive pulmonary disease. *Am J Respir Crit Care Med*; 182: 332–340.
- Seemungal TA, *et al.* (1998). Effect of exacerbation on quality of life in patients with chronic obstructive pulmonary disease. *Am J Respir Crit Care Med*; 157: 1418–1422.
- Sethi S, *et al.* (2010). Pulsed moxifloxacin for the prevention of exacerbations of chronic obstructive pulmonary disease: a randomized controlled trial. *Respir Res*; 11: 10.
- Suissa S, *et al.* (2012). Long-term natural history of chronic obstructive pulmonary disease: severe exacerbations and mortality. *Thorax*; 67: 957–963.
- Tashkin DP, *et al.* (2008). A 4-year trial of tiotropium in chronic obstructive pulmonary disease. *N Engl J Med*; 359: 1543–1554.
- Vogelmeier C, *et al.* (2011). Tiotropium *versus* salmeterol for the prevention of exacerbations of COPD. *N Engl J Med*; 364: 1093–1103.
- Wedzicha JA, *et al.* (2007). COPD exacerbations: defining their cause and prevention. *Lancet*; 370: 786–796.
- Wilkinson TM, *et al.* (2004). Early therapy improves outcomes of exacerbations of chronic obstructive pulmonary disease. *Am J Respir Crit Care Med*; 169: 1298–1303.

Extrapulmonary effects of COPD

Yvonne Nussbaumer-Ochsner and Klaus F. Rabe

COPD is an inflammatory disease of the lungs that is characterised by a fixed airflow limitation. Over the past few years, the understanding of COPD has evolved and it is no longer justified to consider COPD as a disease restricted to the lungs. COPD has become a complex and multicomponent disorder, with the majority of patients dying from cardiovascular diseases or cancer and not primarily from a respiratory disease. Extrapulmonary comorbidities significantly complicate the management of, and influence the prognosis of, patients with COPD. The broad range of clinical presentations, ranging from chronic bronchitis to hyperinflation and severe emphysema, also illustrates that the term 'COPD' describes patients with very different clinical phenotypes.

The main recognised extrapulmonary manifestations include cardiovascular disease and heart failure, musculoskeletal wasting, osteoporosis, metabolic syndrome and depression (table 1). While some of these comorbidities share risk factors with COPD, such as cigarette smoking, other frequently observed comorbidities cannot be attributed to smoking. There is increasing evidence that chronic inflammation is a key factor in COPD and is present in many other chronic diseases associated with COPD. The theory that COPD could be considered part of a 'chronic systemic inflammatory syndrome' takes these different aspects into account.

Local and systemic inflammation

In industrialised countries of the Western world, cigarette smoking accounts for most cases of COPD. Smoking triggers a local inflammatory response throughout the whole tracheobronchial tree. The cellular pattern is rather heterogeneous and inflammatory cells are found in the proximal and peripheral small airways, the lung parenchyma, and the pulmonary vasculature. Apart from these local effects, smoking may significantly contribute to or cause systemic inflammation. COPD patients

> **Key points**
>
> • There is clear evidence that COPD is not simply a disease limited to the airways but should be considered a complex and multicomponent syndrome.
>
> • FEV_1 is not just a lung function parameter for grading COPD severity, but is also a marker for premature death from any cause.
>
> • The course of the disease and the prognosis is influenced by extrapulmonary pathology and accompanying comorbidities.
>
> • Patients with COPD show comorbidities that are not only related to smoking but also to other lifestyle factors, including diet and inactivity; chronic systemic inflammation seems to link them together and might explain why they often occur together.
>
> • Future research is needed to answer the question of whether the successful treatment of comorbidities associated with COPD positively influences the course of the disease itself.

Table 1. Systemic manifestations and comorbidities of COPD

Cardiovascular diseases
Ischaemic heart disease
Hypertension
Pulmonary hypertension
Congestive heart failure
'Metabolic' disorders
Osteoporosis
Skeletal muscle weakness
Cachexia: weight loss and muscle wasting
Diabetes mellitus
Metabolic syndrome
Other comorbid diseases
Lung cancer
Chronic kidney disease
Depression
OSA(S)
Normocytic anaemia

suffering from an acute exacerbation or having severe disease show increased markers of: interleukin (IL)-6, IL-8 and tumour necrosis factor-α (TNF-α); acute-phase proteins, *i.e.* C-reactive protein (CRP) and fibrinogen; and circulating inflammatory cells, such as monocytes, neutrophils and lymphocytes. It is debatable whether this systemic inflammation is the result of: 1) a 'spill-over' of local inflammation in the lungs; 2) a systemic inflammatory effect that affects multiple organ systems; or 3) is attributable to some comorbid conditions that affect the lungs (fig. 1).

Systemic inflammation is actually not only present in patients with COPD, but is also a common feature in various other chronic diseases. Compared to healthy individuals, elevated levels of inflammatory markers, such as CRP and IL-6, are observed in patients with stable coronary artery disease, peripheral arterial disease and diabetes. These findings have to be taken into account when the causative role of COPD in systemic inflammation is investigated, because these conditions often occur together. Systemic inflammation might be the common

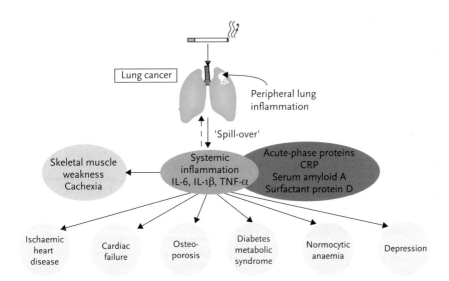

Figure 1. Systemic effects and comorbidities of COPD. Peripheral lung inflammation may cause a 'spill-over' of cytokines, such as IL-6, IL-1β and TNF-α, into the systemic circulation, which may increase the acute-phase proteins, such as CRP. Systemic inflammation may then led to skeletal muscle atrophy and cachexia, and may initiate and worsen comorbid conditions. Systemic inflammation may also accelerate lung cancer. An alternative model is that systemic inflammation causes several inflammatory diseases, including COPD. Reproduced from Barnes et al. (2009).

pathway leading to these chronic diseases and might explain the high prevalence of multiple chronic diseases in the same patient.

Impact on patient care

Comorbidities and systemic effects in patients with COPD not only have prognostic value but also have implications for medical treatment. Medical care should focus on comorbidities that are easier to prevent and treat than COPD itself. A diagnosis of COPD can easily be performed using spirometry, but the severity of the disease is clearly dependent on the presence of comorbidities. Therefore, it has been proposed that any patient aged >40 years with a positive smoking history (>10 pack-years), symptoms, and a lung function compatible with COPD should be carefully evaluated for more general disorders associated with the chronic systemic inflammatory syndrome (table 2).

Therapeutical implications

Pharmacological treatment targeting the lungs has only a minor impact on the course of the disease, and the treatment of COPD should no longer be centred solely on controlling symptoms and reducing exacerbations. Large clinical trials have shown that available drugs for COPD (bronchodilators and inhaled corticosteroids) do not significantly influence the long-term decline in FEV_1.

Table 2. Components of the chronic systemic inflammatory syndrome

Aged >40 years
Smoking >10 pack-years
Symptoms and lung function compatible with COPD
Chronic heart failure
Metabolic syndrome
Increased CRP

At least three components are required for diagnosis. Reproduced from Fabbri et al. (2007) with permission from the publisher.

Another approach would be to target the underlying systemic disease itself. A few observational studies have shown that the treatment of extrapulmonary manifestations (e.g. muscle weakness) and comorbid diseases (e.g. heart disease and peripheral arterial disease) positively influences morbidity and mortality in COPD patients. Even though these studies have clear limitations they so far suggest that statins, angiotensin-converting enzyme inhibitors and angiotensin receptor blockers might all have dual cardiopulmonary properties and, thereby, be able to positively influence the course of the disease. However, these findings have to be confirmed in prospective and carefully controlled trials before any conclusions regarding the management of COPD patients can be drawn.

Assuming that systemic inflammation is a key factor in COPD and other chronic diseases, pulmonary rehabilitation addresses important extrapulmonary components that are not targeted by any pharmacological treatment, and might be the reason for its overwhelming efficacy. Lifestyle interventions in general and more specifically pulmonary rehabilitation are essential components of patient care and should be evaluated in any patient with COPD GOLD stage II or higher (Global Initiative for Chronic Obstructive Lung Disease). Appropriate education about the disease itself, its time course and treatment options, as well as psychosocial support, including smoking cessation and nutritional interventions, are part of a successful rehabilitation programme.

Conclusions

Chronic diseases, including COPD, share common aspects, and chronic systemic inflammation seems to be one of the linking elements. Extrapulmonary effects of COPD not only influence the prognosis but also have an impact on disease management. The treatment of patients with COPD must become truly multidisciplinary and has to move from an organ-specific to a more holistic approach.

Further reading

- Barnes PJ, *et al.* (2009). Systemic manifestations and comorbidities of COPD. *Eur Respir J*; 33: 1165–1185.
- Fabbri LM. (2007). From COPD to chronic systemic inflammatory syndrome? *Lancet*; 370: 797–799.
- Mancini GB, *et al.* (2006). Reduction of morbidity and mortality by statins, angiotensin-converting enzyme inhibitors, and angiotensin receptor blockers in patients with chronic obstructive pulmonary disease. *J Am Coll Cardiol*; 47: 2554–2560.
- Mannino DM, *et al.* (2008). Prevalence and outcomes of diabetes, hypertension and cardiovascular disease in COPD. *Eur Respir J*; 32: 962–969.
- Mortensen EM, *et al.* (2009). Impact of statins and ACE inhibitors on mortality after COPD exacerbations. *Respir Res*; 10: 45.
- Nijm J, *et al.* (2005). Circulating levels of proinflammatory cytokines and neutrophil-platelet aggregates in patients with coronary artery disease. *Am J Cardiol*; 95: 452–456.
- Nussbaumer-Ochsner Y, *et al.* (2011). Systemic manifestations of COPD. *Chest*; 139: 165–173.
- van Gestel YR, *et al.* (2008). Effect of statin therapy on mortality in patients with peripheral arterial disease and comparison of those with *versus* without associated chronic obstructive pulmonary disease. *Am J Cardiol*; 102: 192–196.
- Wisniacki N, *et al.* (2005). Insulin resistance and inflammatory activation in older patients with systolic and diastolic heart failure. *Heart*; 91: 32–37.
- Young RP, *et al.* (2007). Forced expiratory volume in one second: not just a lung function test but a marker of premature death from all causes. *Eur Respir J*; 30: 616–622.

Pharmacology of asthma and COPD

Peter J. Barnes

The pharmacology of asthma and COPD involves understanding the mechanisms and clinical use of bronchodilators and anti-inflammatory or controller therapies.

- Relievers (bronchodilators) give immediate reversal of airway obstruction, largely by relaxing airway smooth muscle.
- Controllers (preventers) suppress the underlying disease process (anti-inflammatory treatments) and provide long-term control of symptoms.
- The most effective therapies are given by inhalation to reduce side-effects.

β_2-adrenergic agonists

Inhaled β_2-agonists are the bronchodilator treatment of choice in asthma because they reverse all known bronchoconstrictor mechanisms and have minimal side-effects when used correctly.

Mode of action
- β_2-agonists produce bronchodilatation by directly stimulating β_2-receptors in airway smooth muscle, leading to relaxation of central and peripheral airways. β_2-agonists are functional antagonists as they reverse bronchoconstriction irrespective of the contractile agent. This is important in asthma as many bronchoconstrictor mechanisms (neural and mediators) contribute, whereas in COPD, their major effect is to reverse cholinergic tone. Activation of β_2-receptors results in the activation of adenylyl cyclase via the stimulatory G-protein (G_s), which increases intracellular cyclic AMP, leading to relaxation of myosin fibrils. β_2-receptors

are localised to several types of airway cell and β_2-agonists may have additional effects.
- β_2-agonists may also have other beneficial effects, by inhibiting the release of mediators from mast cells and of neurotransmitters from airway nerves, as well as reducing plasma exudation from airway blood vessels.
- However, β_2-agonists have no significant long-term effects on chronic inflammation of the airways so in asthma patients they need to be used with a controller therapy.

Short-acting inhaled β₂-agonists (SABAs) (*e.g.* salbutamol and terbutaline) bronchodilate for 3–4 h (less in severe asthma) and used mainly by inhalation as reliever therapy in asthma and COPD. They have a rapid onset and are without significant side-effects. They also protect against bronchoconstrictor stimuli such as exercise, cold air and allergens. SABAs are the bronchodilators of choice in acute severe asthma and COPD, in which the nebulised route of administration is as effective as *i.v.* use. Inhaled delivery is preferable to oral because side-effects are less common and it may be more effective (better access to surface cells such as mast cells). They should not be used on a regular basis; increased use indicates a need for more anti-inflammatory therapy.

Long-acting inhaled β₂-agonists (LABAs) (*e.g.* salmeterol and formoterol twice daily, and indacaterol once daily) have a prolonged bronchodilator and bronchoprotective action. Formoterol has a more rapid onset of action but is a fuller agonist than salmeterol, so tolerance is more likely. Formoterol, but not salmeterol, is more effective as a reliever than SABAs. Inhaled LABAs are added to low or moderate doses of inhaled corticosteroids (ICS) and this is more effective than increasing the dose of ICS but should never be used without an ICS in asthma. Combination inhalers with an ICS and a LABA (fluticasone propionate and salmeterol, budesonide and formoterol, or beclomethasone dipropionate and formoterol) are an effective and convenient way to control asthma and are also useful in COPD. Budesonide/formoterol is very effective as a reliever when added to maintenance treatment with the same drug. LABAs are effective bronchodilators in COPD and reduce exacerbations. Indacaterol has a duration of action >24 h and is approved as a once daily treatment for COPD patients.

Side-effects Unwanted effects result from stimulation of extrapulmonary β-receptors and include muscle tremor, palpitations, restlessness and hypokalaemia. Side-effects are uncommon with inhaled therapy, but more common with oral or *i.v.* administration

Safety A large trial in the USA showed that salmeterol increased mortality and near-death asthma attacks in asthmatic patients, but this was mainly in poor patients who were not using concomitant ICS. This provides a strong argument for prescribing LABAs only in a combination inhaler. There are no safety concerns about LABA use in COPD.

Tolerance Loss of bronchodilator action is minimal, but there is some loss of the bronchoprotective effect against exercise, for example. This is incomplete and not progressive, and does not appear to be a clinical problem.

Anticholinergics

Atropine is a naturally occurring compound that was introduced for the treatment of asthma but, because of side-effects (particularly drying of secretions), less soluble quaternary compounds (*e.g.* ipratropium bromide) were developed.

Mode of action Anticholinergics are specific antagonists of muscarinic receptors and block cholinergic nerve-induced bronchoconstriction. A small degree of resting bronchomotor tone is present because of tonic cholinergic nerve impulses, which release acetylcholine in the vicinity of airway smooth muscle, and cholinergic reflex bronchoconstriction may be initiated by irritants, cold air and stress. Although anticholinergics protect against acute challenge by sulfur dioxide and emotional factors, they are less effective against allergens, exercise and fog. They inhibit reflex cholinergic bronchoconstriction only and have no significant blocking effect on the direct effects of inflammatory mediators, such as histamine and leukotrienes. In COPD, cholinergic tone is the only reversible element of airway narrowing.

Clinical use Ipratropium bromide and oxitropium bromide are inhaled three or four times daily, whereas tiotropium bromide is inhaled once daily. In asthmatics, anticholinergic drugs are less effective bronchodilators than β₂-agonists and offer less protection against bronchial challenges.

Nebulised anticholinergics are effective in acute severe asthma, but less effective than β_2-agonists, so may be added if responses to nebulised β_2-agonists are insufficient. Recent studies have demonstrated that tiotropium may be an effective add-on bronchodilator in some patients with severe asthma. Inhaled anticholinergic drugs are the bronchodilators of choice in COPD and once-daily tiotropium bromide is an effective bronchodilator for COPD, which also reduces exacerbations, mortality and possibly disease progression in early disease.

Side-effects Inhaled anticholinergic drugs are well tolerated, and systemic side-effects are uncommon because very little systemic absorption occurs. Ipratropium bromide, even in high doses, has no detectable effect on airway secretions. Nebulised ipratropium bromide may precipitate glaucoma in elderly patients as a result of a direct effect of the nebulised drug on the eye; this is avoided by use of a mouthpiece rather than a facemask. Dry mouth occurs in about 10% of patients on tiotropium bromide but rarely requires discontinuation of treatment. Urinary retention and glaucoma are rare adverse effects.

Theophylline

Theophylline remains the most widely used asthma therapy worldwide because it is inexpensive, but the greater incidence of side-effects with theophylline and the greater efficacy of β-agonists and ICS have reduced its use. It remains a useful drug in patients with severe asthma and COPD.

Mode of action Theophylline is a weak, nonselective phosphodiesterase (PDE) inhibitor, which causes bronchodilatation by inhibiting PDE3 in airway smooth muscle at concentrations $>$10 mg·L^{-1}. At these concentrations, it is also an antagonist of adenosine receptors and inhibition of A_{2B}-receptors on mast cells could contribute to its beneficial effect in asthma, but blockage of A_1-receptors may lead to serious side-effects, such as cardiac arrhythmias and seizures. At lower concentrations (5–10 mg·L^{-1}) theophylline

may have anti-inflammatory effects in asthma and COPD, either through PDE4 inhibition or, more likely, through inhibition of phosphoinositide-3-kinase-δ. This may also explain how theophylline can reverse corticosteroid resistance in asthma and COPD by increasing histone deacetylase (HDAC)2 activity to allow corticosteroids to switch off activated inflammatory genes.

Clinical use Intravenous aminophylline (a stable mixture or combination of theophylline and ethylenediamine that confers greater solubility in water) is less effective than nebulised β_2-agonists in the treatment of acute severe asthma, and should therefore be reserved for the few patients who fail to respond to β_2-agonists. Theophylline is less effective as a bronchodilator than inhaled β_2-agonists and is more likely to have side-effects. There is increasing evidence that low doses (giving plasma concentrations of 5–10 mg·L^{-1}) may be useful when added to inhaled corticosteroids, particularly in more severe asthma and in COPD, reducing hyperinflation and improving dyspnoea.

Pharmacokinetics Theophylline is reliably absorbed from the gastrointestinal tract, but there are many factors affecting plasma clearance and, thus, plasma concentration. Clearance may be increased by drugs that induce hepatic cytochrome P450 (e.g. rifampicin and ethanol), by smoking and in children, so higher doses may be needed in these cases, whereas clearance is reduced by drugs that inhibit hepatic metabolism (e.g. cimetidine, erythromycin and ciprofloxacin), congestive cardiac failure, liver disease, viral infections, and in the elderly.

Side-effects These are related to plasma concentration and tend to occur when plasma levels exceed 20 mg·L^{-1}, although some patients develop them at lower plasma concentrations. The severity of side-effects may be reduced by gradually increasing the dose until therapeutic concentrations are achieved. The most common side-effects are headache, nausea and vomiting, abdominal discomfort (probably due to PDE4 inhibition), and the dangerous side-effects are cardiac arrhythmias and seizures (due to A_1-receptor antagonism).

Corticosteroids

Corticosteroids are the most effective controller therapy available for asthma, but are poorly effective in COPD.

Mode of action Corticosteroids enter target cells and bind to glucocorticoid receptors in the cytoplasm. The corticosteroid–receptor complex is transported to the nucleus, where it binds to specific sequences on the upstream regulatory element of responsive target genes, resulting in increased or decreased transcription and, subsequently, increased or decreased protein synthesis. Glucocorticoid receptors may also inhibit transcription factors, such as nuclear factor-κB, which activate inflammatory gene expression by a nongenomic mechanism. Corticosteroids inhibit histone acetylation and, thereby, inflammatory gene expression by recruiting HDAC2 to the transcriptional complex. The mechanism of action of corticosteroids in asthma is most related to their anti-inflammatory effects and, particularly, suppression of transcription of activated inflammatory (*e.g.* cytokine) genes. They also have inhibitory effects on many inflammatory and structural cells that are activated in asthma, resulting in reduced airway hyperresponsiveness. By contrast, corticosteroids have no anti-inflammatory effects in COPD and reduced benefit in severe asthma, which may be explained by a reduction in HDAC2 activity as a consequence of oxidative stress.

Clinical use Systemic corticosteroids are used in acute exacerbations of asthma and accelerate their resolution. There is no advantage with high doses of *i.v.* corticosteroids (*e.g.* methylprednisolone, 1 g). Prednisolone (40–60 mg orally) has an effect similar to *i.v.* hydrocortisone and is easier to administer. Maintenance oral corticosteroids are reserved for patients whose asthma cannot be controlled by other therapy (Global Initiative for Asthma (GINA) step 5); the dose is titrated to the lowest that provides acceptable symptom control. Short courses of oral corticosteroids (prednisolone, 30–40 mg daily for 1–2 weeks) are indicated for exacerbations of asthma; the dose may be tapered over 1 week once the exacerbation is resolved.

ICS are currently recommended as first-line therapy in all patients with persistent asthma and may be started in any patient who needs to use a SABA inhaler for symptom control more than twice a week. In most patients, ICS are used twice daily, but once daily use may be possible in patients with mild asthma. If a dose of >800 μg daily *via* a metered-dose inhaler is administered, a spacer should be used to reduce the risk of oropharyngeal side-effects and of absorption from the gastrointestinal tract. ICS in doses of ⩽400 μg daily may be used safely in children. Patients with COPD show a poor response to ICS with no effect on disease progression or mortality, but reduce exacerbations in patients who have severe disease and frequent exacerbations.

Side-effects Corticosteroids inhibit cortisol secretion by a negative feedback effect on the pituitary gland. Hypothalamic–pituitary–adrenal axis suppression is dependent on dose and usually occurs when an oral dose of prednisolone of more than 7.5–10 mg daily is used. Significant suppression after short courses of corticosteroid therapy is not usually a problem but prolonged suppression may occur after several months or years; corticosteroid doses after prolonged oral therapy must therefore be reduced slowly. Symptoms of 'corticosteroid withdrawal syndrome' include lassitude, musculoskeletal pains and occasionally fever.

Side-effects of long-term oral corticosteroid therapy include fluid retention, increased appetite, weight gain, osteoporosis, capillary fragility, hypertension, peptic ulceration, diabetes, cataracts and psychosis. The incidence tends to increase with age.

Systemic side-effects of ICS have been investigated extensively. Effects such as cataract formation and osteoporosis are reported, but often in patients who are also receiving oral corticosteroids. There has been particular concern about growth suppression in children using ICS but, in most studies, doses of $\leqslant 400\,\mu g$ have not been associated with impaired growth and there may even be a growth spurt because asthma is better controlled. In COPD patients, high doses of ICS have been associated with cataracts, diabetes and pneumonia.

The fraction of corticosteroid inhaled into the lungs acts locally on the airway mucosa and may be absorbed from the airway and alveolar surface, thereby reaching the systemic circulation. The fraction of ICS deposited in the oropharynx is swallowed and absorbed from the gut, and then is metabolised in the liver before it reaches the systemic circulation. Budesonide and fluticasone propionate have a greater first-pass metabolism than beclomethasone dipropionate and are therefore less likely to produce systemic effects at high inhaled doses. The use of a spacer reduces oropharyngeal deposition, thereby reducing systemic absorption of corticosteroid.

Antileukotrienes

Antileukotrienes (leukotriene receptor antagonists) are much less effective than ICS in the control of asthma.

Mode of action Elevated concentrations of leukotrienes are detectable in bronchoalveolar lavage fluid and sputum of asthmatic patients. Cysteinyl-leukotrienes (Cys-LTs) are generated from arachidonic acid by the rate-limiting enzyme 5-lipoxygenase. Cys-LTs are potent constrictors of human airways *in vitro* and *in vivo*, cause airway microvascular leakage in animals, and stimulate airway mucus secretion. These effects are all mediated in human airways *via* Cys-LT$_1$ receptors. Montelukast and zafirlukast are potent Cys-LT$_1$ receptor antagonists that markedly inhibit the bronchoconstrictor response to inhaled leukotrienes, reduce allergen-, exercise- and cold air-induced asthma by about 50–70%, and inhibit aspirin-induced responses in aspirin-sensitive asthmatics almost completely. They may also have weak anti-inflammatory effects and may reduce eosinophilic inflammation.

Clinical use Antileukotrienes may have a small and variable bronchodilator effect, indicating that leukotrienes may contribute to baseline bronchoconstriction in asthma. Long-term administration reduces asthma symptoms and the need for rescue β_2-agonists, and improves lung function. However, their effects are significantly less than with ICS in terms of symptom control, improvement in lung function and reduction in exacerbations. They may be useful in some patients whose asthma is not controlled on ICS as an add-on therapy, but are less effective in this respect than a long-acting β_2-agonists or low dose theophylline. They are effective in some but not all patients with aspirin-sensitive asthma. Patients appear to differ in their response to antileukotrienes, and it is impossible to predict which patients will respond best. A major advantage is that they are orally active and may improve compliance with long-term therapy. However, they are expensive, and a trial of therapy is indicated to determine which patients will benefit most.

Side-effects Antileukotrienes are well tolerated and there are no class-specific side-effects. Zafirlukast may produce mild liver dysfunction, so liver function tests are important. Several cases of Churg–Strauss syndrome (systemic vasculitis with eosinophilia and asthma) have been observed in patients on antileukotrienes, but these may be because a concomitant reduction in oral corticosteroids (made possible by the antileukotriene) allows the vasculitis to flare up.

Cromones

Cromones include sodium cromoglycate and the structurally related nedocromil sodium.

Although they protect against indirect bronchoconstrictor stimuli such as exercise, allergens and fog, they are poorly effective compared with low doses of ICS, as they have a short duration of action. Systematic reviews have concluded that they provide little benefit in chronic asthma so they are now rarely used. There is no role for cromones in the management of COPD.

Anti-IgE

Mode of action Omalizumab is a humanised recombinant monoclonal antibody that binds to circulating IgE and, thus, blocks it from activating high-affinity IgE receptors on mast cells and low-affinity IgE receptors on other inflammatory cells, resulting in reduced responses to allergens. Over time, the blocking of IgE reduces its synthesis by B-cells and results in a sustained reduction in IgE.

Clinical use Omalizumab reduces airway inflammation in patients with mild-to-moderate asthma and reduces the incidence of asthma exacerbations, with improved control of asthma in patients maintained on reduced doses of ICS or oral steroids. Omalizumab is most useful in patients with severe asthma who are not controlled on maximal doses of inhaled therapy as it reduces exacerbations and improves asthma control. Only ~30% of patients show a good response and this is not predictable by any clinical features; therefore, a trial of therapy over 4 months is indicated. Omalizumab should be given only to patients with serum IgE levels of 20–700 IU·mL^{-1}; above these levels, it is not possible to give enough antibody to neutralise the IgE. The dose of omalizumab is determined by serum IgE levels and body weight, and is given either once or twice a month. Because of its high cost, only patients at GINA steps 4 and 5 with frequent exacerbations are suitable for this therapy.

Side-effects Occasionally, local reactions occur at the injection sites and, very rarely, anaphylactic reactions have been reported.

Immunosuppressive/corticosteroid-sparing therapy

Immunosuppressive therapy has been considered in asthma when other treatments have been unsuccessful or when a reduction in the dosage of oral corticosteroids is required; it is therefore indicated in very few (<1%) asthmatic patients at present.

Methotrexate Low-dose methotrexate (15 mg weekly) has a corticosteroid-sparing effect in some patients with asthma, but side-effects are relatively common and include nausea (reduced if methotrexate is given as a weekly injection), blood dyscrasia and hepatic damage. Careful monitoring (monthly blood counts and liver enzymes) is essential.

Gold has long been used in the treatment of chronic arthritis. A controlled trial of an oral gold preparation (auranofin) demonstrated some corticosteroid-sparing effect in chronic asthmatic patients maintained on oral corticosteroids, but side-effects (skin rashes and nephropathy) are a limiting factor.

Cyclosporin A Low-dose oral cyclosporin A in patients with corticosteroid-dependent asthma is reported to improve control of symptoms but, in clinical practice, it is unimpressive and its use is limited by severe side-effects (nephrotoxicity and hypertension).

Roflumilast

Roflumilast is a once daily oral PDE4 inhibitor that has anti-inflammatory effects in COPD patients. The dose is limited by side-effects (nausea, vomiting, diarrhoea and headaches) so its clinical efficacy is relatively small. Weight loss may also occur but this is nonprogressive and reversible. COPD patients with severe disease (FEV1 <50% predicted), chronic bronchitis and frequent exacerbations, there is a small improvement in lung function and a reduction in severe exacerbations. It is therefore used as an add-on therapy in this subpopulation of patients with COPD. It should never be co-administered with theophylline, which also has PDE4 inhibitory effects.

Further reading

- Barnes PJ. Pulmonary pharmacology. *In:* Brunton LL, ed. Goodman & Gilman's The Pharmacological Basis of Therapeutics. 12th Edn. New York, McGraw Hill, 2011; pp. 1031–106.

- Chung KF, *et al.*, eds. Pharmacology and Therapeutics of Airway Disease. 2nd Edn. New York, Informa Healthcare, 2009.
- Fanta CH (2009). Asthma. *N Engl J Med*; 360: 1002–1014.
- Global Initiative for Asthma. Global strategy for asthma management and prevention. www.ginasthma.org/uploads/users/files/GINA_Report_2012Feb13.pdf
- Global Initiative for Chronic Obstructive Lung Disease. Global strategy for the diagnosis, management and prevention of COPD. www.goldcopd.org/uploads/users/files/GOLD_Report_2013_Feb20.pdf
- Niewoehner DE (2010). Outpatient management of severe COPD. *N Engl J Med*; 362: 1407–1416.

Bronchiectasis

Nick ten Hacken

Bronchiectasis is a disorder characterised by abnormal bronchial wall thickening and luminal dilation of the central and medium-sized

Key points

- Diagnosis of bronchiectasis is based on the presence of daily production of mucopurulent phlegm and chest imaging that demonstrates dilated and thickened airways. HRCT is the gold standard.

- The diagnosis of bronchiectasis should lead to the investigation and treatment of possible causes and associated conditions.

- Antibiotics form the mainstay of treatment of bronchiectasis. Acute exacerbations should be treated promptly with short courses of antibiotics.

- The efficacy of continuous administration of antibiotics, mucolytics, anti-inflammatory agents and bronchodilators is not clear, but may be considered on an individual basis.

- Bronchopulmonary hygiene physical therapy techniques are widely used, yet there is not enough evidence to support or refute them.

- Surgery may be considered if the area of the bronchiectatic lung is localised and if the patient's symptoms are debilitating or life threatening (e.g. massive haemoptysis).

bronchi, due to a vicious circle of transmural infection and inflammation with mediator release. The prevalence varies between countries but seems to increase with age and is more common in females. Frequent symptoms are chronic cough and production of mucopurulent sputum. Less frequent are haemoptysis, pleuritic pain, recurrent fever, wheeze and dyspnoea. Exacerbations of bronchiectasis are characterised by an increase in symptoms, *i.e.* increase in cough and change in purulence and volume of sputum associated with an increase in malaise. These exacerbations are almost always associated with infections of bronchiectasis. Aetiological agents of bronchiectasis include bacteria (*Haemophilus influenzae*, *Pseudomonas aeruginosa*, *Moraxella catarrhalis*, *Streptococcus pneumoniae* and *Staphylococcus aureus*), mycobacteria (*Mycobacterium avium-intracellulare* complex, *Myobacterium kansasii* and *Myobacterium fortuitum*) and fungi (*Aspergillus fumigatus*). The pattern of microbiology is quite stable; however, resistance to antibiotics may increase in time. *Pseudomonas* is associated with more severe disease. Nontuberculous mycobacteria are frequently associated with *Aspergillus*.

Underlying causes of bronchiectasis may be acquired or inherited, and include post-infective causes, mechanical obstruction, an excessive or deficient immune response, inflammatory pneumonitis, abnormal mucus clearance, and fibrosis. Conditions associated with bronchiectasis include infertility, inflammatory bowel disease, connective tissue disorders, malignancy, diffuse panbronchiolitis, α_1-antitrypsin deficiency and mercury poisoning. In adults, the aetiology is idiopathic in ~50% and in children, 25%; however, these figures may differ in time and between countries due to the availability of diagnostics and antibiotics (including vaccinations). Particularly in patients younger than 40 years of age, CF, primary ciliary dyskinesia (PCD) and common variable immunodeficiency should be considered, and in the presence of suggestive symptoms, further work-up is indicated.

Work-up

The work-up of bronchiectasis comprises the following.

- Blood tests: C-reactive protein, white blood count and differentiation, IgG, IgM, IgA, total IgE, *Aspergillus* serology, and α₁-antitrypsin
- Consider specific antibodies at baseline, and re-assay 21 days after immunisation where screening baseline levels are low
- Specific tests to identify underlying causes or contributing conditions depending on the clinical setting
- Spirometry
- Sputum smear and cultures for bacteria, mycobacteria and fungi
- Radiography of chest and sinus; if necessary, a HRCT scan of the lung

The chest radiograph is abnormal in most patients; however, a normal chest radiograph does not exclude bronchiectasis. HRCT is the 'gold standard' for bronchiectasis. Characteristic findings include internal bronchial diameters 1.5 times greater than that of the adjacent pulmonary artery (signet ring sign) (fig. 1), lack of bronchial tapering, visualisation of bronchi within 1 cm of the costal pleura, visualisation of the bronchi abutting the mediastinal pleura and bronchial wall thickening. The distribution of bronchiectasis on HRCT scan may give diagnostic clues to allergic bronchopulmonary aspergillosis (central/perihilar), CF (upper lobes), PCD (middle lobe) and idiopathic bronchiectasis (lower lobes). Severity of bronchiectasis on HRCT images is poorly correlated with clinical indices.

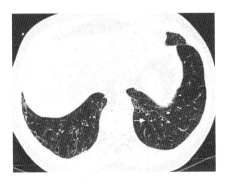

Figure 1. HRCT image demonstrating the signet ring sign (arrow). Reproduced and modified from Perera et al. (2011).

Management

Management of bronchiectasis should aim for:

- fast resolution and prevention of infective exacerbations,
- no sputum infections,
- optimal bronchial clearance,
- minimal respiratory symptoms,
- normal lung function,
- high quality of life, and
- no treatment-related adverse effects.

Obviously, the prompt recognition and treatment of the underlying cause(s) and/or condition(s) is important for both short- and long-term outcomes. Unfortunately, there are only limited high-quality studies on the management of non-CF bronchiectasis. Several reviews list a large number of treatment options; however, due to small study samples, different study populations and outcome variables, and other methodological issues, it is difficult to draw definitive conclusions. A recent extensive guideline of the British Thoracic Society (BTS) has assessed the level of evidence for each referred paper and the grade of each recommendation (Pasteur *et al.*, 2010).

Acute exacerbations Antibiotic treatment is the mainstay of acute exacerbations and is targeted to probable organisms (table 1) or the results of sputum culture(s). A fluoroquinolone is recommended for 7–10 days in outpatients without a history of recurrent exacerbations or sputum cultures. Hospitalised patients may be treated with two intravenous antibiotics with efficacy for *Pseudomonas* (www.uptodate.com). Supportive management may consist of inhaled bronchodilators, systemic corticosteroids and measures to improve bronchial clearance (physical therapy, hydration and mucolytic agents).

Prevention of exacerbations Prolonged use of antibiotics (>4 weeks) may be considered in patients who quickly relapse (three or more times per year according to the BTS guideline) or demonstrate progressive lung function decline. Several treatment strategies have been described:

- oral antibiotic two or three times daily
- oral macrolide three times weekly
- aerosoled tobramycin, gentamycin, colistin, ceftazidime or aztreonam twice daily (aerosoled antibiotics in non-CF bronchiectasis are frequently not licensed or stopped because of side-effects)
- *i.v.* antibiotics, 2–3-week courses with 1–2-month intervals (www.uptodate.com)

A Cochrane review concluded that there is a small benefit in overall clinical response scores but not exacerbation rates. A recent randomised controlled trial (RCT) demonstrated that 500 mg azithromycin three times a week for 6 months significantly improved exacerbation frequency in adult non-CF bronchiectasis patients with a history of at least one exacerbation in the past year (Wong *et al.*, 2012).

Clearly, the indication for prolonged use of antibiotics should be based on a benefit–risk evaluation, also taking possible adverse effects into account.

Sputum and bronchial clearance Inhaled recombinant human DNAse (rhDNAse) administered to stable non-CF bronchiectasis patients has been associated with increased exacerbation frequency and greater FEV_1 decline, and therefore should *not* be given. Oral bromhexine improved expectoration, quantity and quality of sputum, and auscultatory findings during acute infective exacerbations. Macrolides improved sputum production and sputum

inflammatory markers. 12-day inhalation of mannitol improved the tenacity and hydration of sputum. Inhaled fluticasone improved sputum production and sputum inflammation, but not its microbiological profile. Nebulised 0.9% and 7% saline as an adjunct to physiotherapy improved sputum production, sputum viscosity and ease of sputum expectoration; 7% saline was superior to 0.9%. Two systematic reviews found insufficient evidence to support or refute bronchial hygiene physical therapy.

Symptoms and quality of life Haemoptysis is treated with bronchial embolisation; however, surgical resection is sometimes inevitable. Surgical resection may also be considered if the area of the bronchiectatic lung is localised and if the patient's symptoms are debilitating or life threatening. In this case, surgery can even be curative if there is an absence of an ongoing underlying cause. Although surgery is widely used, there have been no RCTs of this. Recent studies reported that selected cases were treated successfully with lobectomy using video-assisted thoracoscopy. Inhaled fluticasone improved dyspnoea, sputum production, days without cough, β_2-agonist use and health-related quality of life. Inhaled medium-dose budesonide combined with formoterol in a single inhaler was more effective than high-dose budesonide (Martinez-Garcia *et al.*, 2012).

Lung function RCTs on short- and long-acting β_2-agonists, anticholinergic therapy, oral methylxanthines, leukotriene antagonists, and oral corticosteroids were not included in Cochrane reviews. Nevertheless, bronchodilator therapy may be considered if a patient has proven airway obstruction. Macrolides may improve methacholine reactivity, airway obstruction and carbon monoxide diffusion. However, if macrolides are considered, nontuberculous mycobacteria must be excluded first and patients must be warned about ototoxicity.

Exercise tolerance Pulmonary rehabilitation is effective in improving exercise capacity and endurance, whereas simultaneous inspiratory muscle training may be important in the longevity of these training effects.

Further reading

- Clinical Evidence Handbook. Bronchiectasis. http://clinicalevidence.bmj.com/ceweb/conditions/rdc/1507/1507.jsp
- The Cochrane Collaboration. The Cochrane Library. www.thecochranelibrary.com
- Ilowite J, et al. (2009). Pharmacological treatment options for bronchiectasis: focus on antimicrobial and anti-inflammatory agents. Drugs; 69: 407–419.
- Lynch DA, et al. (1999). Correlation of CT findings with clinical evaluations in 261 patients with symptomatic bronchiectasis. AJR Am J Roentgenol; 173: 53–58.
- Martinez-Garcia MA, et al. (2012). Clinical efficacy and safety of budesonide-formoterol in non-cystic fibrosis bronchiectasis. Chest; 141: 461–468.
- Nicotra MB, et al. (1995). Clinical, pathophysiologic, and microbiologic characterization of bronchiectasis in an aging cohort. Chest; 108: 955–961.
- Ouellette H (1999). The signet ring sign. Radiology; 212: 67–68.
- Rosen MJ (2006). Chronic cough due to bronchiectasis: ACCP evidence-based clinical practice guidelines. Chest; 129: Suppl. 1, 122S–131S.
- Pasteur MC, et al. (2010). British Thoracic Society guideline for non-CF bronchiectasis. Thorax; 65: Suppl. 1, i1–i58.
- Pasteur MC, et al. (2000). An investigation into causative factors in patients with bronchiectasis. Am J Respir Crit Care Med; 162: 1277–1284.
- Perera PL, et al. (2011). Radiological features of bronchiectasis. Eur Respir Monogr; 52: 44–67.
- Ten Hacken NH, et al. (2011). Bronchiectasis. Clin Evid; 2011: 1507.
- Wolters Kluwer Health. UpToDate. www.uptodate.com
- Wong C, et al. (2012). Azithromycin for prevention of exacerbations in non-cystic fibrosis bronchiectasis (EMBRACE): a randomised, double-blind, placebo-controlled trial. Lancet; 380: 660–667.

Cystic fibrosis

Andrew Bush and Jane C. Davies

Key points

- Adult pulmonologists need to know about CF; it is common across Europe, patients are surviving into middle age and beyond, and new diagnoses of CF are being made even in old age; as diagnosis by newborn screening becomes more widespread across Europe, it is likely that fitter CF patients will be transferred to the adult clinics, and survival will improve further.

- CF is now a true multisystem disease; to the well-known complications of chronic respiratory infection and malabsorption have been added conditions such as cirrhosis, insulin deficiency and diabetes, osteopenia, stress incontinence, and infertility.

- Furthermore, with longevity are coming new complications, including the selection of resistant microorganisms and antibiotic allergy; other organ systems will probably be affected in the aging CF population.

- Treatment of CF thus requires a dedicated multidisciplinary team, comprising physicians, specialist nurses, physiotherapists, dieticians, clinical psychologists and pharmacists.

- The increasing knowledge of the molecular pathophysiology of CF is leading the way in the development of genotype-specific therapies, which will be a paradigm for other diseases.

The autosomal recessive condition CF is the most common inherited disease of white races; its prevalence varies across Europe. Although commonest in white people, it has been found in virtually every ethnic group. The gene, on the long arm of chromosome 7, encodes a multifunctional protein, cystic fibrosis transmembrane regulator (CFTR), which is active at the apical membrane of epithelial cells. The nomenclature of the individual CF genes has recently been revised (table 1). Different classes of mutation have been described (fig. 1); severe mutations (classes I–III) are usually associated with pancreatic-insufficient CF and a worse prognosis, whereas those with milder mutations (IV–VI) are more usually pancreatic sufficient. The combination of a mild and severe gene usually leads to a mild pancreatic phenotype; however, there is only a poor correlation between genotype and pulmonary phenotype. In many parts of Europe, the most common mutation is Phe508del (previously termed ΔF508), but there are marked ethnic differences.

CFTR functions as a chloride channel and regulates other ion channels, such as the epithelial sodium channel (ENaC). Most of the morbidity and mortality of CF is due to chronic bronchial infection, but as adults survive longer, multisystem complications are becoming more important. The airways of the newborn with CF are effectively normal at birth, but from an early age, cycles of infection and inflammation supervene, leading ultimately to severe bronchiectasis and respiratory failure. The most popular hypothesis for the pathophysiology of CF lung disease is airway surface liquid dehydration due to uncontrolled activity of

Table 1. Old and new nomenclature of the 32 common CFTR mutations (ARMS-32 kit)

Old Nomenclature	New nomenclature
ΔF508	p.Phe508del
ΔI507	p.Ile507del
V520F	p.Val520Phe
R117H	p.Arg117His
G542X	p.Gly542X
G551D	p.Gly551Asp
R553X	p.Arg553X
R560T	p.Arg560Thr
S549R	p.Ser549Arg
S549N	p.Ser549Asn
3659delC	p.Thr1176fs
W1282X	p.Trp1282X
3905insT	p.Leu1258fs
N1303K	p.Asn1303Lys
G85E	p.Gly85Glu
A455E	p.Ala455Glu
R334W	p.Arg334Trp
1078delT	p.Phe316fs
R347H	p.Arg347His
R347P	p.Arg347Pro
2183AA>G	p.Lys684fs
1717-1G>A	
621+1G>T	
3849+10kbC>T	
711+1G>T	
1898+1G>A	
2789+5G>A	
R1162X	p.Arg1162X
3876delA	p.Ser1248fs
3120+1G>A	
394delTT	p.Leu88fs
2184delA	p.Lys684fs

ENaC, possibly triggered by viral infection. Median survival for current newborns is predicted to be ~50 yrs, longer for males. In parts of Europe there are now more adult than paediatric CF patients.

Adult physicians will encounter CF patients by two routes:

1. *Referral from a paediatric clinic of an already diagnosed patient.* Transition to a new and strange adult clinic from the familiar staff and surroundings of the paediatric clinic may be a difficult time, and needs to be handled with sensitivity. Increasingly, young adult handover clinics, staffed by paediatricians and adult physicians, are being set up.

2. *A new diagnosis made in adult life.* CF is usually diagnosed in early childhood, increasingly by newborn screening, but mild atypical cases may be missed. Around 10–15% of CF patients present in adult life (table 2). Conversely, always consider the possibility that the diagnosis of CF made in childhood is incorrect and whether a repeat diagnostic work-up should be done. The diagnosis should be considered even in people born in areas where CF newborn screening is offered. Mild cases may be missed by screening; the screening test may not have been performed or the result lost; there may have been a technical issue in the laboratory; and finally, the patient may have moved from an area where screening is not offered.

Diagnostic testing for CF

Once the diagnosis is suspected, it is usually easily confirmed by a sweat test, which must be performed in an experienced centre.

Other diagnostic modalities that are employed include:

- *Genetic testing:* >1,800 variants are described and many rare ones are usually undetected in the routine clinical laboratory, so a negative genotype cannot exclude disease. Furthermore, <50 mutations are definitely accepted as disease-causing, so the presence of rare mutations should always be interpreted with caution. There is an ongoing US CF Foundation project which aims to try to clarify the significance of these rarer mutations (www.cftr2.org).

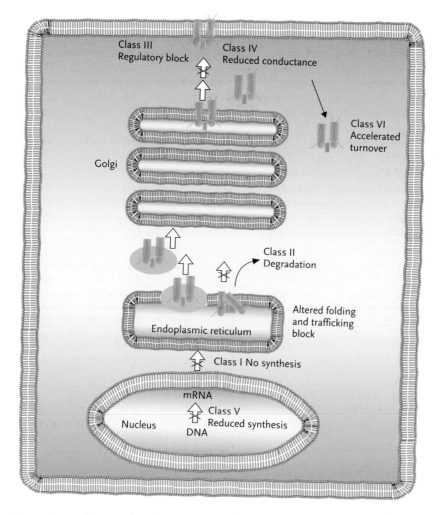

Figure 1. Classes of CF mutation. Class I: no CFTR synthesis (mutation: premature stop codon; G542X, now termed p.Gly542X); class II: CFTR processed incorrectly and does not reach apical cell membrane (Phe508del); class III: CFTR reaches apical membrane, but channel opening time is reduced (G551D, now termed p.Gly551Asp); class IV: CFTR reaches apical membrane, but channel conductance is abnormal (R117H, now known as p.Arg117His); class V: reduced CFTR synthesis (3849 + 10kb C>T, nomenclature unchanged); class VI: CFTR reaches apical cell membrane, but has a shortened half-life due to more rapid turnover (Q1412X, in which the last 70 amino acids are deleted).

- *Nasal transepithelial potential difference measurement:* only available in a few centres.
- *Ancillary testing:* human faecal elastase (pancreatic insufficiency), high-resolution computed tomography for occult bronchiectasis, scrotal ultrasound or

semen analysis for congenital bilateral absence of the vas deferens (CBAVD).

Management of CF

CF has now become a true multisystem disease. Treatment can only be optimally conducted with the help of a full

Table 2. Late presentation of CF

Recurrent respiratory infections	Consider especially with 'suggestive' microorganisms such as *Staphylococcus aureus, Pseudomonas aeruginosa, Burkholderia cepacia* complex
Atypical 'asthma'	Especially if chronic productive cough, and a poor response to standard asthma therapy
Bronchiectasis	Especially if any extrapulmonary features, a positive family history or infection with atypical microorganisms (above)
Nasal polyps, severe sinusitis	Nasal polyps more likely due to aspirin-sensitive asthma, unlike in children, in whom they are virtually diagnostic of CF
Male infertility	Azoospermia due to CBAVD
Electrolyte disturbance	Classically as acute heat exhaustion leading to sodium, chloride and potassium depletion
Atypical mycobacterial infection	Always consider the possibility of CF if these organisms are isolated from sputum
Acute pancreatitis	Typically seen in pancreatic-sufficient CF
CF liver disease	Portal hypertension and variceal haemorrhage; liver cell failure is a late manifestation
Cascade screening	Diagnosis made in a relative leading to extended family screening

Such patients are usually but not invariably pancreatic sufficient. New diagnoses of CF have been made even in old age; CF diagnosis should always be considered.

multidisciplinary team (CF physician, specialist nurse, physiotherapist, dietician, clinical psychologist and pharmacist) and the help of ancillary specialists with expert knowledge of CF (ENT surgeon, obstetrician, and endocrinologist) (table 3). CF patients should be seen at least every 3 months by the core CF team. A large number of treatment guidelines have been published.

Respiratory tract disease The main issues are the prevention of infection where possible by segregation of patients and the aggressive use of antibiotics; although the conventional teaching is that airway infection occurs with a relatively narrow spectrum of microorganisms, recent work based on the use of molecular techniques suggests much greater numbers of infecting organisms including anaerobes. Molecular techniques are still in the research arena and cannot be used to guide clinical decisions. Sputum clearance using a choice of many chest physiotherapy techniques and the identification and aggressive management of late

complications are also important. If the patient has poor lung function, early discussion with the local transplant centre is advisable. Routine respiratory care at every clinic visit should include spirometry and pulse oximetry, and sputum (or cough swab) culture.

Recently, the importance of CF exacerbations has been appreciated. They have more than mere nuisance value, and are termed 'CF lung attacks' by some. There is no uniformly accepted definition, even though time to first exacerbation is a common end-point in clinical trials. Around 25% of patients never return to their pre-exacerbation spirometry values, and frequent exacerbations are a marker of accelerated decline in lung function.

Gastrointestinal disease (table 4) The main issues are to ensure optimal nutrition and be alert to gastrointestinal causes of weight loss that are unrelated to pancreatic insufficiency. Bad nutrition is a very poor prognostic feature. CF patients have higher than normal energy requirements because of

Table 3. Management of CF lung disease

Disease Stage	Pulmonary status	Aim	Management
Early (unusual but seen in adults with milder forms of CF)	Pre-infection	Mucus clearance	Airway clearance techniques (physiotherapy and adjuncts) These include exercise and mucolytics (e.g. rhDNase, hypertonic saline, inhaled mannitol)
		Prevent infection	Segregation and cohorting to prevent cross-infection Prophylactic antibiotics controversial: used against S. aureus in UK but not in USA and other parts of Europe; avoid cephalosporins Prophylaxis against P. aeruginosa with nebulised colomycin has been trialled and is without benefit Influenza vaccination
	Intermittent isolation of Pseudomonas aeruginosa	Eradication of infection; energetic treatment is essential	High doses of appropriate antibiotics P. aeruginosa eradication protocols include both topical (nebulised) and systemic (usually oral ciprofloxacin) Eradication achieved in 80–90%; however, a recent trial has shown no additional benefit from prolonged eradication regimes
Intermediate	Chronic infection with usual organisms (Pseudomonas aeruginosa, eventually present in 80% of patients; Staphylococcus aureus, methicillin resistant and sensitive); less usually Haemophilus influenzae)	Suppression of bacterial load and, thus, limitation of inflammatory response	Depends on organism: P. aeruginosa, nebulised high dose tobramycin (300 mg twice daily) or colomycin Nebulised aztreonam lysine more expensive, but now available, and other nebulised antibiotics are in development Use the new, faster nebuliser devices, e.g. eFlow (PARI GmbH, Starnberg, Germany) and I-neb (Philips Respironics, Murrysville, PA, USA), or the newly available dry powder devices

Table 3. Continued

Disease Stage	Pulmonary status	Aim	Management
		Treat infective exacerbations	Oral or intravenous antibiotics (some centres use regular elective courses, but no evidence to prefer this over symptomatic use) Culture results usually guide choice, but no evidence that this improves outcome
		Reduce inflammation (it is controversial whether the CF airway is intrinsically pro-inflammatory or there is merely a greater airway inflammatory response to infection than normal)	No evidence for a role for corticosteroids except in treating ABPA, because of efficacy but adverse side-effect profile (oral) or lack of benefit (inhaled) Ibuprofen not much used in most of Europe; beware synergistic nephrotoxicity with intravenous aminoglycosides Azithromycin is useful, but mode of action unknown
	Infection with less common organisms (*Burkholderia cepacia* complex, *Stenotrophomonas maltophilia, Achromobacter xylosoxidans*)	Eradication if early; suppression of bacterial load most commonly	Confirm diagnosis in a reference laboratory Treat on an individual basis with specialist microbiological advice
	ABPA	Reduce allergic response Prevent bronchiectasis	Oral corticosteroids (long course often required), consider pulsed methyl prednisolone Addition of an antifungal agent common but evidence limited
	Nontuberculous *mycobacterial* infection	Eradication or suppression (*Mycobacterium abscessus* may be very difficult to eradicate)	Infection with these organisms appears to be becoming more common Diagnosis and management difficult; seek specialist advice, especially for *Mycobacterium abscessus* infection Prolonged courses of multiple chemotherapies will be needed: ethambutol, rifampicin, azithromycin, amikacin, ciprofloxacin, moxifloxacin are among the agents used

Table 3. *Continued*

Disease Stage	Pulmonary status	Aim	Management
	Lobar or segmental atelectasis (may be seen at any stage of CF)	Re-inflation of the lung	Intensive physiotherapy, with rhDNase and hypertonic saline as appropriate Intravenous antibiotics Fibreoptic bronchoscopy; consider endobronchial instillation of rhDNase if conventional management fails
Late	Major haemoptysis (may be seen also in those with well-preserved lung function)	Prevent or halt acute bleeding	Admit for intravenous antibiotics and clotting studies; bronchoscopy not useful Bronchial artery embolisation for ongoing bleeding; can consider the use of tranexamic acid Lobectomy is a last resort
	Pneumothorax (carries a very bad prognosis)	Control air leak Prevent recurrence	Conservative management for trivial pneumothoraces, otherwise tube drainage Early surgery and pleurodesis if does not respond rapidly
	End-stage respiratory failure	Optimise conventional treatment	Oxygen therapy (no survival benefit demonstrated, unlike for COPD) Consider nasal ventilation as a bridge to transplantation
		Refer for lung transplant assessment	
Iatrogenic (usually late unless acquired by cross-infection)	Novel particularly Gram-negative organisms	Prevention by segregation, careful hygiene and targeted use of antibiotics when treating conventional organisms	Seek specialist microbiological advice if treatment is contemplated
	Antibiotic-resistant organisms		

ABPA: allergic bronchopulmonary aspergillosis; rhDNase: recombinant human deoxyribonuclease.

Table 4. Management of gastrointestinal manifestations of CF in the adult

Organ	Manifestation	Management
Pancreas	Exocrine insufficiency: malabsorption, steatorrhoea	High-fat diet Supplementation with enteric coated microsphere pancreatic enzymes and fat-soluble vitamins Fat absorption may be aided by alkaline environment (H_2-blockers or proton pump inhibitors) Gastrostomy feeds if in nutritional failure (parenteral nutrition only rarely required)
	Acute pancreatitis (pancreatic sufficient patients)	As for other causes Oral pancreatin powder (anecdotal evidence only)
Oesophagus	Gastro-oesophageal reflux (especially common post-lung transplant)	Proton pump inhibitors, prokinetic agents Surgery if refractory symptoms
Small bowel	DIOS	Oral Gastrografin (Bracco, Princeton, NJ, USA) or Klean-Prep (Norgine, Amsterdam, the Netherlands) Review dose of, and adherence to, pancreatic enzyme replacement therapy; perform 3-day faecal fat collection Consider pro-kinetic agents Severe acute cases, relieve with colonoscopy; laparotomy a last resort
	Coeliac disease (increased incidence in CF)	Gluten-free diet, as for isolated coeliac disease
	Crohn's disease (any part of the bowel)	Management as for isolated Crohn's disease Seek specialist gastroenterology advice
Colon	Constipation	Laxatives, high-fibre diet Must not be confused with DIOS
Rectum	Rectal prolapse	Rare in adults, usually related to uncontrolled fat malabsorption
Liver	Fatty liver (usually asymptomatic) Macronodular cirrhosis (variceal bleeding, splenomegaly, hypersplenism) Hepatocellular failure a late manifestation	Liver ultrasound at least every 2 years Ursodeoxycholic acid, taurine (seek specialist advice) Severe cases may need transplantation

DIOS: distal intestinal obstruction syndrome.

subclinical malabsorption and a higher energy consumption secondary to infection. Increased metabolic rate is thought by some to be part of the underlying defect. Weight should be measured and BMI calculated at least 3-monthly.

Other organ system disease (table 5) It is important to be aware that new complications are being described as CF patients survive longer. A full systems review is essential at each clinic visit. Finally, the psychological aspects of CF, the effects

Table 5. Treatment of other manifestations of CF in the adult

Organ	Manifestation	Management
Upper airway	Nasal polyps (can cause OSA)	Topical steroids; long courses of antibiotics
		Surgery if medical management fails; re-operation often needed
	Sinusitis	Most patients have asymptomatic changes on radiography or CT scan and require no treatment
		Topical steroids and antibiotics are given initially in prolonged courses if mandated by symptoms
		Surgery if medical management fails, but results often disappointing
		Some use sinus drainage tubes and repeatedly instil antibiotics into the sinuses
Endocrine pancreas	Insulin deficiency, which causes reduced lung function and nutrition before overt hyperglycaemia	Screen regularly with annual glucose tolerance test
		Increasingly, continuous glucose monitoring is used to diagnose this condition
	Frank diabetes; although there may be an element of peripheral insulin resistance, the main root cause is diminished insulin secretion	Have a low threshold for starting insulin, especially in females, who have a worse prognosis if they develop diabetes
		Continue high-fat diet, adjust insulin doses accordingly
		Diabetic ketoacidosis is very rare
		Oral hypoglycaemic agents not to be used outside a randomised controlled trial
Sweat gland	Electrolyte depletion, often leading to acute collapse	Sodium and potassium chloride supplementation
Bones and joints	Osteopenia (CFTR is expressed in bones)	Measure bone mineral density at least every 2 years
	Pathological fracture	Prevention: weight-bearing exercise, high dairy intake, vitamin D and K therapy
		Treat with bisphosphonates if severe
	CF arthropathy (large or small joint)	Nonsteroidal anti-inflammatory agents, prednisolone
		Seek specialist rheumatological advice if more than mild
Male reproductive tract	CBAVD leading to male infertility	Sperm aspiration and *in vitro* fertilisation
		Genetic counselling prior to procedure
Female reproductive tract	Vaginal candidiasis	Topical antifungal agents

Table 5. Continued

Organ	Manifestation	Management
	Stress incontinence	Seek gynaecological advice
	Pregnancy (not an illness, but may be a major therapeutic challenge); females with severe CF may be subfertile, but normal conception is usual	Pre-pregnancy genetic counselling advisable Continue standard CF medications; close collaboration with obstetric unit; may need regular admissions to hospital for intravenous antibiotics. Especially beware if low lung function prior to pregnancy and CF related diabetes on insulin
Late iatrogenic	Antibiotic allergy	Consider desensitisation in hospital
	Chronic renal failure	Cause controversial Variously related to multiple courses of intravenous aminoglycosides, so use these agents appropriately sparingly, and diabetes, so work to ensure good glycaemic control
Miscellaneous	Vasculitis	Rare, usually responds to steroids, but seek specialist rheumatological advice
	Epithelial cancer	Small but definite increase in risk; careful clinical surveillance mandatory

of chronic illness, and the burden of disease and its treatment should not be underestimated; see the poignant stories and poetry on the Breathing Room website.

Future developments

A large number of novel therapies are currently being trialled in CF. Gene therapy, using as vectors either liposomes, viruses or nanoparticles, has been the subject of proof-of-concept trials, and a large therapeutic trial is about to start (www.cfgenetherapy.org. uk). The age of genotype-specific therapy dawned with the use of agents such oral ataluren (PTC_{124}) to override premature stop codons (class I mutations); the results of a large phase III trial have been reported at the US CFF meeting; significance was not reached with the primary end-point but in a planned subgroup analysis, those not receiving nebulised tobramycin, a compound which also overrides premature stop codons, did show significant improvements. More work is needed to determine the role of PTC124 in CF. Other approaches include the use of 'correctors' to allow misfolded protein (class II mutations) to travel to the apical cell membrane (VX-809 and VX-661, currently in early-phase trials) and 'potentiators' to improve activity when they reach this site. The most successful of these has been ivacaftor (Kalydeco, VX-770; Vertex, Cambridge, MA, USA), which has been shown to improve lung function significantly in patients with the commonest class III mutation, p.Gly551Asp (G551D). This agent works by increasing the probability that CFTR will be open and, therefore, may also be useful for other classes of mutations where CFTR reaches the apical membrane including other rare Class III mutations, or in conjunction with correctors for class II mutations. Alternative strategies under investigation include inhibition of ENaC and stimulation of alternative chloride channels; unfortunately, trials with the P2Y2 receptor agonist denufosol, despite showing some early promise, have recently been reported as negative. There is no doubt that we are on the verge of a CF treatment revolution. Most important, however, is to ensure that the basic therapy, which has so greatly improved prognosis, is not neglected here and now.

Further reading

- Amaral MD (2011). Targeting CFTR: how to treat cystic fibrosis by CFTR-repairing therapies. *Curr Drug Targets*; 12: 683–693.
- Becq F (2010). Cystic fibrosis transmembrane conductance regulator modulators for personalized drug treatment of cystic fibrosis: progress to date. *Drugs*; 70: 241–259.
- Bilton D, *et al.* (2011). Inhaled dry powder mannitol in cystic fibrosis: an efficacy and safety study. *Eur Respir J*; 38: 1071–1080.
- Bittar F, *et al.* (2008). Molecular detection of multiple emerging pathogens in sputa from cystic fibrosis patients. *PLoS One*; 3: e2908.
- Breathing Room. Caregiver Stories. www.thebreathingroom.org/cg
- Brenckmann C, *et al.* (2001). Bisphosphonates for osteoporosis in people with cystic fibrosis. *Cochrane Database Syst Rev*; 4: CD002010.
- Brinson GM, *et al.* (1998). Bronchial artery embolization for the treatment of hemoptysis in patients with cystic fibrosis. *Am J Respir Crit Care Med*; 157: 1951–1958.
- Bush A. *In:* European Lung White Book. Sheffield, European Respiratory Society, 2003; pp. 89–95.
- CFTR2. www.cftr2.org
- Chaun H (2001). Colonic disorders in adult cystic fibrosis. *Can J Gastroenterol*; 15: 586–590.
- Clancy JP, *et al.* (2012). Results of a phase IIa study of VX-809, an investigational CFTR corrector compound, in subjects with cystic fibrosis homozygous for the F508del-CFTR mutation. *Thorax*; 67: 12–18.
- Colombo C, *et al.* (2006). Liver disease in cystic fibrosis. *J Pediatr Gastroenterol Nutr*; 43: Suppl. 1, S49–S55.
- Cystic Fibrosis Mutation Database www.genet.sickkids.on.ca/cftr
- Davies JC, *et al.* (2010). Gene therapy for cystic fibrosis. *Proc Am Thorac Soc*; 7: 408–414.
- Dodge JA, *et al.* (2007). Cystic fibrosis mortality and survival in the UK: 1947–2003. *Eur Respir J*; 29: 522–526.
- de Boer K, *et al.* (2011). Exacerbation frequency and clinical outcomes in adult patients with cystic fibrosis. *Thorax*; 66: 680–685.
- Farrell PM, *et al.* (2008). Guidelines for diagnosis of cystic fibrosis in newborns through older adults: Cystic Fibrosis Foundation consensus report. *J Pediatr*; 153: S4–S14.
- Festini F, *et al.* (2006). Isolation measures for prevention of infection with respiratory pathogens in cystic fibrosis: a systematic review. *J Hosp Infect*; 64: 1–6.
- Flume PA, *et al.* (2007). Cystic fibrosis pulmonary guidelines: chronic medications for maintenance of lung health. *Am J Respir Crit Care Med*; 176: 957–969.
- Flume PA, *et al.* (2005). Massive hemoptysis in cystic fibrosis. *Chest*; 128: 729–738.
- Flume PA, *et al.* (2005). Pneumothorax in cystic fibrosis. *Chest*; 128: 720–728.
- Kerem E, *et al.* (2008). Effectiveness of PTC124 treatment of cystic fibrosis caused by nonsense mutations: a prospective phase II trial. *Lancet*; 372: 719–727.
- Kim RD, *et al.* (2008). Pulmonary nontuberculous mycobacterial disease: prospective study of a distinct preexisting syndrome. *Am J Respir Crit Care Med*; 178: 1066–1074.
- Ledson MJ, *et al.* (1998). Prevalence and mechanisms of gastro-oesophageal reflux in adult cystic fibrosis patients. *J R Soc Med*; 91: 7–9.
- Leus J, *et al.* (2000). Detection and follow up of exocrine pancreatic insufficiency in cystic fibrosis: a review. *Eur J Pediatr*; 159: 563–568.
- Matsui H, *et al.* (1998). Evidence for periciliary liquid layer depletion, not abnormal ion composition, in the pathogenesis of cystic fibrosis airways disease. *Cell*; 95: 1005–1015.
- McKone EF, *et al.* (2003). Effect of genotype on phenotype and mortality in cystic fibrosis: a retrospective cohort study. *Lancet*; 361: 1671–1676.
- Nick JA, *et al.* (2005). Manifestations of cystic fibrosis diagnosed in adulthood. *Curr Opin Pulm Med*; 11: 513–518.

- Onady GM, *et al.* (2005). Insulin and oral agents for managing cystic fibrosis-related diabetes. *Cochrane Database Syst Rev*; 3: CD004730.
- Ramsey BW, *et al.* (2011). A CFTR potentiator in patients with cystic fibrosis and the G551D mutation. *N Engl J Med*; 365: 1663–1672.
- Rowe SM, *et al.* (2011). Nasal potential difference measurements to assess CFTR ion channel activity. *Methods Mol Biol*; 741: 69–86.
- Southern KW, *et al.* (2004). Macrolide antibiotics for cystic fibrosis. *Cochrane Database Syst Rev*; 2: CD002203.
- Tarran R, *et al.* (2005). Normal and cystic fibrosis airway surface liquid homeostasis. The effects of phasic shear stress and viral infections. *J Biol Chem*; 280: 35751–35759.
- Tunney MM, *et al.* (2008). Detection of anaerobic bacteria in high numbers in sputum from patients with cystic fibrosis. *Am J Respir Crit Case Med*; 177: 995–1001.
- UK Cystic Fibrosis Gene Therapy Consortium. www.cfgenetherapy.org.uk
- United Kingdom National External Quality Assessment Service. www.ukneqas.org.uk
- Witt H, *et al.* (2007). Chronic pancreatitis: challenges and advances in pathogenesis, genetics, diagnosis, and therapy. *Gastroenterology*; 132: 1557–1573.
- Wood DM, *et al.* (2006). Antibiotic strategies for eradicating *Pseudomonas aeruginosa* in people with cystic fibrosis. *Cochrane Database Syst Rev*; 1: CD004197.
- Yung MW, *et al.* (2002). Nasal polyposis in children with cystic fibrosis: a long-term follow-up study. *Ann Otol Rhinol Laryngol*; 111: 1081–1086.

Work-related and occupational asthma

Eleftherios Zervas and Mina Gaga

Definition

Work-related asthma (WRA) is the most common form of occupational lung disease, causing significant morbidity and disability. WRA accounts for 9–15% of cases of asthma in adults of working age.

WRA may be categorised as:

- occupational asthma (OA), which refers to asthma caused specifically by exposure to an agent present at the workplace; or
- work-aggravated or work-exacerbated asthma (WEA), in which pre-existing asthma is exacerbated by conditions in the work environment.

Thus, the American College of Chest Physicians consensus document and British Occupational Health Research Foundation guidelines define WRA as including OA (*i.e.* asthma induced by sensitiser or irritant work exposures) and WEA (*i.e.* pre-existing or concurrent asthma worsened by work factors).

OA can occur in workers with or without prior asthma and can be subdivided into:

1. sensitiser-induced OA, characterised by a latency period between first exposure to a respiratory sensitiser at work and the development of symptoms

2. irritant-induced OA that occurs typically within a few hours of a high-concentration exposure to an irritant gas, fume or vapour at work

When the causal exposure consists of a single inhalation incident, the condition is commonly called reactive airway dysfunction syndrome.

> **Key points**
>
> - The burden of WRA is still very high, accounting for one in 10 cases of adult asthma, and causing morbidity, disability and high costs.
>
> - Prevention is very important. Health officials, workplace managers and doctors must be aware of the problem, and strict measures for exposures to known sensitisers should always be followed, conditions at work examined and, when necessary, amended.
>
> - Better education of workers and managerial staff as well as medical professionals is key to the prevention and prompt diagnosis and management of WRA and OA. When WRA is diagnosed, prompt management is required and consists of removing or reducing exposure through elimination or substitution of causative agents and, where this is not possible, by effective control of exposure.
>
> - Pharmaceutical treatment of OA follows the general asthma guidelines.

In clinical practice, it is often difficult to differentiate between 'true' OA and aggravation of pre-existing asthma. Conversely, aggravation of symptoms related to work exposure, even in the absence of new sensitisation, requires individual and collective measures in the workplace, similar to OA. A recent consensus definition is that 'OA is defined as asthma induced by exposure in the working environment to airborne dusts, vapours or fumes, with or without pre-existing asthma' (Francis *et al.*, 2007). Physicians involved in adult asthma care need to be aware of the high prevalence of WRA and the importance of inducing or exacerbating factors at work.

Sensitising and triggering agents

More than 250 agents causing OA have been described and are categorised into high molecular weight (HMW) and low molecular weight (LMW) agents, according to whether their molecular weight is above or below 1 kDa. HMW agents are usually proteins of animal and vegetal origin such as flour, laboratory animal proteins and enzymes. LMW agents include a wide variety of chemicals, such as acid anhydrides, platinum salts and reactive dyes. Sensitisation to most HMW and some LMW factors is through an IgE mechanism and can be tested by skin tests. An immunological mechanism is suspected for LMW agents but has not been demonstrated, and an antigen-specific immune response cannot easily be tested in most affected workers.

The most frequently reported agents of occupational asthma are:

- isocyanates
- flour and grain dust
- colophony and fluxes
- latex
- animal and plant proteins
- aldehydes
- wood dust
- metal salts

Epidemiological studies have demonstrated that the level of exposure is the most important determinant of OA. This implies that preventive measures should be aimed at reducing workplace exposure. Prevention through elimination/reduction of exposure is the most effective approach for reducing the burden of OA. However, the relationship between the levels of exposure and the induction of OA is not always clear and the methodology of exposure assessment requires standardisation. Atopy increases the risk of developing OA in workers exposed to various sensitisers including enzymes, bakery allergens, laboratory animals, crab, prawn and acid anhydrides. The latent interval between first exposure and the onset of symptoms varies depending on the agent, the level of exposure/management and biological variability of exposure. The latent interval can extend to many years; however, the risk of OA appears to be highest soon after the first exposure to laboratory animal allergens, isocyanates, platinum salts and enzymes. See table 1 for a list of agents frequently identified by inhalational challenge.

Diagnosis

The clinical presentation and symptoms of OA are no different from nonoccupational asthma. Patients experience attacks of breathlessness, wheezing, cough, chest tightness and limitations in their daily activities. In any working adult patient presenting with such symptoms, the diagnosis of WRA should be considered. In individuals with suspected WRA, the physician should obtain a history of job duties and possible exposures, the use of protective devices and the presence of respiratory disease in co-workers. Table 2 shows examples of occupations/industries with sentinel health events for sensitiser-induced OA.

Symptoms may get worse when the patient enters the work environment but, very often, the patients experience delayed symptoms and therefore may get worse after leaving work. A clinically useful approach, therefore, is not asking whether the patients experience worsening of their symptoms when at work but rather whether they feel better after a weekend or a holiday away from work. However, this is difficult to describe, as most people feel rested and happier at the end of a holiday. The diagnosis requires first spirometry, with a positive bronchodilation test and/or histamine, methacholine or exercise testing of airway hyperresponsiveness for the confirmation of asthma. Furthermore, the

Table 1. LMW and HMW agents frequently identified by inhalational challenge

LMW agents	HMW agents
Isocyanates	Flour
HDI	Plants and grain dust
MDI	Seafood/fish
TDI	Latex
Metals	Animal-derived allergens
Plicatic acid (white or red cedar)	Leather
Wood dust	Enzymes
Hairdressing products	Talc
Epoxy resins	
Gums	
Dyes and fabrics	
Chemicals	
Perfume	

HDI: hexamethylene diisocyanate; MDI: methylene diphenyl diisocyanate; TDI: toluene diisocyanate. Information from Dufour et al. (2009).

Table 2. Examples of occupations/industries with sentinel health events for sensitiser-induced OA

Industry, process or occupation	Selected agents
Jewellery, alloy and catalyst makers	Platinum
Polyurethane, foam coatings, adhesive production and end-use settings (e.g. spray painters, and foam and foundry workers)	Isocyanates
Alloy, catalyst, refinery workers	Chromium, cobalt
Solderers	Soldering flux (colophony)
Plastics industry, dye, insecticide makers, organic chemical manufacture	Phthalic anhydride, trimetallic anhydride (used in epoxy resins)
Foam workers, latex makers, biologists, and hospital and laboratory workers	Formaldehyde
Printing industry	Gum arabic, reactive dyes and acrylates
Metal plating	Nickel sulfate and chromium
Bakers	Flour, amylase and other enzymes
Woodworkers and furniture makers	Red cedar (plicatic acid) and other wood dusts
Laboratory workers and animal researchers	Animal proteins
Detergent formulators	Detergent enzymes such as protease, amylase and lipase
Seafood (crab, snow crab and prawn) workers	Crab, prawn and other shellfish proteins
Healthcare workers and nurses	Psyllium, natural rubber latex, glutaraldehyde, methacrylates, antibiotics and detergent enzymes
Laxative manufacture and packing	Psyllium
Hairdressers and manicurists	Persulfates and acrylates (artificial nails)

Reproduced from Tarlo et al. (2008), with permission from the publisher.

patient should be asked to record symptoms, use of medication and peak expiratory flow (PEF) measurements when working and off work. PEF should be measured at least four times a day for a period of a month while times on and off work should be noted (the recommendation is at least 2 weeks on and 2 weeks off work). The sequential self-measurements of PEF can be complemented by repeated measurements of PC_{20} (the provocative concentration of histamine or methacholine causing a 20% fall in FEV_1). Allergic sensitisation to some inducers, such as animal proteins, can be examined by skin-prick testing or in vitro assays of specific IgE. When the diagnosis cannot be confirmed by serial PEF measurements and skin tests or IgE assays, the 'gold standard' for diagnosing sensitiser-induced OA is a specific bronchial provocation test (specific inhalation challenge), which may demonstrate a direct relationship between exposure to a test agent and an asthmatic response. The response may be early or late and may carry a risk to the patient of a severe reaction. Therefore, these tests should be performed only when necessary and only in specialised centres under medical supervision.

Management

Ideally, causal agents should be eliminated from the workplace, an option that is not often available. The second-best option is to remove the workers from exposure; however, many patients cannot leave their job. In such cases, the early institution of preventive measures, including the replacement of specific reagents where possible, the strict monitoring of exposure levels, and the use of extractor fans and masks, is necessary. The European Union (EU) has allocated a high priority to safeguarding the health and safety of workers. Existing EU health and safety legislation aims to minimise the health risks from dangerous substances in the workplace, placing the emphasis on their elimination and substitution in order to protect workers. There are four important directives in this field, containing the basic provisions for health and safety at work, and further defining the risks related to exposure to chemical agents, biological agents and carcinogens at work. Medical surveillance programmes are very important and may include symptom questionnaires, spirometry and skin-prick testing at regular intervals (e.g. every 6 or 12 months), as well as monitoring of exposure levels.

Once OA has developed, recovery is directly dependent on the duration and level of exposure to the causative agent. Depending on the severity of the case, the condition of the patient can substantially improve during the first year after removal from exposure. Conversely, asthma may persist even after removal from exposure to the causative workplace agent. The likelihood of improvement or resolution of symptoms or prevention of deterioration is greater in workers who have no further exposure to the causative agent, have relatively normal lung function at diagnosis, and have a shorter duration of symptoms prior to diagnosis and prior to avoidance of exposure.

Trigger avoidance is pivotal in preventing asthma symptoms and progression of severity. Nevertheless, pharmacological treatment is also required to control symptomatic patients. Pharmacological treatment follows the general asthma treatment guidelines, and inhaled steroids and β-agonists are the cornerstone of management. Treatment follows a stepwise approach based on asthma control and severity, and the approach is identical to that of nonoccupational asthma.

Socioeconomic impact of WRA

The economic impact of WRA is due not only to direct healthcare costs but also to indirect costs from impaired work productivity and compensation/ rehabilitation costs, as well as to the intangible costs from impaired quality of life. Income loss is more likely when avoidance of exposure leads to a change of job and this income loss is not offset by compensation. In many European countries, compensation does not include rehabilitation or retraining, perhaps accounting for the relatively high proportion (30%) of workers who continue to be exposed to the causative agent.

Moreover, when considering the cost of OA and/or compensation, it is not only lung function impairment and optimal asthma treatment that need to be taken into account, but also psychogenic factors. These can play an important role in the quality of life of OA patients, and significant prevalence of anxiety and depression has been shown in that population.

Further reading

- Ameille J, et al. (1997). Consequences of occupational asthma on employment and financial status: a follow-up study. *Eur Respir J*; 10: 55–58.
- Dufour M-H, et al. (2009). Comparative airway response to high- *versus* low-molecular weight agents in occupational asthma. *Eur Respir J*; 33: 734–739.
- Dykewicz MS (2009). Occupational asthma: current concepts in pathogenesis, diagnosis, and management. *J Allergy Clin Immunol*; 123: 519–528.
- Francis HC, et al. (2007). Defining and investigating occupational asthma: a consensus approach. *Occup Environ Med.*; 64: 361–365.
- Larbanois A, et al. (2002). Socioeconomic outcome of subjects experiencing asthma symptoms at work. *Eur Respir J*; 19: 1107–1113.
- Moscato G, et al. (2003). Diagnosing occupational asthma: how, how much, how far? *Eur Respir J*; 21: 879–885.
- Mullan RJ, et al. (1991). Occupational sentinel health events: an up-dated list for physician recognition and public health surveillance. *Am J Ind Med*; 19: 775–799.
- Nemery B (2004). Occupational asthma for the clinician. *Breathe*; 1: 25–32.
- Newman Taylor AJ, et al., eds. Guidelines for the prevention, identification and management of occupational asthma: evidence review and recommendations. London, British Occupational Health Research Foundation, 2004.
- Newman Taylor AJ (1980). Occupational asthma. *Thorax*; 35: 241–245.
- Tarlo SM, et al. (2008). Diagnosis and management of work-related asthma: American College of Chest Physicians Consensus Statement. *Chest*; 134: Suppl. 3, 1S–41S.
- Tarlo SM, et al. (2009). An official ATS proceedings: asthma in the workplace: the Third Jack Pepys Workshop on Asthma in the Workplace: answered and unanswered questions. *Proc Am Thorac Soc*; 6: 339–349.
- Vandenplas O, et al. (2003). Definitions and types of work-related asthma: a nosological approach. *Eur Respir J*; 21: 706–712.

Respiratory diseases caused by acute inhalation of gases, vapours and dusts

Benoit Nemery

Acute inhalation injury may occur in the workplace, at home or in the community (*e.g.* as a result of fires and explosions, volcanic eruptions, industrial disasters, and accidents involving trains or vehicles transporting chemicals). Inhalation accidents may be of catastrophic proportions, as occurred with the release of methylisocyanate (MIC) in Bhopal, India, in 1984. Mass casualties with inhalation injuries may also result from chemical warfare, and from conventional warfare or terrorist actions involving explosions, fires and building destructions.

The clinical presentation and severity of inhalation injury range from self-limited inhalation fever to life-threatening chemical pneumonitis with lung oedema and

---

Key points

- An influenza-like response (inhalation fever) may follow the inhalation of high quantities of zinc fumes (metal fume fever) or organic aerosols (ODTS).

- After inhalation of poorly water-soluble agents, such as nitrogen dioxide, phosgene or cadmium fumes, pulmonary oedema becomes clinically manifest only 4–12 h after exposure.

- Acute inhalation injury may be followed by various structural lesions in the airways but also by asthma. Such asthma induced by a single inhalation injury is called acute irritant-induced asthma or RADS.

---

evolution to acute respiratory distress syndrome (ARDS) and multiorgan failure. Following inhalation injury, the lesions may heal completely, or there may be persisting structural or functional sequelae.

Inhalation fever

Inhalation fever is the name given to a group of nonallergic, noninfectious, influenza-like clinical syndromes caused by the acute inhalation of metal fumes, organic dusts or some plastic fumes.

Metal fume fever is caused by a single exposure to high amounts of some metallic fumes, most notably those emitted when heating zinc. Organic dust toxic syndrome (ODTS) is caused by the inhalation of large quantities of agricultural and other dusts of biological origin (bio-aerosols), which are generally heavily contaminated with toxin-producing microorganisms. Polymer fume fever occurs after exposure to the fumes of heated fluorine-containing polymers.

The clinical features of the inhalation fevers are similar to those at the beginning of influenza. The actual exposure may or may not have been experienced as irritant to the eyes and respiratory tract. 4–8 h after exposure, the subject begins to feel unwell with fever (up to 40°C), chills, headaches, malaise, nausea and muscle aches. Respiratory symptoms are usually mild and consist mainly of cough and/or sore throat but, occasionally, subjects may have more severe responses with dyspnoea.

The diagnosis of inhalation fever rests essentially on the recent exposure history and the clinical condition, and when these clearly point to inhalation fever, no sophisticated investigations are required. In general, chest auscultation and chest radiography are normal, but in more severe cases, crackles may be heard and there may be transient infiltrates on the chest radiograph. Pulmonary function is often within normal limits; in severe cases, there may be a decrease in diffusing capacity and arterial hypoxaemia. Increased peripheral blood leukocytosis, with a rise in neutrophils, is a consistent finding in the first 24 h after the exposure; other blood tests should be normal, except for indicators of an inflammatory response. Broncho-alveolar lavage studies have shown pronounced and dose-dependent increases in polymorphonuclear leukocytes on the day after exposure to zinc fumes or organic dust.

Inhalation fever must not be confused with other more serious conditions, including chemical pneumonitis, which, in its early phases, could be mistaken for inhalation fever. A differential diagnosis must also be made with various types of infectious pneumonias and with acute extrinsic allergic alveolitis.

Inhalation fever is a self-limited syndrome and recovery normally takes place after a night's rest. Tolerance exists against re-exposures occurring shortly after a bout of metal fume fever or ODTS.

Acute chemical pneumonitis

Major causes The response to acute chemical injury in the respiratory tract is rarely compound-specific (table 1). The main agents that may cause acute inhalation injury are as follows.

Water-soluble irritants, such as ammonia, sulfur dioxide, hydrochloric acid, formaldehyde and acetic acid, have good warning properties and mainly affect the upper respiratory tract, unless massive quantities have been inhaled.

Gases of intermediate water solubility, such as chlorine and hydrogen sulfide, penetrate deeper into the bronchial tree. Accidental release of gaseous chlorine is one of the most frequent causes of inhalation injury, not only in industry but also in the community as a result of transportation accidents, the use of chlorine for disinfecting swimming pools or the mixing of bleach (sodium hypochlorite) with acids; mixing bleach with ammonia leads to the release of volatile and irritant chloramines (including trichloramine). Hydrogen sulfide, which is formed by the putrefaction of organic material in sewage drains, manure pits or the holds of ships, and is also a frequent contaminant in the petrochemical industry, not only causes mucosal irritation but also leads to chemical asphyxia by mechanisms that are somewhat similar to those of cyanide.

Poorly water-soluble agents, such as nitrogen dioxide, phosgene, ozone, mercury vapours and cadmium oxide fumes, are particularly hazardous because they cause little sensory irritation and are, therefore, hardly noticed; they reach the distal airways, thus potentially causing noncardiogenic pulmonary oedema, which develops over the course of several hours.

Exposure to organic solvents is rarely a cause of toxic pneumonitis. However, exposure to very high concentrations of solvent vapours in confined spaces (*e.g.* in chemical tanks) may cause chemical pneumonitis and pulmonary oedema, often in victims who have been unconscious. Pneumonia and respiratory distress syndrome caused by loss of alveolar surfactant may also result from the aspiration of solvents or fuels ingested unintentionally (*e.g.* from siphoning petrol) or intentionally (*e.g.* by fire eaters). Severe acute respiratory illness may also be caused by spraying solvent-propelled, fluorocarbon-containing water-proofing agents and leather conditioners.

Some agrochemicals (such as paraquat and organophosphate or carbamate insecticides) may cause toxic pneumonitis after ingestion or dermal exposure.

The commonest cause of toxic pneumonitis is smoke inhalation caused by domestic, industrial or other fires. Respiratory morbidity is often the major complication in burn victims. It may be caused by direct

Table 1. Possible causes of toxic tracheobronchitis or pneumonitis

Irritant gases
High water solubility: NH_3, SO_2, HCl
Moderate water solubility: Cl_2, H_2S
Low water solubility: O_3, NO_2, $COCl_2$
Organic chemicals
Organic acids: acetic acid
Aldehydes: formaldehyde, acrolein
Isocyanates: MIC, TDI
Amines: hydrazines, chloramines
Riot control agents: CS gas
Vesicants: mustard gas
Organic solvents
Leather treatment sprays
Some agrochemicals: paraquat, cholinesterase inhibitors
Metallic compounds
Mercury vapours
Metallic oxides: CdO, V_2O_5, MnO, Os_3O_4
Halides: $ZnCl_2$, $TiCl_4$, $SbCl_5$, UF_6
$Ni(CO)_4$
Hydrides: B_2H_5, LiH, AsH_3, SbH_3
Complex mixtures
Fire smoke
Pyrolysis products from plastics
Solvent mixtures
Spores and toxins from microorganisms

The agents listed in the table have been documented to cause toxic lung injury; however, other agents with similar properties can also injure the lungs acutely. TDI: toluene diisocyanate.

thermal injury (particularly if hot vapours have been inhaled) but, more generally, the lesions are caused by chemical injury. The toxic components of smoke include gaseous asphyxiants (carbon monoxide and hydrogen cyanide) and irritants, and particulates.

Clinical presentation Depending on the circumstances of the accident, there may be thermal or chemical facial burns. Signs of mucosal irritation include cough, hoarseness, stridor or wheezing, retrosternal pain, and discharge of bronchial mucus, possibly with blood, mucosal tissue and soot. Auscultation of the chest may or may not be abnormal, with wheezing, rhonchi or crepitations. Mucosal oedema, haemorrhage and ulcerations may be visible in the air passages. Victims of inhalation accidents with poorly soluble agents may feel – and look – perfectly well initially but then experience progressive dyspnoea, shallow breathing, cyanosis, frothy pink sputum and, eventually, ventilatory failure. A clinical picture of ARDS may then develop gradually over 4–72 h, even after a period of clinical improvement.

Pulmonary function can be used to monitor ambulatory subjects who have been exposed. Arterial blood gases show varying degrees of hypoxaemia and respiratory acidosis, depending on the severity of the injury. The chest radiograph is usually normal, if only the conducting airways are involved, but there may be signs of peribronchial cuffing. After exposure to deep lung irritants, the chest radiograph is unremarkable in the first hours after presentation but signs of interstitial and alveolar oedema may become visible and, with time, patchy infiltrates, areas of atelectasis and even 'white lungs' may develop. These changes may be due to tissue damage and organisation or they may reflect superimposed infectious (broncho)pneumonia.

In some instances, particularly in the later stages of chemical pneumonitis, there may be pathological (and radiological) features of organising pneumonia with or without bronchiolitis obliterans. Following resolution of the acute pulmonary oedema, a relapse in the clinical condition may occur after 2–6 weeks with dyspnoea, cough, fine crackles, a radiographic picture of miliary nodular infiltrates, arterial hypoxaemia and a restrictive or mixed impairment, with low diffusing capacity. This relapse phase has been attributed to bronchiolar scarring with peribronchiolar and obliterating fibrosis of the bronchioli.

Management At the scene of the accident, appropriate medical intervention includes removal from exposure, resuscitation and supportive treatment. In some instances, emergency personnel must also be protected from chemicals that remain present on victims or their clothes and decontamination procedures must be available. For some types of exposure, asymptomatic persons must remain under observation for 24 h; they should not exercise, nor should they be overfilled with intravenous fluids. Oxygen treatment should be given according to S_aO_2.

The further management of acute inhalation injury will be governed by the severity of the patient's condition, and will involve intensive care treatment with intubation and artificial ventilation, as required. Antibiotics are only to be given if there are signs of infection. In victims of smoke injury, bronchoscopic removal of soot from the airways may be necessary. The administration of (systemic) corticosteroids is probably justified to prevent complications arising from (excessive) inflammation, such as bronchiolitis obliterans, although there are no controlled studies on this issue.

Physicians treating victims in the early days after an incident must accurately document the clinical condition of and all relevant data in these patients. Documentation of the damage by bronchoscopy and HRCT may be justified. Repeated measurements of ventilatory function and arterial blood gases must be carried out, and victims of acute inhalation injury should never be discharged without a comprehensive assessment of their pulmonary function.

Subacute toxic pneumonitis

Although the concept of chemical-induced lung injury is used only for disorders resulting from a single, acute exposure to a toxic chemical, the term subacute toxic pneumonitis may be used to refer to lung injury caused by repeated peaks of toxic exposures or a more prolonged toxic exposure over weeks to months. This is the case with exogenous lipoid pneumonitis,

which may be caused by inhalation of natural or synthetic mineral oils, and with pulmonary alveolar proteinosis, which may be caused by heavy exposure to silica (acute silicoproteinosis) and by other agents, such as indium tin oxide.

The Ardystil syndrome is an example of subacute toxic pneumonitis. This outbreak of severe organising pneumonia occurred in 1992 in Spain, and involved several workers from factories where textiles were air-sprayed with dyes.

Another recently described form of subacute toxic lung injury is popcorn worker's lung. This severe lung disease, characterised as bronchiolitis obliterans, occurred in subjects occupationally exposed to vapours of butter flavouring (containing diacetyl) used for making microwave popcorn and other foods.

Occupational or environmental aetiologies should always be envisaged even in patients presenting with common forms of pulmonary disease, such as asthma, bronchitis, COPD, sarcoidosis or interstitial lung disease (ILD). To discover such aetiologies, a thorough environmental history must be taken in all patients. A high degree of suspicion should exist when the occurrence or presentation of the disease is unusual. This includes severe pneumonia in young, previously healthy subjects, COPD in nonsmokers, or ILD in subjects <40 years of age. Clustering of a rare disease in time or space should also lead to scrutiny. Concomitant skin disease (especially airborne dermatitis) may also point to occupational exposures. Referral to a specialist with expertise in occupational medicine may also be warranted for: patients who report previous or ongoing high exposure to mineral or organic dust, vapours or gases; patients whose work involves burning or heating metals, plastics or solvents, or recycling materials; patients using high-speed mechanical tools for drilling, polishing or crushing; and patients involved in air spraying or aerosolising paints or other agents. Attention should also be given to patients reporting recent changes in procedures, ingredients or suppliers, and those claiming that fellow workers have similar trouble.

Possible sequelae of acute inhalation injury

Following acute inhalation injury, there is often complete recovery. However, this is not always the case. Various persistent anatomical lesions, such as constrictive bronchiolitis, bronchiectases, bronchial strictures or polyps, may be identified by imaging studies or through bronchoscopy.

Moreover, even in the absence of such structural sequelae or in the absence of significant defects in basal spirometry, a state of permanent nonspecific bronchial hyperreactivity may be observed. This condition of adult-onset, nonallergic asthma, known as reactive airways dysfunction syndrome (RADS) or acute irritant-induced asthma, occurs in a proportion of survivors of inhalation injury. Observations in fire-fighters and other personnel involved in rescue operations during and following the collapse of the World Trade Center on September 11, 2001, suggest that RADS may occur even without the occurrence of clinically serious injury.

Further reading

- Blanc P, *et al.* (1993). The lung in metal fume fever. *Semin Respir Med*; 14: 212–225.
- Brusselaers N, *et al.* (2010). Severe burn injury in Europe: a systematic review of the incidence, etiology, morbidity, and mortality. *Crit Care*; 14: R188.
- Das R, *et al.* (1993). Chlorine gas exposure and the lung: a review. *Toxicol Indust Health*; 9: 439–455.
- Douglas WW, *et al.* Fume-related bronchiolitis obliterans. *In:* Epler GR, ed. Diseases of the bronchioles. New York, Raven Press, 1994; pp. 187–213.
- Kreiss K, *et al.* (2002). Clinical bronchiolitis obliterans in workers at a microwave-popcorn plant. *N Engl J Med*; 347: 330–338.
- Langford NJ, *et al.* (2002). Episodes of environmental poisoning worldwide. *Occup Environ Med*; 59: 855–860.
- Malo J-L, *et al.* (2009). Long-term outcomes of acute irritant-induced asthma. *Am J Respir Crit Care Med*; 179: 923–938.
- Moya C, *et al.* (1994). Outbreak of organising pneumonia in textile printing sprayers. *Lancet*; 344: 498–502.
- Nemery B (1996). Late consequences of accidental exposure to inhaled irritants: RADS and the Bhopal disaster. *Eur Respir J*; 9: 1973–1976.
- Nemery B (2003). Reactive fallout of World Trade Center dust. *Am J Respir Crit Care Med*; 168: 2–3.
- Nemery B. Toxic pneumonitis. *In:* Hendrick DJ, *et al.*, eds. Occupational Disorders of the Lung. Recognition, Management, and Prevention. London, WB Saunders, 2002; pp. 201–219.
- Olson KR, *et al.* (1993). Mixing incompatibilities and toxic exposures. *Occup Med*; 8: 549–560.
- Shusterman DJ (1993). Polymer fume fever and other fluorocarbon pyrolysis-related syndromes. *Occup Med*; 8: 519–531.

Hypersensitivity pneumonitis

Torben Sigsgaard and Anna Rask-Andersen

Hypersensitivity pneumonitis (HP), also known as allergic alveolitis, is an immunologically mediated inflammatory lung disease in the lung parenchyma induced by the inhalation of a variety of organic or inorganic antigens and characterised by hypersensitivity to the antigens. The disease is usually named colourfully after the environment in which it occurs (*e.g.* farmer's lung and bird fancier's lung) and has been reported in over 30 different occupations and environments. Regardless of the causative agents or its environmental setting, the pathogenesis and clinical manifestations of the disease are similar. The hallmark of the disease is a massive lymphocytic inflammation with accumulation of activated T-lymphocytes in the lung interstitium.

Epidemiology

In a large, general population-based cohort of HP patients from the UK, the overall incidence rate was approximately 1 per 100 000 population and in Japan the summer-type HP occurs every year in approximately 1 per million population. Most other studies have focused on the risk of developing clinical disease amongst subsets of the population with high levels of exposure to particular antigens. For example, the incidence of farmer's lung in Sweden in the 1980s was 20 per 100 000 person-years. However, there has been a decrease in the incidence of farmer's lung due to changes in farming practice (hay making replaced by silage bags). A recent study from North America showed that the most common causes were bird or hot-tub exposure.

Risk factors

The first reported HP was farmer's lung, caused by inhalation of microorganisms from infested crops. The disease was first described among farmers in the Nordic countries; however, it has since been described in range of farming operations all over the world, making farming-like operations with decaying organic material one of the important exposures to look for when confronted with a case of HP. One of the most common appearances of HP is bird fancier's lung, caused by exposure to birds, *e.g.* pigeons or parakeets. Among pigeon breeder's HP intestinal mucin, a high molecular weight glycoprotein, has been identified as a major antigen.

Key points

- Hypersensitivity pneumonitis (HP) is an immunologically mediated inflammatory lung disease of the parenchyma.

- HP is induced by the inhalation of a variety of organic or inorganic antigens, and is characterised by hypersensitivity to the antigens.

- The main characteristic of HP is massive lymphocytic inflammation with accumulation of activated T-lymphocytes in the lung interstitium.

- The only treatment is to avoid exposure to the offending allergen; if the exposure ceases the symptoms usually subside rapidly, but lung function impairment may persist.

Host factors

Smoking seems to protect towards HP, although the disease has been described in a small number of smokers. The reason behind this protection might be the downregulation of the immune system by tobacco-smoke and nicotine.

In animal models, virus infection seems to increase the susceptibility of mice towards the antigens, and a higher number of virus antigens have been found in the bronchial lavage of HP patients.

Pathological mechanism

Although HP is a well-known disease the pathogenesis still is only partly understood. When Pepys (1978) found precipitating antibodies to mould antigen in many of the cases, it was believed that, for many years, the immune complexes were the basis of the lung changes. It is now believed that the disease is driven by the cellular immune response. Following inhalation of antigen, a complex formed by soluble antigens and IgG antibodies triggers the complement cascade and alveolar macrophage activations is induced resulting in an increase of macrophages. These cells secrete cytokines and chemokines that attract neutrophils in the alveoli and small airways. The number of T-lymphocytes is also increased with a predominance of the $CD8^+$ T-lymphocytes subset resulting in a decrease in the $CD4^+/CD8^+$ ratio (in contrast to observations made in sarcoidosis). Different upregulatory mechanisms result in a stronger interaction between macrophages and T-cells and a more effective antigen-presenting capacity.

Symptoms and findings

The predominant symptoms in HP are tiredness, dyspnoea, fever, shivering, flu-like feeling, cough, muscle and joint aches, and headache. Radiograph of the thorax shows diffuse, fine, nodular shadows, either general or predominantly in the bases. In the early stages the changes can be difficult to detect, but widespread patchy opacities may also be seen. Lung function is decreased with a typical restrictive pattern and decreased diffusing capacity.

Environmental assessment

The origin of the disease is an adverse reaction towards an occupational or environmental factor, so it is imperative to search the patient's environment for this exposure, and to minimise further contact with the offending agent. In many cases it is obvious what the reason might be, for example with a mouldy hay problem occurring after a wet harvest season. In some instances the causal agent might be difficult to find and techniques for the assessment of micro-organisms should be employed in order to assess the exposure to which the patient is exposed.

Diagnosis

The diagnosis of HP relies on an array of nonspecific clinical symptoms and signs developed in an appropriate setting, with demonstration of bilateral patchy infiltrates on chest radiographs, and serum precipitating antibodies against offending antigens. Several different diagnostic criteria for HP have been proposed, all have significant problems that limit their utility. After studying a total of 661 HP patients with a stepwise logistic regression, a panel of clinical experts identified the six significant predictors of HP.

Diagnostic criteria of extrinsic allergic alveolitis are as follows:

- Exposure to a known offending antigen
- Symptoms occurring 4–8 h after exposure
- Positive precipitating antibodies to the offending antigen
- Inspiratory crackles on physical examination
- Recurrent episodes of symptoms
- Weight loss

However, diagnosing HP often pose challenges, even to expert clinicians. Additional investigations (including surgical biopsy) are indicated in patients with interstitial diseases in whom the diagnosis remains unclear after initial assessment.

Table 1. HP types with typical causative exposures and antigens

HP type	Exposure	Antigen
Farmer's lung	Mouldy hay	Saccharopolyspora rectivirgula
Bagassosis	Mouldy bagasse	Thermoactinomyces sacchari
Mushroom worker's lung	Mushroom spores, mushroom compost	Thermophilic actinomycetes
Malt worker's lung	Mouldy barley	Aspergillus clavatus, Faenia rectivirgula
Humidifier/air-conditioner lung	Contaminated water reservoirs	Thermophilic actinomycetes
Grain handler's lung	Mouldy grain	Saccharopolyspora rectivirgula, Thermoactinomyces vulgaris
Cheese worker's lung	Cheese mould	Penicillium casei
Paprika splitter's lung	Paprika dust	Mucor stolonifer
Compost lung	Compost	Aspergillus spp.
Peat moss worker's lung	Peat moss	Monocillium spp., Penicillium citreonigrum
Suberosis	Mouldy cork dust	Penicillium frequentans
Maple bark stripper's lung	Mouldy wood bark	Cryptostroma corticale
Wood pulp worker's lung	Mouldy wood pulp	Alternaria spp.
Wood trimmer's disease	Mouldy wood trimmings	Rhizopus spp.
Japanese summer-type HP	Indoor air	Trichosporon cutaneum
Metal-grinding	Metalworking fluids	Mycobacteria
Hot tub lung	Mist from hot tubs	Mycobacteria
Bird breeder's lung	Pigeons, parakeets, fowl and rodents	Avian or animal proteins
Mollusk-shell hypersensitivity	Sea snail shells	Shell dust
Chemical worker's lung	Manufacture of plastics, polyurethane foam and rubber	Trimellitic anhydride, diisocyanate, methylene diisocyanate

Treatment

The only treatment for allergic diseases is to avoid the exposure to the offending allergen. This can be done in many circumstances, such as when the occurrence is sporadic and not part of the daily work of the patient. However, in some cases, for example in farmers, it might be difficult to completely avoid the exposure for a range of different reasons. Under such circumstances, respiratory protection can be used to minimise the exposure as much as possible.

The effect of medical treatment on the outcome of HP has been discussed. Cortisone has been found to reduce IL-8 synthesis. Cortisone treatment seems to improve the radiological findings and should be given to severely ill patients to ameliorate symptoms, but no apparent benefit is derived from long-term treatment. Cortisone treatment should be given for about 2 months.

Prognosis

If the exposure ceases, the symptoms usually subside rapidly, but lung function impairment may persist for a longer period and become permanent with a restrictive pattern and decreased diffusing capacity. Repeated attacks increase the risk of a poor prognosis. It is therefore important to treat the patient as soon as possible in order to avoid more damage to the lung parenchyma in addition to that already present at the time of diagnosis.

Differential diagnosis

Infectious lung diseases, both of virological and bacteriological origin, as well as other lung diseases such as sarcoidosis have to be ruled out. Another differential diagnosis is the organic dust toxic syndrome (ODTS) also known as 'inhalation fever': acute, febrile, noninfectious, flu-like, short-term reactions that can be produced by inhalation of bio-aerosols and organic dusts. Symptoms are caused by the release of inflammatory cytokines from the lungs caused by an inhalatory overexposure to aerosols. ODTS is quite a common condition, but the prognosis is good and most people have recovered totally without any sequels after 24 h. No treatment is required if the exposure is terminated.

Further reading

- Ando M, et al. (1991). Japanese summer-type hypersensitivity pneumonitis. Geographic distribution, home environment, and clinical characteristics of 621 cases. Am Rev Respir Dis; 144: 765–769.
- Arya A, et al. (2006). Farmer's lung is now in decline. Irish Med J; 99: 203–205.
- Bourke SJ, et al. (2001). Hypersensitivity pneumonitis: current concepts. Eur Respir J Suppl; 32: 81s–92s.
- Hanak V, et al. (2007). Causes and presenting features in 85 consecutive patients with hypersensitivity pneumonitis. Mayo Clinic Proc; 82: 812–816.
- Lacasse Y, et al. (2003). Clinical diagnosis of hypersensitivity pneumonitis. Am J Respir Crit Care Med; 168: 952–958.
- Malmberg P, et al. (1988). Incidence of organic dust toxic syndrome and allergic alveolitis in Swedish farmers. Int Arch Allergy Appl Immunol; 87: 47–54.
- Pepys J (1978). Antigens and hypersensitivity pneumonitis. J Allergy Clin Immunol; 61: 201–203.
- Solaymani-Dodaran M, et al. (2007). Extrinsic allergic alveolitis: incidence and mortality in the general population. QJM; 100: 233–237.

Pneumoconiosis

Allan F. Henderson

Pneumoconiosis is the non-neoplastic reaction of the lung to inhaled dust. Conventionally, asthma, bronchitis and emphysema are excluded from the definition, but these will be included here, where relevant.

Exposure to dusts varies greatly throughout the world, including Europe. The prevalence of pneumoconiosis differs as well, even within countries. Another confounding factor is that dust-related diseases may occur many years after exposure. For example, asbestosis may be seen years after the closure of shipyards. The practicing pneumologist is recommended to become familiar with the industrial history of their locale. Most cases of pneumoconiosis are due to occupational exposure. There are

Key Points

- Pleural plaques indicate exposure to asbestos, but rarely cause problems.

- Asbestos-related diseases (except mesothelioma) are becoming increasingly rare.

- Pleural thickening may result from unrecognised benign asbestos pleurisy.

- CWP and silicosis are much rarer now in Europe but remain significant problems worldwide.

- CWP and silicosis can both be associated with airways obstruction.

- Silicosis and asbestosis increase the risk of lung cancer.

frequently issues of compensation, and the pneumologist working in industrial and post-industrial situations should become familiar with the local arrangements as well as the purely medical issues.

Asbestos

Asbestos is a collective term for a number of silicaceous minerals. The amphiboles crocidolite and amosite are no longer mined or used industrially, but the serpentine chrysotile is still produced and used extensively in Africa, South America and Asia. It is less harmful, but there is frequently contamination with amphiboles. Asbestos was used extensively in construction before its use was curtailed and it is exceedingly persistent. This leads to workers involved with renovation, demolition, *etc.* being at risk of exposure. This may be particularly relevant in the causation of mesothelioma in cohorts not exposed to asbestos at the time of its active importation and use.

Pleural plaques

Hyaline pleural plaques are discrete areas of thickening on the parietal pleura. They are a common manifestation of asbestos exposure. Their development is correlated with cumulative dose exposure to asbestos, but only loosely. They may be absent or profuse in similarly exposed individuals. Their diagnosis is usually an incidental radiographic finding and they are not usually seen on conventional radiology <15 years from the subject's first exposure. However, earlier detection, particularly of small, uncalcified lesions, is possible with CT. Plaques become increasingly calcified over time.

They are generally regarded as asymptomatic but, rarely, grating pleuritic discomfort is reported. Breathlessness is usually due to other causes, but very extensive plaques may exert a cuirass effect. Some series report impaired lung function with plaques, which has been attributed to a number of explanations including subradiographic interstitial fibrosis and peripheral small airway disease.

Plaques are not pre-malignant but they are a marker of asbestos exposure, which implies an increased risk of other asbestos-related diseases. This may cause anxiety. In the UK, this is compensable in Scotland, but not in the rest of the UK.

Benign asbestos pleurisy and diffuse pleural thickening

Once considered separate entities, these conditions are part of a spectrum of inflammatory response to inhaled asbestos fibres that have traversed the lung and lodged in the pleura. Asbestos pleurisy may present as an acute illness with pain, fever and dyspnoea, and may be misdiagnosed as infective. Most, but not all, are characterised by a bloody pleural effusion. Many episodes are asymptomatic. The latency from first exposure is highly variable but may be <10 years. Some episodes may resolve with little legacy, while others progress to diffuse pleural thickening (DPT). Asymptomatic asbestos pleurisy is believed to be the precursor of other cases of DPT. Asbestos pleurisy is frequently recurrent and bilateral, leading to bilateral DPT. Unlike plaques, DPT commonly causes restricted ventilation and, hence, dyspnoea. Plaques and DPT can be difficult to distinguish. Radiologically, the costophrenic angle is obliterated in DPT; pathologically, DPT involves the visceral pleura while plaques are confined to the parietal surface.

Asbestosis

Asbestosis is sometimes erroneously used as a term to describe all types of asbestos-related disease, whereas it is properly defined as interstitial fibrosis due to asbestos. It occurs with significantly heavy exposure to asbestos, such as in shipyard laggers and joiners, not with casual contact. As asbestos use has reduced dramatically, so the incidence of asbestosis has fallen steeply. Cases are virtually confined to older males who encountered asbestos decades ago. There is controversy as to whether asbestosis progresses after removal from exposure or develops many years after exposure. Much of the interest in asbestosis is now medicolegal. The principal issue faced by pneumologists in practice is whether a case of interstitial lung disease is idiopathic pulmonary fibrosis (IPF) or asbestosis. Occupational exposure to asbestos may suggest asbestosis but a working knowledge of industrial processes is needed to assess the relevance of this. The presence of pleural plaques may be supportive but IPF can occur in such patients. Radiological features may help, as does review of progression over time, if such data are available.

The Helsinki criteria were developed in 1997 to assist with evaluating such cases. They include pathological features. A lung biopsy is rarely appropriate as the clinical management is not affected in most cases. *Post mortem* analysis may assist in medicolegal assessment.

There is a high incidence of lung cancer in patients with asbestosis – around 30% in some series. There is controversy as to whether asbestos exposure alone increases the risk of cancer.

Coal

Unlike asbestos, the mining and use of coal continues on a colossal scale, with >7 billion tonnes produced worldwide in 2011. There have been big changes in world demographics, with greatly reduced mining in the UK and huge production in China. Many European countries have significant coal industries. Dust control measures have been successful in reducing coal-related disease but new cases still occur. The number of miners employed in the industry has reduced, serving to reduce the numbers of exposed individuals, but the potential for problems has increased because of higher dust levels produced by increased mechanisation of production.

Coal workers' pneumoconiosis

Simple coal workers' pneumoconiosis (CWP) is the accumulation of coal dust, predominantly in centrilobular macules 2–5 mm in diameter, often more in the upper zones. Despite the dramatic macroscopic appearances observed *post mortem*, and equally marked radiographic findings, simple CWP itself causes no symptoms or lung function abnormality. Symptoms such as dyspnoea require investigation for alternative diagnoses.

Progressive massive fibrosis (PMF) is associated with the presence of larger (>1 cm) nodules pathologically and radiologically. PMF occurs with greater dust exposure, and improved control measures have led to a marked decline in its prevalence. PMF is also associated with impaired lung function, principally restriction.

Caplan's syndrome is the finding of large (0.5–5 cm) nodules in miners with rheumatoid arthritis. The nodules are not profuse and no effect is seen on lung function.

Chronic bronchitis and emphysema are caused by coal dust. Bronchitis is manifested by cough and sputum. Centrilobular emphysema is demonstrated *post mortem* in coal miners, especially when simple CWP is present. Airway obstruction due to this (and compounded by smoking) is the main cause of disability in miners with simple CWP.

Silicosis

Silicon is the second most abundant element on earth. Silica (silicon dioxide) and silicaceous compounds are ubiquitous, and are encountered in a wide variety of industrial processes including mining and quarrying, masonry and construction, and foundry work.

Dust control measures have led to a marked reduction in silicosis in developed countries, with only a few hundred cases in the UK, France and Germany. Many of these date from exposure many years ago. However, this situation is not global, with large numbers of new cases being recorded in China, making silicosis the most prevalent pneumoconiosis worldwide.

Simple silicosis, like simple CWP, causes little physiological disturbance or symptoms despite marked radiological changes, which are characterised by nodule formation with an upper zone predominance. With increased silica load comes an increased fibrotic response, which may become extensive and confluent. Hilar calcification ('egg-shell') is characteristic but not universal. Dyspnoea, accompanied by a dry cough is the usual symptom.

The lung function disturbance is variable. A restrictive defect is common with fibrotic disease but may be accompanied by obstruction that, in the early stages, may be the sole abnormality. Previously attributed to smoking, it is now recognised that silica causes emphysema, which may develop in the absence of nodular change.

Silicosis is associated with an increased risk of lung cancer. As with asbestos, it is currently undetermined as to whether this is due to silica *per se* or whether this is secondary to silicosis.

TB is a common complication in silicosis. Accelerated deterioration in a patient with silicosis should raise suspicion. In the past, diagnosis has often been difficult, but interferon-γ testing has helped. In South Africa, HIV infection has been shown to be synergistic with silicosis in increasing the incidence of TB.

Further reading

- American Thoracic Society Committee of the Scientific Assembly on Environmental and Occupational Health. (1997). Adverse effects of crystalline silica exposure. *Am J Respir Crit Care Med*; 155: 761–768.

- Cassidy A, *et al.* (2007). Occupational exposure to crystalline silica and risk of lung cancer: a multicenter case-control study in Europe.. *Epidemiology*; 18: 36–43.
- Coggan D, *et al.* (1998). Coal mining and chronic obstructive pulmonary disease. *Thorax*; 53: 398–407.
- Copley SJ, *et al.* (2003). Asbestosis and idiopathic pulmonary fibrosis: comparison of thin-section CT features. *Radiology*; 229: 731–736.
- Corbett EL, *et al.* (2000). HIV infection and silicosis: the impact of two potent risk factors on the incidence of mycobacterial disease in South African miners. *AIDS*; 14: 2759–2768.
- Coutts I, *et al.* (1987). Mortality in cases of asbestosis diagnosed by a pneumoconiosis panel. *Thorax*; 42: 111–116.
- Hillerdal G, *et al.* (1987). Benign asbestos pleural effusion: 73 exudates in 60 patients. *Eur J Respir Dis*; 71: 113–121.
- Marine WM, *et al.* (1988). Clinically important respiratory effects of dust exposure and smoking in British coal miners. *Am Rev Respir Dis*; 137: 106–112.
- Tossavainen A (1997). Asbestos, asbestosis, and cancer: the Helsinki criteria for diagnosis and attribution. *Scand J Work Environ Health*; 23: 311–316.

Indoor and outdoor pollution

Giovanni Viegi, Marzia Simoni, Sara Maio, Sonia Cerrai,
Giuseppe Sarno and Sandra Baldacci

Air pollution is a well-established hazard to human health. Air quality is particularly important for subpopulations that are more susceptible (*i.e.* children, the elderly, subjects with cardiorespiratory diseases or those who are socioeconomically deprived) or at higher risk of specific exposures (workers exposed to inorganic dust, wood dust, fumes, gases and cleaning agents). Children are particularly vulnerable since

they inhale a higher volume of air per body weight than adults, their lungs are growing, their immune system is incomplete and defence mechanisms are still evolving. Air pollution can affect the cells in the lung by damaging those that are most susceptible and, if the damaged cells are important in the development of new functional parts of the lung, the lung may not achieve its full growth and function as a child matures to adulthood. This can lead to enhanced susceptibility during adulthood to the effects of ageing and infections, as well as to pollutants. Air pollution has both short-term adverse effects (peak exposures) and long-term adverse effects, and these effects can involve the pulmonary system but also the cardiovascular system.

Air pollution is mostly produced by human activities. Other pollutants derive from natural sources, such as biological allergens (*e.g.* house dust mites, pets dander and moulds) and natural phenomena (*e.g.* volcanic activity and forest fires).

Recent research focuses on two broad sources:

- motor vehicles and industrial plants
- biomass fuels

Traffic-related air pollution is a growing concern in both developed and less-developed countries, and industrial smokestacks continue to be a major source of outdoor air pollution from the burning of fossil fuels throughout the world. However, the most threatened populations live in developing and poor countries, where air pollution reflects a combination of traditional and modern factors. Rapid

Key points

- Recent epidemiological studies have clearly shown that outdoor and indoor air pollution affects respiratory health worldwide, causing an increase in the prevalence of cardiovascular and respiratory symptoms/diseases (*i.e.* COPD, asthma, hay fever and lung function reduction) and of mortality, both in children and in adults.

- Rapid industrialisation and urbanisation have increased air pollution and, consequently, the number of exposed people.

- Conservative estimates show that between 1.5 and 2 million deaths per year could be attributed to indoor air pollution in developing countries.

- The abatement of the main risk factors for respiratory diseases, and the support of healthcare providers and the general community for public health policies improving outdoor/indoor air quality can achieve huge health benefits.

industrialisation, urbanisation and growth in vehicle use increase outdoor air pollution, and, at the same time, traditional indoor burning of solid fuels, such as coal and dung, is still widespread.

With this in mind and in view of the 2013 European 'Year of Air', the European Union is revising its main air pollution control policies, and the European Respiratory Society Environment and Health Committee has developed 10 concise principles for clean air that summarise the scientific state of the art and provide guidance.

Outdoor pollution

The most important outdoor pollutants derive from fossil fuel combustion. Primary pollutants directly emitted into the atmosphere are carbon monoxide, sulfur dioxide, nitrogen dioxide and particulates. Ozone is a secondary pollutant, mainly produced by chemical reaction of nitrogen dioxide and hydrocarbons in the presence of sunlight at warm temperature. Rapid industrialisation and urbanisation in many parts of the world have increased air pollution and, consequently, the number of people exposed to it. In China, for instance, rapid economic development has led to severe environmental degradation, particularly due to coal combustion (which provides 70–75% of all energy in China) and vehicular traffic. Chinese mortality and morbidity associated with outdoor pollution are very high: >300 000 deaths and 20 million cases of respiratory illnesses annually. A more recent study raises the estimate of the death toll in China due to air pollution to 1.2 million.

Today, it is recognised that global warming will increase the effects of outdoor air pollution on health: it will lead to more heat waves, during which air pollution concentrations are also elevated, and during which hot temperatures and air pollutants act in synergy to produce more serious health effects than expected from heat or pollution alone.

The main effects of the more common outdoor pollutants are summarised in table 1.

Exposure–response relationships for outdoor pollutants, especially particulates, have been confirmed by epidemiological studies in recent decades. Short-term exposure, due to acute increase in air pollution, may cause premature mortality and increase hospital admissions for exacerbations of COPD or asthma. Long-term cumulative health effects of chronic exposure comprise an increase in mortality and morbidity for cardiovascular and respiratory diseases, including COPD and lung cancer, and impaired development of the lungs in children. In COPD patients, continued exposure to noxious agents promotes a more rapid decline in lung function and increases the risk of repeated exacerbations. Air pollution can harm the fetus if the mother is exposed to high levels during pregnancy (i.e. intrauterine growth retardation) and can increase respiratory neonatal mortality. Particulates, nitrogen dioxide and ozone are the most important pollutants today. The health effects of particulates are more serious for fine (particular matter with an aerodynamic diameter <2.5 µm ($PM_{2.5}$)) and ultrafine ($PM_{0.1}$) particles, as they penetrate deeper into the airways of the respiratory tract, reaching the alveoli. Vehicular exhausts are responsible for small-sized airborne particulate air pollution in urban areas. Recently, much research has pointed out the negative effects of diesel exhaust exposure; people are exposed not only to motor vehicle exhausts but also to exhausts from other diesel engines (e.g. diesel trains and ships) and from power generators. In June 2012, the International Agency for Research on Cancer (IARC) classified diesel engine exhaust as carcinogenic to humans (Group 1), based on sufficient evidence that exposure is associated with an increased risk of lung cancer.

The role of air pollution in the epidemics of allergies is still debated, even if experimental studies have suggested that the effects of air pollutants on the development and worsening of allergies are biologically plausible. Asthma shows a strong familial association but genetic factors alone are unlikely to account for the rapid rise in its

Table 1. Major outdoor/indoor pollutants and related health effects

Pollutant	Major sources	Health effects

Particulate matter	Outdoor
	  Vehicular traffic
	  Woodstoves
	  Organic matter and fossil fuel combustion
	  Power stations/industry
	  Windblown dust from roadways,
	    agriculture and construction
	  Bushfires/dust storms
	Indoor
	  Woodstoves
	  Organic matter and fossil fuel combustion
	    for heating/cooking
	  ETS
		Lung cancer
		Premature death
		Mortality for cardiorespiratory
		  diseases
		Reduced lung function
		Lower airways inflammation
		Upper airways irritation

Nitrogen dioxide	Outdoor
	  Vehicular traffic
	  Power stations/industry
	Indoor
	  Unvented gas/kerosene appliances
		Exacerbation of asthma
		Airway inflammation
		Bronchial hyperresponsiveness
		Increased susceptibility to
		  respiratory infection

Ozone	Outdoor
	  Sunlight chemical reaction with other
	    pollutants
	  Vehicular traffic
	  Power stations/industry
	  Consumer products
		Lung tissue damage
		Reduced lung function
		Reduced exercise capacity
		Exacerbation of asthma
		Upper airway and eye irritation

Carbon monoxide	Outdoor
	  Organic matter and fossil fuel combustion
	  Vehicular traffic
	  Woodstoves
	Indoor
	  Organic matter and fossil fuel combustion
	    for heating/cooking
	  Woodstoves
	  Unvented gas/kerosene appliances
	  ETS
		Death/coma at very high levels
		Headache, nausea,
		  breathlessness, confusion/
		  reduced mental alertness
		Low birth weight (fetal exposure)

Sulfur dioxide	Outdoor
	  Coal/oil-burning power stations
	  Industry/refineries
	  Diesel engines
	  Metal smelting
		Exacerbation of respiratory
		  diseases including asthma
		Respiratory tract irritation

VOCs	Indoor
	  Building materials and products such as
	    new furniture, solvents, paint,
	    adhesives, insulation
	  Cleaning activities and products
	  Materials for offices
		Lung cancer
		Asthma, dizziness, respiratory
		  and lung diseases
		Chronic eye, lung or skin irritation
		Neurological and reproductive
		  disorders

prevalence seen in recent decades. The rapid increase in the burden of atopic diseases occurred along with rapid urbanisation/industrialisation. Thus, genetic and environmental factors may interact to cause asthma. A growing number of studies shows significant associations of traffic with new-onset asthma, or asthma symptoms/exacerbations, in children.

Some recent studies confirming the association between urban air pollution and health status are described here.

- The Italian EpiAir project, performed in 10 cities on ~300 000 subjects aged ≥35 years, highlighted an increase in mortality from respiratory diseases of 2.29% (95% CI 1.03–3.58%) per 10-μg·m^{-3} increase in PM_{10} (lag 0–3 days); the increase in mortality was higher during summer.
- Data from the Cancer Prevention Study II cohort of the American Cancer Society showed an increase of 4% in mortality for respiratory diseases per 10-ppb increase in ozone concentration.
- Our team in Pisa, Italy, has reported that people living in an urban area are at higher risk of having increased bronchial responsiveness (OR 1.41, 95% CI 1.13–1.76) than people living in a rural area. Moreover, we showed long-term effects of the exposure to traffic air pollution: people residing near a major road (within 100 m) showed significantly higher risks (odds ratios ranging from 1.61 to 2.07) of persistent wheezing, dyspnoea, attacks of shortness of breath with wheezing, asthma, COPD, airway obstruction and atopy. Another Italian study, performed on children (aged 10–17 years) living in Palermo, Italy, confirmed the negative impact of heavy traffic exposure, showing significantly higher risks (odds ratios ranging from 1.39 to 1.84) of asthma, rhinoconjunctivitis and reduced lung function.

Indoor pollution

Indoor environments contribute significantly to human exposure to air pollutants. People spend most of their time indoors: up to 90% in industrialised countries. Furthermore, levels of some pollutants are higher inside than outside buildings. Even at low concentrations, indoor pollutants may have an important biological impact because of long exposure periods (e.g. at home or school, and in workplaces). Conservative

estimates attribute 1.5–2 million deaths per year to indoor air pollution. There is consistent evidence that exposure to indoor pollutants increases the risk of several respiratory/allergic symptoms and diseases (table 1). Relevant indoor pollution sources are environmental tobacco smoke (ETS), a common source of indoor particulates, biomass (wood/coal) fuel use, and mould/damp. Furthermore, within the western countries and in the societies that adopt western lifestyles, consumer products (i.e. computers, televisions, synthetic building materials, etc.) emit large quantities of volatile organic compounds (VOCs) and nonorganic compounds.

ETS is associated with increased risk of acute respiratory or irritation symptoms, infectious diseases, chronic respiratory illnesses, lung function reduction and even lung cancer. In children, ETS also increases the risk of sudden infant death syndrome, middle-ear disease, lower respiratory tract illnesses, wheeze and cough. ETS exposure exacerbates pre-existing asthma and increases symptom burden and morbidity. In nonsmokers, the mortality risk for respiratory diseases is about double for those living with smokers than for those who do not. Studies performed worldwide suggest higher risk for ETS exposure in females than in males. Table 2 shows the results of meta-analyses regarding the associations of ETS exposure with respiratory symptoms/diseases.

About half of the world's population burns biomass for cooking, heating and lighting, in open fires or with inefficient stoves, and in poorly ventilated rooms, especially in developing countries. Indoor air pollution from biomass fuels is strongly poverty-related and represents an important risk factor for acute respiratory illness morbidity and mortality in low-income countries, especially in children and women. In China, indoor air pollution from solid fuel use is responsible for ~420 000 premature deaths annually, more than the nearly 300 000 attributed to urban outdoor air pollution in the country. A more recent study raises the estimate of the death toll in China due to

Table 2. Associations between ETS exposure and respiratory symptoms/disease in never-smokers.

	Population	Estimated pooled risk
Lower respiratory tract infection	<2 years	OR 1.55 (95% CI 1.42–1.69)
	2–6 years	OR 1.71 (95% CI 1.33–2.20)
Cough	Males	OR 1.60 (95% CI 1.22–2.10)
	Females	OR 1.68 (95% CI 1.17–2.34)
Asthma onset	Children	OR 1.32 (95% CI 1.24–1.41)
	Adults	OR 1.97 (95% CI 1.19–3.25)
Lung cancer	Adults	OR 1.21 (95% CI 1.13–1.30)
	Females	RR 1.27 (95% CI 1.17–1.37)
	North America	RR 1.15 (95% CI 1.03–1.28)
	Asia	RR 1.31 (95% CI 1.16–1.48)
	Europe	RR 1.31 (95% CI 1.24–1.52)
OR: odds ratio; RR: relative risk.		

household air pollution to 1 million, close to the 1.2 million due to outdoor air pollution. The evidence that biomass use increases the risk of COPD in females and acute respiratory infections in children is very strong (about three-fold and more than three-fold higher risk in those exposed than in the unexposed, respectively). The IARC has classified the indoor combustion of coal emissions as Group 1, a known carcinogen to humans. There is strong evidence (moderate for males) that females exposed to smoke from coal fires in the home have an elevated risk of lung cancer (OR 1.9, 95% CI 1.1–3.5).

Based on meta-analyses, building dampness and mould are associated with approximately 30–50% increases in respiratory and asthma-related health outcomes. In children, a population attributable risk for asthma of 6.7% has been estimated. In adults, a pooled risk of cough by indoor mould/dampness was estimated at an odds ratio of 2.10 (95% CI 1.27–3.47). There is also evidence for an association of mould exposure with new-onset asthma and worsening of pre-existing asthma (wheezing, cough and shortness of breath) in both children and adults. Allergic symptoms are commonly related to mould exposure (sneezing; nose, mouth or throat irritations; nasal stuffiness or runny nose; and red, itchy or watery eyes).

Finally, exposure to VOCs may result in a spectrum of illnesses ranging from mild (irritations) to very severe effects, including cancer. Such exposure increases the risk for respiratory/allergic effects in infants/children, like asthma, wheeze, chronic bronchitis, reduced lung function, atopy and severity of sensitisation, rhinitis, and pulmonary infections. Many studies indicate that the effects are related to very low levels of exposure. VOC exposure also seems a significant risk factor for asthma (odds ratios ranging from 1.2 to 2.9). Many of the effects observed in children have been shown also in adults.

Biological mechanisms

Many recent studies have shown that oxidative stress, induced by air pollutants, plays a central role in the impact of air pollution. The first contact of inhaled ambient pollutants is with the fluid layer that covers the respiratory epithelium, and the responses following the exposure are mediated through oxidation reactions occurring within this fluid air–lung interface. These reactions can result in oxidative stress and consequent increased production of inflammatory mediators from human airway epithelial cells. Oxidative stress is a situation in which the oxidant–antioxidant balance is disturbed. This imbalance can occur when the generation of oxidant molecules (free radicals) exceeds the available antioxidant defences. The consequence of this oxidative stress can be systemic or local inflammations thus involving the cardiopulmonary system.

The three pollutants of most concern that can cause oxidative stress include nitric oxide, which is a free radical, PM10, and ozone. The majority of human genetic association studies of air pollutants have examined ozone exposure. Ozone is a powerful oxidant and reacts with the bronchial epithelium lining fluid to generate free radicals. It depletes levels of protective antioxidants and increases the production of inflammatory mediators.

The size and the surface of particulates determine the potential to elicit oxidative damage. In general, the smaller the size of the particulates, the higher the toxicity through mechanisms of oxidative stress and inflammation. Nanoparticles (ultrafine particles with diameter <100 nm) are more toxic and inflammogenic than fine particles. They generate reactive oxygen species to a greater extent and exacerbate pre-existing respiratory and cardiovascular disease, also through a dose–response effect.

Pulmonary impairment related to pollutant exposure may be higher in individuals who are genetically at risk for higher susceptibility to oxidative stress. The formation of reactive oxygen species is an important aspect of the inflammatory process of asthma, and genetic aberrations associated with antioxidants might explain the reason why some people with asthma seem at higher risk of exacerbations due to air pollution exposure.

Conclusion

Outdoor and indoor pollution greatly affect respiratory health worldwide, as shown by many recent epidemiological studies.

Patient education about the importance of good indoor air quality in the home and workplace is essential. The support of healthcare providers and the general community for public health policy aimed at improving outdoor air quality through programmes for abating/reducing pollutant emissions is also important. Moreover, there is evidence that increased antioxidant intake may protect against the effects of air pollution. The role of the physician is essential in patient education on the preventive actions to reduce health effects due to pollution.

Hopefully, these actions will reduce the negative effects of air pollution on the respiratory health status and quality of life of the general population, particularly of more susceptible individuals.

Further reading

- Brunekreef B, et al. (2012). Ten principles for clean air. Eur Respir J; 39: 525–528.
- Cibella F, et al. (2011). Proportional Venn diagram and determinants of allergic respiratory diseases in Italian adolescents. Pediatr Allergy Immunol; 22: 60–68.
- Faustini A, et al. (2011). The relationship between ambient particulate matter and respiratory mortality: a multi-city study in Italy. Eur Respir J; 38: 538–547.
- Hulin M, et al. (2012). Respiratory health and indoor air pollutants based on quantitative exposure assessments. Eur Respir J; 40: 1033–1045.
- International Agency for Research on Cancer. Diesel engine exhaust carcinogenic. www.iarc.fr/en/media-centre/pr/2012/pdfs/pr213_E.pdf
- Künzli N, et al. Air quality and health. www.ersnet.org/index.php/publications/reference-books.html
- Lim SS, et al. (2012). A comparative risk assessment of burden of disease and injury attributable to 67 risk factors and risk factor clusters in 21 regions, 1990–2010: a systematic analysis for the Global Burden of Disease Study 2010. Lancet; 380: 2224–2260.
- Maio S, et al. (2009). Urban residence is associated with bronchial hyper-responsiveness in Italian general population samples. Chest; 135: 434–441.
- McGwin G, et al. (2010). Formaldehyde exposure and asthma in children: a systematic review. Environ Health Perspect; 118: 313–317.

- Nuvolone D, *et al.* (2011). Geographical information system and environmental epidemiology: a cross-sectional spatial analysis of the effects of traffic-related air pollution on population respiratory health. *Environ Health*; 10: 12–23.
- Öberg M, *et al.* Second-hand smoke: assessing the environmental burden of disease at national and local levels. Geneva, World Health Organization, 2010.
- Po JY, *et al.* (2011). Respiratory disease associated with solid biomass fuel exposure in rural women and children: systematic review and meta-analysis. *Thorax*; 66: 232–239.
- Valavanidis A, *et al.* (2008). Airborne particulate matter and human health: toxicological assessment and importance of size and composition of particles for oxidative damage and carcinogenic mechanisms. *J Environ Sci Health C Environ Carcinog Ecotoxicol Rev*; 26: 339–362.
- Viegi G, *et al.* (2007). Definition, epidemiology and natural history of COPD. *Eur Respir J*; 30: 993–1013.
- Viegi G, *et al.* (2004). Indoor air pollution and airway disease. *Int J Tuberc Lung Dis*; 8: 1401–1415.
- World Health Organization. Effects of air pollution on children's health and development – a review of the evidence. www.euro.who.int/__data/assets/pdf_file/0010/74728/E86575.pdf
- World Health Organization. WHO guidelines for indoor air quality: dampness and mould. www.euro.who.int/__data/assets/pdf_file/0017/43325/E92645.pdf
- Yang W, *et al.* (2009). Air pollutants, oxidative stress and human health. *Mutat Res*; 674: 45–54.

Smoking-related diseases

Yves Martinet and Nathalie Wirth

Tobacco use is by far the single largest avoidable cause of chronic illness and premature death worldwide. Smokers die of cancer of the lung and other organs as well as of respiratory and cardiovascular diseases. In the European Union (EU), tobacco use kills $\geqslant$650 000 people (more than one in seven of all deaths) each year. Nearly 50% of these deaths involve diseases of the respiratory system, mainly lung cancer and COPD. Given the relatively long period between time of smoking initiation ('first puff') and time of onset of smoking-related lung disease ($\geqslant$10 years), young people who start smoking often disregard the future health risks of tobacco use. Unfortunately, while male smoking is declining in most European countries, female smoking rates are still on the rise in some parts of the EU and in most other countries of the world, due to tobacco industry promotion.

Tobacco smoke

Almost all tobacco-associated lung cancer and respiratory diseases result from smoke inhalation. In this respect, studies have shown that people who only use oral tobacco during their lifetime (such as Swedish snus, for example) are at no greater risk of developing these diseases than nonsmokers; however, the use of oral tobacco is related to several health problems, such as gum and pancreatic cancer and, possibly, cardiovascular diseases. Given that cigarette smoking is by far the most common method of tobacco consumption, the following data mainly concern diseases related to active cigarette smoking.

Cigarette smoke is composed of >4000 substances, including nicotine, chemical

Key points

- Tobacco use is responsible for more than one in seven of all deaths in the EU.

- ~50% of tobacco-related deaths are due to lung cancer and COPD.

- Female smoking is still on the rise in some parts of the EU.

- Preventing tobacco use and treating tobacco addicts should be given top priority.

poisons, toxic gases, small particles and carcinogens. The nicotine present in tobacco leaves is highly addictive but has little toxicity on the respiratory tract. Thus, people smoke for the psychoactive effects of nicotine but die from the high toxicity of the other components present in smoke. Even if tobacco smoke composition varies slightly (due to tobacco type, substances added during manufacturing and filter type), the health risks and effects of tobacco smoking are quite constant from one cigarette brand to another. Furthermore, previously labelled 'low-tar' and 'low-nicotine' cigarettes have been shown to be as hazardous as 'regular' ones. Likewise, hand-rolled cigarette, bidi and water-pipe smoking are at least as dangerous as cigarette smoking. Finally, while pipe and cigar smoke is more toxic than cigarette smoke, cigar and pipe smokers are seldom deep inhalers. This explains the lower incidence of respiratory disease in these 'noninhaling' smokers. However, these smokers have a high incidence of oral cancer. Nevertheless, their rate of respiratory disease is still higher than in nonsmokers.

Cannabis smoke

In respect to effects on the respiratory tract, cannabis smoking is at least as dangerous as tobacco smoking. Moreover, since cannabis is usually smoked mixed with tobacco, young people often become addicted to tobacco for life, even if occasional users merely seek to experience the relaxing effects of tetrahydrocannabinol. This co-consumption of cannabis and tobacco complicates characterisation of the specific health effects of cannabis smoking. Nevertheless, it has been shown that cannabis smoking causes lung cancer and COPD.

Lung cancer

Lung cancer is the most frequent cause of death due to tobacco use: 85–90% of the 225 000 lung cancer deaths occurring each year in the EU are the consequence of tobacco smoking. Lung cancer is one of the deadliest cancers, with 5-year survival rates ranging from 10% to 15%. Lung cancer incidence and mortality increase roughly in proportion to the first power of smoking intensity (number of cigarettes smoked per day) and, most importantly, to the second power of smoking duration (total number of years of smoking). Tobacco smoking results in all major histological types of lung cancer. Over the years, a shift has been observed from squamous cell lung cancer to adenocarcinoma. Lung cancer risk is similar in males and females with comparable smoking histories. With such a highly specific cause and terrible prognosis, the best 'treatment' of lung cancer is to avoid it through tobacco smoking prevention and treatment. Indeed, the relative risk of lung cancer steadily decreases when smokers give up smoking. For example, in the UK, for males who stopped smoking at the ages of 30, 40, 50 and 60 years, the risk of lung cancer by the age of 75 years was 2%, 3%, 6% and 10%, respectively; whereas for males who smoked up to 75 years of age, this cumulative risk reached 16%. In the same way, an increase in overall tobacco consumption by a population is followed by an increase of lung cancer incidence, while a fall in consumption is followed by a drop in lung cancer incidence, as shown for males in France between 1950 and 2006 (fig. 1).

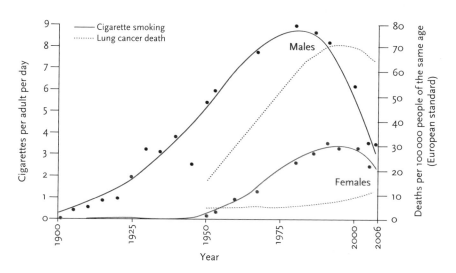

Figure 1. *Trends in cigarette smoking and death from lung cancer by sex in France, 1950–2006. Reproduced and modified from Hill* et al. *(2010) with permission from the publisher.*

COPD and asthma

In 2000, ~30% of the 371 000 deaths from nonmalignant respiratory diseases occurring in the EU were caused by cigarette smoking. Among these cases, COPD was the most frequent cause of death. Nearly two-thirds of these COPD deaths were caused by tobacco smoking. The COPD mortality rate is roughly 20 times higher among heavy smokers (male or female) than nonsmokers. According to international guidelines for COPD classification (American Thoracic Society, European Respiratory Society), up to 60% of current smokers aged >65 years may suffer from COPD. Measurement of FEV_1 and its decline is the best marker of airflow limitation in COPD, and the FEV_1 value is directly related to COPD morbidity and mortality. Physiological decline of FEV_1 with age is accelerated by tobacco smoking, whereas, in contrast, smoking cessation slows lung function decline in smokers (fig. 2). Cessation also improves COPD patient quality of life and is the only measure that definitively improves COPD patient survival. Asthmatic patients who smoke have a higher risk of hospitalisation for their disease and experience more severe symptoms with poor clinical control and poorer quality of life. Finally, active cigarette smoking is a direct cause of asthma onset, and causes more severe symptoms and lung function decline.

Respiratory infectious diseases

Bronchial and lung infectious diseases, including TB, acute bronchiolitis, pneumonia, the common cold and influenza, are more frequent and more severe in smokers.

Interstitial lung diseases

Several interstitial lung diseases, namely respiratory bronchiolitis-associated interstitial lung disease, desquamative interstitial pneumonia and pulmonary Langerhans' cell histiocytosis, are strongly associated with cigarette smoking.

Passive smoking

In addition to its direct harmful effects on active smokers, exposure to tobacco combustion products from smoking is dangerous to nonsmokers, as environmental tobacco smoke is highly toxic. In the EU, in 2002, an estimated 79 449 deaths were attributable to passive smoking from various diseases caused by

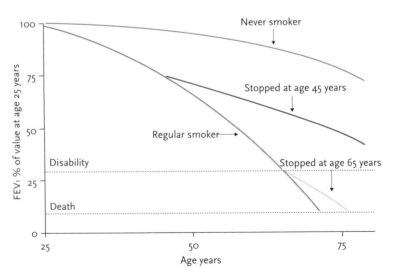

Figure 2. Loss of FEV_1 in never-smokers, regular smokers and smokers giving up at ages 45 and 65 years. Reproduced and modified from Fletcher et al. (1977) with permission from the publisher.

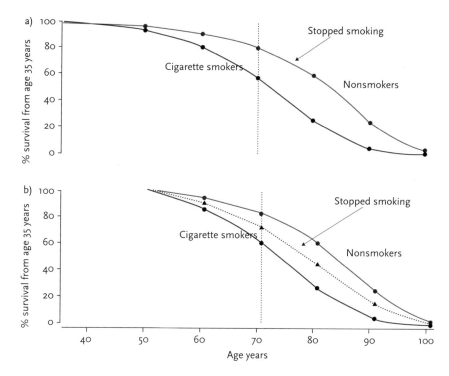

Figure 3. *Survival of male doctors who stopped smoking at ages a) 25–34 years and b) 45–54 years. Reproduced and modified from Doll* et al. *(2004) with permission from the publisher.*

second-hand smoking, including lung cancer (13 241 deaths), chronic non-neoplastic respiratory disease (5 275 deaths), ischaemic heart disease (32 342 deaths) and stroke (28 591 deaths).

Furthermore, COPD, asthma and several infectious diseases are more severe in nonsmokers exposed to passive smoking.

Conclusion

Since current treatments of lung cancer and COPD are poorly efficient, it is obvious that preventing tobacco use through tobacco control and treating tobacco addiction are by far the most efficient means to prevent and 'cure' these respiratory diseases. This conclusion is also true for most other diseases related to cigarette smoking. Indeed, the overall impact of smoking cessation on survival is significant for all smokers at any age, as shown in figure 3.

Further reading

- Arcavi L, et al. (2004). Cigarette smoking and infection. *Arch Intern Med*; 164: 2206–2216.
- The Aspect Consortium. Tobacco or Health In The European Union. Past, Present And Future. Brussels, Luxembourg, Office for Offical Publications of the European Communities, 2004.
- Doll R, et al. (2004). Mortality in relation to smoking: 50 years' observations on male British doctors. *BMJ*; 328: 1519–1528.
- Flanders WD, et al. (2003). Lung cancer mortality in relation to age, duration of smoking, and daily cigarette consumption: results from Cancer Prevention Study II. *Cancer Res*; 63: 6556–6562.
- Fletcher C, et al. (1977). The natural history of chronic airflow obstruction. *Br Med J*; 1: 1645–1648.

- Foulds J, *et al.* (2007). Snus – what should the public-health response be? *Lancet*; 369: 1976–1978.
- Hill C, *et al.* (2010). Le point sur l'épidémie de cancer du poumon dû au tabagisme [Assessment of the lung cancer epidemic due to smoking]. *BEH*; 19–20: 210–213.
- Maio S, *et al.* (2012). The European Respiratory Society spirometry tent: a unique form of screening for airway obstruction. *Eur Respir J*; 39: 1458–1467.
- Mannino DM, *et al.* (2006). The natural history of chronic obstructive pulmonary disease. *Eur Respir J*; 27: 627–643.
- Ryu JM, *et al.* (2001). Smoking-related interstitial lung diseases: a concise review. *Eur Respir J*; 17: 122–132.
- Smoke Free Partnership. Lifting the smokescreen: 10 reasons for a smoke free Europe. Brussels, European Respiratory Society Journals Ltd, 2006.

Treatment of tobacco dependence

Luke Clancy and Zubair Kabir

Tobacco dependence is a disease that would be of little consequence if it were not for the adverse effects of smoking. Instead it causes 30–40% of all cancers and is the principal cause of lung cancer. It is the biggest cause of preventable respiratory disease, even when lung and other respiratory cancers are excluded. Smoking is linked causally or as an important risk factor for: COPD, emphysema, asthma, and respiratory infections that include TB. Nevertheless, to speak of smoking as an occupational or environmental disease is perhaps not entirely accurate. However, without doubt, smoking prevalence has a strong occupational bias. Exposure to second-hand smoke at work is also a significant occupational hazard. This situation has been greatly improved by the enactment of smoke-free laws in many countries, especially within the European Union. However, second-hand smoke remains the most significant indoor pollutant, especially in homes and motorised vehicles.

Treating tobacco dependence is an important issue for respiratory physicians. An interest in the prevention of dependence through tobacco control mechanisms should also be a priority.

Prevention

As always, prevention is the primary intervention to be considered. The mechanisms for tobacco control are well established and have been incorporated in the Framework Convention for Tobacco Control (FCTC), which is the first medical treaty from the World Health Organization (WHO) that has been ratified by 176 countries and the European Community (EC). The WHO has also proposed a strategy, MPOWER as defined in table 1, for the implementation and monitoring of these mechanisms. It is clearly stated in the FCTC that price is the most effective tobacco control measure but that interventions, such as workplace restrictions on smoking and the protection from exposure and product regulation by various means, are also important. Such tobacco control policies were recently modelled to tease out individual effects on current and future trends in tobacco consumption rates and lung cancer death rates, employing previously validated simulation models, e.g. SimSmoke models. It is also agreed that full information, concerning the dangers of smoking, need to be made common knowledge through sustained, mass-media

---

Key points

- Tobacco dependence is a disease and is an important issue for respiratory physicians.

- The prevention of tobacco dependence through tobacco control mechanisms is a priority.

- Effective and cost-effective treatments for tobacco dependence exist in the form of motivational support and pharmacotherapy.

- The treatment of tobacco dependence benefits from knowledge, experience and training, which is not provided in medical schools at the undergraduate level, and should be made a priority.

---

campaigns. The value of health warnings, especially graphical images, is emphasised and there is a realisation that packaging and labelling are important methods of advertising for the tobacco industry. This is especially so in countries where direct advertising, promotion and sponsorship are banned. A step further would be to have plain packaging. However the role of treating smoking in the plan, although regarded as important, is left unclear. The reasons for this are many and include considerations of availability, cost, efficacy and efficiency. This is not surprising, but it is challenging. Even more challenging is the fact that the cost for other evidence-based interventions in the pursuit of tobacco control are usually much less than those for treatment. However, tobacco-dependency treatment is much more cost-effective than other chronic conditions, such as hypercholesterolaemia or hypertension, in terms of quality-adjusted life years (QALYs). Effective treatments are available, are very cost-effective and compare favourably with treatment of other diseases in this regard. Despite this, interest in supplying this service seems low among policymakers. Smoking was, and to some extent still is, not accepted as a disease by many people. This is, in no small part, due to the tobacco industry. For generations, it denied that smoking was harmful and addictive and emphasised the argument for free choice and the apparent glamour of smoking. It is now becoming widely accepted that smoking is a disease and that it is based on addiction. It is very difficult to treat, but the rewards for treating it successfully are enormous.

Table 1. Definition for MPOWER

Monitor tobacco use
Protect people from tobacco use
Offer help to quit tobacco use
Warn about the damages of tobacco
Enforce bans on tobacco advertising, promotion and sponsorship
Raise taxes on tobacco products

One-third of the world's population smokes. If this disease is to be tackled by treating all smokers, the implications are daunting; treatment alone will probably never become the appropriate response to this epidemic, unless much improved and cheaper treatments can be developed to make this possible in the future. A recent controlled trial demonstrated the efficacy of a low-priced product, namely, cytosine in smoking cessation. At present treatment has a defined role. Its importance in tobacco control will vary from time to time and from country to country depending on the stage of implementation of other tobacco control policies. Our first responsibility as doctors is probably to know what treatments exist, then to examine the evidence base for their usefulness and consider how they could be made available to our patients. To achieve such standards, training of health professionals in the treatment of tobacco dependence is crucial.

Evidence-based treatments

Effective and cost-effective treatments for tobacco dependence exist. The two treatment modalities proven to be effective consist of motivational support, in the form of counselling, and pharmacotherapy. Present knowledge suggests that a combination of the two is more effective than either alone. The duration of counselling seems to be important. Within limits, longer seems better – for instance, brief intervention by a general practitioner of some 3 min increases success rates by ~2.5% when compared with those who did not receive such advice. Sessions lasting ~10 min and repeated three to four times at intervals, according to present knowledge, seem to be near the optimal; however, these considerations need to be further defined along with their application.

As regards pharmacological therapies, a number of preparations have been shown to have measurable success rates. These include nicotine replacement therapy (NRT), which approximately the doubles success rate. Varenicline and buproprion also have established success rates. Varenicline seems to be more effective than NRT, while buproprion success rate is similar to that of NRT. The use of these preparations and their safety profiles need to be studied carefully. They provide the clinician with pharmacotherapy, which has proven efficacy and should be used knowledgably by physicians. Tønnesen *et al.* (2007) recently reviewed the evidence for smoking cessation, concluding that with the most optimal drugs and counselling a 1-year abstinence rate of ~25% can be expected for smoking cessation. This compares very favourably with the treatment of any other chronic relapsing disease. Caponnetta *et al.* (2008) recently outlined the predictors of success and failure in treatment. Factors which influence outcomes include: degree of nicotine dependence; age at initiation; how many cigarettes are smoked per day; social support; and family circumstances, such as a nonsmoking partner, sex and comorbidities, *e.g.* alcoholism and depression. They also point out the complex relationship with previous attempts and of course the importance of motivation to quit. The motivational chart in figure 1 clearly

outlines the importance of different stages of motivation before finally quitting smoking.

In addition, evidence suggests that attempts to quit are more frequent in subjects with high baseline BMI and low weight concerns. Innovative approaches, such as brief isometric exercise and the cognitive technique of body scanning, may be effective for reducing the desire to smoke and withdrawal symptoms in temporarily abstaining smokers. The importance of targeting specific groups, such as pregnant women and mentally ill patients, also lack adequate evidence in support of what works and what does not work in treating tobacco dependence.

Conclusion

The treatment of tobacco dependence benefits from the knowledge, experience and training of clinicians. This is not provided in medical schools at the undergraduate level. We expect that the structure of training for the management of this disease, and

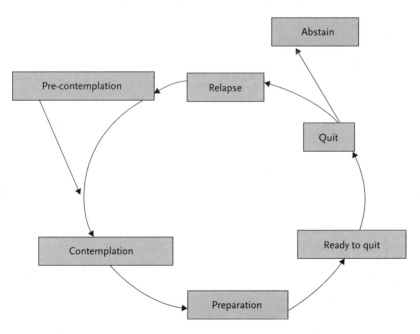

Figure 1. The different stages involved in the process of quitting smoking. Information from DiClemente et al. (1991).

particularly its treatment, will improve and increase in the short term. Knowledge of general tobacco control principles also need to be addressed if we are to succeed in this important endeavour.

Further reading

- Caponnetto P, et al. (2008). Smoking cessation: tips for improving success rates. Breathe; 5: 16–24.
- Currie LM, et al. (2012). The effect of tobacco control policies on smoking prevalence and smoking-attributable deaths in Ireland using the IrelandSS simulation model. Tob Control [In press DOI: 10.1136/tobaccocontrol-2011-050248].
- Cromwell J, et al. (1997). Cost-effectiveness of the clinical practice recommendations in the AHCPR guideline for smoking cessation. JAMA; 278: 1759–1766.
- DiClemente CC, et al. (1991). The process of smoking cessation: an analysis of precontemplation, contemplation, and preparation stages of change. J Consult Clin Psychol; 59: 295–304.
- Fagerström KO, et al. (2008). Pharmacological treatments for tobacco dependence. Eur Respir Rev; 17: 192–198.
- Goodman P, et al. (2007). Effects of the Irish smoking ban on respiratory health of bar workers and air quality in Dublin pubs. Am J Respir Crit Care Med; 175: 840–845.
- Kabir Z, et al. (2011). Attitudes, training and smoking profiles of European Respiratory Society members. Eur Respir J; 38: 225–227.
- Raw M, et al. (2009). A survey of tobacco dependence treatment guidelines in 31 countries. Addiction; 104: 1243–1250.
- Rigotti NA, et al. (2008). Smoking cessation interventions for hospitalized smokers: a systematic review. Arch Intern Med; 168: 1950–1960.
- Tønnesen P, et al. (2007). Smoking cessation in patients with respiratory diseases: a high priority, integral component of therapy. Eur Respir J; 29: 390–417.
- US Department of Health and Human Services. The Health Consequences of Involuntary Exposure to Tobacco Smoke: A Report of the Surgeon General. Atlanta, GA: US Department of Health and Human Services, Centers for Disease Control and Prevention, Coordinating Center for Health Promotion, National Center for Chronic Disease Prevention and Health Promotion, Office on Smoking and Health, 2006.
- Ussher M, et al. (2009). Effect of isometric exercise and body scanning on cigarette cravings and withdrawal symptoms. Addiction; 104: 1251–1257.
- West R, et al. (2011). Placebo-controlled trial of cytosine for smoking cessation. N Engl J Med; 365: 1193–2000.
- World Health Organization. WHO Report on the Global Tobacco Epidemic, 2009: Implementing smoke-free environments. Available from: www.who.int/tobacco/mpower/2009/en/ Date last accessed: July 07, 2012; Date last updated July 7, 2012.

High-altitude disease

Yvonne Nussbaumer-Ochsner and Konrad E. Bloch

Physiological response to altitude

The low barometric pressure at altitude results in a reduced inspiratory oxygen tension and P_aO_2. The immediate physiological response comprises a rise in heart rate and pulmonary arterial pressure. Chemoreceptor-mediated hyperventilation tends to mitigate hypoxaemia but the associated hypocapnia, with P_aCO_2 close to the apnoeic threshold, promotes ventilatory instability with periods of hyperpnoea alternating with central apnoea/hypopnoea. This pattern, termed high-altitude periodic breathing, is observed in healthy subjects at altitudes >1600 m, mostly during sleep. It may cause intermittent dyspnoea and sleep disturbances (figs 1 and 2).

Prolonged altitude exposure triggers various acclimatisation mechanisms including an increased chemoreceptor sensitivity to hypoxia and hypercapnia, enhanced erythropoesis, and alterations in the endocrine system, metabolism and in fluid balance.

The reduced air density at altitude lowers airflow resistance. Vital capacity is slightly reduced due to respiratory muscle weakness and pulmonary congestion. Oxygen uptake through the lungs is affected by a reduced alveolar–capillary oxygen gradient and a reduced transit time of blood through pulmonary capillaries due to increased cardiac output. This causes diffusion limitation leading to hypoxaemia especially during exercise.

High-altitude-related disease

In table 1, different forms of acute and chronic altitude-related illness are summarised. Acute mountain sickness (AMS) is the most common altitude-related illness. It affects 10–40% of lowlanders rapidly ascending to 3000 m and 40–60% at 4500 m. A lack of prior acclimatisation, rapid ascent, high sleeping altitude and individual susceptibility predispose to AMS. Symptoms start within 6–12 h after arrival at altitude and include headache, loss of appetite, nausea or vomiting, weakness, fatigue and insomnia. The diagnosis relies on the constellation of typical symptoms in the setting of altitude exposure. Different scores (*e.g.* the Lake Louise Score) help to establish the diagnosis and to grade AMS severity.

Key points

- A low barometric pressure at altitude results in reduced inspired oxygen tension and P_aO_2.

- Hypoxaemia triggers adaptive physiological repsonses termed acclimatisation.

- Respiratory acclimatisation includes hyperventilation and periodic breathing, which typically prevails during sleep.

- AMS, HACE and HAPE may affect travellers after rapid ascent to altitude. Chronic mountain sickness occurs in long-term residents of high mountain areas.

- Treatment of high-altitude related illness consists of descent, supplemental oxygen and, if necessary, drugs.

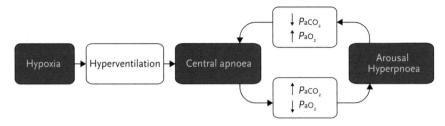

Figure 1. Mechanisms of high-altitude periodic breathing.

If additional neurological signs such as ataxia, cognitive deficits and impaired vigilance develop, a potentially life-threatening high-altitude cerebral oedema (HACE) must be considered. Treatments of AMS include descent to lower altitude, analgesics for headache and acetazolamide. More severe forms of AMS and HACE require dexamethasone and oxygen if available. Inflatable hyperbaric bags simulating descent to 1500–2500 m are also used.

High-altitude pulmonary oedema (HAPE) is a noncardiogenic and noninflammatory oedema resulting from excessive elevation of pulmonary capillary pressure, uneven distribution of blood flow and impaired

alveolar fluid clearance. HAPE is rare below 3500 m but occurs in 2–4% of mountaineers within hours to 4 days after arrival at 4500 m. It is promoted by rapid ascent, physical exertion and individual susceptibility. Manifestations of HAPE include excessive dyspnoea, dry cough, tachycardia, cyanosis, pulmonary crackles and low-grade fever. Chest radiography shows interstitial or alveolar opacities but a normal-sized heart. Descent, supplemental oxygen or both are nearly always successful in HAPE. If oxygen is not available or descent not possible, pharmaceuticals become necessary (table 2). Pulmonary vasodilators such as nifedipine or phosphodiesterase inhibitors (sildenafil)

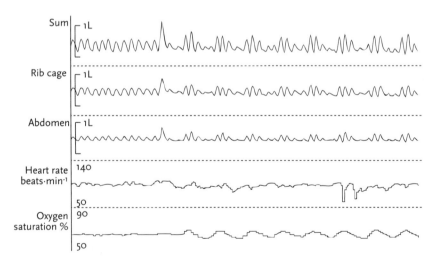

Figure 2. Periodic breathing associated with oscillations in oxygen saturation and heart rate recorded in a 28-year-old female resting after a climb at 6850 m. Reproduced and modified from Bloch et al. (2010) with permission from the publisher.

Table 1. Altitude-related illnesses

Condition	Time of exposure	Main manifestations and diagnostic criteria
AMS	Hours to days	Headache Loss of appetite Insomnia Fatigue
HACE	Hours to days	Severe headache Ataxia Confusion Loss of consciousness
HAPE	Days	Dyspnoea Cough Cyanosis Exercise intolerance Pulmonary hypertension
HAPH, cardiac chronic mountain sickness	Years	Dyspnoea Exercise intolerance Right heart failure $mPpa$ >30 mmHg or $sPpa$ >50 mmHg at altitude of residence Absence of excessive erythrocytosis[#]
CMS, Monge's disease	Years	Headache Dizziness Dyspnoea Sleep disturbances Fatigue Excessive erythrocytosis[#] Pulmonary hypertension[¶] Right heart failure[¶] Hypoventilation[¶]
Subacute mountain sickness, or adult and infantile forms of CSMS	Weeks to months	Dyspnoea Exercise intolerance Pulmonary hypertension Right heart failure

HAPH: high-altitude pulmonary hypertension; $mPpa$: mean pulmonary artery pressure; $sPpa$: systolic pulmonary artery pressure; CMS: chronic mountain sickness; CSMS: cardiac subacute mountain sickness.
[#]: excessive erythrocytosis is defined as haemoglobin concentration $\geqslant$19 g·dL^{-1} in females and $\geqslant$21 g·dL^{-1} in males;
[¶]: in some patients.

lower pulmonary artery pressure. If descent is impossible and oxygen unavailable, a hyperbaric bag may be lifesaving.

Table 2 summarises prevention and treatment of altitude related diseases.

Chronic mountain sickness, a condition observed in long-term high-altitude residents, is characterised by severe hypoxaemia, excessive erythrocytosis and pulmonary hypertension. Affected people suffer from fatigue, dizziness, headache and confusion. Descent to low altitude leads to prompt relief. High-altitude pulmonary hypertension is another condition affecting long-term residents at altitude >2500 m. It causes dyspnoea, exercise intolerance and signs of right heart failure with oedema but erythrocytosis is not a feature.

Table 2. Prevention and treatment of high-altitude disease

Disease	Prevention	Treatment
AMS	Acclimatisation Slow ascent Acetazolamide $2 \times 125-$ 250 mg·day^{-1} starting 24 h before ascent or dexamethasone 2×4 mg·day^{-1} starting 24 h before ascent	Analgesics Antiemetics Acetazolamide 2×250 mg·day^{-1} More severe forms: descent; oxygen 2–6 L·min^{-1}; dexamethasone (initially 8 mg *i.v.*, then 4×4 mg·day^{-1} *p.o.*); acetazolamide (2×250 mg·day^{-1}), eventually in combination with dexamethasone; portable hyperbaric chamber
HACE	As for AMS	Immediate descent If not possible: oxygen (2–6 L·min^{-1}), portable hyperbaric chamber, dexamethasone (initially 8 mg *i.v.*, then 4×4 mg·day^{-1} *p.o.*), check for accompanying HAPE, acetazolamide if descent delayed
HAPE	Acclimatisation Slow accent Avoid overexertion Nifedipine 30–60 mg·day^{-1} (extended-release formulation)	Immediate descent If not possible: oxygen 2–6 L·min^{-1} until oxygen saturation >90% or hyperbaric chamber, nifedipine 10–20 mg initially, switch to an extended-release formulation (nifedipine 30/60 mg) depending on blood pressure, treat accompanying AMS by dexamethasone

Patients with lung disease at altitude

Little is known about the risks of altitude exposure in patients with pre-existing lung disease. Recommendations are largely based on anecdotal evidence.

Chronic obstructive pulmonary disease In patients with impaired gas exchange, PaO$_2$ may drop to low levels at altitude so the use of supplemental oxygen should be considered. It is reasonable that patients with severe disease (FEV$_1$ <50% predicted) with SaO$_2$ <95% at low altitude should have an individual assessment before travelling to altitude. Acetazolamide should be used with caution in patients with severe airflow obstruction, as the metabolic acidosis induced by the drug may further stimulate ventilation thereby worsening dyspnoea and promoting respiratory failure.

Asthma A reduced allergen burden with increasing altitude can be expected at >1500 m. Conversely, inhalation of cold air may worsen asthma, especially in combination with exercise or hypoxia-induced hyperventilation. Asthma patients with controlled disease are advised to take their usual medications when travelling to altitude, to avoid strenuous exercise in a cold environment and to treat any exacerbation appropriately. Patients with uncontrolled, severe asthma should be cautioned against travelling to altitude.

Obstructive sleep apnoea syndrome Untreated OSAS patients residing at sea level and travelling to moderate altitude (>1600 m) experience an exacerbation of sleep apnoea with pronounced hypoxaemia and frequent central events. Sleep quality is worse at altitude and daytime testing shows impaired vigilance and elevated blood pressure. Combined treatment with CPAP and acetazolamide is advisable.

Pulmonary hypertension In general, patients with more than mild pre-existing pulmonary hypertension should be counselled against high-altitude travel because pre-existing pulmonary hypertension may predispose to HAPE. In patients not on medical therapy, prophylaxis with nifedipine and supplemental oxygen should be considered.

Conclusions

Physiological adaptation allows humans to tolerate exposure to even very high altitudes. Rapid ascent, inappropriate time for acclimatisation, strenuous physical exertion and individual susceptibility predispose to high-altitude-related illnesses, which may be prevented with appropriate precautions.

Further reading

- Basnyat B, et al. (2003). High-altitude illness. Lancet; 361: 1967–1974.
- Bloch KE, et al. (2010). Nocturnal periodic breathing during acclimatization at very high altitude at Mt. Muztagh Ata (7546m). Am J Respir Crit Care Med; 182: 562–568.
- Imray C, et al. (2010). Acute mountain sickness: pathophysiology, prevention, and treatment. Prog Cardiovasc Dis; 52: 467–484.
- Latshang TD, et al. (2012). Effect of acetazolamide and autoCPAP therapy on breathing disturbances among patients with obstructive sleep apnea syndrome who travel to altitude. A randomized controlled trial. JAMA; 308: 2390–2398.
- Luks AM, et al. (2007). Travel to high altitude with pre-existing lung disease. Eur Respir J; 29: 770–792.
- Maggiorini M (2010). Prevention and treatment of high-altitude pulmonary edema. Prog Cardiovasc Dis; 52: 500–506.
- Nussbaumer-Ochsner Y, et al. (2010). Exacerbation of sleep apnoea by frequent central events in patients with the obstructive sleep apnoea syndrome at altitude: a randomised trial. Thorax; 65: 429–435.
- Nussbaumer-Ochsner Y, et al. (2007). Lessons from high-altitude physiology. Breathe; 4: 123–132.
- Nussbaumer-Ochsner Y, et al. Air travel and altitude. In: Ayres JG, et al., eds. Environmental Medicine. London, Hodder Arnold, 201.
- Nussbaumer-Ochsner Y, et al. (2012). Effect of short-term acclimatization to high altitude on sleep and nocturnal breathing. Sleep; 35: 419–423.

Diving-related diseases

Einar Thorsen

There are three main groups at risk of diving-related diseases:

- Professional divers are engaged in underwater construction and inspection, and compressed air workers (caisson workers) work at increased ambient pressure in a dry environment, mostly in tunnel construction
- Military forces, police and fire brigades have teams of divers for specialised underwater operations
- Recreational divers make up by far the largest group of divers

The physical environment in which these divers are operating is different, but common to all groups is exposure to increased ambient pressure and the exposure factors associated with pressure.

Pulmonary limitations at depth

Gas density increases proportionately with ambient pressure when air is used as the

---

Key points

- Normal lung function and physical work capacity are required for underwater work.

- Normal lung function is required to reduce the risk of pulmonary barotrauma.

- Cumulative diving exposure is associated with a long-term reduction in lung function of an obstructive pattern, which at some time in the diver's career may preclude further diving.

---

gas breathed. Airway resistance is proportional to gas density and maximal expiratory flow rates are inversely proportional to the square root of gas density. This means that at a depth of 30 m, when relative gas density is four times that of air at atmospheric pressure, maximal expiratory flow rates and maximal voluntary ventilation are reduced by 50%. Most experimental data are close to this theoretical relationship, as illustrated in figure 1.

When diving to depths >50 m, the gas breathed is often a mixture of helium and oxygen to compensate for the mechanical limitations of ventilatory capacity due to gas density. The partial pressure of oxygen in these gas mixtures is usually 30–50 kPa, corresponding to an oxygen fraction of 2–5% at depths of $\geqslant$100 m.

Physical work under water is demanding. It requires evaluation of normal ventilatory capacity and physical work capacity by exercise testing. External resistance and static load related to breathing apparatus and submersion adds to the increased load imposed by gas density. The gas breathed at depth has to be dry to prevent icing in the pressure regulators and evaporative heat loss is high. The gas breathed has the temperature of the ambient water and, because of increased gas density, convective heat loss is increased. Subjects with bronchial hyperreactivity may be at increased risk of bronchoconstriction at depth. There are, however, no definite studies confirming this risk, as subjects with asthma traditionally have been excluded from diving.

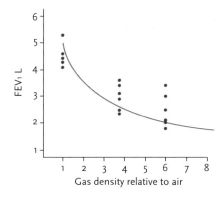

Figure 1. *The theoretical relationship between gas density and FEV₁ and some experimental data. The relative gas density of air at atmospheric pressure is 1.*

Pulmonary barotrauma

Intra-alveolar gas volume will expand during decompression. If there is any obstruction to the free flow of gas out of the alveoli or a decrease in lung compliance, there will be an increase in intra-alveolar pressure, imposing a risk of lung rupture or pulmonary barotrauma. Any processes in the lung associated with airway obstruction or decreased compliance locally or generally are considered to increase the risk. Lung rupture may cause pneumothorax, pneumopericardium, mediastinal emphysema and, most seriously, arterial gas embolism, which may be fatal. A pneumothorax or pneumopericardium encountered at depth may be fatal because of an increase in the transpulmonary pressure difference during decompression that obstructs venous return. The lowest pressure drop associated with diving causing pulmonary barotrauma described in the literature was <20 kPa (200 cmH₂O). The volume expansion for a given pressure reduction is larger close to the surface (Boyle–Mariotte's law).

Pulmonary effects of a single dive

A dive is associated with exposure to hyperoxia and a decompression stress, and both are related to ambient pressure and time. Hyperoxia at partial pressures of oxygen >40 kPa has well known toxic effects on the lung, causing acute reductions in diffusion capacity, vital capacity and maximal expiratory flow rates. The decompression stress is related to the amount of inert gas dissolved in the tissues during the deepest phase of the dive and the rate of decompression. Supersaturation resulting in formation of venous gas bubbles has been demonstrated when the tension of inert gas in the tissues exceeds ambient pressure by ~30 kPa. Venous gas microemboli have been shown to be common with the decompression procedures routinely used in commercial and military diving operations.

The venous gas microemboli are filtered in the pulmonary circulation and are associated with inflammatory responses that add to the toxic effects of hyperoxia. Venous gas microemboli may be shunted over to the systemic circulation through intrapulmonary and intracardiac shunts. A patent foramen ovale is present in 20–30% of the general population. Local circulatory disturbances due to gas bubbles that are either formed *in situ* or transported by the systemic circulation to other areas like joints, skin, brain and spinal cord may cause decompression sickness.

The combination of added static and dynamic respiratory load, immersion and exercise results in a large increase in pulmonary arterial pressure. Undue breathlessness after diving, or even swimming only, may be related to pulmonary oedema.

Long-term effects of diving

The exposure to hyperoxia and the accumulation of gas microemboli in the lung are associated with inflammatory responses. Several cross-sectional studies of divers' lung function indicate that residual effects of single dives accumulate to a long-term effect characterised by an obstructive spirometric pattern and a reduction in diffusion capacity. There are only a few longitudinal studies of divers' lung function, but these studies confirm the findings in the cross-sectional studies by demonstrating a negative relationship between cumulative diving exposure and maximal expiratory flow rates and FEV$_1$.

Treatment of diving related disease and hyperbaric oxygen therapy

Arterial gas embolism and decompression sickness, which are caused by free gas in the tissues, should be treated promptly with recompression and hyperbaric oxygen. The rationale is to reduce bubble radius by increasing ambient pressure and to facilitate diffusion of inert gas out of the bubbles by increasing oxygen tension. The US Navy Treatment Tables are the most commonly used reference. Normobaric oxygen therapy by tight fitting an oronasal mask should always be started immediately and be given during transport to a hyperbaric treatment facility. Restoration of fluid balance is important while other supportive therapy is questionable.

The oxygen exposure during treatment is relatively large and oxygen toxicity with an acute reduction in vital capacity of 10% is acceptable. This is because neurological deficits are the most common manifestations of decompression sickness and the reduction in vital capacity is largely reversible.

Hyperbaric oxygen therapy, most commonly given for 90 min daily at a pressure of 240 kPa for 20–30 days, may be beneficial for late side-effects of radiation therapy for cancer, chronic ischaemic ulcers and chronic osteomyelitis. The oxygen dose is lower than for treatment of decompression sickness but there may be a cumulative oxygen toxicity effect. These patients' lung function should always be evaluated, as lung disease may pose a risk for arterial gas embolism in these patients. Pulmonary radiation injury is a contraindication to hyperbaric oxygen therapy.

Further reading

- Brubakk AO, et al., eds. Bennett and Elliott's Physiology and Medicine of Diving. Edinburgh, Saunders, Elsevier Science Ltd, 2003.
- Lundgren CEG, et al., eds. The Lung at Depth. New York, Marcel Dekker Inc., 1999.
- Tetzlaff K, et al. (2005). Breathing at depth: physiologic and clinical aspects of diving while breathing compressed gas. Clin Chest Med; 26: 355–380.

Radiation-induced lung disease

Robert P. Coppes and Peter van Luijk

Radiotherapy plays an important role in the treatment of tumours located in the thoracic area. The cure rate for these tumours is, however, limited by the low radiation dose that can be tolerated by the lungs. The presently set dose (*e.g.* mean dose <20 Gy) already results in pulmonary complications in about one-fifth of patients.

The primary insults after radiation of the lungs seem to be vascular remodelling and an early inflammatory response termed radiation pneumonitis. These are followed by a late fibroproductive phase (fig. 1). All these pathologies may lead to compromised lung perfusion, increased vascular resistance, reduced gas-exchange interphase between the air and blood, and suboptimal blood oxygenation. Symptoms range from dyspnoea on effort to respiratory failure, oxygen dependency, right heart failure and death.

Almost immediately after irradiation, loss of endothelial cells causes vascular oedema and remodelling. This leads to pulmonary hypertension and right ventricle hypertrophy. Next to this, several inflammatory responses contribute to

radiation pneumonitis. Acute alveolar and interstitial inflammation and loss of type I epithelial cells induce proliferation of type II epithelial cells. This leads to a cascade of induction of inflammatory cytokines (fig. 1), potentially aggravated by chemotherapeutic agents. Subsequently, an influx of inflammatory cells, such as leukocytes, lymphocytes, neutrophils and macrophages, is induced. Though macrophages are a hallmark, T-lymphocytes and mature dendritic cells also play an important role in radiation pneumonitis.

Radiation-induced lung disease is a consequence of:

- loss of endothelial and type I epithelial cells
- malfunction of microvasculature
- inflammatory responses
- lung fibrosis

Increased vascular permeability with protein exudation contributes to the development of radiation pneumonitis. Depending on the irradiated region and volume, the damaged pulmonary blood vessels (low dose and large volumes) or inflammatory parenchymal damage (high dose and low volumes) affect lung function to induce complications.

Following or even without prior symptomatic pneumonitis, chronic radiation-induced pulmonary fibrosis may develop depending on the irradiated lung volume. Radiation fibrosis is caused by accumulation of collagen and other extracellular matrix fibres in the interstitium under persistent cytokine stimuli in combination with arteriocapillary sclerosis.

Key points

- Radiotherapy for tumour treatment results in pulmonary complications in about 20% of patients.

- Radiation-induced lung injury involves vascular damage leading to pulmonary hypertension and develops from an early, inflammatory phase to a late fibrotic phase.

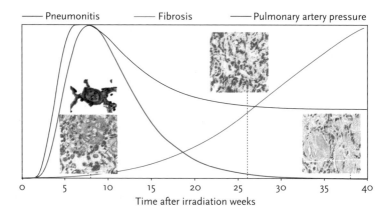

——— Pneumonitis   ——— Fibrosis   ——— Pulmonary artery pressure

Time after irradiation weeks

Figure 1. Radiation-induced lung injury develops in an early vascular damage and inflammation phase, and a late fibrotic phase.

It should be noted that there are other causes of occupational-induced radiation lung disease, for example, resulting from nuclear accidents, and radon and uranium exposure (see Further Reading).

Further reading

- Abu-Qare AW, *et al.* (2002). Depleted uranium – the growing concern. *J Appl Toxicol*; 22: 149–152.
- Al-Zoughool M, *et al.* (2009). Health effects of radon: a review of the literature. *Int J Radiat Biol*; 85: 57–69.
- Ghobadi G, *et al.* (2012). Lung irradiation induces pulmonary vascular remodelling resembling pulmonary arterial hypertension. *Thorax*; 67: 334–341.
- Göransson Nyberg A, *et al.* (2011). Mass casualties and health care following the release of toxic chemicals or radioactive material – contribution of modern biotechnology. *Int J Environ Res Public Health*; 8: 4521–4549.
- Johnston CJ, *et al.* (2004). Inflammatory cell recruitment following thoracic irradiation. *Exp Lung Res*; 30: 369–382.
- Marks LB, *et al.* (2003). Radiation-induced lung injury. *Semin Radiat Oncol*; 13: 333–345.
- McBride WH, *et al.* (2004). A sense of danger from radiation. *Radiat Res*; 162: 1–19.
- Medhora M, *et al.* (2012). Radiation damage to the lung: mitigation by angiotensin-converting enzyme (ACE) inhibitors. *Respirology*; 17: 66–71.
- Novakova-Jiresova A, *et al.* (2007). Changes in expression of injury after irradiation of increasing volumes in rat lung. *Int J Radiat Oncol Biol Phys*; 67: 1510–1518.
- Rodemann HP, *et al.* (1995). Cellular basis of radiation-induced fibrosis. *Radiother Oncol*; 35: 83–90.
- Rübe CE, *et al.* (2004). Increased expression of pro-inflammatory cytokines as a cause of lung toxicity after combined treatment with gemcitabine and thoracic irradiation. *Radiother Oncol*; 72: 231–241.

HRCT in the diagnosis of interstitial lung disease

Giovanni Della Casa, Stefania Cerri, Paolo Spagnolo, Pietro Torricelli and Luca Richeldi

The term interstitial lung disease (ILD) refers to a heterogeneous group of >200 different entities. Because the clinical presentation of most of them is similar (mostly, exertional dyspnoea and dry cough) chest HRCT, a CT technique optimised for high spatial resolution, plays a key role in the assessment of patients who are known to have, or are suspected of having, diffuse lung disease. The study of the HRCT appearance and distribution patterns allows a specific diagnosis to be made in many cases or, at least, is helpful in narrowing the differential diagnosis. For this reason, HRCT has become the imaging modality of choice in ILD. The importance of HRCT is further underlined by the fact that there is no single gold-standard diagnostic test for ILD; instead, a multidisciplinary approach, with integration of radiological, pathologic and clinical data, is considered the optimal approach.

Anatomy of the lung interstitium

Understanding of HRCT patterns of ILD requires knowledge of the anatomy of the normal lung. In the high-contrast environment of the lung, the resolution of HRCT is 0.2–0.3 mm. According to Weibel's concept, the interstitium represents the supporting framework of the lung and is composed of connective tissue fibres that can be divided into two separate, but connected, compartments:

1. the central (or axial) compartment that surrounds the bronchovascular bundles, as they emerge from the pulmonary hila and extend peripherally to the level of respiratory bronchioles
2. the peripheral (or septal) interstitium that includes the interlobular septa and the subpleural interstitium

These two compartments are connected to each other by a fine network of septal connective tissue fibres (the intralobular interstitium).

Interlobular septa can occasionally be visible on HRCT of the normal lung, especially in the periphery of the anterior, lateral, juxtamediastinal regions of the upper and middle lobes, and in the periphery of the anterior and diaphragmatic regions of the lower zones.

The smallest anatomical unit of the lung visible on HRCT is the secondary pulmonary lobule (Miller's lobule), which is the

---

Key points

- Interstitial lung diseases are a heterogeneous group of entities with similar clinical presentations.

- A pattern-based approach to HRCT can help to discriminate between diseases with similar presentations, making a specific diagnosis in many cases or, at least, narrowing the differential diagnosis.

- In controversial cases, surgical biopsy might be necessary and a multidisciplinary approach (integrating clinical presentation and laboratory data, chest imaging, and lung pathology) is considered the best approach to formulate a confident diagnosis.

---

smallest area of lung parenchyma surrounded by connective tissue septa. Secondary pulmonary lobules are irregular polyhedral structures measuring 1.0–2.5 cm in diameter, containing roughly three to five acini and 30–50 primary lobules. Interlobular septa extend perpendicularly from the peripheral interstitium and penetrate the lung to form the boundaries of each secondary lobule. Secondary lobules are clearly demarcated in the periphery of the lung where interlobular septa are thicker, but are poorly demarcated centrally where interlobular septa are thinner and less well defined. Each lobule is supplied at its centre by a bronchiole and pulmonary artery.

Normal lung structures visible on HRCT are bronchi (down to eight generations), pulmonary arteries, pulmonary veins, interlobular septa and the visceral pleura (double layer as lobar fissures). Under normal conditions, structures such as lymphatic vessels, alveoli/acini, capillary vessels and visceral pleura (non-fissural surface) are not visible on HRCT. The centrilobular artery (1 mm in diameter) and the intralobular acinar arteries (0.5 mm in diameter) are identifiable, whereas normal bronchioles supplying a secondary lobule (1 mm in diameter), with a wall thickness of ~0.15 mm, are beyond the resolution of HRCT.

Approach to HRCT

In ILD, the identification of basic HRCT patterns plays a critical role at the beginning of the diagnostic assessment. In fact, the pattern and distribution of the HRCT lung appearance may suggest a specific diagnosis and can help to discriminate among diseases with similar morphology. The same disease may present with different HRCT patterns. This may result from its variable pathological expression (*e.g.* progressive systemic sclerosis with lung involvement may present with a usual interstitial pneumonia (UIP), nonspecific interstitial pneumonia (NSIP) or organising pneumonia pattern), from its temporal phase (*e.g.* hypersensitivity pneumonitis may be detected in its acute, subacute or chronic stage) or from its natural progression (*e.g.*

a NSIP may proceed from minimal changes to end-stage lung). Moreover, the same pattern may be present in several diseases (*e.g.* collagen vascular disorders). This is intuitive, as the lung can respond to injury in a limited and predictable mode, so that many different diseases may lead to similar alterations in pulmonary anatomy, resulting in overlapping imaging findings. These aspects underscore the need for a multidisciplinary approach (clinical presentation and laboratory data, chest imaging, and lung pathology) to formulate a confident diagnosis. Nowadays, the importance of this approach is widely recognised.

Lung parenchymal abnormalities can be grossly divided into those with increased or decreased attenuation (table 1). As a general rule, lung volumes are increased by processes that produce decreased attenuation (*e.g.* air trapping and emphysema) and decreased by processes that produce reticulation and honeycombing.

Increased attenuation

Reticular pattern has several morphological variations, ranging from generalised thickening of the interlobular septa to honeycomb lung. The thickening of interlobular and intralobular septa, thus creating a net-like pattern, can generate this. On HRCT, this pattern is most frequently seen in the periphery extending from and perpendicular to the pleura. Septa can be classified as:

- smooth, where all interstitial compartments are thickened with a smooth profile (*e.g.* pulmonary hydrostatic oedema, lymphangitic carcinomatosis, pulmonary haemorrhage, pulmonary alveolar proteinosis, amyloidosis and a number of rarer conditions)
- irregular (*e.g.* fibrosis, lymphoma or secondary solid tumour)
- nodular, where the interstitial compartments are thickened in nodular form ('beaded appearance') (*e.g.* lymphangitic carcinomatosis,

Table 1. HRCT patterns in different ILDs.

	Increased attenuation			Nodular			Decreased attenuation	
Reticular	GGO	Consolidation	Centrilobular	Paralymphatic	Random		Cystic	Honeycombing
LC	NSIP	COP	RB-ILD	Sarcoidosis	Haematogenous metastases		LCH	UIP/IPF
HP	AIP	AIP	LCH	Silicosis	Miliary TB		LAM	Fibrotic NSIP
Chronic HP	DIP	Sarcoidosis	Subacute HP	LIP	Miliary fungal infection		LIP	Drugs
Sarcoidosis	RB-ILD	Drugs					DIP	Sarcoidosis (stage IV)
Drugs	LIP	Acute/subacute HP					Emphysema	Chronic HP
UIP	COP	Acute exacerbation of ILD						CVD
NSIP	Acute/subacute HP							
CVD	Acute exacerbation of ILD							

LC: lymphangitic carcinomatosis; HP: hypersensitivity pneumonitis; CVD: collagen vascular disease.

sarcoidosis, pneumoconiosis and secondary tumour)

The end-stage fibrotic lung is characterised by a coarse reticular pattern reflecting advanced interstitial fibrosis and architecture destruction, and is commonly associated with honeycombing (*e.g.* UIP, asbestosis, collagen vascular disease and radiation-induced fibrosis).

Ground-glass pattern Ground-glass opacities (GGOs) appear as hazy areas of increased opacity of the lung that are not dense enough to hide the underlying bronchial and vascular structures. It can result from thickening of alveolar septa, or partial alveolar filling with fluid, cells or amorphous material leading to a decrease in the normal ratio between air on the one hand, and blood and soft tissues on the other. In pulmonary fibrosis, GGO can also represent very fine interstitial fibrosis beyond the spatial resolution of the scan obtained. A GGO pattern can be observed in a large number of ILDs, such as:

- NSIP
- acute interstitial pneumonia (AIP)
- desquamative interstitial pneumonia (DIP)
- respiratory bronchiolitis-associated interstitial lung disease (RB-ILD)
- lymphoid interstitial pneumonia (LIP)
- cryptogenic organising pneumonia (COP)
- acute/subacute hypersensitivity pneumonitis
- acute exacerbation of ILD

GGO distribution, ancillary findings and clinical phase (acute *versus* subacute/chronic) may narrow the differential diagnosis or even be suggestive of a specific entity. GGO may be associated in up to one-third of the cases with fibrosis (traction bronchiectasis and honeycombing). In the absence of any of these signs, GGO may, in theory, represent a reversible disease process.

Consolidation pattern A consolidation is an area of increased attenuation where vessels are obscured by consolidated (white) lung; an air bronchogram may or may not be present. This situation typically results from filling of the airspaces with fluid (*e.g.* oedema, blood or pus). Consolidation is a common finding; the following conditions may all manifest with consolidation:

- organising pneumonia
- chronic eosinophilic pneumonia
- lipoid pneumonia
- bronchoalveolar carcinoma (BAC)
- lymphoma

Nodular pattern is characterised by the presence of multiple airspace or interstitial nodules, well or poorly defined, varying in size (up to 3 cm in diameter), with or without presence of cavitation. Low-density nodules with ill-defined margins (nodular GG) may be difficult to recognise. They are commonly seen in patients with diseases primarily affecting the small airways and surrounding areas. High-density nodules with well-defined margins have a solid aspect and obscure the edges of vessels or other adjacent structures. They are more characteristic of diseases primarily affecting the interstitium. The nodular pattern may be classified as:

- centrilobular
- perilymphatic
- random

based on the relationship with the secondary pulmonary lobule. The distribution of the nodules depends on the route of arrival and on the modality of spread. Diseases caused by inhalation show nodules close to the bronchiole in the centre of lobules (centrilobular), while diseases that grow along the lymphatics are more present in the periphery of the lobules and along the fissures (lymphatic). The lesions that spread haematogenously are visible everywhere (random), sometimes in connection with blood vessels.

Centrilobular nodules can be hazy or sharply defined. HRCT features that can help in their discrimination are the distinct central location in the secondary pulmonary lobule, the respect to one another, and the fact that they appear separated by several millimetres from the pleural surfaces, fissures and interlobular septa. Ranging in size from a few millimetres to a centimetre, centrilobular nodules are usually ill defined. They can be further subcategorised on the basis of the presence of an associated 'tree in bud' pattern (*e.g.* centrilobular nodules with a Y-shaped configuration often caused by infection or aspiration). Centrilobular nodules are observed in subacute hypersensitivity pneumonitis, in RB-ILD, and less commonly in pneumoconiosis, pulmonary Langerhans' cell histiocytosis (LCH), LIP and COP.

A perilymphatic distribution of nodules is commonly seen in patients with sarcoidosis, lymphangitic carcinomatosis, LIP and pneumoconiosis. Perilymphatic nodules are subpleural in location but may also be found along interlobular septa, interlobar fissures and bronchovascular bundles, where the lymphatics are most concentrated. Typically, they show a patchy distribution. However, in some patients with perilymphatic nodular disease, nodules can also be found in the centrilobular areas, in association with nodules more typically distributed in subpleural regions and along the interlobular septa (sarcoidosis and lymphangitic carcinomatosis).

Randomly distributed nodules are found diffusely throughout the lung parenchyma without a predominant distribution within either the secondary pulmonary lobules or the lymphatics. They may also be seen at the termination of small pulmonary arterial vessels (feeding-vessel sign). This distribution is typical of haematogenous dissemination (*e.g.* miliary TB, haematogenous metastasis and miliary fungal disease).

Decreased attenuation

Cystic pattern A cyst appears as a round parenchymal lucency or low-attenuating area with a well-defined interface with the normal lung. Cysts have variable wall thickness but usually display an epithelial or fibrous, thin wall (2 mm). The presence of a definable wall and the absence of residual centrilobular artery differentiate cysts from centrilobular emphysema. Cysts in the lung usually contain air but occasionally contain fluid or solid material. The shape of the cysts depends on the mechanism of their formation, the relationship with each other and the concomitance of traction phenomena in the surrounding parenchyma. These 'holes in the lung' may be due to dilation of bronchial structures, abnormal distension of alveolar spaces, focal destruction of lung parenchyma or cavitation of solid lesions. The profusion of the cysts may be variable, from scattered to very numerous. The craniocaudal distribution of the lesions may help in the differential diagnosis of LCH, which usually spares the costophrenic angle while lymphangioleiomyomatosis (LAM) cysts are distributed throughout the lung. A cystic pattern can also be indicative of LIP, DIP and more rare conditions.

Honeycombing consists of cystic airspaces with thick, clearly definable walls lined with bronchiolar epithelium, predominantly in the basal and subpleural areas; the cystic spaces are typically layered along pleural surfaces, in one or more concentric layers. The cyst walls are generally 3–10 mm thick and have a uniform size. Honeycombing represents areas of destroyed and fibrotic lung tissue on histology, where the normal architecture has been lost. Frequently, they are associated with coarse reticulation, architectural distortion and traction bronchiectasis; as such, honeycombing is usually seen in patients with end-stage fibrosis. Diseases that may present with honeycombing include idiopathic pulmonary fibrosis (IPF), fibrotic NSIP, chronic hypersensitivity pneumonitis, sarcoidosis (fibrotic stages) and collagen vascular disease. A subpleural bibasilar honeycombing on HRCT has a high positive predictive value for the histologic diagnosis of UIP.

HRCT features of the most common ILD

Idiopathic interstitial pneumonias (IIPs) are a heterogeneous group of non-neoplastic lung diseases in which the lung parenchyma is damaged by varying patterns of inflammation and/or fibrosis. The American Thoracic Society/European Respiratory Society classification of IIPs, published in 2002 (and currently under revision), defines the morphological patterns on which clinical, radiological and pathological diagnosis of IIPs is based. IIPs include seven entities:

1. IPF, which is characterised by the morphologic pattern of UIP
2. NSIP
3. COP
4. RB-ILD
5. DIP
6. LIP
7. AIP

HRCT has gained an important role in the diagnosis and management of patients with IIP, particularly in distinguishing between UIP and NSIP, the two largest subsets of IIPs.

The typical UIP pattern on HRCT can be found in 50–70% of the biopsy-proven cases. When present, it allows a noninvasive diagnosis to be made with high accuracy, confidence and interobserver agreement. In all of the other IIPs, a confident diagnosis requires biopsy.

Specific diseases

Idiopathic pulmonary fibrosis The term IPF refers to a distinct type of chronic fibrosing pneumonia of unknown cause. It is the most common of the IIPs, accounting for about 50–60% of IIP cases. The prognosis is usually dismal, with a median survival time of 2–4 years from diagnosis.

On chest HRCT, IPF is characterised by the UIP pattern, which is predominantly subpleural with an apical–basal gradient (fig. 1). Specific findings of UIP pattern include honeycombing, peripheral reticular opacities that determine irregular interfaces between the lung and pleura, intralobular interstitial thickening with minimal GGO abnormality, traction bronchiectasis and bronchiolectasis. Lower lobe volume loss is also a common finding. In typical IPF, areas of increased density (GGO) are absent or of limited extension. When GGO is present in IPF, it usually evolves to fibrosis. If the areas of GGO exceed 30% of lung volume, alternative diagnostic hypotheses should be

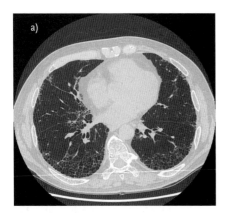

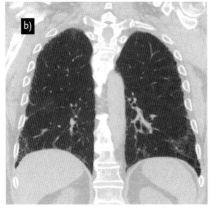

Figure 1. *UIP/IPF. a) Axial and b) coronal HRCT images show stacked, thin-walled cysts in the subpleural portion of the lungs. In definite UIP, honeycombing is most severe in the basilar and peripheral portions of the lungs.*

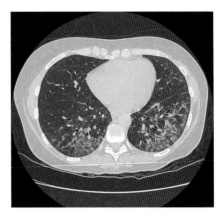

Figure 2. *NSIP. Axial HRCT image shows basilar GGOs, reticulation and traction bronchiectasis consistent with fibrotic NSIP.*

considered, such as NSIP, DIP, COP, hypersensitivity pneumonitis or RB-ILD. Honeycombing can mimic the bullae of emphysema. The association of centrilobular and paraseptal emphysema with lung fibrosis, however, can be observed in heavy smokers. Honeycombing pattern is present in 80–90% of patients with UIP and is considered the strongest predictor of the diagnosis of IPF, even if it can be present in pulmonary fibrosis of other causes. As such, a definite UIP pattern on HRCT, in a patient without clinical evidence of an alternative diagnosis, is sufficient for a confident diagnosis of IPF and carries an accuracy of

80–90%. A UIP pattern can, however, occasionally have other causes, including collagen vascular diseases, chronic hypersensitivity pneumonitis, drugs (*e.g.* bleomycin and amiodarone) and asbestosis. In such cases, a histological confirmation of the diagnosis is required.

Nonspecific interstitial pneumonia is a pathological term used to describe interstitial inflammation and fibrosis with temporal and spatial uniformity that does not fulfil the clinical–pathological criteria of UIP, DIP or AIP. NSIP can be observed in a number of conditions, such as collagen vascular diseases, inhalation of organic/ inorganic antigens, hypersensitivity pneumonitis, drug toxicity or slowly resolving acute lung injury. When no associated process can be found in a patient with a histological and radiological pattern of NSIP, the diagnosis of idiopathic NSIP is established. On HRCT, the disease is usually distributed bilaterally with basal and peripheral predominance (fig. 2). The most common feature is diffuse GGO, occurring in up to 80% of cases. GGO can be the only visible abnormality in ~30% of cases, or can be associated with peripheral irregular linear or reticular opacities in ~50% of cases. Consolidation occurs in 20% of patients. Traction bronchiectasis and micronodules can also be present. Subpleural sparing, if present, is a highly specific feature of NSIP. Honeycombing, a rare finding, which, if present, is usually mild compared with UIP, is only seen in patients with the fibrotic variant of NSIP. Differentiation between fibrotic NSIP and UIP requires surgical lung biopsy. At present, there is no single feature or combination of HRCT features that have high specificity for a histological diagnosis of NSIP. In fact, features of UIP and organising pneumonia may overlap with fibrotic and cellular NSIP, respectively.

Cryptogenic organising pneumonia
Organising pneumonia is often secondary to a known cause such as collagen vascular disease, viral pneumonia or drug reactions. The term COP, which refers to idiopathic organising pneumonia, better defines the disease previously known as bronchiolitis obliterans with organising pneumonia (BOOP), as the main abnormality is the organising pneumonia whereas the bronchiolar obstruction may be absent in up to one-third of the cases. HRCT features of COP are represented by multiple areas of consolidations, which are commonly bilateral, patchy and asymmetric, peripheral, and migrating (in up to 90% of cases) with or without GGOs (fig. 3). The lower lung zones are more frequently affected. Other HRCT findings include small centrilobular nodules, irregular lines, and the 'atoll sign'

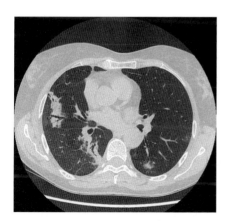

Figure 3. COP. Axial HRCT scan shows multiple bilateral areas of peripheral consolidation with air bronchogram and GGO in the lower lobes.

or 'reversed halo sign' representing peripheral consolidation with inner GGO. A perilobular pattern of increased attenuation has also been described in COP, which can resemble and be confused with interlobular septal thickening. The lung volumes are generally preserved. COP tends to preferentially involve the subpleural and bronchovascular regions of the lung parenchyma. Bronchial dilation and air bronchogram associated with regions of consolidation can also be present. The imaging findings in these cases can often be mistaken for pneumonic consolidation. However, the foci of consolidation generally involve the lower lung zones and have a tendency to migrate, especially in the case of relapses, reported in one-third of cases. Few cases progress to irreversible fibrosis, probably representing the overlap between organising pneumonia and NSIP. Radiological presentation is not pathognomonic but, in the appropriate clinical setting, it allows one to suspect the correct diagnosis. HRCT may also be helpful in identifying a suitable site for biopsy.

Respiratory bronchiolitis-associated ILD
Respiratory bronchiolitis is part of the spectrum of smoking-related lung diseases. It is a distinct histopathological lesion found in the lungs of virtually all cigarette smokers. It usually represents an incidental finding and, as such, is of little clinical significance. Much less often, patients who are heavy smokers develop RB-ILD, a clinical–pathological entity characterised by pulmonary symptoms, abnormal pulmonary function test (PFT) results and imaging abnormalities, with respiratory bronchiolitis being the histological lesion on surgical lung biopsy. It is possible that RB-ILD and DIP are similar processes but at the opposite ends of the disease spectrum. The most common HRCT findings are centrilobular nodules, patchy GGO and thickening of the bronchial walls, which predominate in the upper lobes. The GGO abnormality of RB-ILD has been shown to represent areas of macrophage accumulation in the distal airspaces. Upper lobe emphysema is also commonly present as a result of smoking. Air trapping is frequently seen in expiratory

scans. A small percentage of patients have a reticular pattern in the absence of honeycombing and traction bronchiectasis. The differential diagnosis of RB-ILD includes acute hypersensitivity pneumonitis, DIP and NSIP. An important finding that may help to distinguish RB-ILD from DIP is the presence of centrilobular nodules and unusual presence of cyst formations in RB-ILD.

Desquamative interstitial pneumonia is a rare form of ILD. DIP is strongly associated with cigarette smoking and is considered to represent the end of a spectrum of RB-ILD. Though rarely, DIP may also occur in nonsmokers and has been related to a variety of conditions, including lung infections, exposure to organic dust and marijuana smoke inhalation. For the majority of patients, the onset of symptoms is between 30 and 40 years of age. Males are affected about twice as commonly as females. With smoking cessation and corticosteroid therapy, the prognosis is good. On HRCT, DIP is characterised by diffuse or patchy GGOs, which is caused by diffuse macrophage infiltration of the alveoli, and thickening of alveolar septa with peripheral and basal lung predominance (fig. 4). Other frequent CT findings include spatially limited irregular linear opacities,

also concentrated in the peripheral and basal lung zones, and small (<2 cm) thin-walled cystic spaces, which are indicative of fibrotic changes. Despite differences in the CT appearance, imaging findings of RB-ILD and DIP may overlap and be indistinguishable from each other. Lung biopsy is required for a definite diagnosis.

Lymphoid interstitial pneumonia can be idiopathic, exceedingly rare, or secondary to systemic disorders, in particular Sjögren's syndrome, HIV infection and variable immunodeficiency syndromes. LIP is more common in females than in males, and patients are usually in their fifth decade of life at presentation. HRCT shows bilateral abnormalities that are diffuse or have lower lung predominance. The dominant HRCT feature in patients with LIP is GGO attenuation, which is related to the histological evidence of diffuse interstitial inflammation (fig. 5). Another frequent finding is thin-walled perivascular cysts. They are the only finding that may be irreversible. In contrast to the subpleural, lower lung cystic changes in UIP, the cysts of LIP are usually within the lung parenchyma throughout the mid-lung zones and presumably result from air trapping due to peribronchiolar cellular infiltration. In combination with GGO, these cysts are highly suggestive of LIP. Occasionally,

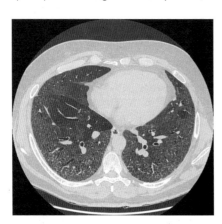

Figure 4. DIP. Axial HRCT scan of heavy smoker shows diffuse and patchy GGO, and thickening of alveolar septa with superimposed small cysts. These findings, suggestive of DIP, were confirmed by surgical lung biopsy.

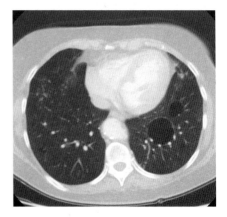

Figure 5. LIP. Axial HRCT image of patient with Sjögren's syndrome shows thin-walled bilateral lung cysts within the lung parenchyma.

centrilobular nodules and septal thickening are seen.

Acute interstitial pneumonia is acute respiratory distress syndrome (ARDS) of unknown cause. The HRCT features of AIP include GGO abnormalities, traction bronchiectasis and architectural distortion. The disease commonly has a symmetric, bilateral distribution with lower lobe predominance. The costophrenic angles are often spared. In the early phase of AIP, prevalent patchy GGOs are the dominant CT features and reflect the presence of alveolar septal oedema and hyaline membranes. Areas of consolidation are also present but usually they are less extensive and limited to the dependent area of the lung (fig. 6). In the early phase, airspace consolidation results from intra-alveolar oedema and haemorrhage. However, consolidations are also present in the fibrotic phase, thus resulting from intra-alveolar fibrosis. In the late phase of AIP, architectural distortion, traction bronchiectasis within areas of GGO consolidation and honeycombing are the most striking CT features and represent fibrotic change. They are more severe in the nondependent areas of the lung. This can be explained by the 'protective' effect of atelectasis and consolidation on the

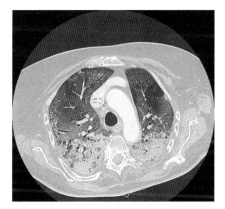

Figure 6. AIP. Axial HRCT image from contrast-enhanced chest CT shows diffuse GGO and reticulation associated with dorsal bilateral consolidations, with relative sparing of the anterior segments.

dependent areas of the lung during the acute phase of disease, which attenuate the potential damage associated with mechanical ventilation.

Although a considerable overlap of HRCT findings exists between AIP and ARDS, the presence of symmetric lower lobe abnormalities with honeycombing may be more suggestive of AIP.

Other diseases

Hypersensitivity pneumonitis is an immunologically induced inflammatory disease involving the lung parenchyma and terminal airways secondary to repeated inhalation of a variety of organic dusts and other agents in a sensitised host. Classically, it can be separated into three phases:

1. acute
2. subacute
3. chronic

depending on the temporality relative to initial exposure. A significant clinical and radiological overlap can often occur between these phases. Acute hypersensitivity pneumonitis presents within a few hours of substantial antigen exposure. HRCT scans, rarely obtained at this stage, demonstrate diffuse or patchy GGO with a geographic distribution, and mosaic perfusion areas due to air trapping (better or only recognised on expiratory scans). Subacute hypersensitivity pneumonitis occurs in response to intermittent or low-dose antigen exposure. HRCT is particularly helpful at this stage of diseases and is characterised by varying proportions of GG, poorly defined centrilobular nodules and areas of decreased attenuation, due to constrictive bronchiolitis with expiratory air trapping (fig. 7). The GGO pattern is general symmetric and diffuse but can be asymmetric. In some cases, reticulation and bronchiectasis may coexist, and may resemble NSIP. Chronic hypersensitivity pneumonitis occurs after long-term, low-dose antigen exposure and usually shows a fibrotic pattern resembling UIP or fibrotic NSIP. HRCT findings include irregular reticular opacities, small nodules, honeycombing and traction bronchiectasis

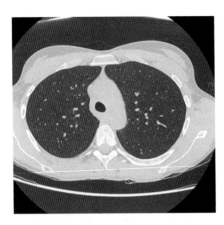

Figure 7. *Subacute hypersensitivity pneumonitis. Axial HRCT image shows multiple centrilobular, hazily defined nodules in both upper lungs. They appear separated from the pleural surfaces, fissures and interlobular septa.*

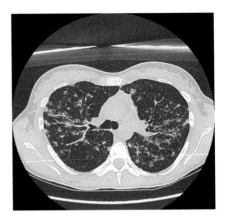

Figure 8. *Sarcoidosis. Axial HRCT image shows multiple coalescent nodules with a perilymphatic distribution in both upper lobes of a young female with a diagnosis of sarcoidosis.*

as well as areas of air trapping and spared lobules, with a heterogeneous appearance, called the 'head cheese sign'. The finding of small centrilobular nodules and the predominant mid-lung zones distribution on HRCT images, with sparing of the bases, help distinguish chronic hypersensitivity pneumonitis from IPF and fibrotic NSIP, which tend to affect more severely the lung bases. Open-lung biopsy is required to make a definite diagnosis in borderline cases.

Sarcoidosis is a systemic disorder of unknown cause characterised histologically by the presence of noncaseating granulomata in affected organs. Thoracic manifestations, the most common cause of morbidity and mortality, occur in 90% of the patients and 20% of them develop chronic fibrotic lung diseases. The classic presentation consists of enlarged hilar and mediastinal lymph nodes, with or without parenchymal involvement. Frequently, the diagnosis is suspected following chest radiography. The radiographic disease staging is as follows:

- Stage 0: no demonstrable abnormality
- Stage I: bilateral hilar lymphadenopathy (BHL) alone
- Stage II: BHL with lung infiltrates

- Stage III: pulmonary infiltrates without BHL
- Stage IV: lung fibrosis

Intrathoracic lymphadenopathy is present in up to 85% of patients at some point during the course of their disease. Hilar and mediastinal lymphadenopathy is better defined on HRCT, which can also allow a more detailed analysis of the nodal calcifications. Sarcoidosis can mimic a number of other diseases. As such, besides a typical manifestation, there may be several less common presentations. The disease preferentially involves the upper lung zones, although in advanced stages, it may display a diffuse distribution. The most common features are multiple nodular opacities with a typical perilymphatic distribution, which correlate with sites of granulomatous inflammation on histology (fig. 8). Nodules are clustered along the bronchovascular bundles, interlobular septa, interlobar fissures, adjacent to the costal pleural (often mimicking pleural plaques) and in the centrilobular regions. Nodules tend to predominate in perihilar and dorsal regions with relative sparing of the lung periphery. Nodules of sarcoidosis typically measure 1–5 mm but, rarely, multiple ill-defined large nodules (ranging in diameter from 1 to 4 cm) can be observed. In addition, multiple coalescent nodules and peripheral ground-glass halos may be seen on HRCT. Occasionally, innumerable small satellite nodules may be adjacent to the large nodules, a finding termed the 'galaxy sign'. In ~10% of patients, a confluence of granulomata may cause a compression of the alveoli and result in poorly defined bilateral parenchymal consolidations with air bronchogram; both parenchymal consolidations and large nodules may also cavitate. Furthermore, innumerable small interstitial granulomas (beyond the resolution of CT) may cause patchy GGOs on HRCT. The parenchymal abnormalities described here are still reversible and often resolve spontaneously, but they may evolve toward pulmonary fibrosis (in 20–25% of cases), which is characterised by linear opacities (radiating laterally from the hilum), fissure displacement, bronchiectasis and honeycombing limited to the upper lung zones, mainly in the dorsal regions. Expiratory CT images can show focal air trapping at any stage of the disease.

Conclusion

The term ILD refers to a large group of entities characterised by radiological findings that often overlap. Chest HRCT is the most important imaging method for the assessment of ILD owing to its sensitivity and specificity. In addition, it plays an important role in the management of specific problems, such as assessment of disease activity and potential reversibility, prediction and evaluation of response to therapy, choice of the most suitable site for lung biopsy, and follow-up. Pulmonologists have to know the basic HRCT patterns of ILD and their distribution because this can help to either make a diagnosis or narrowing the differential diagnosis.

Further reading

- Hansell DM (2010). Thin-section CT of the lungs: the hinterland of normal. *Radiology*; 256: 695–711.
- Jawad H, *et al.* (2012). Radiological approach to interstitial lung disease: a guide for the nonradiologist. *Clin Chest Med*; 33: 11–26.
- Raghu G, *et al.* (2011). An official ATS/ERS/JRS/ALAT statement: idiopathic pulmonary fibrosis: evidence-based guidelines for diagnosis and management. *Am J Respir Crit Care Med*; 183: 788–824.
- Travis WD, *et al.* (2002). American Thoracic Society/European Respiratory Society international multidisciplinary consensus classification of the idiopathic interstitial pneumonias. *Am J Respir Crit Care Med*; 165: 277–304.
- Webb WR (2006). Thin-section CT of the secondary pulmonary lobule: anatomy and the image – the 2004 Fleischner lecture. *Radiology*; 239: 322–338.

Sarcoidosis

Ulrich Costabel

Sarcoidosis is a multisystem granulomatous disorder of unknown aetiology, which commonly affects young and middle-aged adults. The disease frequently presents with bilateral hilar lymphadenopathy, pulmonary infiltration, and ocular and skin lesions. Any organ of the body may be involved. The prevalence rates of sarcoidosis vary widely, from <1 case to 40 cases per 100,000 population. Sarcoidosis is common in Scandinavia, Central Europe, the USA and Japan. It is less frequently seen in other Asian countries, Central and South America,

and Africa. Sarcoidosis in Afro-Americans is more severe, while Caucasians are more likely to present with asymptomatic disease. Overall mortality is 1–5%.

The cause of sarcoidosis remains unknown. Available evidence strongly supports the hypothesis that the disease develops when a specific environmental exposure with antigenic properties occurs in a genetically susceptible individual. Potential aetiological agents include mycobacteria and *Propionibacterium acnes*. Sarcoidosis susceptibility or chronicity has been associated with a number of human leukocyte antigen alleles. Some genetic associations have been found with specific disease subsets, most notably with Löfgren's syndrome. A polymorphism of the *BTNL2* (butyrophilin-like 2) gene has been linked with sarcoidosis. The immunological abnormalities are characterised by the accumulation of activated T-cells of the T-helper cell type 1 and macrophages at sites of ongoing inflammation.

Clinical presentation

The clinical presentation of sarcoidosis varies widely. 30–50% of patients are asymptomatic at the time of diagnosis. Symptoms of sarcoidosis are largely nonspecific. Low-grade fever (sometimes up to 40°C), weight loss (usually limited to 2–6 kg during the 10–12 weeks before presentation), night sweats and arthralgias can be found in about 20–30% of patients. Sarcoidosis is an important and frequently overlooked cause of fever of unknown origin. Fatigue and skeletal muscle weakness are more common, being present in ≤70% of patients when carefully sought. According to

Key points

- Sarcoidosis is a multisystem granulomatous disorder of unknown aetiology, which commonly affects young and middle-aged adults.

- Prevalence of sarcoidosis varies from <1 case to 40 cases per 100 000 population, and overall mortality is 1–5%.

- Clinical presentation varies widely, though fever, fatigue and skeletal muscle weakness are often noted.

- The decision to treat should be carefully assessed based on the benefit to the patient and disease severity; treatment should mainly be considered if symptoms develop or lung function deteriorates.

- The clinical course of sarcoidosis can be unpredictable, so regular monitoring of signs of disease progression is advised.

their initial presentation, sarcoidosis patients can be divided into two distinct subgroups: acute and chronic. The acute form can present as classical Löfgren's syndrome, which is characterised by fever, bilateral hilar lymphadenopathy, ankle arthritis and erythema nodosum. The chronic form shows an insidious onset, and organ-related symptoms predominate, such as cough, dyspnoea, and chest pain.

Diagnostic approach

The criteria of the American Thoracic Society, European Respiratory Society and the World Association of Sarcoidosis and Other Granulomatous Disorders for the diagnosis of sarcoidosis include:

- the presence of a consistent clinical and radiological picture
- histological evidence of noncaseating granulomas
- exclusion of other conditions capable of producing a similar histological or clinical picture

The initial diagnostic work-up for patients with suspected sarcoidosis involves careful baseline assessment of disease distribution and severity by organ, with emphasis on vital target organs (table 1). Specifically, the

Table 1. Initial evaluation for sarcoidosis

| History (occupational and environmental exposure, symptoms) |
| Physical examination |
| Chest radiography |
| Pulmonary function tests: vital capacity, FEV1, TLCO |
| Peripheral blood counts |
| Serum chemistries: calcium, liver enzymes, creatinine, ACE |
| Urine analysis |
| ECG |
| Eye investigation |
| Tuberculin skin test |
| Selection of site for biopsy |
| ACE: angiotensin-converting enzyme. |

diagnostic assessment should attempt to accomplish four goals:

1. provide histological confirmation of the disease
2. assess the extent and severity of organ involvement
3. assess whether the disease is stable or is likely to process
4. determine whether therapy will benefit a patient

Granulomas alone are never diagnostic proof of sarcoidosis.

An important step is the choice of site for a proper biopsy. Transbronchial lung biopsy is the recommended procedure in most cases, with the diagnostic yield reaching 80%. This can be combined with biopsy of the bronchial mucosa. Transbronchial needle aspiration of mediastinal lymph nodes guided by endobronchial ultrasound is useful for diagnosing stage I and II sarcoidosis with a sensitivity of 83–93%. Other easily accessible sites for biopsy are the skin, lip or superficial lymph nodes. In patients without biopsy, clinical and/or radiological features alone may be diagnostic in stage I (reliability of 98%) or stage II (89%), but are less accurate in stage III (52%) or stage 0 (23%). The classical Löfgren's syndrome may not require biopsy proof. Bronchoalveolar lavage and studies of lymphocyte subpopulations showing an increase in the CD4/CD8 ratio may be helpful. Elevated serum angiotensin-converting enzyme and calcium levels may lend support to the diagnosis.

The chest radiogram can be used to classify sarcoidosis into four stages (table 2). CT scanning provides much greater detail of mediastinal and parenchymal abnormalities but is not essential for baseline study. It is indicated when diagnosis is unclear after chest radiography and clinical assessment or to detect complications of the lung disease including bronchiectasis, aspergilloma or superimposed infection.

Pulmonary function tests show only a moderate correlation with the extent of lung involvement detected on imaging. However, it is important to have initial baseline data

Table 2. Chest radiographic stages

Stage	Findings	Frequency %
0	Normal	5–10
I	BHL	50
II	BHL and parenchymal infiltrates	25
III	Parenchymal infiltrates without BHL	15
IB	Signs of fibrosis	5–10
BHL: bilateral hilar lymphadenopathy.		

for evaluating the following clinical course. The most sensitive test is the diffusion capacity. The typical finding is a restriction, but up to 30% of patients show an obstructive impairment that may be associated with the involvement of the bronchial mucosa.

Cardiac involvement is a serious manifestation of sarcoidosis. Cardiac MRI is the preferred diagnostic test as it is a noninvasive and nonradioactive method for diagnosing cardiac sarcoidosis with a high sensitivity.

Pulmonary hypertension is a troublesome complication of sarcoidosis, with increased morbidity and mortality. The frequency is 5–15% in selected patients and 50–60% in patients with dyspnoea out of proportion with the pulmonary function test results. Such patients, most of them in radiographic stage IV, should undergo echocardiography as a screening test and right heart catheterisation for confirmation.

Natural history and prognosis

The disease course is highly variable. Spontaneous remissions occur in nearly two thirds of patients. Serious extrapulmonary involvement (cardiac, central nervous system or hepatic) occurs in 4–7% of patients at time of presentation. Incidence becomes higher as the disease evolves. Adverse prognostic factors include lupus pernio, chronic uveitis, age at onset >40 years, chronic hypercalcaemia, nephrocalcinosis, African ethnic origin, progressive pulmonary sarcoidosis, nasal mucosal involvement, cystic bone lesions, neural sarcoidosis, cardiac sarcoidosis,

pulmonary hypertension and chronic respiratory insufficiency.

Treatment and follow-up

The indication to treat a patient depends on many factors, the most important being whether or not the patients is symptomatic. Except for life- and sight-threatening organ involvement, it should be carefully considered whether the patient might benefit from treatment. For asymptomatic pulmonary patients, a watch-and-wait approach is appropriate; treatment should mainly be considered if symptoms develop or lung function deteriorates. The goal of treatment is to make the patient asymptomatic and to restore or preserve organ function. For patients with symptoms from a single organ, topical therapy may be appropriate for anterior eye or for skin involvement. Otherwise, initial therapy is still based on systemic corticosteroids. For pulmonary sarcoidosis, the initial prednisone dose is 20–40 mg; higher doses may be needed for cardiac or neural sarcoidosis. The dose is slowly tapered to 5–10 mg per day; treatment should be continued for a minimum of 12 months. Patients with Löfgren's syndrome usually do not require therapy with corticosteroids.

For patients with chronic disease requiring years of therapy, alternatives to corticosteroids include methotrexate, azathioprine and hydroxychloroquine, all given usually in combination with low-dose corticosteroids. For refractory sarcoidosis patients, new therapeutic approaches have begun to emerge through the use of immunomodulatory agents. Based on current understanding of pathogenic mechanisms, these are tumour necrosis factor-α-blocking drugs, such as infliximab, thalidomide and pentoxyfylline. Lung transplantation can be considered for severe or end-stage pulmonary sarcoidosis.

Because the clinical course of sarcoidosis can be unpredictable, regular monitoring for signs of disease progression is necessary, using the least invasive and most sensitive tools. For pulmonary sarcoidosis, this is spirometry and diffusion capacity. For stable stage I disease, follow-up every 6–12 months is usually adequate; more frequent evaluations (every 3–6 months) are advised for stage II, III or IV sarcoidosis. All patients should be monitored for a minimum of 3 years after therapy is discontinued. Follow-up needs to be more vigilant after corticosteroid-induced remissions, due to

the high rate of relapses in this context, ranging 15–70%.

Further reading

- Baughman RP, et al., eds. Sarcoidosis. New York, Thieme Medical Publishers, 2010.
- Costabel U, et al. (2010). Diagnostic modalities in sarcoidosis: BAL, EBUS, and PET. Semin Respir Crit Care Med; 31: 404–408.
- Drent M, et al., eds. Sarcoidosis. Eur Respir Monogr; 32. 2005.
- Grutters JC, et al. (2009). Sarcoidosis. Eur Respir Monogr; 46: 126–154.
- Hunninghake GW, et al. (1999). ATS/ERS/WASOG statement on sarcoidosis. Sarcoidosis Vasc Diffuse Lung Dis; 16: 149–173.

Idiopathic interstitial pneumonias

Dario Olivieri, Sara Chiesa and Panagiota Tzani

Idiopathic interstitial pneumonias (IIPs) represent a heterogeneous group of disorders with different clinical and histological features, and different prognosis. They can be considered as inflammatory disorders of the interstitium. Extrapulmonary involvement does not occur. The cause and pathogenetic mechanisms responsible for IIPs have not been elucidated. The first stage of the pathological process consists in the recruitment of inflammatory cells in the interstitium, leading to injury of the epithelial and alveolar cells, and the subsequent abnormal wound healing response, particularly due to the fibroblasts. Nowadays, the dysregulation of fibroblasts and an excessive deposition of extracellular matrix are considered the cardinal points of the pathogenesis of the IIPs.

Because of the poor comprehension of the underlying pathogenetic mechanisms, there is no therapeutic intervention able to affect the cellular and molecular target responsible for the disease and change its course.

The most recent American Thoracic Society (ATS) and European Respiratory Society (ERS) classification of the IIPs includes seven different diseases identified by a typical histological pattern; each histological pattern has precise clinical and radiological features, and a different prognosis (table 1). Here, we discuss the most important clinical aspects of the IIPs, particularly therapeutic possibilities.

Epidemiology

The incidence of the IIPs has been estimated at seven to 11 cases per 100 000 persons and the prevalence ranges between two and 29 cases per 100 000 persons. The disease typically affects adults, with a peak after the sixth decade of life; incidence is higher in males and in smokers (Coultas et al., 1994). There is a familial variant of idiopathic pulmonary fibrosis (IPF)/usual interstitial pneumonia (UIP) that accounts for 0.5–3% of cases of IIP; this form is indistinguishable from the nonfamilial forms except that patients tend to be younger.

Pathogenesis

The pathogenetic mechanisms of the IIPs are not completely clear; there are various

> **Key points**
>
> - IIPs represent a heterogeneous group of disorders with different clinical and histological features and prognoses.
>
> - The most recent ATS and ERS classifications of IIPs include seven different diseases identified by a typical histological pattern: NSIP, cryptogenic organising pneumonia/bronchiolitis obliterans organising pneumonia, acute interstitial pneumonia, respiratory bronchiolitis/interstitial lung disease, desquamative interstitial pneumonia/alveolar macrophage pneumonia and lymphoid interstitial pneumonia.
>
> - The terms IPF and NSIP should only be used for chronic fibrosing interstitial pneumonia of unknown cause limited to the lungs. The prognosis in IPF is worse with a histological pattern of UIP.

Table 1. Classification of IIPs

IPF/UIP
Desquamative interstitial pneumonia/ alveolar macrophage pneumonia
Respiratory bronchiolitis/interstitial lung disease
Acute interstitial pneumonia
Cryptogenic organising pneumonia/ bronchiolitis obliterans organising pneumonia
NSIP
Lymphoid interstitial pneumonia

hypotheses relating to the initial stimulus responsible for the pathogenetic process, such as exposure to toxic substances or viral infections. Independently of the initial cause, the inflammatory–fibrotic process of UIP is characterised by an injury of the alveolar epithelial cells, destruction of the subepithelial basement membrane and subsequent abnormal cicatrisation with an increased fibroblastic response, and excessive deposition of collagen and extracellular matrix.

The interplay between inflammatory and mesenchymal cells is regulated by a number of cytokines produced by fibroblasts and epithelial cells; the most important of these mediators are transforming growth factor (TGF)-β, tumour necrosis factor (TNF)-α, platelet-derived growth factor (PDGF), connective tissue growth factor, integrin-mediated intercellular adhesion molecules, proteases and oxygen radicals. Deficiency of interferon (IFN)-γ may contribute to activation and perpetuation of the fibroblastic process. Histologically, the presence of fibroblastic foci is typical of UIP; the fibroblastic foci are formed by mesenchymal cells similar to myofibroblasts. Under the influence of TGF-β, the cells increase the production of collagen, vimentin and actin, leading to an excessive deposition of extracellular matrix.

In the rare familial form, the mode of transmission is not known; it is probably autosomal dominant with variable penetrance in two-thirds of patients. Familial IPF has been associated with altered α_1-antitrypsin inhibitor alleles on chromosome 14. Genetic polymorphism for interleukin (IL)-1 receptor antagonist or TNF-α may be involved.

Physiology

The physiological aberrations in IIPs are typical of a restrictive pattern and include reduced lung volumes (vital capacity and TLC) and normal or increased expiratory flow rates. TLCO is typically reduced, indicating interstitium damage and, thereby gas exchange impairment (Chetta *et al.*, 2004). A further consequence of this alteration is the hypoxaemia, which is accentuated with exercise. Late in the course of the disease, severe hypoxaemia may also be observed at rest; hypercapnia may be present as well.

Clinical features and diagnosis

The initial symptoms of IIPs are hidden and insidious: persistent nonproductive cough and progressive dyspnoea. In most patients, physical examination reveals end-inspiratory rales (velcro type). The course of the disease may vary depending the variant of IIP; in UIP, the prognosis is extremely severe and the course of the disease is rapid, even if some patients stabilise after an initial period of decline. Respiratory failure appears in 3–8 years and the mean survival from the onset of the disease is around 3–5 years. During the late phases of the disease, patients often show cor pulmonale. Respiratory failure is the main cause of death, followed by pulmonary embolism and heart failure.

Diagnosis of IIP is the result of an integrated and multidisciplinary process, requiring cooperation of the clinician, the radiologist and the pathologist. International guidelines state that histology is useful for diagnosis. Surgical lung biopsy shows higher diagnostic value than transbronchial biopsy and bronchoalveolar lavage. However, it is invasive with potential risks and, sometimes, patients may present clinical and physiological contraindications to surgery. In some cases, an acute exacerbation of the disease may follow surgery, leading to a decline in general condition.

HRCT has become a crucial tool for the diagnostic process and allows an accurate and objective follow-up of the disease. HRCT images consistent with IIP represent one of the most important ATS/ERS/Japanese Respiratory Society (JRS)/Asociación Latinoamericana de Tórax (ALAT) guideline diagnostic criteria. HRCT features are often typical of the disease and, given the high-quality evidence regarding HRCT specificity for the recognition of a histopathological UIP pattern, surgical lung biopsy is not essential. In the appropriate clinical setting, the presence of a UIP pattern on HRCT is sufficient for the diagnosis of IPF (fig. 1).

In particular, in case of UIP, HRCT images show a heterogeneous distribution with a predilection for the peripheral, especially subpleural and basilar, regions of the lung. The main radiologic feature in UIP is honeycombing, *i.e.* cystic radiolucencies as an expression of severe and irreversible fibrotic conversion of the parenchyma.

Secondary features include coarse reticular opacities, thickened bronchial walls, bronchiectasis and bronchiolectasis.

Nonspecific interstitial pneumonia (NSIP) is characterised by the presence of ground-glass areas, as a sign of an active inflammatory process. The main aspects to consider for differential diagnosis of UIP or NSIP are the geographic and temporal histological and radiological heterogeneity, the high concentration of fibroblastic foci and honeycombing in the UIP form.

Cellular analyses of bronchoalveolar lavage (BAL) and transbronchial lung biopsy can be useful in the diagnosis of certain forms of IIPs (Meyer *et al.*, 2012).

Natural history and exacerbations

The course of the disease is characterised by a progressive pulmonary function decline, leading to worsening of general condition and death (fig. 2). A subset of patients develop an accelerated and usually fatal course, showing an extremely rapid decline; this condition is known as acute exacerbation.

The criteria for defining an exacerbation are:

- progressive dyspnoea during the last 30 days
- new pulmonary infiltrates in chest radiographs

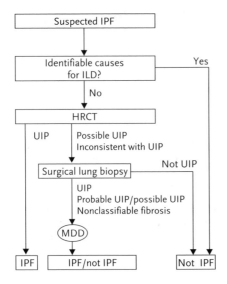

Figure 1. *Diagnostic algorithm for IPF. ILD: interstitial long disease; MDD: multidisciplinary discussion. Reproduced and modified from Raghu et al. (2011) with permission from the publisher.*

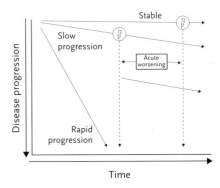

Figure 2. *Natural history of IPF. Reproduced and modified from Raghu et al. (2011) with permission from the publisher.*

- worsening of hypoxaemia with a reduction in oxygen tension >10 mmHg;
- absence of pulmonary infection supported by negative BAL
- absence of any other cause, such as HF, pulmonary embolism or conditions that may cause acute lung damage

Diagnosis of exacerbation may be controversial, despite the codification of the diagnostic criteria; ground-glass opacities are not specific for IIP and may be present in infection. Nonintubated patients in the acute phase of the disease often cannot undergo BAL because of their unstable conditions and they are treated with antibiotics as a precautionary measure. Lung biopsy shows diffuse alveolar damage; however, the invasiveness of the procedure is a limiting factor and only a few well-selected patients undergo surgical lung biopsy. It is our duty to mention the correlation between surgical lung biopsy or lung resection and acute exacerbation, which is not clear yet, as far as causality is concerned. Risk factors involved in this accelerated phase may be a high concentration of oxygen (100%), hyperexpansion of the lung parenchyma and the use of mechanical ventilation in the post-operative phase.

Generally, the factors responsible for the exacerbations are still unknown; clinical presentation in some patients (fever, influenza-like symptoms and neutrophilia in BAL) may be consistent with a viral infection; however, the pathogen has not been identified.

Treatment

IIP treatment is one of the most controversial aspects in the field of the diffuse infiltrative lung diseases. Poor understanding of the pathogenetic mechanisms underlies the ineffectiveness of the current treatment options.

The initial pathogenetic theory considering IIP as an inflammatory process makes reasonable the use of anti-inflammatory drugs, such as corticosteroids, which are considered first-line drugs. Later, cytotoxic and immuno-suppressive agents have been used, usually in combination with corticosteroids.

The most recent developments in the field identify the initial phase of the disease as alveolar epithelial cell injury and destruction of the subepithelial basement membrane, leading to abnormal wound healing with a vigorous fibroblastic response and excessive deposition of collagen and extracellular matrix. This new pathogenetic theory suggests a primary role for fibroblast dysregulation. Thus, the fibroproliferative process becomes the therapeutic target, and new drugs that arrest the proliferation of fibroblasts and the deposition of extracellular matrix are being testing (Bouros et al., 2005).

The increasing clinical awareness of IPF has resulted in the recent publication of guidelines for the accurate diagnosis of IPF and recommendations for its management. The recommendations for diagnosis and treatment intervention in the new ATS/ERS/JRS/ALAT guidelines are evidence-based and eliminate the bias from expert opinions and ongoing practices in the management of IPF.

Anti-inflammatory drugs Although corticosteroids have been considered the mainstay of IPF treatment for decades, there are no randomised placebo-controlled trials using corticosteroids alone. The ATS/ERS international consensus statement concludes that existing therapies are of unproven benefit.

In the past, high doses of prednisone or prednisolone ($1\ mg\cdot kg^{-1}\cdot day^{-1}$, considering ideal body weight) for 4–6 weeks, with a gradual taper, were used. Given the high risk of systemic side-effects and the significant toxicity, especially when used in combination with other drugs, the dose has been re-evaluated and more recent therapeutic regimens recommend low doses of prednisone or prednisolone ($0.5\ mg\cdot kg^{-1}\cdot day^{-1}$ for 4 weeks followed by $0.25\ mg\cdot kg^{-1}\cdot day^{-1}$ for 8 weeks, then $0.125\ mg\cdot kg^{-1}\cdot day^{-1}$). The rate of taper depends on individual characteristics of patients. In the case of responders with clinical and radiological improvement, prolonged maintenance therapy with low-dose, alternate-day prednisone may be established to reduce the chance of recrudescent disease. In the case of exacerbation, $2\,mg \cdot kg^{-1} \cdot day^{-1}$ of methylprednisolone for $\sim$14 days should be administered, depending on individual clinical response.

Given the lack of any scientific evidence of proven benefit, especially a dose–response effect, corticosteroid treatment should not be used in patients at high risk for adverse effects, such as elderly patients.

When the inflammatory component dominates, prompt corticosteroid treatment may lead to a significant improvement and, sometimes, to complete resolution of the disease. Desquamative interstitial pneumonia/alveolar macrophage pneumonia, acute interstitial pneumonia and cryptogenic organising pneumonia/bronchiolitis obliterans organising pneumonia are the IIPs forms with the highest rate of response to steroid therapy.

The new guidelines recommend that patients with IPF should not be treated with corticosteroid monotherapy.

Azathioprine and cyclophosphamide are the most frequently used second-line drugs, alone or in combination with corticosteroids. Currently, there is poor information regarding their efficacy. A possible adjunctive synergic effect is unconfirmed.

Azathioprine is the most frequently used cytotoxic agent and is usually well-tolerated. Its metabolism leads to the production of mercaptopurine, which is similar to purine, and inhibits DNA synthesis. Azathioprine is administered p.o., usually in combination with low-dose corticosteroids; the initial dose is 25–$50\,mg \cdot day^{-1}$ (2–$3\,mg \cdot kg^{-1} \cdot day^{-1}$). If adverse effects do not appear, an increase of $25\,mg$ every 7–14 days is recommended, until a maximum dose of $150\,mg \cdot day^{-1}$ is reached. During treatment with azathioprine, haemachrome and liver function should be monitored; in fact, azathioprine causes bone marrow suppression and hepatotoxicity. There are

no clinical trials that confirm a certain benefit of combination (corticosteroids plus azathioprine) therapy. Given the minor toxicity compared with cyclophosphamide, azathioprine should be administered in patients with symptomatic or progressive disease for 6 months unless adverse effects that suggest interruption or modification of the treatment appear. A more prolonged treatment is reserved only in patients with a clinical response or complete remission of the disease.

Cyclophosphamide is usually used as a second-line drug for patients who presented adverse effects from high-dose corticosteroid therapy. It is an alkylating agent that activates the liver microsomal system and inhibits DNA synthesis; it has a marked effect on lymphocyte, thus it is used as an immunosuppressive agent. The route of administration is usually oral or intravenous but it can also be administered by intramuscular injection. Generally, cyclophosphamide is used combined with low-dose corticosteroids. Principal adverse effects are bone marrow suppression, haemorrhagic cystitis, nausea and vomiting. Scientific evidence confirming the efficacy of cyclophosphamide in IIP treatment is lacking; no clinical benefit regarding survival and progression of the disease has been reported.

Cyclosporine is a fungal peptide that exerts potent immunosuppressive effects; it inhibits T-lymphocyte proliferation by inhibiting the release of IL-2. It causes some important adverse effects, especially renal, hepatic and gastrointestinal effects. Cyclosporine is rarely used for IIP treatment and its use is limited for selected patients awaiting lung transplantation. There are no clinical trials showing that cyclosporine therapy is of benefit.

The new guidelines recommend that patients with IPF should not be treated with cyclosporine. Moreover, combination therapy with corticosteroid and immunomodulator therapy should not be recommended in IPF patients.

Novel therapeutic strategies The use of novel drugs in IIP treatment is suggested by the new pathophysiological theory that recognises the fibroproliferative process plays a central role.

IFN-γ is a novel biological antifibrotic drug with a number of inhibitory effects on fibroblasts. In the literature, there are only few studies relating to the real efficacy of IFN-γ, either alone or in combination therapy with low-dose corticosteroids. Neither Ziesche et al. (1999) nor Raghu et al. (2004) reported any statistically significant differences in the primary outcome variables, such as disease progression, mortality and functional deterioration. However, patients with mild-to-moderate disease presented better, statistically significant survival. Although IFN-γ may represent a useful therapeutic tool in selected patients, additional data supporting its efficacy are needed.

The new guidelines recommend that patients with IPF should not be treated with IFN-γ.

Colchicine inhibits the synthesis of collagen and suppresses some growth factors that are necessary for fibroblast proliferation. On the basis of these properties, the use of this drug is being tested. Data are limited, although there is no evidence that colchicine improves the progression of the disease and survival. The new guidelines recommend that patients with IPF should not be treated with colchicine.

D-penicillamine is a thiolic compound that interferes with collagen turnover, inhibiting collagen synthesis and deposition by interrupting cross-linking of collagen molecules. There are no clinical controlled trials showing any benefit of D-penicillamine therapy. Given the frequency adverse effects, D-penicillamine does not appear to be a treatment choice in IIPs.

Pirfenidone (5-methyl-1-phenyl-2[1H]-pyridone) attenuates pulmonary fibrosis in animal models. It reduces synthesis of collagen (I and III) and TNF-α, and inhibits TGF-β-stimulated collagen synthesis. Moreover, it decreases synthesis of extracellular matrix and blocks the mitogenic effect of profibrotic cytokines.

Azuma et al. (2005) published the results of a double-blind, randomised, placebo-controlled trial but no statistically significant difference in desaturation during the 6-min walk test (6MWT) was found; however, a positive treatment effect with pirfenidone was demonstrated in secondary end points, such as vital capacity and prevention of acute exacerbation of the disease. In fact, successive studies showed that pirfenidone preserves vital capacity and improves progression-free survival time better than placebo. The new guidelines recommend that the majority of patients with IPF should not be treated with pirfenidone but this therapy may be a reasonable choice in a minority of patients.

Experimental models in vitro and in vivo showed that angiotensin-converting enzyme inhibitors and statins possess antifibrotic properties. However, there is no evidence of survival improvement in treated patients.

There is evidence that oxidant agents production increases in IIP. In particular, neutrophils, macrophages and fibroblasts release oxidant agents, such as reactive oxygen species, hydrogen peroxide and superoxide anions. These factors, added to the reduction of antioxidants, facilitate fibroblast dysregulation and deposition of extracellular matrix.

N-acetylcysteine (NAC) is derived from the amino acid cysteine. It is considered a precursor of glutathione (GSH) and stimulates GSH synthesis. GSH has strong antioxidant properties, as it removes free oxygen radicals and decreases hydrogen peroxide. The route of administration is oral at a dose of 1800 mg·day^{-1} added to conventional therapy with corticosteroids and azathioprine. A significant difference in the rate of decline of FVC and T_{LCO} has been described in patients treated with NAC; however, no difference was observed in mortality.

A recent study showed that increased risks of death and hospitalisation were observed in patients with IPF who were treated with a combination of prednisone, azathioprine, and NAC, as compared with placebo.

The new guidelines recommend that the majority of patients should not be treated with NAC monotherapy or with combination corticosteroid, azathioprine and NAC therapy, but this therapy may be reasonable in a minority of patients.

Endothelin 1 (ET-1) is a potent mitogen for endothelial and smooth muscle cells. ET-1 is strongly upregulated in patients with IIP and is mainly expressed in epithelial cells. Some studies have suggested that inhibition of ET-1 could have antifibrotic effects. Bosentan is a nonselective ETA and ETB receptor antagonist which is used in patients with pulmonary hypertension, and it could delay the progression of IIPs. The Bosentan Use in Interstitial Lung Disease (BUILD)-1 trial showed that bosentan was not superior to placebo in the 6MWT, and the effects of bosentan treatment on health-related quality of life and dyspnoea in the all-treated population were minimal. Similarly, in the BUILD-3 trial, no treatment effects were observed on health-related quality of life or dyspnoea (King et al., 2011). The new guidelines recommend that patients with IPF should not be treated with bosentan.

TNF-α has been found to be significantly elevated in bleomycin-induced pulmonary fibrosis. TNF-α stimulates a series of cytokines, such as TGF-β and IL-5, and modifies eosinophil recruitment in the parenchyma. Antibodies against TNF-α and soluble TNF-α receptor antagonists have been found to reduce the fibrotic process in animals. A recent study of etanercept for patients with IPF failed to show a difference in the primary end-point of change in FVC. Nonsignificant trends were observed in T_{LCO} and 6MWT parameters. The new guidelines recommend that patients with IPF should not be treated with etanercept.

Tyrosine kinase receptors have been shown to be involved in lung fibrosis. BIBF 1120 is a potent intracellular inhibitor of tyrosine kinases; its targets include PDGF receptors α and β, vascular endothelial growth factor receptors 1–3, and fibroblast growth factor receptors 1–3. A recent study showed that BIBF 1120 at a dose of 150 mg twice daily was associated with a trend toward a reduction in the decline in lung function compared with placebo, with fewer acute exacerbations and preserved quality of life (Richeldi et al., 2011).

The typical fibroproliferative process in IIP seems to be related to inflammation and vascular injury. Indeed, endothelium damage causes exposition of the intimal tissue to the circulation and this is strongly pro-thrombotic. Pulmonary embolism is one of the most common causes of death in IIP patients and D-dimer levels often increase in exacerbations of the disease (Castro et al., 2001). In a prospective study, Kubo et al. (2005) evaluated the role of thrombotic events in the natural history of the disease and survival improvement in IIP patients receiving oral anticoagulant therapy. Patients treated with warfarin added to corticosteroids had significantly higher survival after exacerbation when compared to patients treated with corticosteroids alone. D-dimer levels and number of exacerbation-free days did not differ between the two groups. The mechanisms underlying better survival in patients treated with anticoagulant therapy are unclear. Certainly, extravascular deposition of fibrin and thrombotic events play a main role in the fibroproliferative process and acute lung injury.

The new guidelines recommend that the majority of patients with IPF should not be treated with anticoagulants but this therapy may be a reasonable choice in a minority of patients.

The study by Lee et al. (2011) showed an apparent survival benefit associated with medications to suppress the acidity of the gastric juice, given as gastro-oesophageal reflux (GOR) therapy. This observation is consistent with an increasing body of evidence supporting the concept of silent microaspiration as a result of abnormal GOR in the pathogenesis of IPF. If GOR therapy improves survival in patients with IPF, then other treatment interventions to decrease and/or control GOR should include aggressive conservative measures with altered eating, drinking and sleep habits/behavioural patterns, decrease in abdominal girth, and/or laparoscopic anti-reflux

For referral	Radiographic or histological evidence of UIP irrespective of vital capacity
	Histological evidence of fibrotic NSIP
For listing	Radiographic or histological evidence of UIP and any of the following:
	TLCO $<$39% pred
	$>$10% reduction in FVC in the last 6 months
	Oxygen saturation $<$88% during 6MWT
	Honeycombing on HRCT (fibrosis score $>$2)
	Histological evidence of NSIP and any of the following:
	TLCO $<$ 35% predicted
	$>$10% reduction in FVC or
	$>$15% in TLCO in the last 6 months

surgery. However, further studies are needed to confirm these data.

Lung transplantation is the only option that definitely improves survival in IIP patients and the only option for patients who respond poorly to medical therapy. IIPs represent the second most frequent disease that requires lung transplantation. It is extremely important to decide when to list a patient for transplantation. Given the legal complexity of the process, early listing is urged. Recently, the International Society for Heart and Lung Transplantation published guidelines for establishing the characteristics and the criteria for transplantation and listing (table 2). The new guidelines recommend that appropriate patients with IPF should undergo lung transplantation.

Unfortunately, many patients die while awaiting transplantation because of the poor availability of donor organs. Post-operative mortality in transplanted patients is high, because of rejection, infections and other complications. 2- and 5-year survival rates following single lung transplantation are ~70% and ~50%, respectively.

Stem cell-based therapy Given the recent advances in IPF pathogenesis, new therapeutic models are being investigated, focusing on the cellular and molecular mechanisms underlying the disease. In particular, alveolar epithelial cell injury arises from an abnormal accumulation of fibroblasts and deposition of extracellular matrix, resulting in distortion of lung parenchyma architecture. Therefore, lung tissue regeneration, remodelling and repair mechanisms could represent new potential therapeutic targets.

The discovery that stem cells can contribute to the formation of differentiated cell types, especially after injury, justifies the experimental use of stem cells in tissue regeneration. It is believed that stem cells play a central role in cell injury and fibrotic process; however, their role is still controversial. In particular, the mechanisms of cell recruitment to site in case of tissue damage are not completely clear. Therefore, embryo or adult stem cells transplantation could be a valid novel therapeutic option in pulmonary fibrosis. Official data confirming the efficacy and applicability of this treatment are lacking; furthermore, the importance of immunosuppressive therapy before stem cells transplantation is unclear, as the data are poor.

Further reading

- American Thoracic Society, European Respiratory Society. (2002). International multidisciplinary consensus classification of the idiopathic interstitial pneumonias. *Am J Respir Crit Care Med*; 165: 277–304.
- Azuma A, *et al.* (2005). Double-blind, placebo-controlled trial of pirfenidone in patients with idiopathic pulmonary fibrosis. *Am J Respir Crit Care Med*; 171: 1040–1047.

- Bouros D, *et al.* (2005). Current and future therapeutic approaches in idiopathic pulmonary fibrosis. *Eur Respir J*; 26: 693–703.
- Castro DJ, *et al.* (2001). Diagnostic value of D dimer in pulmonary embolism and pneumonia. *Respiration*; 68: 371–375.
- Chetta A, *et al.* (2004). Pulmonary function testing in interstitial lung diseases. *Respiration*; 71: 209–213.
- Coultas DB, *et al.* (1994). The epidemiology of interstitial lung diseases. *Am J Respir Crit Care Med*; 150: 967–972.
- King TE Jr, *et al.* (2011). BUILD-3: a randomized, controlled trial of bosentan in idiopathic pulmonary fibrosis. *Am J Respir Crit Care Med*; 184: 92–99.
- Kubo H, *et al.* (2005). Anticoagulant therapy for idiopathic pulmonary fibrosis. *Chest*; 128: 1475–1482.
- Lee JS, *et al.* (2011). Gastroesophageal reflux therapy is associated with longer survival in idiopathic pulmonary fibrosis. *Am J Respir Crit Care Med*; 184: 1390–1394.
- Meyer KC, *et al.* (2012). An Official American Thoracic Society clinical practice guideline: The clinical utility of bronchoalveolar lavage cellular analysis in interstitial lung disease. *Am J Respir Crit Care Med*; 185: 1004–1014.
- Raghu G, *et al.* (2004). A placebo-controlled trial of interferon γ-1b in patients with idiopathic pulmonary fibrosis. *N Engl J Med*; 350: 125–133.
- Raghu G, *et al.* (2011). An official ATS/ERS/JRS/ALAT statement: Idiopathic pulmonary fibrosis: evidence-based guidelines for diagnosis and management. *Am J Respir Crit Care Med*; 183: 788–824.
- Richeldi L, *et al.* (2011). Efficacy of a tyrosine kinase inhibitor in idiopathic pulmonary fibrosis. *N Engl J Med*; 365: 1079–1087.
- The Idiopathic Pulmonary Fibrosis Clinical Research Network. (2012). Prednisone, azathioprine, and N-acetylcysteine for pulmonary fibrosis. *N Engl J Med*; 366: 1968–1977.
- Ziesche R, *et al.* (1999). A preliminary study of long-term treatment with interferon γ-1b and low-dose prednisolone in patients with idiopathic pulmonary fibrosis. *N Engl J Med*; 341: 1264–1269.

Eosinophilic diseases

Andrew Menzies-Gow

The exact role of the eosinophil in health has yet to be determined. It is believed to play a role in combating helminthic parasitic infections and, in health, eosinophils primarily reside within the gastrointestinal mucosa. Eosinophilic lung diseases cover a wide spectrum of pathology ranging from airways disease, such as eosinophilic bronchitis, to parenchymal disease, such as eosinophilic pneumonia, and systemic diseases, such as hypereosinophilic syndrome (HES) (table 1).

Nonasthmatic eosinophilic bronchitis

Eosinophilic bronchitis is a common and treatable form of chronic cough that was first identified in 1989. Nonasthmatic eosinophilic bronchitis is a condition that presents with a corticosteroid-responsive chronic cough in nonsmokers. These patients have evidence of eosinophilic airway inflammation without the variable airflow obstruction or airway hyperresponsiveness characteristic of asthma.

Eosinophilic bronchitis accounts for 10–30% of cases of chronic cough referred for specialist investigation. Eosinophilic bronchitis is defined as a chronic cough in patients with no symptoms or objective evidence of airflow obstruction, a histamine/methacholine PC20 (provocative concentration causing a 20% fall in FEV1) of $>16\,mg \cdot mL^{-1}$ and >3% sputum eosinophilia.

It is unclear why eosinophilic inflammation leads to asthma in some individuals and eosinophilic bronchitis in others. Studies by Brightling (2006) suggest that the key may be mast cell localisation. In asthmatics, mast cells infiltrate airways smooth muscle, resulting in airflow obstruction and hyperresponsiveness. In eosinophilic bronchitis, mast cells infiltrate the airway epithelium, leading to bronchitis and cough.

Anti-inflammatory therapy with inhaled corticosteroids is the mainstay of the treatment of eosinophilic bronchitis. Inhaled corticosteroids produce a significant improvement in symptoms as well as fall in sputum eosinophilia. There is no evidence to suggest that any one inhaled corticosteroid is more effective. Data is also not available to guide the dose or duration of inhaled corticosteroid therapy. Logically, antileukotrienes may be of benefit, but this hypothesis has not been tested in clinical trials. In very resistant cases, oral corticosteroids may be required for symptom control.

Little is known about the natural history of the condition, but it can be transient, episodic or persistent unless treated.

Key points

- Eosinophilic lung disease covers a wide spectrum of pathology from airways to parenchymal lung disease.

- Always exclude secondary causes of eosinophilia before diagnosing acute or chronic eosinophilic pneumonia.

- Novel therapies are being introduced for eosinophilia, including tyrosine kinase inhibitors and monoclonal antibodies against IL-5.

Table 1. The causes and associations of eosinophilic lung disease

Eosinophilic lung disease	Cause/association
Eosinophilic bronchitis	Unknown
HES	Idiopathic Lymphoproliferative variant with clonal expansion of T-cells and IL-5 production Myeloproliferative variant with fusion tyrosine kinase FIP1L1–PDGFRA
Pulmonary eosinophilic syndromes	Acute eosinophilic pneumonia Chronic eosinophilic pneumonia Löffler's syndrome Tropical eosinophilia
Allergic bronchopulmonary aspergillosis	*Aspergillus* proliferation in airway lumen induces Th2-mediated, IgE-driven bronchial inflammation
Churg–Strauss syndrome	Eosinophilic vasculitis of small to medium-sized vessels
Drug-induced pulmonary eosinophilia	Antibiotics Antifungals NSAIDS Antiepileptics Antipsychotics Anticoagulants Allopurinol Methotrexate
Helminthic infections	*Ascaris lumbricoides* *Strongyloides* Schistosomiasis Filariasis *Toxocara canis*

Th: T-helper cell; NSAID: nonsteroidal anti-inflammatory drugs.

Acute and chronic eosinophilic pneumonia

Acute eosinophilic pneumonia presents as an acute febrile illness of <1 month's duration and predominately affects cigarette smokers. The average age at presentation is 30 years with symptoms of dyspnoea, cough, myalgia and fever. Patients often present with severe type I respiratory failure requiring ventilation. Unlike other pulmonary eosinophilic syndromes, the blood eosinophil count is usually normal. The chest radiograph demonstrates diffuse alveolar and interstitial infiltrates. The diagnosis is confirmed by the presence of a bronchoalveolar lavage eosinophilia of >25% in the absence of parasitic, fungal or other infections, and no history of drug hypersensitivity. Acute eosinophilic pneumonia responds quickly to oral corticosteroids with no relapse after stopping therapy.

Chronic eosinophilic pneumonia typically presents in middle-aged asthmatic females but it can also develop in nonasthmatic individuals. The symptoms are gradually progressive and include shortness of breath, cough, fever and weight loss. Clinical examination demonstrates wheezing and hypoxia. Patients usually have a raised blood eosinophil count along with elevated inflammatory markers. The majority of patients have infiltrates visible on chest radiography and they are peripherally distributed in about two-thirds of cases (fig. 1).

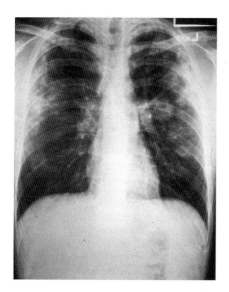

Figure 1. Chest radiograph of a patient presenting with chronic eosinophilic pneumonia demonstrating the characteristic peripheral infiltrates.

HRCT is more sensitive at demonstrating infiltrates and ~50% of patients also have mediastinal adenopathy. Patients respond well to oral corticosteroids but tend to relapse on discontinuation of therapy. Many patients require long-term, low-dose oral corticosteroids to control the condition; in a small minority, alternative, steroid-sparing agents have been used. This condition is frequently misdiagnosed as asthma. Blood eosinophilia and pulmonary infiltrates respond to corticosteroids within 24–48 h, making it easy to miss this condition if the relevant investigations are not performed prior to starting steroids.

Both acute and chronic eosinophilic pneumonia are idiopathic conditions. It is important to exclude secondary causes of eosinophilia before diagnosing either condition. In clinical practice, this requires a careful travel history asking about residence in areas of endemic parasitic infection and a careful drug history including illicit substances. The other main causes of a pulmonary eosinophilic syndrome are allergic bronchopulmonary aspergillosis,

HES and Churg–Strauss syndrome, which should be excluded at the time of diagnosis.

Hypereosinophilic syndrome

HES is a heterogeneous group of disorders characterised by the presence of marked blood and tissue eosinophilia resulting in a variety of clinical manifestations. The following criteria are used to define idiopathic HES:

- blood eosinophilia >1500 cells per mm^3 for ⩾6 months
- absence of an underlying cause for the eosinophilia
- end organ damage due to the eosinophilia

Idiopathic HES can occur at any age but tends to develop in the 30s or 40s with a male predominance. Nonspecific systemic symptoms are common. More specific symptoms will depend upon which organs are affected. The lungs are involved in ~40% of patients, and present with cough and airflow limitation. Pulmonary function tests demonstrate an obstructive pattern in patients with cough. In patients with cardiac involvement, concomitant pulmonary fibrosis can occur, leading to a restrictive or mixed pattern. The chest radiograph can be normal or demonstrate spontaneously clearing airspace shadowing in early disease. At a later stage, with multi-organ involvement, up to one-third of cases will have diffuse, nonsegmental interstitial infiltrates.

Dulohery et al. (2011) reported the frequency of pulmonary HES and associated clinical and radiologic features. In their case series of 49 patients, 24% had parenchymal lung involvement, which most commonly consisted of patchy ground-glass opacities and consolidation; one patient exhibited numerous pulmonary nodules. 27% had asthma. Most patients with pulmonary involvement of HES improved and no deaths were observed.

The most important cause of morbidity and mortality in idiopathic HES is cardiovascular involvement. Thromboembolic disease and involvement of the nervous system are also common presentations.

Until recently, oral corticosteroids have been the mainstay of treatment. Better understanding of eosinophil biology has led to the use of more logical targeted therapies. Distinct HES subtypes are now recognised. The myeloproliferative variant is associated with the presence of a fusion tyrosine kinase, FIP1L1–PDGFRA (FIP1-like protein 1–platelet-derived growth factor receptor-α). Historically, these patients had a poor prognosis with poor steroid responsiveness. The use of the tyrosine kinase inhibitor imatinib in this group of patients has significantly improved their outcome.

The lymphoproliferative variant is a consequence of increased production of eosinophilopoietic cytokines by clonal populations of phenotypically abnormal, activated T-lymphocytes. Identification of interleukin (IL)-5 as a key mediator of eosinophilopoiesis led to the use in clinical trials of an anti-IL-5 monoclonal antibody (mepolizumab) for HES. Mepolizumab is an effective corticosteroid-sparing agent in patients with HES negative for FIP1L1–PDGFRA.

Further reading

- Allen J (2006). Acute eosinophilic pneumonia. *Semin Respir Crit Care Med*; 27: 142–147.
- Brightling CE (2006). Chronic cough due to nonasthmatic eosinophilic bronchitis: ACCP evidence based clinical practice guidelines. *Chest*; 129: Suppl. 1, 116S–121S.
- Dulohery MM, *et al.* (2011). Lung involvement in hypereosinophilc syndromes. *Respir Med*; 105: 114–121.
- Klion AD, *et al.* (2006). Approaches to the treatment of hypereosinophilic syndromes: a workshop summary report. *J Allergy Clin Immunol*; 117: 1292–1302.
- Marchand E, *et al.* (2006). Idiopathic chronic eosinophilic pneumonia. *Semin Respir Crit Care Med*; 27: 134–141.
- Rhee CK, *et al.* (2013). Clinical characteristics and corticosteroid treatment of acute eosinophilic pneumonia. *Eur Respir J*; 41: 402–409.
- Rothenberg ME, *et al.* (2008). Treatment of patients with the hypereosinophilic syndrome with mepolizumab. *N Engl J Med*; 358: 1215–1228.

Drug-induced respiratory disease

Philippe Camus and Philippe Bonniaud

Key points

- DIRD is not uncommon, and can involve the larynx, major and lower airways, lung, pleura, pulmonary circulation, neuromuscular system and haemoglobin. Chemotherapy agents, amiodarone, ACE inhibitors, NSAIDs and β-blockers pose particular risk of adverse respiratory effects.

- Some DIRDs cause acute life-threatening respiratory distress, requiring immediate management.

- The clinical, imaging and pathological expression of DIRD may closely resemble that of illnesses of other causes or that occur idiopathically. Pathology is rarely specific for drug aetiology.

- Diagnosing DIRD requires a high degree of awareness, up-to-date knowledge and ruling out of other causes, particularly infection, using BAL and appropriate tests.

- Stopping the drug is often followed by improvement in symptoms, signs and imaging. Care should be taken to avoid relapse of the condition for which the drug was given.

- Corticosteroid therapy is reserved for severe cases and where dechallenge does not produce satisfactory improvement; duration varies with drug and pattern.

- Generally, rechallenge with the drug is discouraged as severe relapse can occur.

Drug-induced respiratory disease (DIRD) is a relatively common, generally unpredictable set of complications of therapy with or exposure to one of >700 distinct drugs (www.pneumotox.com). Drugs account for about 3% of all interstitial lung disease (ILD) cases and about 8–10% of acute lung injury (ALI) cases are due to drugs, mainly chemotherapy and amiodarone. The biologics (erlotinib, dasatinib, gefitinib, imatinib and nilotinib), monoclonal antibodies (abciximab, adalimumab, bevacizumab, cetuximab and infliximab) and etanercept can cause mechanism-based or idiosyncratic adverse respiratory reactions. Irradiation, inhaled or injected substances of abuse, excipients and vehicles, herbals, and vaccines can also cause respiratory injury. Iatrogenic non-drug-induced complications include the adverse consequences of catheters, and medical, imaging and surgical procedures (these are not covered here). The diagnosis of DIRD is mainly one of exclusion (table 1). Aetiologies other than drugs must be carefully excluded, including the pulmonary manifestations of the underlying illness when present, and opportunistic infections due to *Pneumocystis jiroveci* or other fungi, parasites, viruses or bacteria. Patients exposed to methotrexate, chemotherapy agents or immunosuppressive drugs including prolonged corticosteroid therapy, tumour necrosis factor (TNF)-α antagonists, rituximab, and those who have received radiation therapy to the chest, or are stem cell or lung transplant recipients are particularly exposed to the risk of developing opportunistic respiratory infections.

ERS Handbook: Respiratory Medicine

399

Table 1. Checklist for diagnosing and managing DIRDs

Emergent management should be placed ahead of causality assessment while managing acute drug-induced emergencies such as anaphylaxis, bronchospasm, asphyxia, diffuse white-out, bleeding, tamponade, pulmonary hypertension, respiratory muscle paralysis or methaemoglobinaemia.

Maintain a high degree of **awareness**. Two main questions arise:

1) Could new and otherwise unexplained signs and symptoms (respiratory and/or nonrespiratory) be due to a drug or drugs? Check Pneumotox by drug names.

2) Which pattern of involvement may result from the drug the patients is on? Check Pneumotox by patterns.

Take complete **history** and list current or past exposure to any medication, abused substance, or herbal, chemical or physical agent.

Retrieve and review any **pre-therapy imaging** and pulmonary function, if available.

Review the possibility of **respiratory involvement from any underlying disease** present (connective tissue disease including rheumatoid arthritis, malignant conditions, *etc.*).

Correlate time on each specific drug and **timing of exposure** (delay between first exposure and onset of signs and symptoms). This can vary from minutes with anaphylaxis or bronchospasm, to months or years with ILD.

Attempt to define the **pattern of involvement** (using clinical features, imaging, HRCT, BAL and diuresis) in a noninvasive, conservative way. A lung biopsy is rarely indicated as the procedure carries its own morbidity/mortality and may yield nonspecific findings. A matching table of drugs and pathology patterns is available on Pneumotox (pattern XV) and in table 2.

Correlate each drug with pattern of involvement in the patient (see Further Reading and Pneumotox)

Differential: evaluate the possibility of underlying disease or coincidental illness (including heart failure or an opportunistic infection in the immunodepressed) *versus* drug-induced disease

Most **in vitro tests** have fallen out of favour except the unusual drug-induced ANA, ANCA and anti-HNE.

Discontinue drug, underlying condition permitting. Cover with a substitute drug if needed. Expect improvement in hours, weeks or more depending on drug and pattern.

Decide on corticosteroid therapy. Corticosteroid therapy is indicated depending on severity, extensity of involvement and response to drug discontinuance.

Organise follow-up for resolution of signs, symptoms, pulmonary physiology and imaging.

Consider **rechallenge** only if drug is vital, or with the purpose of desensitisation or induction of tolerance, preferably if documented in the literature. Make sure the patient will never get re-exposed to the culprit drug.

HNE: human neutrophil elastase.

Drugs history is now included in the workup of any patient with ILD and the same should apply to other patterns of drug-induced respiratory involvement (table 3). Overall, the greatest incidence is with chemotherapy agents including bleomycin (up to 50%, depending on the drug regimen and which diagnostic test is used to diagnose it), angiotensin-converting enzyme inhibitors (ACEIs), amiodarone (2-4%), methotrexate (0.5–1%), mineral lipids (paraffin) in the elderly, mammalian target of rapamycin (mTOR) inhibitors, nitrofurantoin, TNF-α antagonists, tyrosine kinase inhibitors (TKIs),

Table 2. Main imaging–pathological patterns of DIRDs

Pattern on chest radiograph or CT	Causal drugs	Pathology correlate
Diffuse haze Ground-glass opacity	Drugs that cause interstitial pneumonia (NSIP-like)	Interstitial inflammation
	Chemotherapy agents	Early/mild pulmonary oedema, alveolar haemorrhage or DAD
Localised ground-glass opacity	Radiation therapy	Early mild radiation lung injury (interstitial oedema, cell sloughing, cell debris)
Diffuse white-out	Drugs that produce acute ILD, pulmonary oedema, eosinophilic pneumonia, DAD or DAH[#]	Dense cellular interstitial pneumonitis with or without eosinophilia Acute pulmonary oedema Alveolar haemorrhage
Disseminated ground-glass opacity with a mosaic pattern of distribution	Drugs that cause interstitial pneumonia	Cellular interstitial pneumonia DIP
Bilateral perihilar alveolar opacities with a batwing pattern of distribution	Drugs that cause pulmonary oedema, DAD or DAH	Pulmonary oedema DAD DAH
Subpleural areas of consolidation	Drugs that cause pulmonary eosinophilia or OP	Eosinophilic pneumonia OP
Opacities with a recognisable segmental or lobar pattern of distribution	Amiodarone	Phospholipidosis OP
	Statins	OP
	Paraffin	Exogenous lipoid pneumonia
Miliary pattern	BCG therapy Methotrexate Sirolimus	Granulomatous reaction
Area of consolidation A mass	Drugs that cause OP or eosinophilic pneumonia	OP Eosinophilic pneumonia
	Amiodarone	Phospholipidosis Amiodaronoma
	Paraffin	Paraffinoma
Wandering opacities	Drugs that cause OP or PIE	OP Eosinophilic pneumonia
	Irradiation for breast carcinoma	OP
Multiple nodular opacities	Amiodarone	APT features
	Bleomycin	OP
	Bleomycin	Areas of nodular fibrosis
Pulmonary fibrosis Low lung volumes	Chemotherapy agents Amiodarone Nitrofurantoin Irradiation	Pulmonary fibrosis NSIP-fibrotic or UIP pattern

NSIP: nonspecific interstitial pneumonia; DIP: desquamative interstitial pneumonia; OP: organising pneumonia; BCG: bacille Calmette–Guérin; UIP: usual interstitial pneumonia. [#]: see appropriate pattern at www.pneumotox.com

radiation therapy, drugs of abuse including heroin and cocaine, levamisole, and liquid silicone. As drugs may target any subsystem of the respiratory apparatus, varied clinical and imaging presentations may ensue. DIRD can be in the form of ILD, noncardiogenic pulmonary oedema, ALI/acute respiratory distress syndrome (ARDS), alveolar haemorrhage, lung nodules, stridor and asphyxia, catastrophic bronchospasm,

Table 3. Patterns and mechanisms of DIRD

Pattern	Pathophysiology
Parenchymal lung disease	Interstitial/alveolar inflammation/filling
Interstitial lung diseases[#]	Influx/persistence of inflammatory cells Interstitial oedema
Endogenous lipoid pneumonia (phospholipidosis)	Disordered phospholipid catabolism[¶]
Exogenous lipid pneumonia	Accumulation of nondigestible oil and oil-laden macrophages in alveolar spaces
Pulmonary fibrosis	Scarring
Diffuse pulmonary calcification	Precipitation of calcium in pulmonary interstitium
Foreign body reaction	Granulomas around drug or excipients
Pulmonary nodules	Circumscribed areas of OP or fibrosis
Pulmonary oedema	
Noncardiogenic pulmonary oedema	Increased permeability of alveolar barrier to fluid
Cardiogenic pulmonary oedema	Raised pulmonary venous pressure due to myocardial injury
ALI/ARDS	Increased permeability of alveolar capillary barrier to fluid and proteins
Transfusion-related ALI	Immune-mediated blood reaction to anti-HLA antibodies of donor origin. Neutrophil sequestration
Pulmonary haemorrhage	
DAH	Synchronous capillary bleeding usually from disordered coagulation, low platelets or capillaritis
ANCA-associated DAH	ANCA/activated neutrophil-mediated capillaritis and consequent bleeding
Airway involvement	
Bronchospasm/asthma	Subverted prostaglandin/leukotriene handling
Obliterative bronchiolitis	Acceleration of bronchiolitis from the underlying disease?
Cough	Bradykinin-mediated?
Foreign body bronchiolitis	Airway-centred reaction against drug or vehicle
Large airway involvement or closure	
Angio-oedema	Bradykinin-mediated?
Haematoma causing UAO	Localised bleeding causing compression
Pulmonary vasculopathy	
Pulmonary thromboembolism	Excessive coagulation
Pulmonary arterial hypertension	Serotonin-based?
Pulmonary vasculitis/capillaritis	Drug-induced ANCAs
Fat/lipid/silicone embolism	Increased capillary permeability Bypass of foreign fluid through the lung, causing brain injury
Foreign body vasculopathy	Granulomatous reaction around foreign drug-associated material

Table 3. Continued

Pattern	Pathophysiology
Cement/mercury embolism	Lodging of acrylate or metallic mercury in the distal pulmonary circulation
Pleural/pericardial involvement	
Pleural effusion	Pleural inflammation
Pleural thickening/fibrosis	Scarring/fibrosis
Pleural effusion and drug lupus	Autoimmune-mediated?
Haemothorax	Drug-induced disordered coagulation
Chylothorax	PDGFR inhibition?
Serositis	Autoimmune-mediated?
Haemopericardium	Drug-induced disordered coagulation
Pleuritic chest pain	Pleural inflammation
Pleuroparenchymal fibroelastosis	Scarring, elastic fibre type
Pleural mass or masses	Scarring around foreign material (talc)
Mediastinal involvement	
Lymphadenopathy	Unknown
Mediastinal lipomatosis	Central fat distribution[+]
Fibrosing mediastinitis	Scarring, usually radiation induced
Neuromuscular involvement	
Respiratory muscle weakness/paralysis	Myoneural presynaptic blockade of acetylcholine release
Ventilatory depression/apnoea	Opiate effect on central ventilatory oscillator
Respiratory muscle/myopathy	Corticosteroid-induced muscle wasting Statin-induced myopathy
Acquired haemoglobinopathy	
Methaemoglobinaemia	Haemoglobin poisoning *via* iron oxidation
Systemic syndromes	
DRESS	T-cells, HHV6 or HHV8
Antiphospholipid antibody syndrome	Unknown
Drug-induced lupus	Drug-triggered autoimmunity
Anaphylaxis	Some due to drug-induced IgE release
Hypersensitivity reactions	Reaction to foreign (*e.g.* murine) proteins
Eosinophilic granulomatosis with polyangiitis (Churg–Strauss)	Unknown
Immune reconstitution syndrome	Exaggerated reaction to microorganisms once immune cells repopulate tissues
Polymyositis/dermatopolymyositis	Unknown
Sarcoidosis	Unknown
Systemic vasculitis	Drug-induced ANCA-mediated?

Table 3. Continued

Pattern	Pathophysiology
Miscellaneous	
Vertebral compression fracture	Osteoporosis Radiation-induced damage
Rib fracture	Osteoporosis Radiation-induced damage
Chest deformity/platythorax	Pleuropulmonary fibrosis in childhood
Fire-eater's lung	Aspiration of liquid hydrocarbon

See also www.pneumotox.com UAO: upper airway obstruction; OP: organising pneumonia; HLA: human leukocyte antigen; PDGFR: platelet-derived growth factor receptor; HHV: human herpesvirus. #: including pulmonary infiltration with eosinophilia and OP; ¶: amiodarone is the typical causal drug; +: common with corticosteroid therapy.

cough, pulmonary hypertension, pleural effusion, cardiac tamponade, haemothorax, neuromuscular blockade, or haemoglobinopathy.

Life-threatening presentations include anaphylaxis, acute laryngeal angio-oedema (usually from ACEIs), catastrophic bronchospasm (typically from nonsteroidal anti-inflammatory drugs (NSAIDs) or β-blockers), acute methotrexate pneumonitis, minocycline- or tobacco-related acute eosinophilic pneumonia, tocolytic- or chemotherapy-induced pulmonary oedema, chemotherapy-induced ALI or ARDS, anticoagulant-induced diffuse alveolar haemorrhage (DAH), large volume-occupying pleural effusions, cardiac tamponade, methaemoglobinaemia, neuromuscular paralysis and systemic conditions such as DRESS (drug reaction with eosinophilia and systemic symptoms). These presentations, particularly when they occur in the emergency room or intra- or perioperatively, portend immediate severity and require prompt evaluation. Management is aimed at restoring airway patency, maintaining oxygenation and reversing drug-induced inflammation and oedema using drug withdrawal and corticosteroid therapy. Further compounding these issues, drugs can cause cardiac injury, which may cause heart failure and can impact the lung and pleura (table 3).

Pathophysiology: mechanisms

Mechanisms in DIRD are summarised in table 3. With a few drugs (e.g. chemotherapy agents and amiodarone), reactions may correspond to a dose-related cytopathic mechanism. Identification of a threshold dosage may then enable risk reduction. However, most drug reactions are idiosyncratic and unpredictable, occurring in only a few predisposed individuals, possibly with a predilection in those who harbour a distinct pharmacokinetic trait. Several drugs in a given family produce a stereotyped pattern of involvement (e.g. β-blockers, NSAIDs and bronchospasm, NSAIDs and eosinophilic pneumonia, chemotherapy and pulmonary oedema or ALI-ARDS/diffuse alveolar damage (DAD), anticoagulants and DAH, and ergots and pleural involvement), suggesting a reaction linked to the pharmacological effect of the drug, even though the pharmacophores differ. Drug disposition in the lung may be a relevant factor for toxicity. Amiodarone and its metabolite concentrate in lung, causing toxicity to lung cells. The slow efflux of these compounds from the lung may explain both the slow resolution of amiodarone pulmonary toxicity (APT) and relapses of the condition even when amiodarone is discontinued, at a time when corticosteroid therapy is being tapered. The pulmonary metabolism of nitrofurantoin, cyclophosphamide, mitomycin, bleomycin and paraquat in designated lung cells generates reactive oxygen species, which cause cell stress and death, pulmonary inflammation, and/or fibrosis. The heterogeneous distribution of activating enzymes in lung may account for the selective targeted alveolar or bronchiolar injury seen with certain drugs. Drug-induced asthma is largely non-IgE-dependent. Small incremental doses of NSAIDs or aspirin can be given to asthmatics who are intolerant to these drugs to induce a state of tolerance that can be maintained on continued exposure to the medication. Unusual cases of respiratory injury result from deposition of drug excipients in the small airways and pulmonary arterioles, causing reactive foreign body obstructive granulomas that cause obstruction to airflow or pulmonary hypertension. Amiodarone, radiation and chemotherapy agent toxicity is potentiated by molecular oxygen. Patients must be spared unnecessary association of these factors. Patients on chemotherapy for malignant conditions or who receive amiodarone in the long term may exhibit a time- or dose-related decrease in TLCO thought to reflect subclinical toxicity, without necessarily annunciating the development of clinical disease. In that setting, risk-to-benefit evaluation of drug discontinuation or maintenance is indicated in each patient.

Clinical presentation

Drugs can cause injury when administered by the oral, intravenous, intramuscular, inhaled, pleural, dermal, intrathecal, intracoronary or gynaecological route. DIRD can also develop following delivery in organs situated upstream of the lung (e.g. vertebrae, brain, liver and oesophagus). A high index of suspicion is warranted. Drugs should be a diagnostic consideration in any patient with otherwise unexplained symptoms, abnormal pulmonary physiology or new radiographic findings while being treated with a compatible drug or set of drugs. Some adverse reactions develop within minutes of exposure, suggesting causality (e.g. β-blocker-induced bronchospasm, and chemotherapy- or tocolytic-induced pulmonary oedema).

For many drugs, there may be a delay of weeks, months or years before symptom presentation. Presenting symptoms include a nonproductive cough, dyspnoea, wheezing, cyanosis, fever, rigors and malaise. Acute bronchospasm, angio-oedema, cardiovascular collapse, shock, stridor, hoarseness, wheezing, haemoptysis or acute chest pain are less common presentations. Other features include a cutaneous rash, lymph-node enlargement, myositis, livedo reticularis, skin necrosis, hepatitis or other deep-seated organ involvement. Rare patients present with a systemic picture reminiscent of the lupus erythematosus (lupus-inducing agents), granulomatous polyangiitis (propylthiouracil), eosinophilic granulomatous polyangiitis (leukotriene receptor antagonists) or dermatopolymyositis (statins). Severity of DIRD is linked to the acuteness of presentation, extent and location of the pathological process, and reversibility upon drug discontinuance or under the influence of therapy. Life-threatening presentations include anaphylactic shock, upper airway angioedema and closure, acute ILD, pulmonary infiltration with eosinophilia (PIE), organising pneumonia, noncardiogenic pulmonary oedema or alveolar haemorrhage, catastrophic bronchospasm, large pleural effusions, tamponade, methaemoglobinaemia, apnoea, and respiratory paralysis. Drug withdrawal, if followed by abatement of signs and symptoms, supports the drug aetiology. The risk of rechallenge should be balanced against the merit of securing the diagnosis, as fatal reactions may ensue.

Many clinical situations are inextricably complex, particularly in ILD patients who are exposed to several possible causal drugs, who have received radiation therapy, or in whom DIRD cannot be confidently separated from underlying disease-related pulmonary involvement or from an infection. Oncology patients who are receiving chemotherapy, TKIs, mTOR inhibitors and/or radiation therapy, or those with rheumatoid arthritis who receive combination therapy with corticosteroids and/or anti-TNF antibody therapy exemplify these difficulties. Careful assessment of each drug's causality and meticulous exclusion of an infection are required using molecular techniques on bronchoalveolar lavage (BAL) fluid. Notwithstanding that, patients may progress without a firm diagnosis despite exclusion of an infection, withdrawal of the suspect drug, corticosteroids and empiric antibiotic therapy. Diagnosing drug-induced ILD is also difficult in patients with autoimmune conditions, or in recipients of solid organ or stem cell transplants who receive long-term treatments with cytotoxic agents, immunosuppressive drugs, rituximab and corticosteroids.

Imaging

Imaging is most useful in patients presenting with pulmonary opacities. Patterns and correlates are shown in table 2.

The extent of involvement seen on imaging roughly correlates with gas exchange. HRCT discloses inter- and intralobular septal thickening, disseminated lobular opacities, faint or dense ground-glass shadowing, or alveolar filling. Pleural effusion denotes severe ILD or pulmonary oedema, or occurs in isolation as a complication of therapy with one or more of ~60 different drugs. Amiodarone pulmonary toxicity takes the form of asymmetric pulmonary opacities, areas of condensation that may be electron-dense due to the two iodine atoms per amiodarone molecule, a density with recognisable segmental distribution or, rarely, shaggy lung nodules. Early 'chemotherapy lung' corresponding to DAD and ALI is in the form of a diffuse haze or ground glass. Late chemotherapy lung resembles pulmonary fibrosis. Eosinophilic pneumonia can manifest with lung opacities, having a preferentially subpleural distribution. Acute nitrofurantoin lung is in the form of diffuse haze and small pleural effusions, while the chronic form of the disease shows scattered peribronchovascular zonal consolidation. Organising pneumonia may present with characteristic migratory opacities on serial chest films or diffuse involvement.

Mediastinal or hilar lymphadenopathy characterises those cases with a drug-induced sarcoid-like reaction. Pulmonary opacities in exogenous lipoid pneumonia exhibit low attenuation numbers, and pulmonary arteries and their branches are discernible within the involved area. Radiation pneumonitis develops preferentially in the area of the radiation beam, although current stereotactic body irradiation tends to produce circumscribed whorled foci of radiation pneumonitis. Inferring pathology from the pattern seen on imaging should be interpreted with caution. Fatty mediastinal deposits suggest corticosteroid therapy. Embolism of acrylate cement or mercury can be visualized as branched vascular densities on unenhanced CT. An air–fluid level or pneumothorax can be a complication of chemotherapy-induced tumoural cavitation.

BAL, pathology and other tests

BAL is indicated to rule out an infection (particularly *P. jiroveci*) *via* stains, cultures and reverse transcriptase PCR. BAL can also indicate which cell type (*i.e.* lymphocytes, eosinophils or neutrophils) is increased, and whether atypical cells or phospholipid-laden (foamy) alveolar macrophages are present. BAL is useful to diagnose methotrexate pneumonitis, drug-induced eosinophilic pneumonias, APT and chemotherapy lung. BAL cell numbers normalise as patients improve. The BAL in exogenous lipoid pneumonia contains stainable mineral lipids free in the BAL fluid and within vacuoles in alveolar macrophages.

Drugs can cause virtually any known pattern of ILD, including: cellular or fibrotic nonspecific interstitial pneumonia; eosinophilic pneumonia; ALI or DAD; classic or acute fibrinous organising pneumonia; interstitial granulomas; alveolar haemorrhage; pulmonary capillaritis or vasculitis; desquamative, giant-cell or lymphocytic-interstitial pneumonia; a usual interstitial pneumonia or pulmonary alveolar proteinosis pattern; and diffuse pulmonary calcification. These are not specific to the drug aetiology. Only phospholipidosis and exogenous lipoid pneumonia are suggestive enough to point to the drug aetiology. While examination of a lung biopsy sample helps eliminate a condition other than drugs, including an infection, a risk–benefit analysis is not available and mortality is significant, especially in the hypoxaemic or immunodepressed. A conservative approach is advised, where drug dechallenge is the usual first step.

No *in vitro* test of monocyte cell migration in the presence of a drug or metabolite has demonstrated utility in DIRD, and these can be misleading. Certain phenotypic traits may indicate an increased risk of developing DIRD. However, these tests are not widely available.

Monitoring of drug levels in plasma can be helpful to track aspirin over-dosing, or exposure to illicit opiates or levamisole.

Specific reactions

Parenchymal lung disease Methotrexate pneumonitis typifies acute fulminant drug-induced ILD, a condition that can be produced by ~70 other drugs. The condition develops with no forewarning symptoms in patients on long-term methotrexate, typically those with rheumatoid arthritis. A background of pre-existing ILD is a risk factor. The disease manifests with cough, fever, dyspnoea and diffuse pulmonary opacities, sometimes with rapidly progressive white-out and hypoxaemic respiratory failure. Lymphocytes dominate in the BAL. The main differential is *Pneumocystis* or another opportunistic infection that needs be ruled out using the BAL. Methotrexate pneumonitis may also follow less severe a course with faint pulmonary opacities on imaging. Rarely, pulmonary fibrosis develops following an episode of methotrexate lung. Corticosteroid therapy is indicated in severe cases.

Pulmonary eosinophilia is a common pattern of reaction to one of >150 drugs. Other causes of pulmonary infiltrates and eosinophilia must be ruled out, including parasitic infestation. There is bilateral shadowing in the context of peripheral and BAL eosinophilia. Acute eosinophilic pneumonia is a severe form of PIE with acute respiratory failure. Characteristic

causal drugs include NSAIDs, antibiotics (*e.g.* minocycline), abused drugs and recent uptake of tobacco smoking. Rechallenge is contraindicated, as relapse will almost inevitably occur. Severe systemic presentations characterised by a cutaneous rash and deep-seated organ involvement are termed DRESS or anticonvulsant syndrome.

APT is a distinctive condition that develops insidiously over months or years into treatment with amiodarone in ~3% of patients. High dosages and advanced age increase the risk of developing the condition. APT takes the form of asymmetric areas of pneumonitis or consolidation that can be electron-dense on HRCT, as is liver tissue. Pulmonary function is restrictive in nature. Foamy cells in the BAL are suggestive but not diagnostic of APT. Other APT presentations include ground-glass shadowing, lung nodules, pulmonary fibrosis or pleural effusion. Amiodarone withdrawal may not be sufficient for APT to resolve due to the high affinity and persistence of amiodarone in lung tissue. Corticosteroid therapy often is indicated to speed up recovery. Severe APT can occur after thoracic surgery, particularly in oxygen-exposed patients in the form of an ARDS picture. Prognosis is guarded.

About 150 drugs can cause NCPE (noncardiogenic pulmonary oedema), including the chemotherapeutic agents taxanes and gemcitabine, blood products, tocolytics, and aspirin. Severity ranges from transient pulmonary infiltrates following each course with the drug to acute pulmonary oedema or an ARDS picture.

Chemotherapy lung takes the form of pulmonary infiltrates during or shortly after completion of treatment with the drug. Bleomycin, cyclophosphamide, gemcitabine, nitrosoureas and taxanes are classic causal drugs, with more recent evidence implicating TKIs (cetuximab, erlotinib, gefitinib and pemetrexed). On pathology, there is modest interstitial inflammation and oedema, a reactive epithelium, and areas of ALI or DAD. The condition may improve upon drug discontinuance and corticosteroid therapy. In more advanced cases, an ARDS picture develops. Late cases present irreversible pulmonary fibrosis.

Drug-induced organising pneumonia resembles cryptogenic organising pneumonia or organising pneumonia of other causes. It is in the form of migratory opacities, a fixed opacity or mass, or diffuse shadowing with respiratory failure. Main causal agents include amiodarone, interferons, minocycline, rituximab, statins and breast radiation therapy. Drug withdrawal is followed by improvement while failure to recognise the drug aetiology exposes to the risk of relapses. Corticosteroid therapy is reserved for severe organising pneumonia cases or those with equivocal effect of drug dechallenge.

Interferons, anti-TNF agents and a few other drugs may cause pulmonary infiltrates and lymphadenopathy, and a granulomatous pattern of reaction mimicking sarcoidosis. A confirmatory biopsy and interferon-γ test for TB may be indicated to rule out an infection.

Drug-induced DAH is best diagnosed by BAL, which shows bloodier return on sequential aliquots. Anticoagulants, thrombolytic agents, abciximab and other antiplatelet agents, propylthiouracil, and cocaine (among 70 other drugs) can cause the syndrome. DAH is with or without capillaritis. Rarely, alveolar haemorrhage occurs as a manifestation of drug-induced anti-neutrophil cytoplasmic antibody (ANCA) vasculitis (mainly propylthiouracil- or levamisole-induced).

Pulmonary fibrosis can occur as a complication of treatments with chemotherapy agents, amiodarone and irradiation (then conforming to the radiation portal). Patients present with dyspnoea, diffuse linear or streaky opacities and volume loss on imaging. In contrast to interstitial pulmonary fibrosis, honeycombing is unusual. The condition may stabilise with or progress despite drug discontinuance. Response to corticosteroid therapy is often limited. A few patients have received a lung transplant.

Corticosteroid therapy is indicated in severe drug-induced ILD, preferably if an infection

is reasonably excluded and wherever drug withdrawal is not followed by improvement.

Airway involvement Angio-oedema classically occurs with ACEIs and it is more common in middle-aged or elderly African-American women. The condition may develop within hours of the first administration of the drug or it occurs months or years into an uneventful treatment, in the form of rapidly progressive breathing difficulty due to upper airway oedema and narrowing. Oedema of the lips, tongue, mouth floor, arytenoids and larynx has been reported, but the thoracic trachea is typically spared. Yearly incidence is ~1%, which makes it a significant cumulative risk in patients treated with these medications over the long term. Some patients develop the condition after airway manipulation or the trauma of intubation. About 40% of the patients are admitted to an intensive care unit (ICU) and mechanical ventilation is indicated in about 10%. Emergent identification and maintenance of upper airway patency is essential. Orotracheal intubation is indicated in severe cases. Short of stabilising the airway, emergent tracheostomy may be required, with significant attending risks. Although patients improve upon drug discontinuance, close follow-up is necessary as a rebound phenomenon can occur in the first 24-48 h. Patients should not be re-exposed to any ACEI, or grave relapse can occur. Angiotensin receptor II blockers should be given prudently, as a few patients will cross-react.

Catastrophic bronchospasm may follow exposure to as little as one tablet of NSAID, aspirin or nonselective β-blockers (among 120 other drugs). The accident occurs within minutes, with a predilection for aspirin-sensitive individuals, atopics and asthmatics. About 15% of ICU-admitted asthma attack cases are triggered by exposure to such drugs. Insufflated heroin has recently emerged as a significant cause of severe bronchospasm and urine drug screening is indicated. Rechallenge with the culprit drug inevitably leads to relapse with a risk of hypoxic brain damage and death.

Lone, chronic, annoying cough is a common complication of treatments with ACEI.

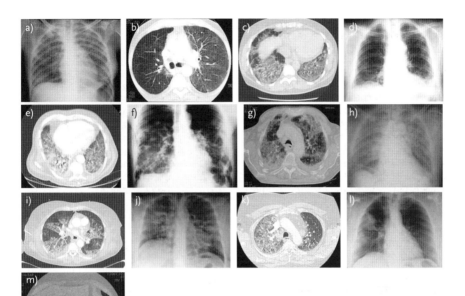

Figure 1. Radiographic patterns of a–c) drug-induced parenchymal injury, d and e) bleomycin pulmonary toxicity, f and g) drug-induced eosinophilic pneumonia, h and i) acute pulmonary oedema, j and k) amiodarone pulmonary toxicity, and l and m) organising pneumonia.

Incidence depends on which ACEI is used. It may be difficult to make sure when exactly the cough started with respect the when the ACEI was started. When in doubt, dechallenge is indicated. The cough remits with drug discontinuance, except if it was revealing an underlying lung condition.

Rare cases of penicillamine-induced obliterative bronchiolitis have been reported. These may reflect acceleration of underlying small airway disease related to the background connective tissue disease. Obliterative bronchiolitis can complicate herbal therapy with the Asian *Sauropus* shrub leaf, or be a manifestation of graft *versus* host disease or lung rejection in stem-cell and lung transplant recipients, respectively.

Foreign-body bronchiolitis has been described in a few subjects who intentionally inhaled cosmetic talc.

Pleura Nearly 60 drugs can injure the pleura, including ergolines and dasatinib. Involvement is in the form of a free-flowing exudate with or without eosinophilia, or a serosanguineous effusion. Lupus-inducing drugs can cause drug lupus, which manifests with pleuritis, pleural or pleuropericardial effusion, and circulating and pleural antinuclear antibody (ANA). Anti-TNF agents (infliximab, etanercept and adalimumab) and interferons may also cause lupus. Sometimes, anti-double stranded DNA antibodies are present as well. Signs, symptoms and ANA resolve upon discontinuation of the drug

All ergots are notable for the insidious development of bilateral pleural thickening with or without an effusion, causing dyspnoea, chest pain, audible friction rubs and restrictive lung dysfunction. There is definite but slow improvement upon discontinuance of the drug.

Pulmonary vasculopathy This condition is mostly is in the form of pulmonary hypertension analogous to primary pulmonary hypertension. Iatrogenic pulmonary hypertension may follow treatments with amphetamine-like anorectics (fenfluramine and benfluorex) or dasatinib. Pulmonary hypertension in drug abusers stems from injection of crushed tablets, or results from stimulant (amphetamine) use or abuse.

Methaemoglobinaemia is a drug-induced state of ferric (rather than ferrous) iron oxidation in haemoglobin. Methaemoglobin is a poor oxygen carrier. Clinical presentation is slate-grey cyanosis, a low S_{pO_2}, and a normal measured P_{aO_2} and calculated S_{aO_2}. Actual measurement of methaemoglobin is indicated in patients exposed to a causative drug, mainly benzocaine, dapsone, nitrites and nitric oxide.

Further reading

- Barclay JA, *et al.* (2011). Dapsone-induced methemoglobinemia: a primer for clinicians. *Ann Pharmacother*; 45: 1103–1315.
- Cacoub P, *et al.* (2011). The DRESS syndrome: a literature review. *Am J Med*; 124: 588–597.
- Camus P. The Drug-Induced Respiratory Disease Website. www.pneumotox.com
- Chin KM, *et al.* (2006). Is methamphetamine use associated with idiopathic pulmonary arterial hypertension? *Chest*; 130: 1657–1663.
- de Jesus Perez V, *et al.* (2011). Drugs and toxins-associated pulmonary arterial hypertension: lessons learned and challenges ahead. *Int J Clin Pract Suppl*; 169: 8–10.
- Hadjinicolaou AV, *et al.* (2011a). Non-infectious pulmonary complications of newer biological agents for rheumatic diseases – a systematic literature review. *Rheumatology (Oxford)*; 50: 2297–2305.
- Hadjinicolaou AV, *et al.* (2011b). Non-infectious pulmonary toxicity of rituximab: a systematic review. *Rheumatology (Oxford)*; 51: 653–662.
- Hamblin MJ, *et al.* (2011). Rheumatoid arthritis-associated interstitial lung disease: diagnostic dilemma. *Pulm Med*; 2011: 872120.

- Khasnis AA, *et al.* (2010). Tumor necrosis factor inhibitors and lung disease: a paradox of efficacy and risk. *Semin Arthritis Rheum*; 40: 147–163.
- Lara AR, *et al.* (2010). Diffuse alveolar hemorrhage. *Chest*; 137: 1164–1171.
- Marchiori E, *et al.* (2011). Exogenous lipoid pneumonia. Clinical and radiological manifestations. *Respir Med*; 105: 659–566.
- Min JH, *et al.* (2011). Drug-induced interstitial lung disease in tyrosine kinase inhibitor therapy for non-small cell lung cancer: a review on current insight. *Cancer Chemother Pharmacol*; 68: 1099–1109.
- Newsome BR, *et al.* (2011). Diffuse alveolar hemorrhage. *South Med J*; 104: 269–274.
- Papiris SA, *et al.* (2010). Amiodarone: review of pulmonary effects and toxicity. *Drug Saf*; 33: 539–558.
- Rubin RL (2005). Drug-induced lupus. *Toxicology*; 209: 135–147.
- Saito Y, *et al.* (2012). Current status of DILD in molecular targeted therapies. *Int J Clin Oncol*; 17: 534–541.
- Sanchez-Borges M, *et al.* (2010). Angiotensin-converting enzyme inhibitors and angioedema. *Allergy Asthma Immunol Res*; 2: 195–198.
- Sarzi-Puttini P, *et al.* (2005). Drug-induced lupus erythematosus. *Autoimmunity*; 38: 507–518.
- Schreiber J (2011). Drug-induced lung diseases. *Dtsch Med Wochenschr*; 136: 631–634.
- Schwaiblmair M, *et al.* (2012). Drug induced interstitial lung disease. *Open Respir Med J*; 6: 63–74.
- Slavenburg S, *et al.* (2010). Pneumonitis as a consequence of (Peg)-interferon-ribavirin combination therapy for hepatitis C: a review of the literature. *Dig Dis Sci*; 55: 579–585.
- Torrisi JM, *et al.* (2011). CT findings of chemotherapy-induced toxicity: what radiologists need to know about the clinical and radiologic manifestations of chemotherapy toxicity. *Radiology*; 258: 41–56.

Pulmonary embolism

Massimo Pistolesi

Despite the recent advances in prevention and diagnostic imaging, pulmonary embolism remains a major health problem. The incidence of this pathological condition is as high as one in 1000 cases per year in the general population. Early diagnosis is fundamental as early treatment is highly effective. However, due to the low specificity of its clinical presentation, this common disease is still underdiagnosed and it is estimated that in the USA >100 000 people die each year of pulmonary embolism.

Several points are summarised below concerning the diagnostic strategies to be adopted in patients with clinical suspicion of pulmonary embolism that have been highlighted and brought to the attention of the scientific community by recent scientific publications, expert reviews and international guidelines.

Key points

- Although early treatment is highly effective, pulmonary embolism is underdiagnosed and, therefore, remains a major health problem.

- Diagnostic strategy should be based on clinical evaluation of the probability of pulmonary embolism.

- The NPVs and PPVs of diagnostic tests for pulmonary embolism are high when the results are concordant with the clinical assessment.

- Additional testing is necessary when the test results are inconsistent with clinical probability.

General rules for the diagnostic work-up of patients clinically suspected of pulmonary embolism

- Pre-test clinical probability of pulmonary embolism should be objectively assessed in each patient.
- D-dimer should be determined if pre-test probability of pulmonary embolism is low or intermediate.
- Diagnostic imaging of the chest should be used to assess post-test probability of pulmonary embolism in most patients. Further testing is necessary when the post-test probability of pulmonary embolism is neither sufficiently low nor sufficiently high to permit therapeutic decisions.
- Diagnostic strategies of pulmonary embolism can differ significantly in different clinical contexts and special conditions.

Pre-test clinical probability of pulmonary embolism

A thorough clinical evaluation is the key step in raising the suspicion of the disease and setting up appropriate diagnostic strategies. A recent study has shown that the vast majority of patients with pulmonary embolism has at least one of four symptoms which, in decreasing order of frequency, are:

1. sudden onset dyspnoea
2. chest pain
3. fainting (or syncope)
4. haemoptysis

Although the diagnostic yield of individual clinical symptoms, signs and common laboratory tests is limited, the combination of these variables, either by empirical assessment or by a prediction rule, can be used to stratify patients by risk of pulmonary embolism (low, intermediate or high). The results of two broad prospective studies in the 1990s (Prospective Investigation of Pulmonary Embolism Diagnosis (PIOPED) and Prospective Investigative Study of Acute Pulmonary Embolism Diagnosis (PISA-PED)) indicate that physicians' estimates of the clinical likelihood of pulmonary embolism, even if based on empirical assessment, do have predictive value.

Three objective scoring systems have been tested prospectively and validated in large-scale clinical trials:

- Wells score
- Geneva score
- Pisa score

The three scoring systems perform reasonably well in objectively assessing the clinical probability of pulmonary embolism in outpatients or emergency room patients. The Pisa score seems to perform better than other scoring systems in hospitalised patients. It appears that fully standardised scoring systems, such as the Wells and Geneva scores, with no implicit evaluation of symptoms (*e.g.* dyspnoea and chest pain) or simple instrumental findings (*e.g.* ECG and chest radiograph), did not perform better than subjective clinical judgment of experienced physicians in the PIOPED and the PISA-PED studies. Conversely, interpretation of ECG and chest radiographs in these patients, as in the Pisa score, necessitates a certain level of clinical experience and is hard to standardise. The three scoring systems are reported in table 1.

Nevertheless, several prospective studies have shown that, whatever scoring method is used, pre-test clinical probability categorises patients into subgroups with different prevalences of pulmonary embolism, and that the positive and negative predictive value (NPV) of various objective tests is strongly conditioned by the independently assessed pre-test clinical probability. Accordingly, recent international guidelines recommend that the clinical probability of the disease should be

assessed in each patient with suspected pulmonary embolism before any further objective testing occurs. Future research is needed to develop standardised models, of varying degrees of complexity, which may find applications in different clinical settings to predict the probability of pulmonary embolisms.

D-dimer

Plasma D-dimer levels are elevated in the presence of simultaneous activation of coagulation and fibrinolysis. Consequently, a normal D-dimer level has a high NPV for pulmonary embolism or deep vein thrombosis (DVT). However, endogenous fibrin production may be increased in a wide variety of conditions including, cancer, inflammation, infection, pregnancy and chronic illnesses. Elevated plasma D-dimer levels have, for this reason, a low positive predictive value (PPV) for pulmonary embolism and DVT.

The value of D-dimer measurement in the diagnostic work-up of each patient must be considered according to the determined clinical probability of pulmonary embolism and the sensitivity of the particular method of D-dimer measurement employed. A negative D-dimer test result, measured by any method, in combination with a low probability clinical assessment, excludes pulmonary embolism with accuracy. An intermediate clinical probability also would exclude pulmonary emlbolism with reasonable certainty if D-dimer was measured by a high-sensitivity ELISA. It has been shown that the 3-month risk of pulmonary emlbolism or DVT in untreated patients with a negative D-dimer and a low or intermediate clinical probability is <1%. Conversely, if clinical assessment results in a high probability of pulmonary embolism, a concomitant negative D-dimer test does not exclude pulmonary embolism.

The number of patients with suspected pulmonary embolism in whom D-dimer must be measured to exclude one pulmonary embolism episode ranges between three in the emergency department and ⩾10 in hospitalised patients. It then

Table 1. Clinical probability scoring systems

Wells score		Geneva score		Pisa score	
Signs and symptoms of DVT	3.0	Recent surgery	2	High	One or more of three symptoms (sudden onset of dyspnoea, chest pain and fainting), not explained, and one or more of three chest X-ray findings (amputation of hilar artery, focal oligaemia and pleural-based consolidation)
Heart rate >100 beats·min⁻¹	1.5	Previous PE or DVT	2	Intermediate	One or more of the above symptoms, alone or with ECG findings of acute right ventricular overload
Immobilisation of surgery	1.5	Older age	2	Low	None of the above symptoms is present or an alternative diagnosis that may account for their presence is identified
Previous DVT or PE	1.5	Hypocapnia	2		
Haemoptysis	1.5	Hypoxaemia	2		
Malignancy	1.5	Tachycardia	2		
PE more likely than an alternative diagnosis	3.0	Plate-like atelectasis	2		
		Hemidiaphragm elevation	2		
Low	<2	Low	≤4		
Intermediate	2–6	Intermediate	5–8		
High	>6	High	≥9		
PE: pulmonary embolism.					

appears recommendable to consider D-dimer measurement in the diagnostic work-up of pulmonary embolism only in outpatients or in patients in the emergency department with low or intermediate levels of clinical probability.

The sensitivity of D-dimer testing for pulmonary embolism increases with the extent of pulmonary embolism. D-dimer concentrations are the highest in patients with pulmonary embolism involving the pulmonary trunk and lobar arteries and with perfusion scan defects involving >50% of the pulmonary circulation.

In recent years, the contribution of CT angiography (CTA) to the diagnosis of pulmonary embolism has greatly increased as a consequence of the extraordinary advancement in CTA technology. Multidetector CTA has become the most widely used technique for the diagnosis or exclusion of pulmonary embolism, and has almost replaced lung scanning as a screening test and conventional pulmonary angiography as the reference standard for the diagnosis of acute pulmonary embolism. CTA, however, does not escape the simple rule that the combined use of the estimated clinical probability and the results of one noninvasive test substantially increases the accuracy of confirming or ruling out a disease, as compared with either assessment alone. As shown by the PIOPED II trial, the predictive value of CTA is high with a concordant clinical assessment, but additional testing is necessary when clinical probability is inconsistent with the imaging results. Several recent papers have shown a positive yield rate of CTA of <10% in patients who are clinically suspected of pulmonary embolism. This may indicate that the wide availability of CTA has led to an overuse of the technique as a screening procedure for pulmonary embolism in the emergency department. It has been suggested that a substantial number of CTAs could be avoided by adhering to the information derived from clinical evaluation and D-dimer testing.

Perfusion (Q') lung scanning was introduced 40 years ago as the first chest imaging method for the diagnosis of pulmonary embolism. A normal Q' scan excludes pulmonary embolism (high sensitivity and high NPV), whatever the pre-test clinical probability. However, Q' scanning was thought to be poorly specific (low PPV) for pulmonary embolism because all common pulmonary diseases (infections, neoplasms and COPD) can produce decreased blood flow to the affected regions.

Ventilation (V') scanning was added to Q' scanning to increase the specificity of scintigraphy. This diagnostic approach is based on the flawed expectation that regions of the lung excluded from perfusion by emboli maintain normal ventilation, thus giving rise to V'/Q' mismatch. This criterion for diagnosing pulmonary embolism is at variance with the notion that ventilation is shifted away from embolised lung regions. The concept that deadspace ventilation is not significantly increased in the course of pulmonary embolism was widely held in respiratory pathophysiology before the V'/Q' scanning approach was developed, as asserted by Comroe (1966), who foresaw that 'decrease in wasted ventilation [ventilation to unperfused or poorly perfused lung] helps the patient but hinders the physician in diagnosis'. This is in keeping with the results of the PIOPED trial, in which it was shown that a high-probability V'/Q' scan (Q' defects without matching V' abnormalities) lacks sensitivity in diagnosing pulmonary embolism, as it fails to identify 59% of pulmonary embolism patients (sensitivity 41%, specificity 97%). The combination of clinical probability and V'/Q' scan results either confirms or excludes pulmonary embolism in <30% of patients. The diagnostic value of the Q' scan (without V' imaging) was reappraised in the PISA-PED study, in which Q' scans were read either as compatible with pulmonary embolism when featuring wedge-shaped (segmental) perfusion defects or not compatible with pulmonary embolism when featuring defects other than wedge-shaped or normal perfusion. When compared with the original PIOPED protocol, the PISA-PED approach has several advantages:

1) Q' scanning either confirms or excludes the clinical suspicion of pulmonary embolism (thus virtually eliminating nondiagnostic examinations)

2) the sensitivity of lung scintigraphy is greatly increased (86% *versus* 41%) but with minor reduction of specificity (from 97% to 93%)

3) the combination of clinical probability and Q' scanning results confirms or excludes pulmonary embolism in ~80% of patients.

More recently, the diagnostic performance of Q' scanning for pulmonary embolism was confirmed by examining 889 scans from the PIOPED II. PIOPED II data were used to test the hypothesis that reading Q' scans without V' scans, and categorising the Q' scan as 'pulmonary embolism present', 'pulmonary embolism absent' or 'nondiagnostic' can result in clinically useful sensitivity and specificity in a high proportion of patients. The study has confirmed that Q' scan and CTA have comparable positive and NPVs, with no nondiagnostic readings for the Q' scan (table 2). Accordingly, in 2012, the Society of Nuclear Medicine revised the practice guidelines for lung scintigraphy, reporting that 'The modified PIOPED II and PISAPED criteria using information from chest radiograph and perfusion scans have been shown to perform equivalently to those including ventilation scintigraphy, with fewer nondiagnostic studies'.

Diagnostic strategies in different clinical contexts and special conditions

Most clinicians and diagnostic radiologists feel more comfortable with an anatomical demonstration of whether a clot is present than assessing the probability of pulmonary embolism by looking at V'/Q' mismatches (PIOPED) or evaluating the shape of a perfusion defect (PISA-PED). Furthermore, contrary to scintigraphy, in most hospitals, CTA is available 24 h a day, 7 days a week. However, CTA cannot be performed in the whole population of patients suspected of pulmonary embolism. As shown in the PIOPED II trial, 50% of the recruited patients did not undergo CTA because of documented contraindications, such as renal failure, abnormal creatinine levels, allergy to the

contrast agent, possible pregnancy, critical illness, requirement of ventilator support or recent myocardial infarction. In all these conditions, Q' scanning could be the preferred alternative approach to the diagnosis of pulmonary embolism. This approach is particularly important for reproductive-age female patients in whom the breast irradiation dose from CTA can be minimised by using the Q' scan as the first imaging test. It has been recently shown that contrast medium-induced nephropathy is at least as common as a diagnosis of pulmonary embolism after CTA.

Under circumstances in which clinical probability and imaging test (CTA or scintigraphy) results are discordant and further testing, such as lower limb compression ultrasonography, is required to either confirm or exclude the diagnosis. Another practical approach could be to image the pulmonary circulation with CTA if Q' scan was the first imaging test used or *vice versa*.

Conclusions

The choice of a diagnostic strategy for pulmonary embolism depends on the pre-test clinical probability of pulmonary embolism, the condition of the patient, the availability of the necessary test, the risks of testing, the risk of an inaccurate positive or negative diagnosis, and the cost. Clinical evaluation makes it possible to classify patients into probability categories corresponding to an increasing prevalence of pulmonary embolism, whether assessed by implicit clinical judgment or by a validated prediction rule. Structured models to assess clinical probability so far developed have different performances in patients of the emergency department and those who are hospitalised. Exclusion of pulmonary embolism by clinical probability assessment and D-dimer spares the cost and radiation of an imaging evaluation. CTA has become the method of choice for imaging the pulmonary vasculature when pulmonary embolism is suspected in routine clinical practice. Scintigraphy can be considered the preferred alternative chest imaging technique for patients with

Table 2. Predictive value of multidetector CTA and Q' scanning from retrospective evaluation of PIOPED II data

Imaging test	PPV	NPV	Nondiagnostic
Q' scan	85	96	0
CTA	86	95	6
Data are presented as %.			

contraindication to CTA. If scintigraphy is used, eliminating the V' scan can reduce cost and radiation load with gain in diagnostic yield.

Further reading

- Comroe JH Jr (1966). The main function of the pulmonary circulation. *Circulation*; 33: 146–158.
- Eisner MD (2003). Before diagnostic testing for pulmonary embolism: estimating the prior probability of disease. *Am J Med*; 114: 232–234.
- Mamlouk MD, *et al.* (2010). Pulmonary embolism at CT angiography: implications for appropriateness, cost, and radiation exposure in 2003 patients. *Radiology*; 256: 625–632.
- Miniati M, *et al.* (1996). Value of perfusion lung scan in the diagnosis of pulmonary embolism: results of the Prospective Investigative Study of Acute Pulmonary Embolism Diagnosis (PISA-PED). *Am J Respir Crit Care Med*; 154: 1387–1393.
- Miniati M, *et al.* (2012). Clinical presentation of acute pulmonary embolism: survey of 800 cases. *PLoS One*; 7: e30891.
- Mitchell AM, *et al.* (2012). Prospective study of the incidence of contrast-induced nephropathy among patients evaluated for pulmonary embolism by contrast-enhanced computed tomography. *Acad Emerg Med*; 19: 618–625.
- Parker AJ, *et al.* (2012). SNM practice guideline for lung scintigraphy 4.0. *J Nucl Med Technol*; 40: 57–65.
- PIOPED Investigators. (1990). Value of the ventilation/perfusion scan in acute pulmonary embolism: results of the Prospective Investigation of Pulmonary Embolism Diagnosis (PIOPED). *JAMA*; 263: 2753–2759.
- Pistolesi M (2010). Pulmonary CT angiography in patients suspected of having pulmonary embolism: case finding or screening procedure? *Radiology*; 256: 334–337.
- Remy-Jardin M, *et al.* (2007). Management of suspected acute pulmonary embolism in the era of CT angiography. A statement from the Fleischner Society. *Radiology*; 245: 315–329.
- Sostman HD, *et al.* (2008). Sensitivity and specificity of perfusion scintigraphy for acute pulmonary embolism in PIOPED II. *J Nucl Med*; 49: 1741–1748.
- Stein PD, *et al.* (2011). Controversies in diagnosis of pulmonary embolism. *Clin Appl Thromb Hemost*; 17: 140–149.
- Stein PD, *et al.* (2006). Multidetector computed tomography for acute pulmonary embolism. *N Engl J Med*; 354: 2317–2327.
- Tsai J, *et al.* (2012). Correlates of in-hospital deaths among hospitalizations with pulmonary embolism: findings from the 2001–2008 National Hospital Discharge Survey. *PLoS One*; 7: e34048.

Pulmonary vasculitis

Georgios Margaritopoulos and Athol U. Wells

The principles of diagnosis and management are broadly similar across the individual pulmonary vasculitides, subdivided into primary systemic and secondary disorders (table 1). The main challenges for the clinician are:

- to recognise that vasculitis is a possible diagnosis
- to make the diagnosis in nonclassical disease
- to select a level of treatment appropriate to disease severity

Granulomatosis with polyangiitis (GPA) (the entity formerly known as Wegener's granulomatosis) and Churg–Strauss syndrome (CSS) are the most frequent exemplars of life-threatening anti-neutrophil cytoplasmic antibody vasculitides (AAVs).

Epidemiology and pathogenesis

GPA is the third most prevalent systemic vasculitis (after giant cell arteritis and

vasculitides in rheumatoid arthritis), with an annual incidence of 3–11 per million, largely affecting adults aged 30–50 years. CSS has an annual incidence of ~3 per million and mainly affects adults aged 30–50 years. In neither disorder is there a strong sex predilection.

Anti-neutrophil cytoplasmic antibodies (ANCAs) are often present in systemic vasculitides involving the small and medium-sized vessels, including CSS, GPA and microscopic polyangiitis (MPA). ANCAs are subcategorised as cytoplasmic, perinuclear or atypical, and are directed primarily against proteinase-3 in GPA (cytoplasmic) and against myeloperoxidase in CSS (perinuclear), although all ANCA patterns have been reported in both disorders. In vitro and animal data suggest that ANCAs interact with primed neutrophils, leading to endothelial damage and further neutrophil recruitment. Both diseases are generally considered to be triggered by foreign agents, including drugs and infections, with the most suggestive data relating to chronic nasal carriage of *Staphylococcus aureus* in GPA.

Clinical presentation

Vasculitis should be suspected in diffuse alveolar haemorrhage. Haemoptysis is often absent or scant. Diffuse alveolar haemorrhage should be suspected when unexplained infiltrates on chest imaging are associated with a fall in haemoglobin over a day or two or, in chronic low-grade haemorrhage, with an iron-deficiency anaemia. Bronchoalveolar lavage is usually diagnostic of haemorrhage. Vasculitis should also be suspected: 1) in patients

Key points

- Haemoptysis is often scant or absent in diffuse alveolar haemorrhage.

- Vasculitis must often be treated empirically, in the absence of full diagnostic clinical criteria or a histological diagnosis.

- Initial treatment should be definitive, even when the diagnosis is tentative.

- Chronic infection and malignancy are the most frequent differential diagnosis.

Table 1. *Classification of pulmonary vasculitis*

Vasculitis	Frequency of lung involvement
Primary[#]	
Large vessel	
Giant-cell arteritis	Rare
Takayasu's arteritis	Frequent
Medium-sized vessel	
Polyarteritis nodosa	Rare
Kawasaki disease	No
Small vessel[¶]	
Granulomatosis with polyangiitis (Wegener's)	Frequent
Churg–Strauss syndrome	Frequent
Microscopic polyangiitis	Frequent
Henoch–Schönlein purpura	No
Essential cryoglobulinaemia	No
Secondary	
Rheumatological	
Pulmonary–renal (*e.g.* Goodpasture's syndrome)	
Relapsing polychronditis	
Behçet's syndrome	
Chronic infection	
Lymphoma	
Drugs	

[#]: Chapel Hill international consensus nomenclature; [¶]: with variable medium-sized vessel involvement.

presenting with breathlessness on exertion and an unexplained isolated or disproportionate reduction in T_{LCO}); 2) in patients with features of an underlying systemic vasculitis, such as GPA, CSS or a pulmonary–renal syndrome (of which Goodpasture's disease is the best-known example). Investigations that tend to be useful in suspected vasculitis are shown in table 2.

Churg–Strauss syndrome

The American College of Rheumatology (ACR) definition of CSS requires the satisfaction of at least four of six criteria (table 3). There is typically a prodrome of rhinitis with nasal polyps and the eventual development of late-onset asthma, followed by eosinophilia in tissue or peripheral blood and, ultimately, systemic vasculitis. Other frequent sites of involvement include the nervous system (especially mononeuritis multiplex) in 75%, skin (60%), heart (50%), joints and, less frequently, the kidneys and gastrointestinal tract. The classical triad at lung biopsy is necrotising angiitis, granulomata and tissue eosinophilia. Pulmonary infiltrates on chest imaging are more common than pulmonary nodules (which very seldom cavitate). Pleural disease is present in 50%. The diagnostic role of ANCA continues to be debated. ANCAs, usually perinuclear ANCAs (p-ANCAs), are present in up to two-thirds of patients, but also occur in many other nonvasculitic autoimmune and infectious conditions.

Table 2. *Useful investigations for suspected pulmonary vasculitis*

Imaging
Chest radiography
HRCT
Lung function tests
Pulmonary function tests
Arterial gases
Renal function
Urine dipstick testing and microscopy for proteinuria, haematuria and cellular casts
Estimation of renal function
Consider renal biopsy (if evidence of nephritis)
Immunology
ANCAs
Anti-GBM antibodies
Immune complexes
Rheumatoid factor
ANAs
Antiphospholipid antibodies
Bronchoalveolar lavage
Iron-laden macrophages
Biopsy
Renal
Skin
Lung (surgical)
GBM: glomerular basement membrane; ANA: anti-nuclear antibody.

Table 3. *ACR diagnostic criteria for CSS (four out of six required)*

Presence of asthma
Peripheral blood eosinophilia (>10%)
Evidence of a neuropathy in a vasculitic pattern (*e.g.* mononeuritis multiplex)
Transient pulmonary infiltrates
A history of sinus disease
Evidence of extravascular eosinophilia on biopsy

Thus, neither the presence nor the absence of p-ANCAs is diagnostically definitive and is no more than a useful ancillary finding increasing or decreasing the diagnostic likelihood.

Granulomatosis with polyangiitis

The classic historical GPA triad consisted of renal, lower respiratory tract and upper respiratory tract involvement. Most often, chronic rhinitis, sinusitis or mastoiditis progresses to generalised disease over months to years, with lower respiratory tract involvement in 65–85%, including diffuse alveolar haemorrhage, which may be life-threatening and tends to occur before specific pulmonary manifestations of GPA are apparent. Fever and weight loss are frequent. There is a wide range of extrapulmonary organ involvement. Lung involvement is asymptomatic in a third of cases. The cardinal histological features are granulomatous inflammation and necrotising vasculitis, affecting small to medium-sized vessels. Chest imaging may show one or more nodules that can cavitate, localised or diffuse infiltrates (which may represent alveolar haemorrhage), or evidence of large and small airway disease. As in CSS, the diagnosis should never be dependent upon ANCA positivity: cytoplasmic ANCAs (c-ANCAs) are not present in all cases (especially when GPA is confined to the lungs), and are also found in other vasculitides, chronic bacterial infections and cryoglobulinaemia.

Among vasculitides, MPA, a necrotising vasculitis affecting small to medium-sized vessels, is the main clinical mimic of GPA. Although pulmonary involvement is less frequent than in GPA, this disorder also often presents with diffuse alveolar haemorrhage, which can have a poor prognosis. Necrotising glomerulonephritis, mononeuritis multiplex and skin lesions are variably present. The cardinal histological distinction is the absence of granulomas, which are characteristically present in GPA.

Diagnosis of vasculitis

A confident diagnosis requires histological confirmation or satisfaction of the requisite number of clinical criteria. However, many patients with vasculitis have features overlapping between diagnostic entities with transient or non-fulfilment of diagnostic criteria. Thus, a versatile diagnostic approach is required. When vasculitis is suspected but full clinical criteria are not satisfied, a histological diagnosis should made, if possible. However, a negative biopsy does not exclude vasculitis, which may be patchy or give rise to nonspecific inflammatory change (as in upper airway biopsies in GPA patients).

Thus, the diagnosis of a vasculitic syndrome is sometimes necessarily empirical, with chronic infection and malignancy the most frequent differential diagnoses. In such cases, initial treatment and monitoring should be as for the vasculitic syndrome most closely corresponding to the clinical presentation in that patient. Initial treatment should be definitive as a clear response provides important support for the diagnosis, whereas a tentative therapeutic approach often prolongs diagnostic uncertainty.

Prognosis

The poor historical outcome of the vasculitic syndromes has been transformed by more aggressive therapy but also by the increasing detection of milder disease, including patients with limited involvement. In localised pulmonary GPA and CSS alike, the outcome is much better outcome than with multiorgan involvement. In CSS, the prognosis worsens strikingly with two or more extrapulmonary complications (5-year survival 54%). Mortality is largely ascribable to sepsis (as a complication of treatment) or disease progression. Death from progressive disease is most commonly due to renal failure or lung involvement in GPA, and to renal failure, cerebrovascular involvement and gastrointestinal disease in CSS (with 10% of deaths accounted for by lung disease).

Treatment

Remission induction therapy of AAVs should be dictated by disease extent and severity (table 4).

In limited disease there are limited data supporting the use of oral steroids as monotherapy and/or a single cytotoxic agent such as methotrexate, azathioprine and mycophenolate mofetil.

In early generalised disease, oral cyclophosphamide and steroids are the cornerstones of treatment. Methotrexate ($0.3\ mg \cdot kg^{-1} \cdot week^{-1}$) is as effective as daily oral cyclophosphamide in the induction of remission, although relapse is more likely with cessation of treatment at 12 months.

In generalised active disease, oral cyclophosphamide and intravenous methylprednisolone have generally been used. However, oral cyclophosphamide ($2.0\ mg \cdot kg^{-1} \cdot day^{-1}$) and intravenous cyclophosphamide ($600\ mg \cdot m^{-2}$, at three to four weekly intervals, depending on disease severity) are equally successful in inducing remission. Intravenous therapy is associated with a slightly higher relapse rate but is much less toxic in the short term and is

Table 4. EUVAS classification clinical features

Limited isolated upper airway disease
Early generalised end-organ involvement that lacks a clear or immediate threat to organ function
Generalised active end-organ involvement with clinically significant impairment of organ function
Severe immediate threat of organ failure or death
Refractory disease that has failed to respond to conventional therapies
Remission (maintenance): no evidence of ongoing vasculitic activity
EUVAS: European Vasculitis Study Group.

much less likely to provoke haemorrhagic cystitis and subsequent malignancy, based on long-term systemic lupus erythematosus data. Importantly, in multicentre controlled trials, rituximab given weekly for 4 weeks was found to be as efficacious as oral cyclophosphamide in inducing remission (including a patient with alveolar haemorrhage) and has a particular role in patients with relapsing disease that is poorly controlled by traditional immuno-suppressive therapy.

In severe disease with diffuse alveolar haemorrhage or renal failure, plasma exchange should be considered early together with high doses of intravenous methylprednisolone and oral cyclophosphamide. The early use of rituximab is strongly recommended in this difficult clinical scenario and if disease is overtly life-threatening at presentation, initial combination therapy using all three agents should be considered, especially when plasma exchange is not readily available.

In refractory disease, intravenous immunoglobulin and anti-thymocyte globulin have been variably efficacious.

Following initial treatment, less intense long-term therapy is almost invariably required. Standard maintenance treatment has consisted of azathioprine ($2.0 \, mg \cdot kg^{-1} \cdot day^{-1}$), usually with in combination with low-dose corticosteroid therapy. Methotrexate (25 mg per week) is as efficacious as azathioprine. However, relapse is more prevalent with the use of mycophenolate mofetil and this agent should, therefore, be considered only in patients intolerant of azathioprine and methotrexate. Maintenance therapy should be continued for a $\geqslant 18$ months but in many cases, prolonged maintenance therapy is required, sometimes for decade or longer.

Prophylactic co-trimoxazole (trimethoprim 160 mg/sulphamethoxazole 800 mg three times a week) is often used with prolonged intense immunosuppression, to reduce the risk of opportunistic *Pneumocystis jiroveci* infection. In GPA, co-trimoxazole therapy has been efficacious in localised respiratory tract disease and may have an ancillary role in maintaining remission.

Further reading

- Conron M, et al. (2000). Churg–Strauss syndrome. *Thorax*; 55: 870–877.
- Falk RJ, et al. (2011). Granulomatosis with polyangiitis (Wegener's): an alternative name for Wegener's granulomatosis. *Arthritis Rheum*; 63: 863–864.
- Frankel SK, et al. (2012). The pulmonary vasculitides. *Am J Respir Crit Care Med*; 186: 216–224.
- Guillevin L, et al. (1996). Prognostic factors in polyarteritis nodosa and Churg–Strauss syndrome. A prospective study in 342 patients. *Medicine*; 75: 17–28.
- Jayne D, et al. (2003). A randomized trial of maintenance therapy for vasculitis associated with antineutrophil cytoplas-mic autoantibodies. *New Engl J Med*; 349: 36–44.
- Jennette JC, et al. (1994). Nomenclature of systemic vasculitides. Proposal of an International consensus conference. *Arthritis and Rheumatism*; 37: 187–192.
- Lanham JG, et al. (1984). Systemic vasculitis with asthma and eosinophilia: the clinical approach to the Churg–Strauss syndrome. *Medicine (Baltimore)*; 63: 65–81.
- Lhote F, et al. (1998). Polyarteritis nodosa, microscopic polyangiitis and Churg–Strauss syndrome. *Semin Respir Crit Care Med*; 19: 27–46.
- Pagnoux C, et al. (2008). Azathioprine or methotrexate maintenance for ANCA-associated vasculitis. *N Engl J Med*; 359: 2790–2803.
- Specks U. Pulmonary vasculitis. In: Schwarz MI, et al., eds. Interstitial Lung Disease. Hamilton, B.C. Dekker, 1998; pp. 507–534.
- Stone JH, et al. (2010). Rituximab *versus* cyclophosphamide for ANCA-associated vasculitis. *N Engl J Med*; 363: 221–232.

Pulmonary hypertension

Marc Humbert and Gérald Simonneau

Classification

Pulmonary hypertension is defined as an increase in mean pulmonary arterial pressure (mP_{pa}) $\geqslant$25 mmHg at rest as assessed by right heart catheterisation. According to values of pulmonary wedge pressure (P_{pw}), pulmonary hypertension can be pre-capillary (P_{pw} $\leqslant$15 mmHg) or post-capillary (P_{pw} >15 mmHg).

Pulmonary hypertension can be classified into five groups according to pathological, pathophysiological and therapeutic characteristics. Despite comparable elevations of mP_{pa} in the different clinical groups, the underlying mechanisms, diagnostic approaches, and prognostic and therapeutic implications are completely different.

The clinical classification of pulmonary hypertension is shown in table 1. Group 1 relates to pulmonary arterial hypertension (PAH), corresponding to idiopathic, heritable and associated PAH. The term familial PAH has been replaced by heritable PAH because specific gene mutations have been identified in sporadic cases with no family history, mainly because of the low penetrance of the causal mutations. Heritable forms of PAH include clinically sporadic idiopathic PAH with germline mutations (mainly in the bone morphogenetic protein receptor II (*BMPR2*) gene as well as the activin receptor-like kinase type-1 (*ALK1*) or endoglin genes) and clinical familial cases with or without identified mutation. Associated PAH includes conditions that can have a similar clinical presentation to that seen in idiopathic PAH with comparable histological findings. Associated PAH accounts for approximately half of the patients followed at specialised centres. Pulmonary veno-occlusive disease (PVOD) and pulmonary capillary haemangiomatosis remain difficult disorders to classify since they share some characteristics with PAH but also demonstrate a number of differences.

> **Key points**
>
> - Pulmonary hypertension is defined as an increase in mP_{pa} $\geqslant$25 mmHg at rest as assessed by right heart catheterisation.
>
> - PAH is a rare condition characterised by chronic pre-capillary pulmonary hypertension leading to right heart failure and death.
>
> - PAH can be sporadic (idiopathic PAH), heritable, induced by drugs or toxins, or associated with other conditions such as connective tissue diseases.
>
> - Doppler echocardiography is the investigation of choice for noninvasive screening but measurement of haemodynamic parameters during right heart catheterisation is mandatory to confirm pre-capillary pulmonary hypertension (mP_{pa} $\geqslant$25 mmHg and P_{pw} $\leqslant$15 mmHg).
>
> - Recent advances in the management of PAH include prostaglandins, ERA and PDE5 I.
>
> - Lung transplantation is an option for severe patients deteriorating despite medical treatment.

Table 1. *Updated clinical classification of pulmonary hypertension (PH)*

1 PAH
1.1 Idiopathic PAH
1.2 Heritable
1.2.1 BMPR2
1.2.2 ALK1, endoglin (with or without hereditary haemorrhagic telangiectasia)
1.2.3 Unknown
1.3 Drug and toxin induced
1.4 APAH
1.4.1 Connective tissue diseases
1.4.2 HIV infection
1.4.3 Portal hypertension
1.4.4 Congenital heart disease
1.4.5 Schistosomiasis
1.4.6 Chronic haemolytic anaemia
1.5 Persistent PH of the newborn
1' PVOD and/or pulmonary capillary haemangiomatosis
2 PH due to left heart disease
2.1 Systolic dysfunction
2.2 Diastolic dysfunction
2.3 Valvular disease
3 PH due to lung diseases and/or hypoxia
3.1 COPD
3.2 Interstitial lung disease
3.3 Other pulmonary diseases with mixed restrictive and obstructive pattern
3.4 Sleep-disordered breathing
3.5 Alveolar hypoventilation disorders
3.6 Chronic exposure to high altitude
3.7 Developmental abnormalities
4 CTEPH
5 PH with unclear and/or multifactorial mechanisms
5.1 Haematological disorders: myeloproliferative disorders, splenectomy.
5.2 Systemic disorders, sarcoidosis, pulmonary Langerhans' cell histiocytosis, lymphangioleiomyomatosis, neurofibromatosis, vasculitis
5.3 Metabolic disorders: glycogen storage disease, Gaucher disease, thyroid disorders
5.4 Others: tumoural obstruction, fibrosing mediastinitis, chronic renal failure on dialysis
APAH: associated PAH. Reproduced from Simonneau *et al.* (2009) with permission from the publisher.

Given the current evidence, these conditions have been individualised as a distinct category but not completely separated from PAH, and have been designated as clinical group 1'. Chronic thromboembolic pulmonary hypertension (CTEPH) is an important subcategory of pulmonary hypertension, which may be cured by surgical pulmonary endarterectomy. It was decided to maintain only a single category of CTEPH without attempting to distinguish between proximal and distal forms. The most frequent causes of pulmonary hypertension are those complicating left heart diseases (group 2) and pulmonary diseases (group 3).

All forms of pulmonary hypertension have some common pathological features regardless of their aetiology:

- medial hypertrophy of muscular and elastic arteries
- dilation and intimal atheromas of elastic pulmonary arteries
- right ventricular hypertrophy

In addition to the aforementioned pathological changes common to all forms of pulmonary hypertension, PAH is characterised by constrictive and complex arterial lesions involving to varying degrees the pre- and intra-acinar pulmonary arteries. The plexiform lesion is a focal proliferation of endothelial channels lined by myofibroblasts, smooth muscle cells and connective tissue matrix. The lesion is located within pre- and intra-acinar pulmonary arteries, and is associated with expansion and partial destruction of the arterial wall with extension of the plexiform lesion into the perivascular connective tissue. The plexiform lesion is often located at an arterial branching point (fig. 1).

Epidemiology and survival

PAH is a rare condition with a prevalence ranging 15–50 per million in western Europe. In the early 2000s, the prevalence of idiopathic PAH was about 6 per million in the French Registry and its incidence was 2 per million per year. Median survival of idiopathic PAH was 2.8 years in the National Institutes of Health Registry before the recent development of PAH-specific therapies. Despite improvements in recent years, idiopathic, familial and anorexigen-associated PAH remains progressive, fatal diseases in the modern management era. Mortality is most closely associated with male sex, right ventricular haemodynamic function and exercise limitation.

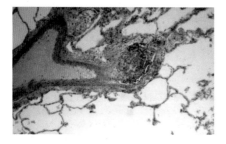

Figure 1. A typical plexiform lesion in a patient with idiopathic PAH. The lesion is located at an arterial branching point.

Diagnosis

The diagnostic process starts with the identification of the more common clinical groups of pulmonary hypertension (group 2: left heart diseases; group 3: pulmonary diseases), distinguishing group 4 (CTEPH) and, finally, making the diagnosis and recognising the different types of group 1 (PAH) and the rarer conditions of group 5.

PAH should be considered in the differential diagnosis of exertional dyspnoea, syncope, angina and/or progressive limitation of exercise capacity, particularly in patients without apparent risk factors, symptoms or signs of common cardiovascular and respiratory disorders. Special awareness should be directed towards patients with associated conditions and/or risk factors for development of PAH, such as family history, connective tissue diseases, congenital heart diseases, HIV infection, portal hypertension, haemolytic anaemia, or a history of drug and toxin intake known to induce PAH. In everyday clinical practice, such awareness may be low. More often, pulmonary hypertension is found unexpectedly on transthoracic echocardiography requested for another indication.

If noninvasive assessment is compatible with pulmonary hypertension, clinical history, symptoms, signs, ECG, chest radiograph, transthoracic echocardiogram, pulmonary function tests (including nocturnal oximetry if required) and HRCT of the chest are requested to identify the presence of group 2 (left heart diseases) or group 3 (pulmonary diseases). If these are not found or if pulmonary hypertension seems 'out of proportion' to their severity, less common causes of pulmonary hypertension should be sought. Ventilation/perfusion lung scanning should be considered. If the ventilation/perfusion scan shows multiple segmental perfusion defects, a diagnosis of group 4 (CTEPH) should be suspected. The final diagnosis of CTEPH (and the assessment of suitability for pulmonary endarterectomy) will require helical CT of the chest, right heart catheterisation and selective pulmonary angiography. HRCT of the chest may also

Table 2. *Functional assessment of pulmonary hypertension (PH) modified after the NYHA classification*

Functional class	Description
I	Patients with PH but without resulting limitation of physical activity Ordinary physical activity does not cause undue dyspnoea or fatigue, chest pain or near syncope
II	Patients with PH resulting in slight limitation of physical activity They are comfortable at rest Ordinary physical activity causes undue dyspnoea or fatigue, chest pain or near syncope
III	Patients with PH resulting in marked limitation of physical activity They are comfortable at rest Less than ordinary activity causes undue dyspnoea or fatigue, chest pain or near syncope
IV	Patients with PH with inability to carry out any physical activity without symptoms These patients manifest signs of right heart failure Dyspnoea and/or fatigue may even be present at rest Discomfort is increased by any physical activity

show signs suggestive of group 1' (PVOD). If the ventilation/perfusion scan is normal or shows only subsegmental 'patchy' perfusion defects, a tentative diagnosis of group 1 (PAH) or the rarer conditions of group 5 is made. Performing a right heart catheterisation will be necessary to confirm the diagnosis and assess haemodynamic severity. Additional specific diagnostic tests, including haematology, biochemistry, immunology, serology and ultrasonography, will allow the final diagnosis to be refined. 6-min walk distance is an important marker of exercise limitation with prognostic value in PAH. New York Heart Association (NYHA) functional class is a simple clinical parameter of major prognostic value (table 2).

Treatment

A treatment algorithm for PAH patients is shown in figure 2. The grades of recommendation and levels of evidence for the PAH treatments are derived from European guidelines published jointly by the European Respiratory Society and the European Society of Cardiology in 2009. The treatment algorithm does not apply to patients in other clinical groups and, in particular, not to patients with pulmonary hypertension associated with group 2 (left

heart disease) or with group 3 (pulmonary diseases). In addition, the different treatments have been evaluated by randomised control trials mainly in idiopathic PAH, heritable PAH, PAH due to anorexigen drugs and in PAH associated with connective tissue diseases or with congenital heart diseases (surgically corrected or not). The grades of recommendation and levels of evidence for the other PAH subgroups are lower.

The suggested initial approach, after the diagnosis of PAH, is the adoption of general measures, the initiation of supportive therapy and referral to an expert centre. Acute vasoreactivity testing with inhaled nitric oxide or intravenous prostacyclin or adenosine should be performed in all patients with group 1 (PAH), although patients with idiopathic PAH and PAH associated with anorexigen use are the most likely to exhibit an acute positive response and to profit from long-term calcium channel blocker therapy. Vasoreactive patients should be treated with optimally tolerated doses of calcium channel blockers; adequate response should be confirmed after 3–4 months of treatment. Nonresponders to acute vasoreactivity testing who are in NYHA functional class II

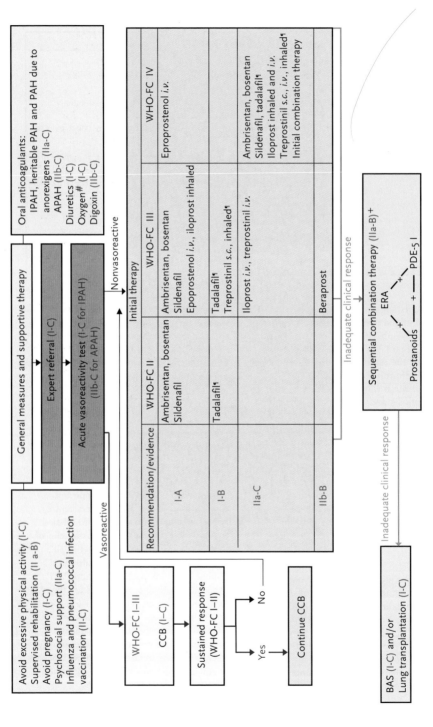

Figure 2. Evidence-based treatment algorithm for PAH patients (for group 1 patients only). Level of recommendation and evidence have been evaluated in the European Society of Cardiology/European Respiratory Society European Guidelines and a shown in red. IPAH: idiopathic pulmonary arterial hypertension; APAH: associated pulmonary arterial hypertension; WHO-FC: World Health Organization functional class; CCB: calcium channel blockers; i.v.: intravenous; s.c.: subcutaneous; BAS: balloon

should be treated with an endothelin receptor antagonist (ERA) or a phosphodiesterase-5 inhibitor (PDE5 I). Nonresponders to acute vasoreactivity testing or acute responders who do not respond to chronic calcium channel blocker therapy should be considered candidates for treatment with either an ERA, a PDE5 I or a prostanoid. As head-to-head comparisons between different compounds are not available, no evidence-based first-line treatment can be proposed. In this case, the choice of drug is dependent on a variety of factors, including the approval status, the route of administration, the side-effect profile, patients' preferences and physicians' experience. Some experts still use first-line *i.v.* epoprostenol in NYHA functional class III patients, because of its survival benefits. Continuous *i.v.* epoprostenol may be considered as first-line therapy for NYHA functional class IV PAH patients because of the survival benefit in this subset.

In case of inadequate clinical response, sequential combination therapy should be considered. Combination therapy can either include an ERA plus a PDE5 I, a prostanoid plus an ERA, a prostanoid plus a PDE5 I or a triple combination therapy. Appropriate protocols for timing and dosing to limit possible side-effects of the combination have still to be defined.

Balloon atrioseptostomy and/or lung transplantation are indicated for PAH with inadequate clinical response despite optimal medical therapy or where medical treatments are unavailable. These procedures should be performed only in experienced centres.

Further reading

- D'Alonzo GE, *et al.* (1991). Survival in patients with primary pulmonary hypertension. *Ann Int Med*; 115: 343–349.
- Galiè N, *et al.* (2009). Guidelines for the diagnosis and treatment of pulmonary hypertension. The task force for the diagnosis and treatment of pulmonary hypertension of the European Society of Cardiology (ESC) and the European Respiratory Society (ERS), endorsed by the International Society of Heart and Lung Transplantation (ISHLT). *Eur Respir J*; 34: 1219–1263.
- Humbert M, *et al.* (2006). Pulmonary arterial hypertension in France: results from a national registry. *Am J Respir Crit Care Med*; 173: 1023–1030.
- Humbert M, *et al.* (2010). Survival in patients with idiopathic, familial, and anorexigen-associated pulmonary arterial hypertension in the modern management era. *Circulation*; 122: 156–163.
- Rich S, *et al.* (1987). Primary pulmonary hypertension: a national prospective study. *Ann Int Med*; 107: 216–223.
- Simonneau G, *et al.* (2009). Updated clinical classification of pulmonary hypertension. *J Am Coll Cardiol*; 54: Suppl. 1, S43–S54.

Pleural effusion

Robert Loddenkemper

<table>
<tr><td>

Key points

- Pleural effusions may present as primary manifestations of many diseases. However, most often, they are observed as secondary manifestations or complications of other diseases.

- Cardiac failure is the main cause of pleural effusions. Of noncardiac causes, parapneumonic effusions are commonest, followed by malignant pleural effusions and pleural effusions due to pulmonary embolism.

- Small pleural effusions can be detected best by ultrasound (or CT).

- Pleural effusion can, in the majority of cases, be diagnosed by case history, clinical presentation, imaging techniques and examination of pleural fluid.

- The most important laboratory parameter of pleural fluid is total protein, distinguishing trans- from exudates.

- Biopsy procedures such as closed-needle biopsy or medical thoracoscopy/pleuroscopy may be necessary to confirm or exclude malignant or tuberculous causes.

- Treatment depends upon the underlying disease.

- Local treatment options include therapeutic thoracentesis, chest-tube drainage, chemical pleurodesis and, rarely, surgical interventions.

</td></tr>
</table>

Pleural effusion is defined as accumulation of fluid in the pleural space that exceeds the physiological amounts of 10–20 mL. Pleural effusion develops either when the formation of pleural fluid is excessive or when fluid resorption is disturbed. Pleural effusions may represent a primary manifestation of many diseases, but most often they are observed as secondary manifestations or complications of other diseases.

Pleural effusion is found in almost 10% of patients who have internal diseases and the main cause in 30–40% of these is cardiac failure. Among the noncardiac effusions, parapneumonic effusions are the most common at 36%, of which ~75% are of bacterial and 25% of viral origin. Malignant pleural effusions follow in 18% of cases, half of which are caused by lung or breast cancer. Pleural effusion is secondary to pulmonary embolism in 14% of cases, to liver cirrhosis in 5% and to gastrointestinal diseases, mainly pancreatitis, in 2% of cases. Many other possible causes, such as collagen vascular diseases like rheumatoid arthritis and systemic lupus erythematosus as well as several drugs (www.pneumotox. com), play an important role in differential diagnosis. Often, pleural effusions are observed after abdominal surgery, liver transplantation or coronary artery bypass surgery/pericardiectomy.

Pleural effusion may result from a number of pathophysiological mechanisms, all of which disturb the physiological balance between the formation and removal of pleural fluid (normal production estimated at 15 mL·day^{-1} in a 60-kg person). Most effusions develop from both an increase in the entry rate of liquid into the pleural space and a decrease in the maximal exit rate of liquid from the pleural space. Transudative effusions are caused either by increased hydrostatic pressure (*e.g.* in cardiac failure) or by reduced plasma oncotic pressure because of protein deficiency (*e.g.* liver cirrhosis or nephrotic syndrome). The pleura itself remains intact. Rarely, transudates may arise from the entry of liquids with low protein concentrations (*e.g.* urine, cerebrospinal fluid or iatrogenic intrapleural infusion of fluids). In contrast, pathological changes in the pleura result in exudation caused by a diffuse increase of capillary permeability, due to localised ruptures (*e.g.* blood vessels, lymphatic vessels, lung abscess or oesophagus) or to disturbed absorption (*e.g.* lymphatic blockage).

Pleural effusion may present at all ages, but is mainly found in adults. Malignant pleural effusions are observed predominantly in patients aged >60 yrs.

The most common clinical presentations are dyspnoea and chest pain, and those of the individual underlying diseases. Physical examination reveals dullness on percussion, usually at the base of the thorax, and decreased breath sounds.

Pleural effusion may be demonstrated by a number of techniques with different sensitivities. The demonstration by percussion requires at least 300–400 mL of fluid, whereas at least 200–300 mL is necessary for standard chest radiography. Smaller amounts can be recognised by lateral decubitus radiography, which also demonstrates whether the fluid is moving freely. Ultrasound is able to demonstrate small effusions, and the sensitivity is almost 100% for volumes of ⩾100 mL. CT and MRI have very similar sensitivities, but require more advanced technology and are therefore much more expensive. However, if pulmonary embolism is suspected, CT angiography is the preferred test.

In the majority of cases, the aetiology is based on the case history, clinical presentation, imaging techniques and examination of the pleural fluid.

The presence of a pleural effusion is established only by thoracentesis. The site should be selected according to the results of the diagnostic procedures. At least if the effusion is small, thoracentesis should be performed under ultrasound guidance. Thoracentesis is indicated in all cases of pleural effusion of unknown origin and in effusions that do not resolve after appropriate treatment. Additional biopsy procedures, such as closed-needle biopsy or medical thoracoscopy/pleuroscopy, may be necessary to confirm or exclude malignant or tuberculous causes. These are performed in a stepwise diagnostic approach (fig. 1).

In many cases, evaluation of the pleural fluid yields valuable diagnostic information or

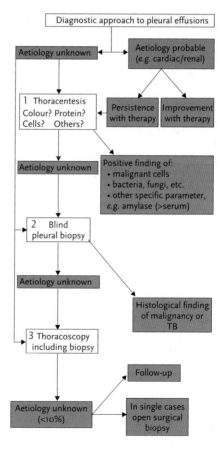

Figure 1. *Diagnostic approach to pleural effusions.*

Table 1. *Investigative parameters of pleural effusion*

Obligatory
Appearance
Total protein
Cell differentiation (cytology)
Optional
Glucose (pH)
Lactate dehydrogenase
Cholesterol
NT-proBNP
Triglycerides
Amylase
Bilirubin
Creatinine
Haematocrit
Immunocytology
Tumour markers
Adenosine deaminase
Interferon-γ release assay
Antinuclear factor, rheumatoid factors, *etc.*
Search for infecting organisms
Tubercle bacilli
Gram staining
Anaerobic, aerobic bacteria
Fungi and parasites

even permits a clear diagnosis. The most important criteria are appearance, protein content and cellular components. In the case of more specific diagnostic questions, routine measurement of the glucose content is supplemented by determination of further laboratory parameters and search for infecting organisms (table 1).

The most important laboratory parameter is the total protein content in the effusion, for which a threshold value of 30 g·L^{-1} differentiates a transudate from an exudate. However, this value is not exclusive, and additional parameters such as lactate dehydrogenase (>200 U·L^{-1}) or cholesterol (>0.55 mmol·L^{-1} (60 mg·dL^{-1})) may be helpful (table 2). The simultaneous determination of serum values is important, because these may strongly influence the values in the pleura. Low glucose values may indicate rheumatoid pleuritis, lupus pleuritis, empyema, TB or malignant effusion, or oesophageal perforation. Elevated levels of N-terminal pro-brain natriuretic protein (NT-proBNP) (in pleural fluid and/or blood) are characteristic of effusions caused by cardiac failure.

Markedly elevated amylase values are observed in acute pancreatitis and pancreatic pseudocysts, oesophageal perforation and, occasionally, in malignant effusions.

Haemothorax is characterised by purely bloody effusions and haematocrit values that exceed those in peripheral blood by >50%.

In chylothorax, increased triglycerides distinguish chylous from pseudochylous effusions. Although nonspecific, adenosine deaminase and T-cell-based interferon-γ release assays may allow support the diagnosis of TB as the cause of lymphocytic pleural effusions.

Diagnostic testing for the infecting organisms that cause pleural effusion is indicated in parapneumonic effusions/empyemas with aerobic and anaerobic cultures, and in suspected tuberculous, fungal or parasitic effusions.

Therapeutic aims in patients with pleural effusion are palliation of symptoms (pain and dyspnoea), treatment of the underlying diseases, prevention of pleural fibrosis with

Table 2. *Light's criteria for exudates*

	Effusion concentration	Effusion/serum concentration ratio	Sensitivity %	Accuracy %
Total protein	>3 g·dL^{-1}	>0.5	89.5	95.4
Lactate dehydrogenase	>200 U·L^{-1}	>0.6	91.4	94.7

reduction of pulmonary function, and prevention of recurrences. The therapeutic approach depends on the availability of options for causal or only symptomatic treatments.

Empyema usually requires, besides antibiotic treatment, additional pleural drainage. Resolution may be further facilitated by instillation of a fibrinolytic agent. In malignant pleural effusions, therapeutic thoracentesis or chest-tube drainage combined with chemical pleurodesis, or medical thoracoscopy with talc poudrage are the preferred options for local treatment. In those resulting from tumours likely to respond to chemotherapy or hormonal treatment, systemic treatment should be started and may be combined with therapeutic thoracentesis or pleurodesis.

Further reading

- Antony VB, et al. (2001). Management of malignant pleural effusions. Eur Respir J; 18: 402–419.
- Chegou NN, et al. (2008). Evaluation of adapted whole-blood interferon-γ release assays for the diagnosis of pleural tuberculosis. Respiration; 76: 131–138.
- Colice GL, et al. (2000). Medical and surgical treatment of parapneumonic effusions: an evidence-based guideline. Chest; 118: 1158–1171.
- Heffner JE (2006).Discriminating between transudates and exudates. Clin Chest Med; 27: 241–252.
- Hooper C, et al. (2010). Investigation of a unilateral pleural effusion in adults: British Thoracic Society pleural disease guideline 2010. Thorax; 65: Suppl. 2, ii4–ii17.
- Koegelenberg CF, et al. (2008). Parapneumonic pleural effusions and empyema. Respiration; 75: 241–250.
- Kolditz M, et al. (2006). High diagnostic accuracy of NT-proBNP for cardiac origin of pleural effusions. Eur Respir J; 28: 114–150.
- Light RW (2002). Diagnostic approach in a patient with pleural effusion. Eur Respir Monogr; 22: 131–145.
- Light RW, ed. Pleural Diseases. 5th Edn. Philadelphia, Lippincott Williams & Wilkins, 2007.
- Roberts ME, et al. (2010). Management of malignant pleural effusion. British Thoracic Society pleural disease guideline 2010. Thorax; 65: Suppl. 2, ii32–ii40.
- Rodriguez-Panadero F, et al. (2006). Thoracoscopy: general overview and place in the diagnosis and management of pleural effusion. Eur Respir J; 28: 409–422.
- Trajman A, et al. (2008). Novel tests for diagnosing tuberculous pleural effusion: what works and what does not? Eur Respir J; 31: 1098–1106.

Pneumothorax and pneumomediastinum

Paul Schneider

Pneumothorax is defined as an accumulation of air in the pleural space with secondary lung collapse. This accumulation is of diverse derivation, but visceral pleural rupture with air leakage is the most common cause. An original possibly ruptured oesophagus with diminished chest wall integrity can cause free air in the pleural space, as can, more rarely, a gas-forming organism.

In most instances, the pneumothorax presents with minor symptoms without any physiological changes. Rarely, a simple

Key points

- The most likely cause of a primary spontaneous pneumothorax is the rupture of small subpleural bulla.

- Pneumothorax usually present with acute chest pain and dyspnoea.

- Pneumothorax can be complicated by persistent air leak for >3 days, pneumomediastinum and haemopneumothorax.

- Recurrence is the most common indication for surgery in patients with a primary spontaneous pneumothorax.

- Surgery is accomplished by a video-assisted thoracoscopy mechanical abrasion, or by parietal apical pleurectomy in association with resection of the lung.

- In secondary pneumothorax, the mortality rate for surgery may reach 10% and the morbidity is significant.

pneumothorax progresses and develops with significant haemodynamic and respiratory instability, hypoxia and shock. This clinical presentation is accompanied by a tension pneumothorax and demands emergency treatment.

The pneumothorax can be classified according to cause or clinical presentation, or according to spontaneous, traumatic or iatrogenic aetiology (table 1). The first category includes primary and secondary causes. A primary spontaneous pneumothorax occurs in individuals with no known pulmonary disease. A secondary pneumothorax occurs in patients with clinical or radiographic evidence of underlying lung disease. Traumatic pneumothorax occurs as a result of penetrating or blunt trauma with disruption of the bronchus, the lung or the oesophagus. A traumatic pneumothorax is defined as 'open' with an associated disruption of the chest wall. Iatrogenic pneumothorax includes the diagnostic and therapeutic pneumothorax, which are relatively common in the hospital environment but will not be considered in this discussion.

Primary spontaneous pneumothorax

Clinical features The most likely cause of a primary spontaneous pneumothorax is the rupture of small subpleural bulla (fig. 1), occuring at rest or during exercise. It is seen most often in young, tall male patients with admitted cigarette or cannabis smoking habits. Hereditary aspects have been described.

In the North American population, incidence varies from 6–7 per 100 000

Table 1. *Classification of pneumothorax*

Spontaneous

  Primary (healthy individuals)

  Secondary (underlying pulmonary disease)

    COPD

    Infection

    Neoplasm

    Catamenial

    Miscellaneous

Traumatic

  Blunt

  Penetrating

Iatrogenic

  Inadvertent

  Diagnostic

  Therapeutic

males to 1–2 per 100 000 females. Bilateral pneumothoraces occur in <10% of patients. Recurrences are observed in 42% of patients, usually within 2 years. After the second pneumothorax, the chances of having a third episode increase to >50%.

The clinical presentation usually relates to the degree of pulmonary collapse. Although some patients have an asymptomatic pneumothorax, more often they present with acute chest pain and dyspnoea.

Physical findings may be totally absent if the collapse is minimal, while substantial

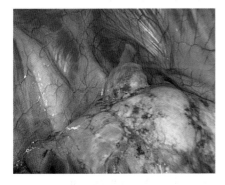

Figure 1. *Bulla on the apex.*

collapse is defined in decreased chest wall movement on the affected side. Percussion of the chest cavity is hyperresonant and tympanic, and on auscultation breath sounds are decreased or absent. A pleural friction rub can sometimes be heard. Tachycardia is found in most patients.

Diagnosis The clinical diagnosis of a pneumothorax is best confirmed by erect posteroanterior and lateral chest radiographs. Expiration posteroanterior chest radiography may be useful to demonstrate a small pneumothorax not seen on standard film.

CT imaging is generally not necessary unless abnormalities are noted on the plain chest radiograph or further evaluation is required (*e.g.* of suspected secondary pneumothorax), or if an aberrant chest drain emplacement is suspected.

Complications Air leakage may persist for >48 h after the treatment of a pneumothorax. Often the air leak is seen in patients with a secondary pneumothorax, but occasionally patients with a primary spontaneous pneumothorax develop this complication. In this instance, surgery must be considered.

Pneumomediastinum (fig. 2) is secondary to the dissection of air along the bronchial and pulmonary vessel sheets or as a complication of a spontaneous pneumothorax. It is generally of no clinical consequence, but other causes of pneumomediastinum, such as injury to major airways or oesophagus perforation, may need to be excluded. Pneumoperitoneum secondary to a pneumothorax is rare, and it must be differentiated from a pneumoperitoneum associated with a perforated abdominal organ. Interstitial and subcutaneous emphysema are usually of no consequence.

Haemothorax (fig. 3) is a rare complication of a pneumothorax and most often results from the rupture of a small vessel located in adhesions between the visceral and the parietal pleura. Often, re-expansion of the lung with a chest drain helps to tamponade the bleeding point. Occasionally, the patient becomes hypotensive and requires emergency surgery.

Bilateral pneumothorax happens in <1% of cases and can be simultaneous or, more commonly, sequential.

Management The different clinical situations in spontaneous pneumothorax require different therapeutic approaches. The nonoperative approach includes observation, simple aspiration, and thoracostomy with ambulatory chest drainage. Chemical pleurodesis with tetracycline or talc are options that can be used to reduce the risk of recurrence. Surgical intervention entails apical bullectomy with or without pleurodesis by pleurectomy or gauze abrasion.

Observation Asymptomatic patients in good health (<20%) with a small pneumothorax and no evidence of radiographic progression may be treated per observation. To ensure no complications develop, it is recommended that these patients be observed in hospital for 24–48 h. Before discharge, patients must be warned of a potential tension pneumothorax development. A weekly follow-up with clinical examination and chest radiograph is to be carried out until the pneumothorax has been completely resolved. The main inconvenience in this form of therapy is the duration, which far exceeds what is seen with conventional pleural drainage plus the added risk of a tension pneumothorax development. Therefore, observation only is inappropriate in most cases.

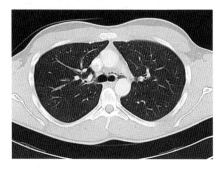

Figure 2. Pneumomediastinum.

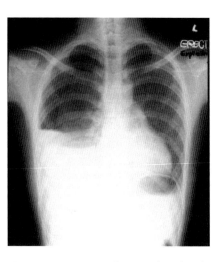

Figure 3. Haemopneumothorax on the right side.

Aspiration and small chest tube drainage
Simple aspiration of air with a 16-gauge intravenous cannula connected to a three-way stopcock and a 60-mL syringe is an option.

Small 9-Fr. chest tubes with or without flutter valves have also been used as an alternative to larger and more conventional thoracostomy tubes. The success rate is high, but problems associated with kinking and occlusion of the drains have been described. Treatment is still controversial. Simple aspiration is recommended by the British Thoracic Society – but not by the American College of Chest Physicians – as first-line treatment for the primary pneumothorax requiring intervention. Acceptance by medical staff is seemingly modest.

Conventional tube thoracostomy
Conventional tube thoracostomy remains the procedure of choice for the management of moderate-to-large pneumothoraces. The drain allows for rapid and complete evacuation of air from the pleural space. Although underwater-seal drainage is sufficient for most cases of pneumothorax, the current author prefers the use of negative intrapleural pressure to maintain lung re-expansion over a period of 5 days.

Table 2. Indications for surgery in primary spontaneous pneumothorax

First episode
Prolonged air leak
No re-expansion of the lung
Bilateral pneumothoraces
Haemopneumothorax
Occupational hazard (flight personnel, divers)
Absence of medical facilities in isolated area
Tension pneumothorax
Associated single large bulla
Individual indication
Second episode
Ipsilateral recurrence
Contralateral recurrence after a first pneumothorax

Nonsurgical therapy of recurrences Most surgeons are concerned about the routine use of chemopleurodesis in the treatment of spontaneous pneumothorax. Being a benign disease occurring in young people who may require surgery in later life (for other disease development) the important symphysis which follows chemopleurodesis complicates and multiplies the risk in association with high morbidity rates, especially if lung resection or transplantation is considered. Chemical pleurodesis should therefore be used only in selected cases.

Indications for surgery Surgery may be indicated in the first instance, if the pneumothorax is complicated by a persisting air leak over 3 days. Furthermore, haemothorax development, failure to re-expand the lung, bilateral involvement and tension hazard are indications. Patients with an occupational risk hazard are a classic indication. Some authors have proposed that all young patients with a diagnosed spontaneous pneumothorax should be spared a drain thoracostomy and proceed directly to surgical intervention. This approach is not standard treatment, though

many patients are operated on as a result of complication or disease recurrence. Indications for surgery in primary spontaneous pneumothorax are presented in table 2.

Surgical therapy The principles of surgical intervention for spontaneous pneumothorax consist of bulla or bleb resection (fig. 4) and obliteration of the pleural space to prevent recurrence. Recurrence is the most common indication for surgery in patients with a primary spontaneous pneumothorax. Multiple wedge resections may also be required when the disease is present at several sites. Segmentectomy and lobectomy are usually unnecessary and are contraindicated.

Obliteration of the pleural space is thought to be necessary to prevent recurrences. It is accomplished by mechanical abrasion, or by parietal apical pleurectomy (fig. 5), which is performed in association with resection of the lung during a video-assisted thoracoscopy.

The operation is carried out under general anaesthesia with a dual-lumen endotracheal tube. Only two thoracic incisions are made for the thoracoscope and dissecting or stapling instruments.

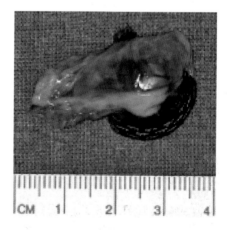

Figure 4. Specimen of an apical bulla resected by stapler.

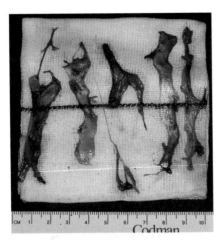

Figure 5. *Specimen of apical parietal pleurectomy.*

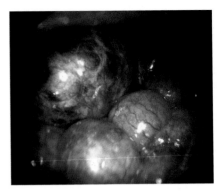

Figure 6. *Thoracoscopic view of bullous emphysema with pneumothorax.*

Apical parietal pleurectomy can be performed easily using this technique with modern endo-scissors and forceps. However, a single-centre randomised study of 787 patients shows that pleurodesis can be achieved with talc poudrage even in young patients with a lower morbidity, less surgical time and no significant differences concerning recurrence of pneumothorax.

Video-assisted surgery is recommended as the first-line surgical treatment for patients with recurrent primary spontaneous pneumothorax. This recommendation is based on its favourable early postoperative course without major complication and the long-term outcome with 3% recurrence, and patient satisfaction.

Secondary pneumothorax

Spontaneous pneumothorax can be secondary to a variety of pulmonary and nonpulmonary disorders.

COPD is the most common cause of secondary pneumothorax (fig. 6 and table 3). It occurs typically in patients aged >50 years and is the result of a bulla rupture into the pleural space.

Most patients with COPD and pneumo-thorax present with chest pain and acute sudden respiratory distress. These patients show little tolerance to even a small

pneumothorax because of their limited pulmonary function. Diagnosis is difficult due to physical findings associated with COPD (*e.g.* hyperresonance on percussion and diminished breath sounds at auscultation). In most cases, the diagnosis is made by chest radiographs, which are also difficult to interpret because of the increased radiolucency of the diseased lung. For these difficult cases, CT may be necessary to confirm the diagnosis, localise the pneumothorax and facilitate distinction between a large bulla and a pneumothorax.

The emergency treatment of patients with a secondary pneumothorax is similar to that described for primary spontaneous pneumo-thorax, except that observation alone is seldom justified. If the pleural space is adequately drained and the lung maintains a re-expanded state, the air leak eventually closes. In some patients, however, a bronchopleural fistula persists for 10–15 days, and surgical repair must be considered.

When surgery is required, the procedure must be individualised and based on the extent and disease infiltration, as well as the air leak location.

Staple resection of the bullae should be carried out, followed by a subtotal parietal pleurectomy or pleural abrasion.

The mortality rate for this surgery may reach 10% and morbidity is significant in those individuals with a poor overall physical

Table 3. Causes of secondary pneumothorax

Airway and pulmonary disease
COPD (bullous or diffuse emphysema)
Asthma
CF
Intersitial lung disease
Pulmonary fibrosis (fig. 7)
Sarcoidosis
Infectious disease
Tuberculous and other mycobacterial
Bacterial
Pneumocystis jiroveci
Parasitic
Mycotic
AIDS
Neoplasic
Bronchogenic carcinoma
Metastatic (lymphoma or sarcoma)
Catamenial
Endometriosis
Miscellaneous
Marfan's syndrome
Ehlers–Danlos syndrome
Histiocytosis X
Scleroderma
Lymphangiomyomatosis
Collagen disease

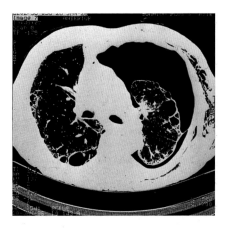

Figure 7. Severe pulmonary fibrosis with pneumothorax on the left side.

surgery is the safest approach with excellent long-term results.

Further reading

- Abolnik IZ, *et al.* (1991). On the inheritance of primary spontaneous pneumothorax. *Am J Med Genet*; 40: 155–158.
- Aguinagalde B, *et al.* (2010). Percutaneous aspiration versus tube drainage for spontaneous pneumothorax: systematic review and meta-analysis. *Eur J Cardiothorac Surg*; 37: 1129–1135.
- Baumann MH, *et al.* (2001). Management of spontaneous pneumothorax: an American College of Chest Physicians Delphi consensus statement. *Chest*; 119: 590–602.
- Ben-Nun A, *et al.* (2006). Video-assisted thoracoscopic surgery for recurrent spontaneous pneumothorax: the long-term benefit. *World J Surg*; 30: 285–290.
- Beshay M, *et al.* (2007). Emphysema and secondary pneumothorax in young adults smoking cannabis. *Eur J Cardiothorac Surg*; 32: 834–838.
- Chambers A, *et al.* (2009). In patients with first-episode primary spontaneous pneumothorax is video-assisted thoracoscopic surgery superior to tube thoracostomy alone in terms of time to resolution of pneumothorax and incidence of recurrence? *Interact Cardiovasc Thorac Surg*; 9: 1003–1008.

condition. Other options, such as chemical pleurodesis, autologous blood injection and permanent fistula drainage can be considered in individual cases.

Conclusion

Primary spontaneous pneumothorax occurs in young patients with no evidence of coexisting lung disease, while secondary pneumothorax is mostly seen in emphysema patients. Unless there is a complication, most surgeons will manage the first episode by conventional tube drainage. Recurrences are treated by bulla or bleb resection with apical parietal pleurectomy. Video-assisted

- Chen JS, *et al.* (2009). Management of recurrent primary spontaneous pneumothorax after thoracoscopic surgery: should observation, drainage, redo thoracoscopy, or thoracotomy be used? *Surg Endosc*; 23: 2438–2444.
- Henry M, *et al.* (2003). BTS guidelines for the management of spontaneous pneumothorax. *Thorax*; 58: Suppl. 2, ii39–ii52.
- Moreno-Merino S, *et al.* (2012). Comparative study of talc poudrage *versus* pleural abrasion for the treatment of primary spontaneous pneumothorax. *Interact Cardiovasc Thorac Surg*; 15: 81–85.

Mediastinitis

Pierre-Emmanuel Falcoz, Nicola Santelmo and Gilbert Massard

The majority of acute mediastinal infections results from oesophageal perforation or infection following a trans-sternal cardiac procedure. Occasionally, acute mediastinitis results from oropharyngeal abscesses with severe cervical infection spreading along the fascial planes into the mediastinum. This particularly virulent form of mediastinal infection is described as descending necrotising mediastinitis (DNM).

DNM is a potentially lethal condition especially if diagnosis or treatment is delayed or inappropriate. Despite the introduction of modern antimicrobial therapy and CT imaging, DNM has continued to produce high mortality rates (reported between 25% and 40%).

Criteria for diagnosis of DNM

Criteria for diagnosis of DNM have been accurately defined as follows.

- Clinical manifestations of a severe infection
- Establishment of a relationship between an oropharyngeal or cervical infection and subsequent mediastinitis
- Demonstration of radiographic features characteristic of DNM
- Documentation of a necrotising mediastinal infection at the time of operative debridement or necropsy

Epidemiology

Primary sites of infection are periodontal, retropharyngeal and peritonsillar abscesses. According to Wheatley et al. (1990), the most common primary oropharyngeal infection is odontogenic (25 out of 43 cases), with mandibular or molar abscesses

> **Key points**
>
> - DNM is a particularly virulent and potentially lethal mediastinal infection.
>
> - Initial presentation is toxic shock and respiratory difficulty, sometimes with other signs such as erythema and oedema of the neck and upper chest.
>
> - DNM is an emergency, and should be treated with broad-spectrum intravenous antibiotics as well as early and aggressive surgical drainage.

being the second and third most common primary infections, respectively.

Route of diffusion

Familiarity with the cervical fascial planes is essential in understanding the propagation pathways, symptoms and thoracic complications of cervical infections. The infection spreads from neck to mediastinum along three primary routes: via the retropharyngeal space, the perivascular space and the pre-tracheal space. The retropharyngeal space has been thought to be the most important route by which a cervical infectious disease spreads to the mediastinum (70% of cases in the series of Moncada et al. (1978)). Rapid spread of infection is facilitated by tissue necrosis (loss of anatomical structure), gravity and negative intrathoracic pressure.

Pathogens involved

DNM is a polymicrobial process with anaerobic organisms being the most predominant. Freeman et al. (2000) reviewed the English literature and found 96 patients with DNM between 1990 and 1999. All but four (4%) had mixed aerobic and anaerobic infection, with those pathogens often acting synergistically; in the four exceptions, the sole pathogen was β-haemolytic Streptococcus. Chow et al. (1978) reported that anaerobes had been recovered from 94% of patients with DNM; 52% had mixed infections and 88% had polymicrobial infections.

Clinical and radiological signs

The anamnesis of mediastinitis is as follows.

- Phase I: periodontal or peritonsillar abscess treated by simple antibiotherapy
- Phase II: erythema and oedema of the neck with or without associated with subcutaneous emphysema
- Phase III: acute aggravation of the infectious syndrome; onset of cough, dyspnoea, sternal pain and painful dysphagia

Patients with DNM usually present with toxic shock and respiratory difficulty. Other presenting signs may include erythema and oedema of the neck and upper chest. In severe infections, frank necrosis of the skin, fascia and muscle may be present. In the chest, DNM may produce abscesses and empyemas, pleural and pericardial effusions, intrathoracic haemorrhage, and cardiac tamponade, and frequently results in the death of the patient.

Delay of diagnosis is one of the primary reasons for high mortality in DNM. Diagnosis of DNM from conventional radiographic studies may be difficult, principally because the signs appear late in the course of the disease. Cervicothoracic CT imaging is currently considered the diagnostic study of choice for patients in whom DNM is suspected. Indeed, CT scan findings have been proven to confirm the diagnosis of DNM with high accuracy in these patients who often have a nonspecific constellation of symptoms. Various CT imaging findings are increased attenuation of mediastinal fat, air fluid levels, pleural and pericardial effusions,

oesophageal thickening and enlarged lymph nodes. Brunelli et al. (1996) found cervicothoracic CT imaging to be immediately diagnostic in all patients in whom it was used.

Treatment

The principles of treatment are:

- emergency
- intravenous broad-spectrum antibiotic therapy: probabilistic and secondarily adapted to the pathogen(s)
- early and aggressive surgical drainage: extensive debridement, excision of necrotic tissue, bacteriological sampling, mediastinal and pleural irrigation, and feeding jejunostomy

The decision on the type of surgical drainage to be employed is a crucial one. Classically, four approaches have been reported:

1. transcervical
2. standard posterolateral thoracotomy
3. median sternotomy
4. transthoracic via subxyphoid or clamshell incision

A thoracoscopic approach and video-assisted mediastinoscopic drainage can also be found. Although each of these techniques offers potential advantages and disadvantages, the posterolateral thoracotomy incision (sometimes bilateral) remains the standard by which other transthoracic approaches should be measured.

The optimal surgical approach for mediastinal drainage is theoretically dependent on the level of diffusion of necrotising process. Several studies have reported that mediastinal drainage is best accomplished through a transthoracic approach when the necrotising process extends below the level of the fourth thoracic vertebra posteriorly or the tracheal bifurcation anteriorly. However, because of the rapid spread of this type of infection, other investigators have advocated mandatory transthoracic mediastinal exploration regardless of the level of infection. This latter point was confirmed in a meta-analysis, where a statistically significant difference ($p < 0.05$) in survival was found between patients undergoing transcervical mediastinal drainage (53%) *versus* those receiving transthoracic mediastinal drainage (81%).

Close-watch care Recurrent abscesses and collections are common after first operative drainage (50%) and they should be drained promptly. Ideally, CT or, failing that, ultrasound-guided percutaneous drainage of recurrent abscesses and collections may decrease the need for recurrent surgical procedures in these critically ill patients. Surveillance should be continued until no evidence of progressive infection is found on CT imaging and the patient displays no clinical signs of infection. Hyperbaric oxygen therapy has not shown any real proof of effectiveness in this particular framework, when looking at evidence-based medicine. It should not take the place of or delay surgical treatment.

Mediastinal fibrosis Fibrosing mediastinitis is an uncommon chronic sequela of prior infectious mediastinal involvement. A chronic, noninfectious inflammatory process results in progressive mediastinal fibrosis. The fibrosis may constrict or obstruct virtually any of the mediastinal organs (in particular, the superior vena cava, oesophagus, and pulmonary vein or artery). CT scans demonstrate a localised (or less frequently diffuse) mass infiltrating the mediastinum and constricting the structure; extensive calcification is associated with the fibrotic mass in a vast majority of the cases. This appearance is pathognomonic of the disorder.

Conclusions

DNM is caused by downward spread of neck infections and constitutes a highly fatal complication of oropharyngeal lesions. CT imaging should be performed in all patients with persistent symptoms of septicaemia after being treated for oropharyngeal infections. Prompt surgical drainage of the mediastinum should be performed. The optimal mediastinal drainage method should be tailored to each

patient's condition and extension of the mediastinitis (posterolateral thoracotomy is frequently required). In the post-operative period, progression of the disease and effectiveness of surgical therapy should be monitored by CT. Further drainage should be carried out if necessary either surgically or by percutaneous drainage.

Further reading

- Brunelli A, *et al.* (1996). Descending necrotizing mediastinitis: cervicotomy or thoracotomy? *J Thorac Cardiovasc Surg*; 111: 485–486.
- Chow AW, *et al.* (1978). Orofacial odontogenic infections. *Ann Intern Med*; 88: 392–402.
- Corsten MJ, *et al.* (1997). Optimal treatment of descending necrotizing mediastinitis. *Thorax*; 52: 702–708.
- Devaraj A, *et al.* (2007). Computed tomography findings in fibrosing mediastinitis. *Clin Radiol*; 62: 781–786.
- Estera AS, *et al.* (1983). Descending necrotizing mediastinitis. *Surg Gynecol Obstet*; 157: 545–552.
- Freeman RK, *et al.* (2000). Descending necrotizing mediastinitis: an analysis of the effects of serial surgical debridement on patient mortality. *J Thorac Cardiovasc Surg*; 119: 260–267.
- Marty-Ané CH, *et al.* (1999). Management of descending necrotizing mediastinitis: an aggressive treatment for an aggressive disease. *Ann Thorac Surg*; 68: 212–217.
- Kocher GJ, *et al.* (2012). Diffuse descending necrotizing mediastinitis: surgical therapy and outcome in a single-centre series. *Eur J Cardiothorac Surg*; 42: e66–e72.
- Moncada R, *et al.* (1978). Mediastinitis from odontogenic and deep cervical infection: anatomic pathways of propagation. *Chest*; 73: 497–500.
- Shimizu K, *et al.* (2006). Successful video-assisted mediastinoscopic drainage of descending necrotizing mediastinitis. *Ann Thorac Surg*; 81: 2279–2281.
- Wheatley MJ, *et al.* (1990). Descending necrotizing mediastinitis: transcervical drainage is not enough. *Ann Thorac Surg*; 49: 780–784.

- Haremza C, *et al.* (2011). Successfully treated descending necrotizing mediastinitis through thoracotomy using a pedicled muscular serratus anterior flap. *Interact Cardiovasc Thorac Surg*; 13: 456–458.

- Erkmen CP, *et al.* (2012). Use of cervicothoracic anatomy as a guide for directed drainage of descending necrotizing mediastinitis. *Ann Thorac Surg*; 93: 1293–1294.

Neuromuscular disorders

Andrea Vianello

Various neuromuscular diseases (NMDs) can progress to the point where they cause pulmonary complications (table 1); a careful respiratory follow-up adapted to the variable time course of each disease is therefore mandatory. Although the diseases have different causes and clinical courses, common principles apply to their management.

Evaluation of patients with suspected respiratory impairment

Clinical evaluation As the first step, a systematic clinical evaluation is essential to detect the subtle respiratory symptoms and signs related to respiratory muscle failure. Symptoms are frequently nonspecific, including fatigue, lethargy or difficulty concentrating. Dyspnoea and orthopnoea are often late findings in patients with usually severe functional impairment due to peripheral muscle weakness. Patients with sleep-disordered breathing (SDB) often seem to have symptoms such as an unrefreshed feeling upon awakening, morning headaches, disappearance of snoring, daytime tiredness, and irritability as a result of repeated arousals and carbon dioxide retention. Physical evaluation is essential and may reveal an increase in respiratory rate, followed by alternating abdominal and rib cage breathing (respiratory alternans), the absence of outward excursion of the abdomen during inspiration or even paradoxical inward inspiratory movement due to diaphragm weakness (abdominal paradox), accessory muscle recruitment, and mucous encumbrance of upper or lower airways. Indicators of bulbar muscle involvement include dysarthria, trouble swallowing liquids, aspiration manifesting as a new-onset cough, or frank choking.

Pulmonary function testing Pulmonary function tests (PFTs) should be performed routinely during the evaluation of patients with NMD. Because of the inadequacy of inspiratory muscle function, PFTs generally reveal the pattern of a restrictive ventilatory defect, with the following characteristics:

- preserved TLC until a far-advanced stage of the disease;
- elevated residual volume;
- reduced vital capacity (VC); and
- preserved functional residual capacity.

When VC falls below 55% predicted, the onset of insidiously progressive hypercapnia is likely. A significant difference between upright and recumbent lung volumes has been reported frequently for patients with NMD; in particular, a fall in VC of $\geqslant 25\%$ has been considered a sensitive indicator of diaphragmatic weakness. A specific evaluation of respiratory muscle strength is mandatory as these tests are both sensitive and highly prognostic. A high negative maximal inspiratory pressure (MIP) result ($< $ -80 cmH$_2$O) or a high positive maximal

Key points

- NMD have a range of causes, but common principles apply to their treatment.
- Treatment focuses on ventilatory assistance and assisted coughing techniques.

Table 1. NMDs affecting respiratory function

Site of lesion	Specific disorders
Anterior horn cell	Amyotrophic lateral sclerosis Poliomyelitis Type I SMA, intermediate SMA
Peripheral nerve and/or nerve roots	Guillain–Barré syndrome Charcot–Marie–Tooth disease
Neuromuscular junction	Congenital myasthenia
Muscle	Duchenne/Becker muscular dystrophy Limb-girdle muscular dystrophy (especially types 2C-2F-2I) Facioscapulohumeral muscular dystrophy Congenital muscular dystrophy Congenital myotonic dystrophy Acid maltase deficiency Congenital myopathy Mitochondrial myopathy Bethlem myopathy

SMA: spinal muscular atrophy.

expiratory pressure result ($> +90$ cmH$_2$O) excludes clinically relevant inspiratory or expiratory muscle weakness. Cough peak expiratory flow (CPEF) is the single most important factor in determining whether the ability to eliminate bronchial secretions is well preserved. Patients who, either alone or with assistance, are able to generate a CPEF >270 L·min^{-1} can effectively remove bronchial secretions, whereas those with a CPEF <160 L·min^{-1} usually require tracheal suctioning at the onset of respiratory infections. The frequency of pulmonary function monitoring depends on the rapidity of progression of the neuromuscular syndrome and may range from every 1– 2 months to yearly. Once the VC drops below 40–50% pred or MIP below 30% pred, daytime arterial blood gas analysis should be performed.

Sleep study All patients with NMD should be monitored carefully for the presence of SDB. Nocturnal oximetry alone is inadequate to detect sleep apnoea and hypoventilation. In addition, criteria defining significant desaturations remain controversial. Overnight polysomnography (PSG) or respiratory polygraphy is advisable for patients who develop symptoms and

signs of sleep–wake abnormality or nocturnal respiratory failure. It has been suggested that PSG or respiratory polygraphy should be performed in all NMD patients as early as possible to take a baseline recording. It should be repeated according to the course of the disease to detect abnormalities during sleep and subsequent indication for long-term ventilatory treatment.

Management

Long-term noninvasive positive pressure ventilation In recent years, the approach to care in neuromuscular respiratory failure has been revised, due to two new critical developments:

1) technology has advanced and several new types of ventilatory aids have been introduced, which deliver effective mechanical ventilation, even noninvasively; and

2) the majority of severely disabled ventilator users have expressed satisfaction with their lives, even though they are usually unable to achieve some of the goals associated with acceptable quality of life in the 'normal' population.

As a consequence, increasing numbers of NMD patients with advanced respiratory impairment are now being successfully treated by long-term noninvasive positive pressure ventilation (NPPV), usually in the home setting. The noninvasive administration of positive pressure ventilation requires a positive pressure ventilator delivering pressurised gas to the lungs through an interface via the nose or mouth, or both. In recent years, manufacturers have developed a new generation of microprocessor-controlled ventilators aimed at combining a minimum warranted alveolar ventilation with maximal patient comfort. Also, special features have been incorporated that are designed to facilitate the application of noninvasive techniques and are simple, reliable and easy for the patient to use.

Long-term NPPV is required when spontaneous respiratory muscle effort is unable to sustain adequate alveolar ventilation, causing chronic-stable or slowly progressive respiratory failure.

Indications for NPPV therapy in chronic NMD are symptoms (such as fatigue, dyspnoea, morning headache) and one of the following physiological criteria.

- Significant daytime carbon dixoide retention ($PaCO_2$ >50 mmHg)
- Nocturnal oxygen desaturation (SaO_2 <88% for at least five consecutive minutes)

- FVC <50% pred or MIP <60 cmH$_2$O (only for rapidly progressive disease)

The following complications are considered to be contraindications for the noninvasive ventilatory approach.

- Severely impaired swallowing, leading to chronic aspiration and repeated pneumonia
- Ineffective clearing of tracheobronchial secretions, despite the use of noninvasive manual or mechanical expiratory aids
- The need for round-the-clock (>20 h) ventilatory support

These conditions usually require an invasive application of mechanical ventilation via tracheostomy. There is no consensus on the optimal interface to use in delivering NPPV: nasal masks are usually preferable for nocturnal ventilation, due to the fact that they are more comfortable and permit better speech; conversely, oronasal interfaces may be a suitable alternative for subjects who have excessive air leaking through the mouth or nose. Mouthpiece interfaces have also been successfully used to deliver NPPV for up to 24 h·day^{-1}. Finally, the choice of ventilator and interface in most cases is individualised according to patients' preference and physicians' intuition and experience, rather than based on standardised evidence-based guidelines. Administration of NPPV to NMD patients with chronic respiratory failure may be expected to allow some individuals with nonprogressive pathology to live to nearly normal life expectancy, extend survival by many years in patients with other conditions, improve physiological lung function and quality of life (QoL), and decrease the frequency of exacerbations requiring acute care facilities. Although ineffective for prolonging survival in patients with rapidly progressive conditions and advanced bulbar muscle involvement, such as amyotrophic lateral sclerosis/motor neurone disease, NPPV may be added with the aim of improving some aspects of the QoL, in particular energy, vitality and symptoms related to SDB, being considered as an important part of the total palliative care plan for terminally ill cases.

Approach to acute respiratory illness The onset of acute respiratory failure, due to the combination of inspiratory, expiratory or bulbar innervated muscle dysfunction leading to inadequate cough and inability to handle oropharyngeal secretions, is a crucial event in the advanced stage of most NMD and a major cause of death, unless mechanical ventilation is used. Respiratory tract infection is the most common precipitating factor, potentially aggravating inspiratory muscle weakness and promoting atelectasis and pneumonia. A list of potential precipitating factors is presented in table 2.

A noninvasive approach to the management of respiratory tract infections causing acute respiratory failure, based on the combination of expiratory muscle aid and NPPV, has been proposed. This treatment strategy may result in a reduced need for nasal suctioning and conventional intubation, and/or tracheostomy. Among noninvasive expiratory aids, manually assisted coughing techniques have been demonstrated to be effective in facilitating the elimination of airway secretions. Additionally, mechanical insufflation–exsufflation has been shown to effectively mobilise mucous secretions and has been proposed as a complement to manually assisted coughing techniques in the prevention of pulmonary morbidity (fig. 1).

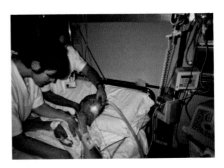

Figure 1. Application of mechanical insufflation–exsufflation combined with manually assisted coughing during respiratory tract infection.

Mechanical insufflation–exsufflation can be administered by a device consisting of a two-stage axial compressor that provides positive pressure to the airway, then rapidly shifts to negative pressure, thereby generating a forced expiration. For NMD patients who still require endotracheal intubation and invasive mechanical ventilation, preventive application of NPPV after extubation may provide a clinically important advantage by averting the need for re-intubation or tracheostomy, and shortening their stay in the intensive care unit.

Conclusion

It is now clear that life can be greatly prolonged for most individuals with NMD by the availability of noninvasive aids and that the great majority of severely disabled patients submitted to ventilatory assistance are satisfied with their lives. Clinicians with a special competence in the management of such patients have the responsibility of offering these treatment options, encouraging the patients to decide in advance whether or not these measures would be acceptable.

Further reading

- Bach JR, *et al.* (1997). Prevention of pulmonary morbidity for patients with Duchenne muscular dystrophy. *Chest*; 112: 1024–1028.

Table 2. *Potential causes of acute respiratory failure in NMD patients*

Common
Upper respiratory tract infection/acute bronchitis
Pneumonia
Atelectasis
Cardiac failure
Less common
Pneumothorax
Pulmonary embolism
Sedatives and hypnotics
Tracheal haemorrhage (patients with tracheostomy)

446

- Bourke SC, et al. (2006). Effects of non-invasive ventilation on survival and quality of life in patients with amyotrophic lateral sclerosis: a randomised controlled trial. *Lancet Neurol*; 5: 140–147.
- Braun NM, et al. (1983). Respiratory muscle and pulmonary function in polymyositis and other proximal myopathies. *Thorax*; 38: 616–623.
- Clinical indications for noninvasive positive pressure ventilation in chronic respiratory failure due to restrictive lung disease, COPD, and nocturnal hypoventilation – a consensus conference report. *Chest*; 116: 521–534.
- Gomez-Merino E, et al. (2002). Duchenne muscular dystrophy: prolongation of life by noninvasive ventilation and mechanically assisted coughing. *Am J Phys Med Rehabil*; 81: 411–415.
- Hill NS (2002). Ventilator management for neuromuscular disease. *Semin Respir Crit Care Med*; 23: 293–305.
- Hull J, et al. (2012). British Thoracic Society guidelines for respiratory management of children with neuromuscular weakness. *Thorax*; 67: i1–i40.
- Kohler M, et al. (2005). Quality of life, physical disability, and respiratory impairment in Duchenne muscular dystrophy. *Am J Respir Crit Care Med*; 172: 1032–1036.
- Lofaso F, et al. (2002). Polysomnography for the management of progressive neuromuscular disorders. *Eur Respir J*; 19: 989–990.
- Mellies U, et al. (2003). Daytime predictors of sleep disordered breathing in children and adolescents with neuromuscular disorders. *Neuromusc Disord*; 13: 123–128.
- Polkey MI, et al. (1999). Respiratory aspects of neurological disease. *J Neurol Neurosurg Psychiatry*; 66: 5–15.
- Simonds A, et al. (1998). Impact of nasal ventilation on survival in hypercapnic Duchenne muscular dystrophy. *Thorax*; 53: 949–952.
- Simonds AK (2006). Recent advances in respiratory care for neuromuscular disease. *Chest*; 130: 1879–1886.
- Vianello A, et al. (1994). Long-term nasal intermittent positive pressure ventilation in advanced Duchenne's muscular dystrophy. *Chest*; 105: 445–448.
- Vianello A, et al. (2000). Non-invasive ventilatory approach to treatment of acute respiratory failure in neuromuscular disorders. A comparison with endotracheal intubation. *Intensive Care Med*; 26: 384–390.
- Vianello A, et al. (2005). Mechanical insufflation–exsufflation improves outcomes for neuromuscular disease patients with respiratory tract infections. *Am J Phys Med Rehabil*; 84: 83–88.
- Vianello A, et al. (2011). Prevention of extubation failure in high-risk patients with neuromuscular disease. *J Crit Care*; 26: 517–524.

Chest wall disorders

Pierre-Emmanuel Falcoz, Nicola Santelmo and Gilbert Massard

There is a large and diverse group of congenital abnormalities of the thorax that manifest as deformities and/or defects of the anterior chest wall. Depending on the severity of the case, there may be cardiopulmonary (tolerance to exercise) or psychological implications.

This diverse group includes:

- pectus excavatum or 'funnel chest'
- pectus carinatum or 'keel chest'
- Poland syndrome
- cleft sternum

Among these, pectus excavatum and pectus carinatum are the two most common chest wall abnormalities.

Key points

- The two most common chest wall abnormalities are pectus excavatum and pectus carinatum.

- The two most common surgical procedures for pectus excavatum repair are the modified Ravitch technique and the Nuss procedure.

- Careful pre-operative evaluation on the basis of clinical and psychological symptoms is required to select potential candidates for surgical remodelling.

- The optimal timing of surgical repair would be after the main growth has stopped (late teens or early 20s).

Pathogenesis

Over the years, the theories concerning the pathogenesis of pectoral deformities evolved from substernal ligament traction to overgrowth of the rib cartilage and later to a stress–strain imbalance. The genetic aspects of pectus deformities have just started to emerge and, hopefully, will answer many questions.

Pectus excavatum is a recessively inherited chest wall deformity with an occurrence of 0.3% of all births (9:1 predominance in males). In patients with pectus excavatum, the normally moderately convex contour of the anterior chest wall is replaced by precordial depression. Depending on the severity of the anomaly, the sternovertebral space is narrowed, there is a shift of the heart into the left hemithorax and pulmonary expansion is confined.

The indications for surgery may be summarised as follows.

- Aesthetic (psychological repercussion)
- Symptom
- Exercise intolerance, decreased endurance or exercise-induced asthma
- Body images issues (CT scan)
- Pain
- Abnormal/low FVC, FEV_1 or maximum voluntary ventilation
- Decreased oxygen pulse, oxygen uptake or V'_E
- Echocardiogram: compression of right atrium/right ventricle (rare)
- CT Haller index >3.0
- Calliper measurement depth >2.5 cm

Pectus carinatum In pectus carinatum, the clinical aspect includes a variety of protrusion deformities of the anterior chest wall. The most common variety consists of anterior displacement of the sternal gladiolus with the appropriate cartilages in tow. In severe forms, there is also a narrowing of the transverse diameter of the chest, which seems to further exaggerate the anomaly.

The indications for surgery may be summarised as follows.

• Aesthetic (psychological repercussion)
• Pain
• Frequent injury
• Body image issues
• Abnormal pulmonary function testing

Surgical treatment

Pectus excavatum Although there are a number of different techniques utilised by surgeons, most repairs performed today will be either the modified Ravitch technique or the Nuss procedure (note that the Wada procedure of sternal turnover is no longer used).

The Ravitch technique requires the exposition of the thorax's anterior region (horizontal inframammary fold incision preferred) with resection of costal cartilages affected bilaterally, the performance of a cross-sternal osteotomy with the placing of a temporary stabiliser (support bar anterior to the sternum), and the development of a muscular flap.

The Nuss technique is an alternative and new technique performed by means of minimally invasive surgery, and based on the skeleton's malleability and the remodelling capacity of the thorax. The technique consists of the implantation of a retrosternal steel bar that modifies the concavity of the sternum while maintaining the contour of the reformed thorax, all by means of two small incisions on each side of the thorax. In terms of chest wall kinematics, the Nuss procedure increases chest wall volume by 11% without affecting chest wall displacement or rib cage configuration.

Pectus carinatum The repair of pectus carinatum, including exposure, detachment of the pectoralis muscles, transverse osteotomy and resection of the deformed cartilages, is largely identical to that described in pectus excavatum. Operative correction requires double bilateral chondrotomy parasternally and at points of transition to the normal ribs, followed by detorsion of the sternum, retrosternal mobilisation and correction of the everted sternum, as well as of the everted and inverted ribs. After incomplete wedge osteotomy, the mobilised sternum is finally stabilised by a temporary support bar anterior to the sternum and cartilages (in place for $\geqslant 6$ months).

Controversies

Some controversies do need to be mentioned. First, concerning pectus excavatum, there has never been a randomised controlled trial comparing the results of the two most common surgical procedures. The meta-analysis by Nasr *et al.* (2010) comparing the Nuss procedure and the Ravitch technique repair suggested no differences with respect to overall complications, length of hospital stay or time to ambulation. Secondly, concerning the optimal timing of surgical repair, it seems that the best time for repair would be after the main growth has stopped (*i.e.* after adolescence in the late teens or early 20s), as opposed to early repair. Although the operation is more traumatic after adolescence, the results are far better with minimal recurrence. Thirdly, the goal of such an approach remains elusive. Not only are we unable to reach an agreement on such simple issues as how to measure the clinical or even the anatomical severity of pectoral deformities, but we are still engaged in a seemingly endless debate with the insurance companies as to whether these often physiologically and psychologically crippling abnormalities should be even considered a 'disease' at all.

Conclusion

Chest wall abnormalities (pectus excavatum and pectus carinatum) are a relatively rare problem but are commonly seen in the practice of general thoracic surgery. Careful pre-operative evaluation on the basis of clinical but also psychological symptoms is required to select potential candidates for surgical remodelling. Surgical procedures, based on the surgeon's personal expertise, are currently relatively well codified and provide satisfactory results with a low rate of complications.

Further reading

- Binazzi B, et al. (2012). Effects of the Nuss procedure on chest wall kinematics in adolescents with pectus excavatum. *Respir Physiol Neurobiol*; 183: 122–127.
- Colombani PM (2009). Preoperative assessment of chest wall deformities. *Semin Thorac Cardiovasc Surg*; 21: 58–63.
- Emil S, et al. (2012). Pectus carinatum treatment in Canada: current practices. *J Pediatr Surg*; 47: 862–826.
- Feng J, et al. (2001). The biomechanical, morphologic, and histochemical properties of the costal cartilages in children with pectus excavatum. *J Pediatr Surg*; 36: 1770–1776.
- Fonkalsrud EW, et al. (2004). Less extensive techniques for repair of pectus carinatum: the undertreated chest deformity. *J Am Coll Surg*; 198: 898–905.
- Gurnett CA, et al. (2009). Genetic linkage localizes an adolescent idiopathic scoliosis and pectus excavatum gene to chromosome 18 q. *Spine (Phila Pa 1976)*; 34: E94–E100.
- Haller JA, et al. (1989). Evolving management of pectus excavatum based on a single institutional experience of 664 patients. *Ann Surg*; 209: 578–583.
- Huddelston CB (2004). Pectus excavatum. *Semin Thorac Cardiovasc Surg*; 16: 225–232.
- Nasr A, et al. (2010). Comparison of the Nuss and the Ravitch procedure for pectus excavatum repair: a meta-analysis. *J Pediatr Surg*; 45: 880–886.
- Nuss D, et al. (1998). A ten-year review of minimally invasive technique for the correction of pectus excavatum. *J Pediatr Surg*; 33: 545–552.
- Ravitch MM (1949). The operative treatment of pectus excavatum. *Ann Surg*; 129: 429–444.
- Robicsek F, et al. (2009a). Surgical repair of anterior chest wall deformities: the past, the present, the future. Introduction. *Semin Thorac Cardiovasc Surg*; 21: 43.
- Robiscek F, et al. (2009b). Surgical repair of pectus excavatum and carinatum. *Semin Thorac Cardiovasc Surg*; 21: 64–75.
- Saxena AK, et al. (1999). Surgical repair of pectus carinatum. *Int Surg*; 84: 326–330.
- Shamberger SC, et al. Congenital deformities. *In:* Pearson FG, et al., eds. Thoracic Surgery. New York, Churchill Livingstone, 1995; pp. 1189–1209.
- Shu Q, et al. (2011). Experience in minimally invasive Nuss operation for 406 children with pectus excavatum. *World J Pediatr*; 7: 257–261.

Pathology and molecular biology of lung cancer

Sylvie Lantuéjoul, Lénaïg Mescam-Mancini, Barbara Burroni and Anne McLeer-Florin

Lung cancer prognosis is poor, with a global survival rate, all stages combined, of ~15%, mainly because most cases are surgically unresectable at the time of diagnosis. However, the discovery in 2004 of EGFR (epidermal growth factor receptor) mutations in a subset of adenocarcinomas, leading to a specific clinical response to tyrosine kinase inhibitors (TKIs), has raised high hopes towards development of targeted therapies (Travis et al., 2011). Lung tumours in nonsmokers are the seventh cause of death by cancer worldwide and are more readily observed in women, especially in Asia. These tumours are characterised by the presence of a 'driver' mutation – translocation or amplification of an oncogene – leading to constitutive stimulation of cell proliferation and anti-apoptotic signalling pathways in the tumour cells (fig. 1) (Weinstein et al., 2008).

ErbB family

The ErbB family comprises EGFR (also known as ErbB1 or HER1), ErbB2 (HER2 or Neu), ErbB3 (HER3) and ErbB4 (HER4).

> **Key points**
>
> - Lung cancer prognosis is poor, most cases being surgically unresectable at the time of diagnosis.
>
> - Driver mutations, translocations or amplifications are involved in lung oncogenesis, and have led to a molecular classification of lung tumours.

EGFR gene mutations lead to activation of the Ras/mitogen-activated protein kinase (MAPK) and phosphatidylinositol-3-kinase (PI3K)/AKT downstream pathways. These mutations are found in 50% of adenocarcinomas in Asian patients and in only 15% of Caucasian patients (West et al., 2012). They mostly arise in nonsmoking women with papillar or lepidic adenocarcinomas, according to the new World Health Organization (WHO) classification of lung adenocarcinoma (Travis et al., 2011), that are thyroid transcription factor (TTF)1 positive (Shigematsu et al., 2006). In 85% of cases, these activating mutations correspond to a deletion in exon 19 (39%) or a point mutation (L858R) in exon 21 (46%), and confer sensitivity to the EGFR TKI gefitinib (marketed as Iressa by AstraZeneca, London, UK) and erlotinib (Tarceva; Genentech–Roche, San Francisco, CA, USA), which are US Food and Drug Administration (FDA)-approved for the treatment of mutated metastatic non-small cell lung carcinomas (NSCLCs) (Uramoto et al., 2007). Conversely, insertion in exon 20 is correlated with primary resistance to EGFR TKIs, and the T790M mutation is associated with secondary resistance (Cheng et al., 2012). Antibodies raised against the exon 19-deleted form (del746–750) (clone 6B6; Cell Signaling Technology (Danvers, MA, USA) monoclonal antibody (mAb) 2085) and the exon 21-mutated form (L858R) (clone D38B1; Cell Signaling Technology mAb 3197) are in development for diagnosis by immunohistochemistry, with sensitivities ranging from 40% to 100% and specificities from 88% to 100% (Kitamura et al., 2010).

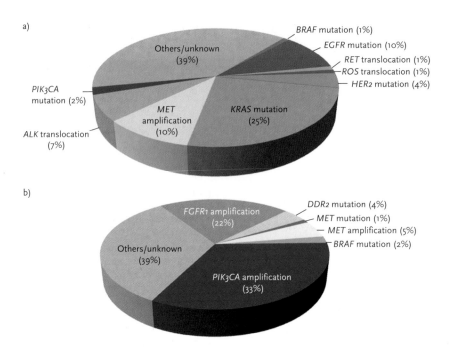

Figure 1. Druggable genetic abnormalities (mutation, amplification and rearrangement) in pulmonary a) adenocarcinomas and b) squamous cell carcinomas in Caucasian patients.

Mutations of *HER2* and *HER4* are rare (2–4%). *HER2* mutations (exon 20) arise in nonsmoking Asian women, and could confer sensitivity to trastuzumab and pan-EGFR/HER2 inhibitors (lapatinib, BIBW29952, neratinib, *etc.*) (Brabender *et al.*, 2001).

KRAS and *BRAF*

KRAS mutations are observed in up to 30% of adenocarcinomas. *KRAS* and *EGFR* mutations are mutually exclusive (Shigematsu *et al.*, 2006), and *KRAS* mutations are associated with a resistance to EGFR TKIs.

BRAF is a downstream effector of *RAS*. The *BRAF* V600E mutation is the most frequent (50%), before G469A (39%) and D594G (11%). They are observed in 3% of NSCLCs. Mutations other than V600E are more common in smokers; V600E is more common in women with micropapillar adenocarcinoma of poor prognosis. These mutations could confer sensitivity to MEK (MAPK kinase) inhibitors (Paik *et al.*, 2011).

ALK

In 2007, *ALK* (anaplastic lymphoma kinase) (chromosome 2p23) and *EML4* (echinoderm microtubule-associated protein-like 4) (2p21) gene rearrangement was identified in NSCLC (Soda *et al.*, 2007). Other *ALK* partners have been reported, such as *TFG* (TRK-fused gene), *KIF5B* (kinesin family member 5B) and *KLC1* (kinesin light chain 1) (Takeuchi *et al.*, 2012; Togashi *et al.*, 2012). These rearrangements are observed in 3–7% of NCSLCs and are mutually exclusive with *EGFR* and *KRAS* mutations. Patients with *ALK* rearrangement are often young, light smokers or nonsmokers at an advanced stage with frequent pleural localisations (Soda *et al.*, 2007). *ALK*-positive tumours are mostly TTF1-positive adenocarcinomas with signet-ring cells (Rodig *et al.*, 2009). A favourable response with the FDA-approved small molecule ALK and Met inhibitor crizotinib (PF-02341066) has been obtained in phase I/II clinical trials. FISH (fluorescence *in situ* hybridisation) remains the gold-standard technique for diagnosis but this technique is costly and time-consuming, and several authors have suggested pre-screening by immunohistochemistry (fig. 2a and b) with two antibodies (clone 5A4 (Abcam, Cambridge, UK) and D5F3 (Cell Signaling Technology)) presenting high sensitivities and specificities (92–100% and 99–100%, respectively) (McLeer-Florin *et al.*, 2012).

ROS1 and RET

ROS1 (c-Ros oncogene 1, 6q22) rearrangements have been detected in 0.9–1.7% of NSCLCs (Bergethon *et al.*, 2012; Takeuchi *et al.*, 2012) and *RET* (Ret proto-oncogene, 10q11.2) rearrangements are observed in 1.2% of adenocarcinomas. Both types of rearrangements arise in young light smoking or nonsmoking patients with adenocarcinomas, and seem to be mutually exclusive with *EGFR* mutations or *ALK* rearrangements. Crizotinib could target *ROS1* rearranged tumours and vandetanib, a VEGFR (vascular endothelial growth factor receptor), EGFR and Ret inhibitor, could inhibit *RET*-rearranged tumour cell proliferation (Takeuchi *et al.*, 2012).

MET

In lung cancer, the c-Met pathway, including PI3K/AKT/mammalian target of rapamycin (mTOR), Ras/MEK/MAPK, Src and STAT (signal transducer and activator of transcription), is activated either *via* ligand (hepatocyte growth factor (HGF)) or receptor overexpression, *MET* gene

amplification, mutations, or alternative splicing (Feng *et al.*, 2012). Various scores for c-Met overexpression and *MET* amplification have been proposed (fig. 2c and d). *MET* amplification seems to be correlated with a poor outcome (Cappuzzo *et al.*, 2009), and c-Met phosphorylation with the development of brain metastases and primary and acquired resistance to EGFR TKIs (Benedettini *et al.*, 2010).

PIK3CA

The *PIK3CA* gene is mutated in 3.6% of squamous cell carcinomas (SCCs) and 2% of adenocarcinomas with an acinar or papillary histology (Samuels *et al.*, 2005). Mutations affect exons 9 and 20, and amplification of the 3q25–27 genomic region containing *PIK3CA* (3q26) is detected in 10% NSCLC. In SCC, 3q26 amplification is reported in 40% of cases. These mutations or amplifications are not exclusive with those of *EGFR* and *KRAS*. Various PI3K inhibitors are under development, some also targeting mTOR (Heist *et al.*, 2012).

FGFR1

Amplification of *FGFR1* (fibroblast growth factor receptor 1, 8p12) has recently been discovered in 20% of SCCs and 3.4% of adenocarcinomas (Weiss *et al.*, 2010). Inhibition of FGFR1 by a pan-FGFR TKI, PD173074, is being evaluated in a phase I trial (www.clinicaltrials.gov identifier NCT00979134).

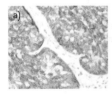 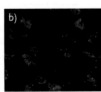 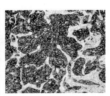 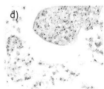

Figure 2. Examples of ALK and c-Met changes in NSCLC. a) Immunohistochemical expression of ALK fusion protein (Abcam clone 5A4). b) ALK gene rearrangement demonstrated by break-apart FISH (Vysis LSI ALK Dual-Color Break Apart Rearrangement Probe; Abbott Molecular, Des Plaines, IL, USA) showing typical split signals (red and green) in the same ALK-rearranged tumour as in a). c) Immunohistochemical expression of c-Met protein (clone SP44; Ventana Medical Systems, Oro Valley, AZ, USA). d) MET gene amplification demonstrated by SISH (silver in situ hybridisation) (black: MET gene; red: chromosome 7 centromere) (Ventana Medical Systems).

Conclusion

Historically, lung cancer classification and treatment were based on tumour histology. Recent discovery of driver mutations in genes encoding tyrosine kinases have led to a molecular classification of lung tumours, allowing the emergence of a personalised, targeted therapy, and improved outcomes.

Further reading

- Benedettini E, *et al.* (2010). Met activation in non-small cell lung cancer is associated with *de novo* resistance to EGFR inhibitors and the development of brain metastasis. *Am J Pathol*; 177: 415–423.
- Bergethon K, *et al.* (2012). *ROS1* rearrangements define a unique molecular class of lung cancers. *J Clin Oncol*; 30: 863–870.
- Brabender J, *et al.* (2001). Epidermal growth factor receptor and HER2-neu mRNA expression in non-small cell lung cancer is correlated with survival. *Clin Cancer Res*; 7: 1850–1855.
- Cappuzzo F, *et al.* (2009). Increased *MET* gene copy number negatively affects survival of surgically resected non-small-cell lung cancer patients. *J Clin Oncol*; 27: 1667–1674.
- Cheng L, *et al.* (2012). Molecular pathology of lung cancer: key to personalized medicine. *Mod Pathol*; 25: 347–369.
- Feng Y, *et al.* (2012). MET signaling: novel targeted inhibition and its clinical development in lung cancer. *J Thorac Oncol*; 7: 459–467.
- Heist R, *et al.* (2012). Genetic changes in squamous cell lung cancer: a review. *J Thorac Oncol*; 7: 924–933.
- Kitamura A, *et al.* (2010). Immunohistochemical detection of *EGFR* mutation using mutation-specific antibodies in lung cancer. *Clin Cancer Res*; 16: 3349–3355.
- McLeer-Florin A, *et al.* (2012). Dual IHC and FISH testing for *ALK* gene rearrangement in lung adenocarcinomas in a routine practice: a French study. *J Thorac Oncol*; 7: 348–354.
- Paik PK, *et al.* (2011). Clinical characteristics of patients with lung adenocarcinomas harboring *BRAF* mutations. *J Clin Oncol*; 29: 2046–2051.
- Rodig SJ, *et al.* (2009). Unique clinicopathologic features characterize *ALK*-rearranged lung adenocarcinoma in the western population. *Clin Cancer Res*; 15: 5216–5223.
- Samuels Y, *et al.* (2005). Mutant PIK3CA promotes cell growth and invasion of human cancer cells. *Cancer Cell*; 7: 561–573.
- Shigematsu H, *et al.* (2006). Somatic mutations of epidermal growth factor receptor signaling pathway in lung cancers. *Int J Cancer*; 118: 257–262.
- Soda M, *et al.* (2007). Identification of the transforming *EML4–ALK* fusion gene in non-small-cell lung cancer. *Nature*; 448: 561–566.
- Takeuchi K, *et al.* (2012). *RET, ROS1* and *ALK* fusions in lung cancer. *Nat Med*; 18: 378–381.
- Togashi Y, *et al.* (2012). *KLC1–ALK*: a novel fusion in lung cancer identified using a formalin-fixed paraffin-embedded tissue only. *PLoS One*; 7: e31323.
- Travis WD, *et al.* (2011). International association for the study of lung cancer/american thoracic society/european respiratory society international multidisciplinary classification of lung adenocarcinoma. *J Thorac Oncol*; 6: 244–285.
- Uramoto H, *et al.* (2007). Which biomarker predicts benefit from EGFR-TKI treatment for patients with lung cancer? *Br J Cancer*; 96: 857–863.
- Weinstein IB, *et al.* (2008). Oncogene addiction. *Cancer Res*; 68: 3077–3080.
- Weiss J, *et al.* (2010). Frequent and focal *FGFR1* amplification associates with therapeutically tractable FGFR1 dependency in squamous cell lung cancer. *Sci Transl Med*; 2: 62–93.
- West L, *et al.* (2012). A novel classification of lung cancer into molecular subtypes. *PLoS One*; 7: e31906.

Lung cancer: diagnosis and staging

Johan Vansteenkiste, Sofie Derijcke and Inge Hantson

Lung cancer is the most common cause of cancer-related mortality worldwide for both males and females, with a global incidence of about 1.3 million cases per year. The term lung cancer, or bronchogenic carcinoma, refers to malignancies that originate in the airways or pulmonary parenchyma.

Epidemiology

Lung cancer occurs through a complex multistage process that results from the combination of carcinogen exposure and genetic susceptibility (fig. 1).

A number of lifestyle and environmental factors have been associated with the development of lung cancer, of which cigarette smoking is the most important. Cigarette smoking accounts for approximately 80–90% of all lung cancers. Compared with nonsmokers, smokers have an ~20-fold increase in lung cancer risk, depending on the duration of smoking and the number of cigarettes smoked per day. Cigarette smokers can benefit at any age

from smoking cessation: as the period of abstinence from smoking increases, the risk of lung cancer decreases, although it remains elevated compared with never-smokers. However, in recent years, an increasing number of never-smoking patients present with a lung cancer, often females with adenocarcinoma histology. A number of other factors may affect the risk of developing lung cancer, such as underlying acquired lung diseases (COPD and pulmonary fibrosis) and environmental exposures, often synergistically with smoking (asbestos, radon, metals, ionising radiation including previous radiotherapy, fine dust air pollution and polycyclic aromatic hydrocarbons).

Several molecular genetic abnormalities have been described in lung cancer, including chromosomal aberrations (*e.g.* chromosome 3p or 8p deletions), overexpression of oncogenes (*EGFR*, *KRAS*, *c-MET*, *BCL2*, *etc.*), deletions and/or mutations in tumour suppressor genes (*TP53*, *RB1* and genes on chromosome 3p) or altered telomerase activity.

Clinical manifestations

The majority of patients with lung cancer have advanced disease at clinical presentation, which reflects the frequent asymptomatic course of early-stage lung cancer.

Symptoms due to the intrathoracic effects of the tumour are cough (central airway or pleural involvement), haemoptysis, chest pain, dyspnoea, hoarseness (laryngeal nerve involvement), superior vena cava syndrome (dilated neck veins and facial oedema), Pancoast syndrome (pain, Horner sign and hand muscle atrophy).

Key points

- The pulmonologist has a crucial role in obtaining tissue for diagnosis and molecular analyses.

- Lung cancer staging is a stepwise process of more general tests for all, and more dedicated tests for patients with a prospect of radical treatment.

- Functional assessment is key for patients with a prospect of radical treatment.

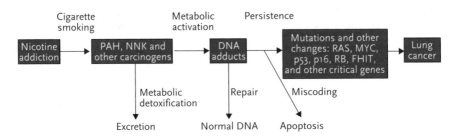

Figure 1. The multistep process leading from nicotine addiction to lung cancer. PAH: polyaromatic hydrocarbons; NHK: nicotine-derived nitrosamine ketone. Reproduced from Hecht (1999) with permission from the publisher.

In addition, paraneoplastic effects of lung cancer are common: hypercalcaemia (nausea, lethargy and dehydration), syndrome of inappropriate antidiuretic hormone (hyponatraemia), hypertrophic osteoarthropathy (clubbing and periosteal proliferation of tubular bones), dermatomyositis, haematological manifestations (anaemia, leukocytosis and thrombocytosis), hypercoagulability, Cushing's syndrome and neurological syndromes (Lambert–Eaton). It is important to distinguish paraneoplastic effects from symptoms due to metastasis, as only the latter impede a radical approach.

As for extrathoracic disease, the most frequent sites of distant metastases are the liver (pain and constitutional symptoms), adrenal glands, bones (pain) and brain (headache, paresis and seizures). General symptoms such as anorexia, weight loss and asthenia are often also present.

Diagnosis

Bronchoscopy is the appropriate test for centrally located tumours, where a pathological diagnosis will be obtained in ~90% of cases, by means of forceps biopsy, bronchial brushing or washing.

Peripheral lesions, especially solitary pulmonary nodules, can be a diagnostic challenge. Noninvasive techniques are positron emission tomography (PET) with ^{18}F-2-fluoro-2-deoxy-D-glucose (FDG) (enhanced uptake of FDG is seen in tumours) or contrast-enhanced CT. For most lesions, pathological documentation is needed: peripheral

sampling of tissue by bronchoscopy (nowadays assisted by endobronchial ultrasound), fine-needle aspiration by CT guidance or, sometimes, surgical sampling by video-assisted thoracoscopy.

Historically, very small diagnostic samples were sufficient to make the pathological diagnosis of either non-small cell lung cancer (NSCLC) or small cell lung cancer (SCLC). One of the major recent advances in chemotherapy and molecular targeted therapy has been the use tissue-based predictive factors for treatment efficacy (e.g. nonsquamous histology for pemetrexed, activating EGFR mutation for gefitinib or erlotinib and EML4–ALK translocation mutation for crizotinib). This has largely changed the role of the pulmonologist in the diagnostic process and reversed the evolution of diagnosis based on ever smaller samples to one based on ever less invasive techniques. In order to respond to the increasing demand for larger amounts of tissue to perform additional immunohistochemistry, fluorescence in situ hybridisation or mutation testing, it now important to maximise the number of biopsies at bronchoscopy, to make cell blocks of the cytological samples obtained at endobronchial ultrasound-guide transbronchial needle aspiration (EBUS-TBNA) or to use larger core needles when taking a CT-guided transthoracic biopsy.

Staging

Staging, the process of determining the extent of lung cancer, is crucial for the prognosis and choice of treatment. The stage is defined by the international TNM (tumour, node, metastasis) classification. The most recent version, adopted since 2010, is applicable to NSCLC, SCLC and carcinoid tumours. The combination of T, N, and M descriptors determines the overall disease stage: stage I (localised tumour and no lymph node spread); stage II (spread to hilar nodes); stage III (more advanced tumour and/or mediastinal lymph node spread); and stage IV (distant metastasis) (table 1).

Staging is a stepwise process. For all patients, the minimal noninvasive staging will include a detailed medical history (smoking habits, occupational history, intra- and extrathoracic and paraneoplastic symptoms, and performance status), a physical examination (e.g. careful auscultation and percussion may suggest the presence of atelectasis, pleural effusion or large airway obstruction, liver enlargement may indicate hepatic metastases, etc.), blood testing and a contrast-enhanced CT from the adrenal gland to the lung apex. According to symptoms and locoregional spread, CT or MRI of the brain, bone scintigraphy, or other tests may be appropriate.

Patients with a potential for radical treatment (i.e. no evident metastatic disease or major comorbidity) will usually need additional tests. They will benefit from FDG-PET or fusion FDG-PET-CT, which improve staging of locoregional lymph node and distant spread (e.g. PET may indicate unexpected metastases in up to 20% of patients).

In nonmetastatic patients, the exact definition of locoregional spread will help to choose the best type of multimodality treatment (i.e. how to combine chemotherapy, surgery and radiotherapy). Detailed invasive locoregional staging often is indicated for that purpose, as the value of CT to ascertain the nature of mediastinal lymph nodes is limited: pooled positive predictive value 50% and negative predictive value 80%. Addition of PET has improved these figures to 80% and 90%, respectively. Based on a recent landmark randomised trial, endoscopic staging has taken over the role of mediastinoscopy as initial test in most patients. Endoscopic lymph node staging consists of EBUS-TBNA (for paratracheal nodes 2R, 2L, 4R and 4L, subcarinal node 7, and hilar nodes 10R, 10L, 11R and 11L) and/or oesophageal ultrasound-guided fine-needle aspiration (for left paratracheal nodes 4L and 5, subcarinal node 7, paraoesophageal nodes 8 and 9, and hilar nodes 10R and 10L) (fig. 2). These techniques can reduce the need for baseline surgical staging by 70%. Endoscopic staging

Table 1. Major staging groups, preferred treatment patterns and expected 5-year survival rates for NSCLC

Stage	Treatment	5-year survival %
Early		
I	Surgical resection (adjuvant chemotherapy for large tumours) Radiotherapy if medically inoperable	58–73
II	Surgical resection and adjuvant chemotherapy Radiotherapy if medically inoperable	36–46
Locally advanced		
IIIA	Surgical or nonsurgical combined-modality treatment	24
IIIB	Nonsurgical combined-modality treatment	9
Advanced		
IV	Chemotherapy and/or targeted agents	<5
Data from Goldstraw *et al.* (2007).		

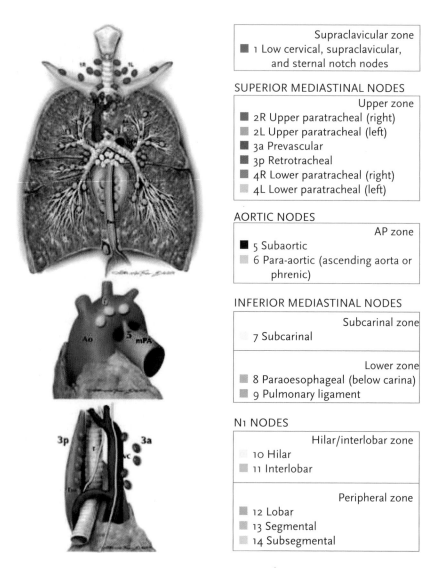

	Supraclavicular zone
■	1 Low cervical, supraclavicular, and sternal notch nodes

SUPERIOR MEDIASTINAL NODES

	Upper zone
■	2R Upper paratracheal (right)
▨	2L Upper paratracheal (left)
■	3a Prevascular
■	3p Retrotracheal
■	4R Lower paratracheal (right)
▢	4L Lower paratracheal (left)

AORTIC NODES

	AP zone
■	5 Subaortic
▢	6 Para-aortic (ascending aorta or phrenic)

INFERIOR MEDIASTINAL NODES

	Subcarinal zone
▢	7 Subcarinal

	Lower zone
▨	8 Paraoesophageal (below carina)
▨	9 Pulmonary ligament

N1 NODES

	Hilar/interlobar zone
▢	10 Hilar
▨	11 Interlobar

	Peripheral zone
▨	12 Lobar
▨	13 Segmental
▢	14 Subsegmental

Figure 2. Map of locoregional lymph nodes. Reproduced and modified from Rusch et al. (2007) with permission from the publisher.

may lead to false-negative results in ~20% of the cases; therefore, a negative test result in a patient suspected of having lymph node disease should be completed by an adequate surgical procedure. Another important advantage of using endoscopic techniques upfront is that mediastinoscopic staging can be reserved as the most

accurate technique for assessment of lymph node staging after induction treatment.

Functional assessment

All patients need an ECG and basic pulmonary function tests, such as FEV_1 and FVC. In patients scheduled for radical treatment (surgical or nonsurgical combined-modality treatment), a more detailed functional evaluation is needed, especially as many patients have co-existing smoking-related cardiopulmonary disease. To determine the volume of lung that can be removed and to identify patients at risk of post-operative complications, each patient should undergo pulmonary function testing: lung volumes and TLCO. Post-operative respiratory failure rarely occurs if the predicted post-resection FEV1 and TLCO are more than 30–40% of the normal values.

Additional cardiopulmonary exercise testing with ergospirometry is indicated when baseline FEV1 or TLCO values are <80% predicted. In this group, patients who reach their target heart rate and exercise capacity and who have a maximal oxygen uptake (V'_{O_2}max) >15 mL·kg^{-1}·min^{-1} are less likely to have post-operative complications or mortality. If the V'_{O_2}max is between 10 and 20 mL·kg^{-1}·min^{-1}, quantitative pulmonary perfusion scanning may be used to calculate more precisely the estimated post-operative values and the proportion of lung that can be removed. Moreover, patients with a baseline oxygen saturation of <90%, those who desaturate more than 4% during exercise testing or those with PaCO$_2$ >45 mmHg have a greater likelihood of post-operative complications.

Apart from pulmonary function evaluation, assessment of other comorbid conditions, such as heart disease (echocardiography and coronary tests), renal insufficiency and diabetes, may be warranted. ·

Further reading

- Alberg AJ, et al. (2007). Epidemiology of lung cancer: ACCP evidence-based clinical practice guidelines (2nd edition). Chest; 132: Suppl. 3, 29S–55S.
- Annema JT, et al. (2010). Mediastinoscopy versus endosonography for mediastinal nodal staging of lung cancer. A randomized trial. JAMA; 304: 2245–2252.
- Brunelli A, et al. (2009). ERS/ESTS clinical guidelines on fitness for radical therapy in lung cancer patients (surgery and chemo-radiotherapy). Eur Respir J; 34: 17–41.
- Goldstraw P, et al. (2007). The IASLC Lung Cancer Staging Project: proposals for the revision of the TNM stage groupings in the forthcoming (seventh) edition of the TNM Classification of malignant tumours. J Thorac Oncol; 2: 706–714.
- Hecht SS (1999). Tobacco smoke carcinogens and lung cancer. J Natl Cancer Inst; 91: 1194–1210.
- Rusch VW, et al. (2007). The IASLC lung cancer staging project: proposals for the revision of the N descriptors in the forthcoming seventh edition of the TNM classification for lung cancer. J Thorac Oncol; 2: 603–612.
- Toh CK, et al. (2006). Never-smokers with lung cancer: epidemiologic evidence of a distinct disease entity. J Clin Oncol; 24: 2245–2251.
- Vansteenkiste J, et al. (2010). Early stage NSCLC: challenges in staging and adjuvant treatment: evidence-based staging. Ann Oncol; 21: Suppl. 7, 189–195.

Chemotherapy and molecular biological therapy

Amanda Tufman and Rudolf M. Huber

Most patients with lung cancer present in advanced stages of disease and cannot be cured by surgery or radiation therapy. In metastatic disease, the focus of treatment is palliation of symptoms and maintenance of quality of life. Systemic treatment with chemotherapy and with newer 'targeted' therapies form the basis of treatment in stage IV, and can significantly improve symptoms, and improve both progression-free and overall survival. Whereas chemotherapy involves the use of substances with nonspecific cytotoxic and antiproliferative properties, molecular biological therapy aims at more specific targets that are usually more active than normal.

Depending on the clinical situation, either a single chemotherapeutic agent or a doublet may be given. If the patient is fit enough for chemotherapy, a platinum-based doublet is used. Differences in tumour histology and molecular biology are increasingly taken into account when planning systemic therapy, in particular for non-small cell lung cancer (NSCLC).

In earlier stages of disease, systemic chemotherapy can be curative when combined with local irradiation (radiochemotherapy) or surgery. Chemotherapy given after surgery is known as adjuvant chemotherapy; that administered before surgery is neoadjuvant or induction chemotherapy. Generally, chemotherapy is administered intravenously, although some agents may be given orally. There are also circumstances in which chemotherapeutic agents may be administered locally (intrathecally or in the pleural space). Although most modern chemotherapeutic agents have milder side-effects than the older agents, side-effects remain problematic and include neutropenia, neuropathy, nephropathy, fatigue, hair loss, and nausea and vomiting (table 1).

Key points

- Due to the interdisciplinary nature of lung cancer treatment, decision-making should take place in structured tumour boards.

- Performance status is an important parameter in treatment decision-making.

- The side-effects of chemotherapy vary between agents and should be taken into account during treatment planning.

- Endobronchial techniques are an important tool in the palliation of lung cancer patients.

- First-line treatment of advanced NSCLC, adjuvant chemotherapy and chemotherapy for radiochemotherapy is mostly a platinum-based doublet.

- The individualisation of treatment based on histology and molecular biology, in particular the EGFR mutation and EML4–ALK fusion, is of increasing importance in NSCLC.

- SCLC generally responds well to initial chemotherapy.

- Prophylactic cranial irradiation has an important role in the treatment of SCLC.

Table 1. *The major side-effects of chemotherapeutic agents*

Nausea and vomiting	Cisplatin is highly emetogenic Prophylactic antiemetics should be given to all patients receiving chemotherapy Delayed nausea and vomiting may occur days after administration Commonly used antiemetics include dexamethasone, serotonin antagonists and neurokinin-1 inhibition
Neutropenia	Severe neutropenia refers to peripheral neutrophil counts <500 cells·μL^{-1} Reverse isolation in hospitalised patients with severe neutropenia may reduce the risk of nosocomial infections Febrile neutropenia refers to elevated oral or axillary temperature (>38°C for >1 h or >38.2°C one-time measurement) in the setting of severe neutropenia, and should be treated with intravenous antibiotics The prophylactic use of granulocyte colony-stimulating factors can be considered in those at increased risk of developing febrile neutropenia
Anaemia	Consider transfusion in symptomatic patients or those with very low haemoglobin The use of erythrocyte-stimulating factors (*e.g.* erythropoietin) is generally not recommended; however, it can reduce the number of transfusions and improves fatigue
Neuropathy	Most commonly caused by the taxanes and vinorelbine
Fatigue	Multifactorial Malnutrition, anaemia and depression commonly play a role

How to treat a patient is dependent not only on the diagnosis itself but on the patient's comorbidities and overall medical condition, as well as on the overall prognosis and goal of treatment (table 2). Performance status scales attempt to standardise the assessment of a patient's general state of health; the Karnofsky scale and the World Health Organization (WHO)/Eastern Cooperative Oncology Group (ECOG) scale are commonly used (table 3).

In most cases, the overall management of lung cancer involves a combination of chemotherapy, radiation, bronchoscopic intervention and surgery. For this reason, interdisciplinary tumour boards are an important forum for discussion and decision-making in the care of lung cancer patients.

Chemotherapy in small cell lung cancer

First line Small cell lung cancer (SCLC) is almost always a systemic disease and, in most cases, the initial response to chemotherapy is quite good.

Cisplatin plus etoposide is a frequently used first-line combination, although carboplatin can be used instead of cisplatin in patients with poor prognosis/performance status or contraindications to cisplatin. Another commonly used but less effective regimen is adriamycin, cyclophosphamide and vincristine. In SCLC, chemotherapy offers a clear survival benefit, from 4–6-week survival in untreated patients with extensive disease, to 12-month survival in extensive disease with chemotherapy.

Second line The second-line treatment of SCLC has been shown to increase survival and quality of life compared with best supportive care alone. Here, the choice of medications depends on the length of time since the initial remission. For patients whose tumours initially respond well to chemotherapy and then go on to recur or progress >3–6 months later, the medications used in first-line treatment can be given again. Tumours that progress <3 months after the end of first-line therapy should be treated with different agents: in this setting, topotecan monotherapy is a common choice and can be given intravenously or orally. If the tumour does not respond to first-line therapies or

Table 2. Considerations for individual chemotherapeutic agents

Cisplatin	Highly emetogenic (appropriate use of anti-emetics is essential) Nephrotoxic: avoid in patients with reduced GFR Pre-hydration ($\geqslant$500 mL NaCl 0.9% per 50 mg cisplatin) reduces the risk of nephrotoxicity
Carboplatin	Consider as alternative to cisplatin in elderly patients or those with contraindications to cisplatin, dosed at AUC
Vinorelbine	May cause neuropathy or neutropenia Available in pill form for oral administration
Gemcitabine	30-min infusion time (more toxicity with slower infusion), avoid combination with radiotherapy due to increased side-effects
Pemetrexed	Short (10-min) infusion time Effective in patients with nonsquamous cell NSCLC and mesothelioma The risk of myelosuppression can be significantly reduced by vitamin B_{12} (1000 IU *i.m.* every 9 weeks) and folate (0.35–1 mg·day^{-1})
Paclitaxel	Premedication to prevent allergic reaction is required (dexamethasone and antihistamine)
Docetaxel	Premedication to prevent allergic reaction is required (dexamethasone)

GFR: glomerular filtration rate; AUC: area under the curve; *i.m.*: intramuscular.

progresses quickly after chemotherapy, second-line treatment is usually recommended. Inclusion in clinical trials or best supportive care alone are also reasonable options.

Multimodal therapy Studies have shown that adjuvant chemotherapy improves survival in SCLC patients with completely resected, very limited disease. In patients with limited disease, local radiation is generally combined with chemotherapy. Concurrent chemoradiation regimens including cisplatin are the most effective. In extensive SCLC, thoracic radiation may be considered in patients who have responded well to chemotherapy.

Prophylactic cranial irradiation has been shown to improve survival in SCLC patients who reach good remission after chemotherapy, including those with extensive disease at the time of diagnosis.

Nonsmall cell lung cancer

Chemotherapy is the treatment of choice for most NSCLC patients with metastases or malignant pleural effusion, although its

Table 3. The WHO/ECOG scale

WHO/ECOG performance status	Description
0	Patient is fully active and unrestricted in daily activities
1	Patient cannot carry out physically strenuous activities but is able to care for self and carry out light work
2	Patient is ambulatory and can care for self but is unable to work Up and about for >50% of waking hours
3	Patient is limited in self-care activities and confined to bed or chair for >50% of waking hours
4	Completely disabled Cannot care for self Totally confined to bed or chair

efficacy is limited. In fit patients, first-line treatment should consist of cisplatin (or carboplatin) paired with one of gemcitabine, docetaxel, paclitaxel, pemetrexed or vinorelbine, administered over four to six cycles. The increase in survival offered by platinum-based chemotherapy is in the range of several months, although some patients experience durable remissions, and there is evidence that chemotherapy improves patients' quality of life and performance status. Unfortunately, ~40% of NSCLC tumours do not respond to chemotherapy and only 20% of NSCLC patients experience significant regression of their tumours. In earlier randomised trials with platinum-based chemotherapy doublets (cisplatin/paclitaxel, cisplatin/gemcitabine, cisplatin/docetaxel, vinorelbine/cisplatin or carboplatin/paclitaxel), there were no significant differences in response rate or overall survival. More recent studies show that histology plays a role in the response of NSCLC to various chemotherapeutic medications. In particular, nonsquamous histology (adenocarcinomas and large cell NSCLC) is predictive for better activity of pemetrexed.

Patients with poor performance status may not tolerate platinum-based doublet chemotherapy but can often be treated with a single chemotherapeutic agent, for instance gemcitabine or paclitaxel, or in some cases with a carboplatin-based doublet. First-line treatment with targeted therapies (see later) is an option for some patients.

Second/third-line chemotherapy in NSCLC generally involves monotherapy with a chemotherapeutic agent (docetaxel for all NSCLC histologies and pemetrexed for nonsquamous histology) or the epidermal growth factor receptor (EGFR) tyrosine kinase inhibitor (TKI) erlotinib. Participation in phase II or III clinical trials with newer targeted agents may offer patients the option of treatment with medications not yet available on the market. There is some recent evidence that early second-line or maintenance therapy with an alternative medication (switch maintenance) or with

one of the original substances (continuation maintenance) may be beneficial, perhaps especially for patients who did not respond particularly well to first-line chemotherapy (stable disease patients compared to partial/ complete responders).

Targeted therapies The role of targeted therapies in NSCLC is growing rapidly. At the moment, especially in adenocarcinoma, in ~50 % of the tumours, we can detect a so-called driving mutation. Unlike traditional chemotherapeutics, which interfere with cell division in all rapidly dividing cells, targeted therapies attempt to inhibit cell activity more selectively at the level of growth factor receptors and intracellular signalling cascades.

EGFR is involved in signalling cascades leading to cell division and proliferation. In tumour cells, mutations in and overexpression of the *EGFR* gene or downstream components of the EGFR pathway increase proliferation, survival and metastasis. Several targeted therapies attempt to interfere with this abnormal EGFR activity: erlotinib and gefitinib are both TKIs that inactivate the intracellular portion of EGFR, whereas cetuximab, as an antibody, binds to the extracellular domain of the receptor. EGFR inhibitors do not cause typical chemotherapy side-effects, but commonly cause clinically significant rash, diarrhoea and liver enzyme elevation.

There is evidence that *EGFR* mutations in exon 19 and 21 (activating mutations) predict a good response to EGFR TKIs, whereas other mutations, such as T790M, may cause resistance. Response to EGFR inhibitors is also associated with certain clinical characteristics (female patients, nonsmokers, adenocarcinoma and Asian ethnicity). Erlotinib is approved as a second- or third-line therapy in NSCLC regardless of *EGFR* mutation status but should only be given in the first line if an activating *EGFR* mutation is present. Gefitinib is only approved for use in patients with a documented activating mutation in *EGFR*. First-line treatment with erlotinib has been demonstrated to improve progression-free survival in European patients harbouring

EGFR mutation compared with first-line chemotherapy.

Usually, a secondary resistance develops during treatment with erlotinib or gefitinib, which is, among others, caused by *MET* amplification or resistance mutations in *EGFR*. For this situation, further treatment in clinical trials would be possible.

Further treatable growth-activating targets are *ALK* (anaplastic lymphoma kinase) gene rearrangements, which occur in approximately 3–5% of NSCLC, especially in adenocarcinoma. *EML4* (echinoderm microtubule-associated protein-like 4)–*ALK* fusion is especially found in patients with NSCLC. Crizotinib is a TKI of MET, c-Ros and ALK. Phase II data have shown these tumours to be highly sensitive to the ALK TKI crizotinib. Crizotinib is approved for the treatment of *EML4–ALK*-positive NSCLC in the USA and Europe.

Because tumours are dependent on the growth of new blood vessels, inhibition of angiogenesis is of major therapeutic interest. Bevacizumab is a monoclonal antibody against vascular endothelial growth factor. In stage IIIB and IV NSCLC patients, there is evidence that the addition of bevacizumab to platinum-based doublets is beneficial. The combination of bevacizumab with carboplatin plus paclitaxel was shown to provide a survival benefit, whereas the combination of bevacizumab with cisplatin plus gemcitabine only showed a benefit in progression-free survival.

Bevacizumab can cause severe haemoptysis, seen in a randomised phase II trial, mostly in patients with squamous cell histology. Thereafter, most studies have excluded patients with brain metastases, previous haemoptysis, cavitary lung lesions or concurrent anticoagulation.

Malignant mesothelioma

If systemic treatment is applied, usually cisplatin plus pemetrexed is given. The data in the literature are not adequately elaborated; in practice, more than six cycles are often used. In patients with contraindications to cisplatin, the off-label use of carboplatin can be considered. There is evidence supporting off-label second-line treatment with vinorelbine, gemcitabine or, in some cases, pemetrexed.

Palliative treatments

In advanced lung cancer, progressive tumour growth in the central airways can produce haemoptysis, cough and airway obstruction leading to shortness of breath or pneumonia. In these situations, quality of life may primarily be improved through the palliative use of endoscopic tumour debulking techniques or prosthetic measures. Brachytherapy is also an effective option for the local treatment of tumour growth in or around the central airways, and stents may be used to maintain airway patency in patients with compression due to tumour. The general supportive/palliative measures are applied additionally as needed.

Palliative radiation provides symptomatic relief in patients with brain and bone metastases. Pleurodesis is an option for patients with recurrent malignant pleural effusions.

Further reading

- American College of Chest Physicians. www.chestnet.org.
- American Society of Clinical Oncology. www.asco.org.
- Azzoli CG, *et al.* (2011). American society of clinical oncology clinical practice guideline update on chemotherapy for stage IV non-small-cell lung cancer. *J Clin Oncol*; 29: 3825–3831.
- D'Addario G, *et al.* (2010). Metastatic non-small cell lung cancer: ESMO clinical practice guidelines for diagnosis, treatment and follow-up. *Ann Oncol*; 21: Suppl. 5, v116–v119.
- International Association for the Study of Lung Cancer. www.iaslc.org.
- Keedy VL, *et al.* (2011). American Society of Clinical Oncology provisional clinical opinion: epidermal growth factor receptor (*EGFR*) mutation testing for patients with advanced non-small cell lung cancer considering first-line EGFR tyrosine-kinase inhibitor (TKI) therapy. *J Clin Oncol*; 29: 2121–2127.

- Scherpereel A, *et al.* (2010). Guidelines of the European Respiratory Society and the European Society of Thoracic Surgeons for the management of malignant pleural mesothelioma. *Eur Respir J*; 35: 479–495.
- Sørensen M, *et al.* (2010). Small-cell lung cancer: ESMO clinical practice guidelines for diagnosis, treatment and follow-up. *Ann Oncol*; 21: Suppl. 5, v120–v125.
- Spiro SG, *et al.*, eds. Thoracic Malignancies. Sheffield, European Respiratory Society, 2009.
- Stahel RA, *et al.* (2010). Malignant pleural mesothelioma: ESMO clinical practice guidelines for diagnosis, treatment and follow-up. *Ann Oncol*; 21: Suppl. 5, v126–v128.

Surgical treatment for lung cancer

Gilbert Massard, Nicola Santelmo and Pierre-Emmanuel Falcoz

Despite the progress made in thoracic oncology over the past 30 years, surgical treatment based on anatomical resection with complete mediastinal lymph node dissection remains the mainstay of cure for nonsmall cell lung cancer (NSCLC). Although combined modality treatments based on neoadjuvant or adjuvant chemotherapy are credited with a slight advantage in survival, the area under the survival curve proves that the most substantial part of cure is owed to surgery. Contemporary alternatives to surgery for small tumours are stereotaxic radiotherapy

and radiofrequency ablation; these treatments are not yet scientifically validated and ignore lymphatic spread (see later). In the N2 category, surgery has been challenged by exclusive radiochemotherapy in a recent multicentre trial by Van Meerbeeck *et al.* (2007), whose conclusions are not acceptable: the surgical arm comprised an incomplete resection rate of nearly 50%. Most patients nowadays are subjected to combined treatments, but the scientific evidence remains ambiguous and controversial. It is unclear whether neoadjuvant therapies are more beneficial to the N2 population or to those with incipient disease. Meta-analysis demonstrated a benefit for patients undergoing adjuvant therapy; this is of weak clinical relevance for the individual patient, given that treatment of 20 patients is needed to save one at 2 years. The result deteriorates in the long term, and long-term complications of chemotherapy appear in survivors. In summary, to date, the best possible surgery needs to be performed in operable patients. Classic resection by open thoracotomy is increasingly challenged by VATS (video-assisted thoracoscopic surgery) in the case of small tumours. Generalisation of screening programmes with low-dose CT is expected to increase considerably accrual of small, T1 tumours in the future (National Lung Screening Trial Research Team, 2011).

Work-up of the patient should include a check-up of fitness according to European Respiratory Society/European Society of Thoracic Surgeons (ESTS) guidelines.

The aim of this section is to describe the quality requirements of contemporary oncologic thoracic surgery, based on

Key points

The following recommendations are evidence based.

- Optimal results are obtained by specialised surgeons working in high-volume units.

- Anatomical resection combined with a complete lymph node dissection is the gold standard. Increasingly VATS is becoming an alternative to open surgery in patients with small tumours.

- Bronchoplastic and angioplastic lobectomies are viable alternatives to pneumonectomy, provided that a complete resection can be achieved.

- Segmentectomies could be applied to high-risk patients with tumours <2 cm in diameter; wedge excisions may be recommended for very small bronchoalveolar carcinoma (ground-glass opacity).

recommendations issued by a working group of the French Society for Thoracic and Cardiovascular Surgery.

How can we define early-stage lung cancer?

Although there is no clear definition of early-stage lung cancer, it seems adequate to restrict this label to patients with reasonable chances of survival. Since lymph node invasion at the N2 level is a marker of poor prognosis, the medical oncologist would certainly restrict the definition to stages No and N1.

For the surgeon, resectable disease offers an advantage over nonresectable disease. Minimal N2, defined as microscopic metastasis to a single N2 node, is credited with a survival rate of 30–35% at 5 years, which is comparable to the worst N1. Furthermore, resectable T4No disease, such as selected cases of Pancoast tumours or main carinal invasion, may achieve a 5-year survival of >40%.

Any marginal situation needs to be discussed with a qualified thoracic surgeon, and any decision not to operate should be validated by a qualified thoracic surgeon in a multidisciplinary discussion.

What are the usual survival figures?

The following figures drawn from the classic surgical literature apply to surgical treatment, regardless of any neoadjuvant or adjuvant treatment.

For stage I, the usual figures vary from 55% to 75% with a substantial difference between T1 and T2. Survival is further influenced by the type of resection (lobectomy *versus* pneumonectomy) and the comorbidity, which accounts for half of late deaths (table 1).

For stage II, reported 5-year survival rates vary between 35% and 50%. Besides a difference between T1N1 and T2N1, there is a very dissimilar survival pattern according to the intra- or extralobar location of the N1 node. Intralobar N1 is credited with 5-year survival close to 55%, whereas in extralobar N1 it reaches only 35% (table 2).

For stage IIIA-N2, survival rates at 5 years are considerably lower and range from 15% to 25%. However, minimal N2 is a subgroup with a possible survival rate of 35% at 5 years. There is a small subset of completely resectable IIIA-T4No disease (Pancoast tumours, main carina involvement) that can achieve a survival of close to 50% at 5 years.

The large majority of patients with stage IIIB are inoperable and global survival at 5 years is <5%.

Quality requirements: the surgeon and the institution

Thoracic oncologic surgery is a specialised medical activity. Well-trained thoracic surgeons working in high-volume units obtain the best results.

Qualification of the individual surgeon A comparison of the results of lung resections performed by either general or well-trained thoracic surgeons in a cohort of 1583 cases of resection for lung cancer performed between 1991 and 1995 showed that operative mortality was twice as high when resection was performed by general surgeons. It is remarkable that 75% of general surgeons performed <10 resections during the observation period.

Hospital volume and its impact on post-operative mortality A review of data from the Medicare registry between 1994 and 1999

Table 1. Survival following stage I disease: independent factors of prognosis

	Yes %	No %	p-value	Relative risk
Pneumonectomy	53	62.7	0.031	1.55
Angio-invasion	54.5	61.9	0.029	1.85
Atherosclerosis	46.3	64.3	0.017	1.55
Data from Thomas *et al.* (2002).				

Table 2. Comparison of 5-year survival for intralobar and extralobar N1

| First author | Patients n | 5-year survival % | |
		Intralobar N1	Extralobar N1
Yano	78	64	39
Van Velzen	391	57	30
Riquet	256	53	38

revealed that operative mortality following lobectomy varied from 6.4% in a low-activity centre (fewer than nine cases per year) to 4.2% in a high-activity centre (>46 cases per year); following pneumonectomy, the range extended from 17% to 10.6%, respectively.

We may conclude that a high hospital volume warrants the necessary routine not only of the operating surgeon, but also of the surrounding team.

Hospital volume and its impact on long-term survival It has been confirmed that hospital volume affects not only early outcome but also long-term survival, in a study that included 2118 patients operated upon in one of 76 hospitals over a 10-year period, divided into quintiles according to hospital volume. Operative mortality ranged from 3% at high- to 6% at low-volume units; operative morbidity ranged 20–44%. The 5-year survival decreased from 44% at high- to 33% at low-volume centres.

This study suggests that appropriate decision-making is enhanced by routine.

Qualification of thoracic surgeons depends on national rules in the different European countries. In an attempt at harmonisation over the European territory, the European Union of Medical Specialists has created the European Board of Thoracic Surgery certification, which may be obtained by an examination conducted every year by the ESTS.

Basic principles of surgical treatment: complete anatomic resection and complete lymph node dissection.

The basic principles described here are based on recommendations issued by a working group of the French Society for Thoracic and Cardiovascular Surgery. A complete cancer operation requires anatomic resection of the primary lesion and complete homolateral lymph-node dissection.

Complete anatomic resection Anatomic resection means either lobectomy or pneumonectomy with precise hilar dissection, according to the locoregional extent of the tumour. The rule is to privilege lobectomy whenever it enables a complete resection. Standard lobectomy is not possible if the tumour extends across the fissure, invades the main pulmonary artery or involves the bronchial tree proximal to the lobar take-off; a double location in different lobes is also an indication for pneumonectomy.

Lobectomy is preferred to pneumonectomy because of a substantially lower operative risk. Operative mortality is ~2% following lobectomy, and ranges from 6% to 10% following pneumonectomy. Mortality after pneumonectomy may be >10% in patients aged >70 years, or in case of extended resection. There is an ongoing debate whether mortality of pneumonectomy is increased after induction chemotherapy, especially on the right side. We have recently demonstrated a similar risk when compared to standard operations and a survival advantage even if the patient remains stage N2. Other disadvantages of pneumonectomy are decreased quality of life owing to loss of respiratory function and decreased possibilities of repeated curative resection should a metachronous primary cancer occur (~10% of stages I and II).

Resection of less than a pulmonary lobe is not recommended as routine. The Lung

Cancer Study Group (Ginsberg et al., 1995) compared lobectomy and segmentectomy (or wedge excision) for T1N0 cancer in a randomised trial. There was a drop in 5-year survival of 20% for patients subjected to segmentectomy and a three-fold increase of local recurrence following segmentectomy or wedge excision. More recent investigations from Japan conclude that wedge excisions are valuable in small bronchoalveolar carcinoma; similarly, segmentectomies could be applied to stage I tumours <2 cm.

When the tumour is invading surrounding anatomical structures, an enlarged *en bloc* R-0 resection may achieve satisfactory long-term results; this should be carried out in specialised institutions so that an excessive operative mortality does not erase the survival benefit of resection.

Complete homolateral lymph node dissection
The goals of lymph node dissection are:

1. to ascertain staging

2. to ensure complete resection of the disease

Staging is important at the individual level to set prognosis and to define the mostappropriate treatment strategy. At the collective level, adequate staging facilitates comparison of different treatment modalities or results from different institutions.

Leaving unrecognised lymph node metastases obviously leads to 'local recurrence'. Medical imaging has serious pitfalls. CT underestimates N2 stage in one patient out of five and overestimates in one patient out of two. A negative positron emission tomography (PET) scan matches with mediastinoscopy, but the latter is subject to 10–15% failures; a positive PET requires histological assessment because the false-positive rate is >40%. Furthermore, >30% of patients with N2 disease have no apparent disease at the N1 level (so-called skip metastases). Even among patients with T1 disease, 22% have mediastinal lymph node involvement.

As such, intraoperative exploration of the mediastinum is mandatory and can be achieved by two different procedures:

• random sampling of nodes
• complete node dissection

Obviously, only complete dissection appears to be serious and reliable. The arguments are as follows.

In patients with pathological stage I-N0 disease, survival increases with the number of dissected nodes. This demonstrates that the more lymph nodes are harvested, the lower the risk of ignoring an invaded node and the more reliable the staging.

In a cross-sectional analysis, we compared sampling and dissection in each single case of 248 resections. Sampling identified 52% of resections as N2; multilevel N2 was identified in 42% of events only. Resection based on sampling alone would have been complete in only 12%.

The standard lymph node dissection is defined as an *en bloc* dissection of all lymphatic tissue along its anatomical borders (tracheobronchial tree, sheets of major vessels and oesophagus). On the right side, it includes lower oesophageal nodes within the pulmonary ligament, subcarinal space and paratracheal space. On the left side, it includes the pulmonary ligament, subcarinal space, aortopulmonary window, phrenic nodes and subaortic nodes up to the left tracheobronchial angle.

Formal lymph node dissection does not increase the post-operative complication rate. There is increasing evidence for a positive effect on survival. An initial nonrandomised study compared sampling to dissection in stage II and III, and concluded that there is a survival advantage following dissection.

A randomised study including >500 patients demonstrated a survival advantage of node dissection without relation to a stage migration effect: it was observed not only stage-by-stage but also when comparing the two investigated groups as a whole (table 3).

A meta-analysis concluded that 4-year survival was increased in patients having undergone node dissection, with a hazard ratio of 0.78.

Are there alternatives to pneumonectomy?

Given the high operative mortality rate of pneumonectomy, it is meaningful to look for alternatives. Bronchoplastic operations (sleeve lobectomy) are indicated:

1) when the tumour involves the lobar take-off on the endobronchial side

2) when positive N1 nodes with capsular disruption are identified at the origin of the lobar bronchus

Angioplastic lobectomies are indicated when the lobar branches destined for the upper lobe cannot be divided safely with tumour-free margins; this situation is much more frequent on the left side for anatomical reasons.

The operative risk of bronchoplastic lobectomy is comparable to standard lobectomy, with a mortality of $\leqslant 2\%$. Long-term survival and rate of local recurrence match with reported data per stage (table 4). A meta-analysis by Ma et al. (2007) showed that mortality was almost half that after pneumonectomy in experienced teams; 1-year survival was improved after bronchoplastic resection.

What is the impact of minimally invasive surgery?

Minimally invasive major resections, such as lobectomy and, more recently,

Table 4. Survival following bronchoplastic lobectomy

First author	Stage I	Stage II	Stage III
Tedder	63	37	21
Mehran	57	46	0
Van Schil	62	31	31
Massard	70	37	8
Icard	60	30	27
Tronc	63	48	8

Data are presented as %.

segmentectomy, performed by VATS, are increasingly offered to patients with small tumours. The common end-points are that, while operative mortality is similar to that of open procedures, there is a significant decrease of complication rate and length of hospital stay. Post-operative pain is considerably lower, recovery is faster and the social cost is decreased (Whitson et al., 2008; Paul et al., 2010; Yang et al., 2012).

Oncologic concerns may be addressed as follows. Minimally invasive resection can be recommended for T1 and small T2 tumours, and achieves equivalent long-term survival rates when compared with open surgery . Evidence for N1 or N2 disease primarily orientates towards classic open surgery, except for very experienced teams. There is no doubt that a precise anatomical dissection of the hilar structures (artery, vein and bronchus) can be safely performed. A negative PET lowers the risk for mediastinal lymph node involvement; furthermore, there is a shift towards less invasive histology in the case of small tumours (adenocarcinoma with lepidic growth in particular). Nevertheless, a careful evaluation of the mediastinum with mediastinoscopy and/or lymph node dissection is still recommended.

The demand for minimally invasive surgery will certainly be increased if lung cancer screening programmes with low-dose CT are generalised.

Table 3. Lymph node dissection increases survival: results of a randomised study

	5-year survival	
	268 dissections	264 samplings
Stage I	82.2	57.5
Stage II	50.4	34.0
Stage III	27.0	6.2
Global	48.4	36.9

Date are presented as %. Reproduced from Wu et al. (2002), with permission from the publisher.

Further reading

- Allen MS, *et al.* (2006). Mortality and morbidity of major pulmonary resections in patients with early stage lung cancer: initial results of the randomized prospective ACOSOG Z0030 trial. *Ann Thorac Surg*; 81: 1013–1019.
- American College of Chest Physicians (2013). Diagnosis and management of lung cancer, 3rd ed: American College of Chest Physicians evidence-based clinical practice guidelines. *Chest*; 143: Suppl., 1S–e512S.
- Berghmans T, *et al.* (2005). Survival improvement in respectable non-small cell lung cancer with (neo)adjuvant chemotherapy: results of a meta-analysis of the literature. *Lung Cancer*; 49: 13–23.
- Brunelli A, *et al.* (2009). ERS/ESTS guidelines on fitness for radical therapy in lung cancer patients (surgery and chemo-radiotherapy). *Eur Respir J*; 34: 17–41.
- Cerfolio RJ, *et al.* (2003). The role of FDG-PET scan in staging patients with non-small cell carcinoma. *Ann Thorac Surg*; 76: 861–866.
- Ginsberg RJ, *et al.* (1995). Randomized trial of lobectomy versus limited resection for T1N0 non-small cell lung cancer. *Ann Thorac Surg*; 60: 615–623.
- Mansour Z, *et al.* (2007). Induction chemotherapy does not increase the operative risk of pneumonectomy! *Eur J Cardiothorac Surg*; 31: 181–185.
- Martinod E, *et al.* (2002). Management of superior sulcus tumors: experience with 139 cases treated by surgical resection. *Ann Thorac Surg*; 73: 1534–1540.
- Massard G (1999). Local control of disease and survival following broncho-plastic lobectomy for non-small cell lung cancer. *Eur J Cardiothorac Surg*; 16: 276–282.
- National Lung Screening Trial Research Team. (2011). Reduced lung cancer mortality with low-dose computed tomographic screening. *N Engl J Med*; 365: 395–409.
- Paul S, *et al.* (2010). Thoracoscopic lobectomy is associated with lower morbidity than open lobectomy: a propensity-matched analysis from the STS database. *J Thorac Cardiovasc Surg*; 139: 366–378.
- Riquet M, *et al.* (1997). Prognostic value of T and N in non small cell lung cancer three centimeters or less in diameter. *Eur J Cardiothorac Surg*; 11: 440–444.
- Thomas P, *et al.* (2002). Stage I non-small cell lung cancer: a pragmatic approach to prognosis after complete resection. *Ann Thorac Surg*; 73: 1065–1070.
- Van Meerbeeck JP, *et al.* (2007). Randomized controlled trial of resection versus radiotherapy after induction chemotherapy in stage IIIA-N2 non-small cell lung cancer. *J Natl Cancer Instit*; 99: 442–450.
- Whitson BA, *et al.* (2008). Surgery for early-stage non-small cell lung cancer: a systematic review of the video-assisted thoracoscopic surgery versus thoracotomy approaches to lobectomy. *Ann Thorac Surg*; 86: 2008–2018.
- Wright G, *et al.* (2006). Surgery for non-small cell lung cancer : systematic review and meta-analysis of randomized trials. *Thorax*; 61: 597–603.
- Wu YL, *et al.* (2002). A randomized trial of systematic nodal dissection in respectable non-small cell lung cancer. *Lung Cancer*; 36: 1–6.
- Yang C-FJ, *et al.* (2012). Thoracoscopic segmentectomy for lung cancer. *Ann Thorac Surg*; 94: 668–681.

Radiotherapy for lung cancer

Luigi Moretti and Paul Van Houtte

While surgery remains the treatment of choice for early-stage disease, radiotherapy is the commonest treatment modality for lung cancer, with >50% of patients receiving radiation at some point in their disease history, either for cure or palliation. In the past, conventional radiotherapy yielded poor outcomes for early-stage patients or locally advanced disease due to the radiation techniques available. However, today, major technical advances (positron emission tomography (PET)/CT-based treatment plans, three-dimensional treatment planning, multileaf collimators, gating techniques, *etc.*) allow us to overcome the challenge of delivering an effective radiation dose while protecting vital organs or structures (lungs, oesophagus, heart, spinal cord, *etc.*). This is well illustrated by the breakthrough of stereotactic body radiation therapy (SBRT) for early-stage disease leading to impressive local control and survival (table 1).

Furthermore, the management of locally advanced non-small cell lung cancer (NSCLC) has moved to a multimodality approach including a platinum-based chemotherapy delivered concurrently with high-dose radiotherapy and surgery for selected cases. Systemic treatments (chemotherapy and targeted agents) are taking a more and more important place either for stage IV disease or in association with radiotherapy and surgery for earlier cases. Today, NSCLC is no longer considered a single disease, and pathological subtypes or receptor mutations (epidermal growth factor receptor, *etc.*) should be identified.

For small cell lung cancer (SCLC), definitive chemoradiotherapy is usually used for limited- or extensive-stage SCLC with a good response to chemotherapy, although surgical resection for early-stage SCLC (T1-2N0) may be considered.

Mechanism of action

At the cellular level, the most important effects of radiation are linked to double-stranded breaks in nuclear DNA, either by direct ionisation or by indirect formation of free radicals, formed by water radiolysis, that subsequently interact with DNA. Radiation

---

Key points

- For early-stage NSCLC patients, surgery (lobectomy or an anatomical segmentectomy with lymph node dissection) remains the standard treatment, while SBRT is indicated for medically inoperable patients.

- In locally advanced NSCLC, definitive concurrent chemoradiotherapy is preferred while surgery is used for selected cases (with induction or adjuvant chemotherapy).

- Although still controversial, post-operative radiotherapy is recommended for patients with positive surgical margins and/or pathologic N2 disease.

- The current management of SCLC includes chemoradiotherapy with or without induction chemotherapy.

- PCI is indicated for all stages of SCLC after response to primary therapy.

Table 1. Overall survival based on stage at presentation and treatment applied

Disease stage	Overall survival	Median survival	Treatment
NSCLC			
I–II (early)	53–80% at 5 years 68–77% at 5 years	20–60 months	Surgery SBRT
III (locally advanced)	9–16% at 5 years 15–22% at 3 years	13–17 months	Chemoradiation
IV (advanced)	30–40% at 1 year	8–10 months	Chemotherapy
SCLC			
Limited	20–30% at 5 years 30–40% at 3 years 50% at 1 year	18 months	Chemoradiation
Extensive	0–2% at 3 years 27–40% at 1 year	7–10 months	Chemotherapy

can also affect the processes of the cell cycle and alter cell growth. When not able to repair the damage, cell undergo several types of death, *i.e.* apoptosis or senescence, and are ultimately cleared by physiological normal mechanisms. Similarly, adverse effects of radiation are mainly the consequence of radiation damage to surrounding normal tissues, which were not able to repair adequately.

Tumour radiobiology

Tumour radiobiology is complex, as response depends not only on dose but also on individual radiosensitivity, timing, total dose, fraction size and other agents given concurrently (*i.e.* chemotherapy). It allows the optimisation of a radiotherapy schedule and therapeutic ratio for individual patients in regards to maximising tumour control probability and minimising normal tissue complication probability.

The biological factors that influence the response of normal and neoplastic tissues to fractionated radiotherapy are repair, redistribution, repopulation, reoxygenation and intrinsic radiosensitivity (the 'five Rs' of radiotherapy).

Radiotherapy indications

- Definitive treatment for medically inoperable stage I NSCLC using hypofractionated SBRT

- Definitive treatment for locally advanced (stage III) NSCLC and limited-stage SCLC with concurrent chemotherapy
- Prophylactic cranial irradiation in all stages of SCLC after response to primary treatment
- Post-operative radiation after surgical resection with pathologic N2 disease and T4 disease except for separate nodules in the same lobe, close/positive surgical margins and gross residual disease
- Palliation for pain, bleeding, superior vena cava syndrome, brain metastasis and cord compression

Techniques of radiotherapy

- External beam radiation with three-dimensional conformal radiation (3D-CRT), intensity-modulated radiotherapy or SBRT
- Intraoperative high dose rate brachytherapy (used after wedge resection, this may improve local control rates)
- Endobronchial brachytherapy (for palliation of endobronchial disease or to boost treatment after initial course of definitive 3D-CRT for primary cancer with endobronchial component or for small endobronchial-only tumour)

Radiotherapy planning

NSCLC For definitive radiotherapy, the prescribed dose depends on the target volumes and the presence of organs at risk in the region that needs to be treated. In addition, local tumour control is correlated with total dose delivered and the delivery time, with a potential impact on survival.

Traditionally, the mediastinum or elective nodal area were treated with 45–50 Gy in conventional fractions (once-daily doses of 1.8–2.0 Gy), and the primary or gross tumour boosted to a total dose of $\geqslant$60 Gy. The tumour dose of 60 Gy was established as the standard of care in the old Radiation Therapy Oncology Group (RTOG) 73-01 randomised trial. Nevertheless, there was still a high rate of local failure and distant relapse. Thus, higher radiation doses have been advocated in an attempt to improve local control, either by increasing the total dose with conventional daily dose of 2 Gy or using an accelerated radiation schedule. This was only possible by changing the old concept of elective nodal irradiation to limit the radiotherapy fields to the primary tumour and involved nodes (biopsy-proven, or based on CT scan and fluorodeoxyglucose PET imaging). Another important step was the use of induction chemotherapy, which was showed to improve survival by reducing distant metastases. A concurrent schedule has been established to be superior to the induction approach both in long-term survival and local control, but with an increase in acute toxicities. Different regimens are used, usually a platinum-based doublet with a third-generation drug (*i.e.* paclitaxel or vinorelbine). The optimal sequence must still be defined: concurrent *versus* induction followed by a concurrent chemoradiation strategy. The later approach may be of interest in the case of bulky disease for the downsizing of tumour and the subsequent volume reduction in normal tissue irradiated. The place of maintenance chemotherapy, targeted agents or pemetrexed for adenocarcinoma is currently not known.

In the particular case of superior sulcus tumours, neoadjuvant concurrent chemoradiation (45 Gy) followed by surgery and adjuvant chemotherapy is the preferred approach. If initially unresectable (or after restaging), definitive concurrent chemoradiation to a dose of 63–66 Gy is indicated.

Although it remains globally controversial, post-operative radiation is generally recommended after surgical resection when a pathological report demonstrates N2 disease, extracapsular nodal extension (ECE), T4 disease, positive surgical margins or macroscopic residual disease. When post-operative radiation is indicated, the mediastinum is commonly treated with 50 Gy in 25 fractions, with an additional boost of 10 Gy on areas of ECE or bulky nodal disease. Similarly, regions of gross residual disease should be treated with 66 Gy if the normal surrounding structures allow it.

SBRT or stereotactic ablative radiation therapy (SABR) is a novel form of high-precision, image-guided radiotherapy for stage I NSCLC. This technique requires accurate patient positioning, breathing control, four-dimensional target definition and the use of multiple non-coplanar radiation beams, subsequently allowing steep dose gradients and major hypofractionation (delivering a high dose in a few fractions, approximately three to eight treatments). Indeed, high biological effective doses ($>$100 Gy) are required to achieve a significant improvement in local tumour control and survival in medically operable or inoperable NSCLC patients. At this moment, concurrent chemotherapy should be avoided with dose-escalated radiotherapy or SBRT until further clinical data are available.

SCLC The treatment of limited-stage SCLC includes chest radiotherapy delivered concurrently with cisplatin and etoposide during the first cycles if possible. The optimal radiation dose or schedule (one or two fractions daily) is still not known (trials are ongoing). Hyperfractionation, with fraction of 1.5 Gy twice daily to a total dose of 45 Gy, was shown to be superior to a classical 45 Gy in 5 weeks with one fraction a day, but with an increase in acute toxicities. Currently, chest radiotherapy for SCLC is similar to NSCLC, increasing the total radiation dose ($\geqslant 60$ Gy) and avoiding elective mediastinal irradiation.

Prophylactic cranial irradiation (PCI) should be given for all stages of SCLC after any degree of favourable response to primary treatment. The current standard total dose is 25 Gy given in 10 fractions. No benefit was demonstrated from the use of higher doses.

Despite the fact that the rate of brain metastases is similar to that in limited-stage SCLC, the role of PCI in NSCLC remains more controversial since it was shown to reduce brain metastases but does not improve overall survival in randomised studies. Nevertheless, the development of brain metastases is common in patients with locally advanced NSCLC treated with chemoradiation and, therefore, a subgroup of patients (especially younger patients) may still benefit from either PCI or an aggressive cranial treatment after early detection of brain metastases.

Palliative radiotherapy

For relief of symptoms such as pain, haemoptysis, dysphagia and dyspnoea, different dose schedules are being used and proven adequate: 1×10 Gy, 10×3 Gy, 5×4 Gy, 2×8.5 Gy (with a 1-week interval), $13–15 \times 3$ Gy (daily) and 20×2.5 Gy (daily).

Selection of treatment should be tailored to the needs of patients, usually being centred on quality of life, and based on age, performance status, tumour burden and specific symptoms.

One schedule (10 fractions of 3 Gy) seems to be favoured among radiation oncologists, with a good balance between palliation, 1-year survival and treatment time commitment.

For patients with good performance status and limited distant disease (*e.g.* oligometastatic), a definitive dose of radiation concurrent with chemotherapy may be preferred to have a sustained symptomatic improvement, and continuing good performance status.

Radiotherapy side-effects

Radiotherapy-induced toxicity is related to the volume of normal tissues surrounding the target tumour. The dose-limiting organs for chest radiation are the spinal cord, lung, oesophagus and heart. Classically, side-effects are divided into early/acute and late/chronic toxicity. These unwanted effects can be reduced using dose–volume constraints, which are modified by multiples factors, such as concurrent chemotherapy or surgery. Most of the toxicity data are derived from conventionally fractionated radiation and may not apply with SBRT in which large doses per fractions are used. Although the results are not mature yet, several studies suggested limited early toxicity after SBRT for early-stage NSCLC not close to the central structures. Toxicities should be graded using the Common Terminology Criteria for Adverse Events system (CTCAE) from the National Cancer Institute (NCI).

Common acute side-effects seen in radiotherapy for lung cancer include oesophagitis, skin irritation (dermatitis), cough, fatigue and nausea/vomiting. Most of these are resolved 2–4 weeks after radiotherapy. Acute pneumonitis can occur 1–6 months after radiation.

Delayed complications include radiation pneumonitis, pulmonary fibrosis, pericarditis, pericardial effusion, coronary artery disease, oesophageal stricture/fistula, Lhermitte's syndrome, brachial plexopathy, rib fracture and second cancers.

Radiation pneumonitis typically occurs approximately 6–10 weeks after radiotherapy. Most patients have only radiographic changes without any clinical symptoms or functional end-point modifications. Clinical symptoms are cough, dyspnoea, hypoxia and fever. Symptomatic radiation pneumonitis can be treated with steroids after excluding an infection. Pulmonary fibrosis usually evolves 6 months to several years after treatment. Several dosimetric parameters can be used to help predict the risk of pulmonary toxicity, commonly the V_{20} (the total lung volume receiving at least 20 Gy) and the mean lung dose (MLD). Current guidelines recommend a V_{20} below 30–35% and a MLD below 18–20 Gy. Additionally, the use of systemic chemotherapy as well as the sequencing of therapies may have a significant impact on the toxicity.

Oesophageal toxicity is globally the most common acute toxicity during chest/mediastinal radiotherapy. While oesophagitis can be severe, it is rarely a reason to stop treatment if managed adequately. Dosimetric factors that influence oesophageal toxicity include the length of oesophagus receiving beyond 40–50 Gy and the mean oesophageal dose. Again, the use of concurrent chemotherapy with thoracic radiation significantly increases severe esophagitis compared to radiation alone.

Since patients treated for locally advanced lung cancer typically have pre-existing cardiopulmonary disease, the risk of radiation-induced cardiovascular disease is rather difficult to define, especially among the few long-term survivors. After mediastinal irradiation with at least a portion of the heart receiving a relatively high dose, the most common complications are pericarditis, coronary artery disease and, less frequently, myocardial infarction. The new advances in radiotherapy techniques allow the reduction of heart volume irradiated and subsequently potentially reduce the risk of cardiac toxicity.

While rare and sometimes spectacular, Lhermitte's syndrome (sudden electric-like shocks extending down the spine with head flexion) usually resolves spontaneously, and is not predictive for chronic myelopathy. Spinal cord radiation injury is a very rare but serious complication of radiotherapy. Accordingly, most centres use conservative spinal cord dose constraints and limit the maximum dose to 45–50 Gy.

Caution should be used in treating central lesions with SBRT as they are at increased risk of toxicity compared to peripheral lesions. In addition, tumour volume is a significant predictor of severe toxicity, which suggests limiting the use of SBRT for early-stage NSCLC. Reported complications include pneumonitis, pleural effusion, haemoptysis and rib fracture depending on initial tumour location. Accordingly, SBRT for apical lesions carries a risk of brachial plexus toxicity. Specific dose constraints are recommended for SBRT, allowing for the prediction of the risk of toxicity as well as the potential to lower this risk before treatment. Clinical data with a longer follow-up are needed to better quantify the risk of late complications associated with SBRT.

Further reading

- Aupérin A, et al. (2010). Meta-analysis of concomitant versus sequential radiochemotherapy in locally advanced non-small-cell lung cancer. J Clin Oncol; 28: 2181–2190.
- Blanchard P, et al. (2010). Prophylactic cranial irradiation in lung cancer. Curr Opin Oncol; 22: 94–101.
- Chi A, et al. (2010). Systemic review of the patterns of failure following stereotactic body radiation therapy in early-stage non-small-cell lung cancer: clinical implications. Radiother Oncol; 94: 1–11.
- Graves PR, et al. (2010). Radiation pulmonary toxicity: from mechanisms to management. Semin Radiat Oncol; 20: 201–207.
- Le Péchoux C (2011). Role of postoperative radiotherapy in resected non-small cell lung cancer: a reassessment based on new data. Oncologist; 16: 672–681.
- MacManus M, et al. (2009). Use of PET and PET/CT for radiation therapy planning: IAEA expert report 2006–2007. Radiother Oncol; 91: 85–94.
- Pantarotto JR, et al. Radiotherapy for locally advanced lung cancer: stages IIIA and IIIB. In: Pass HI, et al., eds. Principles and Practice of Lung Cancer. 4th Edn. Philadelphia, Lippincott Williams & Wilkins, 2010; pp. 579–558.
- Timmerman RD, et al. Stereotactic techniques for lung cancer treatment. In: Pass HI, et al., eds. Principles and Practice of Lung Cancer. 4th Edn. Philadelphia, Lippincott Williams & Wilkins, 2010; pp. 589–600.

Metastatic tumours

Elisabeth Quoix

The thorax is a common site of metastasis from various cancers, which may affect the hilar or mediastinal lymph nodes, bone (chest wall and vertebrae), lung, pleura, muscle, or heart and pericardium. These metastases may induce mediastinal compression syndromes (Pancoast, superior vena cava syndrome, dysphagia, *etc.*), just like locoregional extension of a primary lung cancer.

Pleural metastases

They occur commonly in patients with haematological or solid tumours. In a series of 133 patients (Anderson *et al.*, 1974), the most common primary sites appeared to be breast carcinoma (35 patients), lung cancer (32 patients), lymphomas (20 patients), Hodgkin's disease (12 patient), ovary carcinoma (nine patients), adenocarcinoma of unknown primary tumour (six patients) and melanoma (four patients). In females specifically, 37% of malignant pleural effusions are due to breast cancer, 20% to gynaecological cancers and 15% to lung cancer (Kreisman *et al.*, 1983). Probably, with the increase in the frequency of lung cancer in females, in the next few years, there will be a higher percentage of malignant pleural effusions secondary to lung cancer (fig. 1).

Pericardial effusions

Of 55 patients admitted in an intensive care unit with malignant pericardial effusion, 30 had a lung carcinoma as primary site, nine a breast cancer, five haematological malignancies and 11 other solid tumors (Dequanter *et al.*, 2008).

Pulmonary metastases

The lung is a prominent site of metastasis of breast, colon, kidney, uterus, and head and neck tumours. Some otherwise rare tumours (choriocarcinoma, osteosarcoma, testicular tumour, melanoma, Ewing tumour and thyroid carcinoma) frequently metastasise to the lung. Endothoracic metastases of breast cancer are essentially pleuropulmonary (figs 2 and 3). In a review of 660 cases of breast cancers followed for a period of 5 years between 1975 and 1979, 119 endothoracic metastases were recorded.

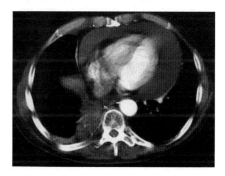

Figure 1. Neoplastic pericardial effusion in a patient with lung cancer.

> **Key points**
>
> • The thorax is a common site of metastasis from several cancers.
>
> • It is sometimes difficult to distinguish between primary lung cancer and metastases from other primaries.
>
> • Prognosis is linked to the underlying primary.

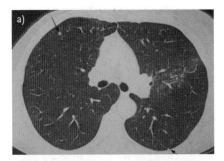

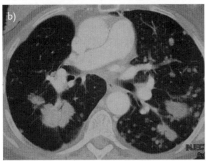

Figure 2. a) Multiple micronodules in a female who developed chronic cough 2 years after a breast cancer. b) The same patient 6 years later. Multiple nodules are present, some of them displaying a pneumonic pattern.

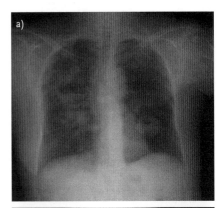

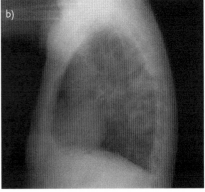

Figure 3. Multiple excavated pumonary metastases. a) Posteroanterior chest radiograph. b) Lateral chest radiograph.

Among them, 79 were pleural or pleuroparietal, 80 were pulmonary (lymphangitis, n=41; multiple nodules, n=34; solitary nodules, n=9; endobronchial, n=7; tumoural emboli, n=2; alveolar metastasis, n=1), 46 were hilar or mediastinal, and two were myocardial metastases (Kreisman *et al.*, 1983). Pulmonary metastases are also frequent in lung cancer and their prognosis appears to be of intermediate value if there is no other site involved; they are now classified as M1a in the new staging classification (Ou *et al.*, 2008). Sometimes, pulmonary metastases may be excavated (fig. 3) and may induce pneumothorax. Some may be calcified either spontaneously (osteosarcoma, bone giant cell tumour or papillary carcinoma of the thyroid) or after treatment (Seo *et al.*, 2001).

Endobronchial metastasis is an infrequent feature (table 1), the most frequent primary site being the head and neck (although it might be difficult to distinguish them from a primary lung cancer) and the next most common being the breast and kidney (Sorensen, 2004; Milleron *et al.*, 1986).

It may be quite difficult if not impossible to distinguish a primary lung cancer from endobronchial metastasis on a CT image. Endobronchial metastases from melanoma often appear black on CT images. Endobronchial metastases of a kidney cancer display strong enhancement on contrast-enhanced CT images (Park *et al.*, 2004). Whenever bronchofibroscopy is performed, there may be quite severe bleeding from the biopsy attempt; cough with haemoptysis is the most frequent symptom.

Table 1. Endobronchial metastases: frequency by primary site

Primary tumour	Metastases n (%)
Head and neck	71 (31)
Breast	32 (14)
Kidney	31 (13)
Colon/rectum	25 (11)
Melanoma	18 (8)
Sarcoma	10 (4)
Thyroid	9 (4)
Bladder	6 (3)
Ovarian	5 (2)
Prostate	4 (2)
Oesophagus	3 (1)
Testis	3 (1)
Pancreas	3 (1)
Adrenal gland	2 (1)
Stomach	2 (1)
Other	3 (1)
Data from Seo *et al.* (2001).	

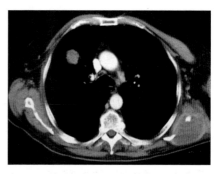

Figure 4. Left scapula osteolytic metastasis of a right upper lobe adenocarcinoma.

Tumoural emboli may provide similar clinical and radiological features as thromboemboli; however, peripheral tumoural microemboli are characterised by normal imaging but respiratory failure (Dizon *et al.*, 2008; Chatkin *et al.*, 2007). Diagnosis may be obtained by transbronchial biopsy or by videothoracoscopy; on histological examination, multiple carcinomatous emboli are visible in distal pulmonary arteries, veins and lymphatics.

Hilar and mediastinal metastatic lymph nodes

Metastatic hilar and mediastinal lymph nodes are mostly linked to an intrathoracic carcinoma. Among 565 patients, only 37 had a history of extrathoracic carcinoma in a surgical series (Riquet *et al.*, 2009). The primary cancer was most frequently breast, with others being from the kidney, testis, prostate, thyroid and other sites. Metastasis of breast cancer to intrathoracic nodes seems to occur quite frequently. In an autopsy series by Thomas *et al.* (1979) of females who had died of disseminated breast cancer, metastatic involvement of intrathoracic lymph nodes was found in 71% of cases. Lymph node involvement was more extensive in the mediastinum ipsilateral to the primary breast cancer than in the contralateral mediastinum.

Bone metastases in the chest

The bones of the chest are common sites of secondary lesions of lung, prostate and breast cancer, in which bone is the most common metastatic site (Costelloe *et al.*, 2009).

Bone metastases affect 8% of patients with breast cancer. Bone scanning remains the

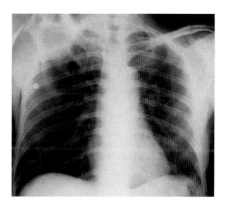

Figure 5. Osteolytic metastasis of the second right rib.

mainstay for detection of bone metastases. In a meta-analysis of six studies comparing bone scanning and positron emission tomography (PET) without CT in breast cancer, a pooled lesion-based sensitivity of 88% and specificity of 87% was found for bone scanning, and a sensitivity of 69% and a specificity of 98% for PET (Shie *et al.*, 2008).

Bone is a frequent metastatic site in lung cancer (fig. 4). In a recent study of 1000 patients, 105 (10.5%) had bone metastases at diagnosis (Song *et al.*, 2009). The sensitivity of PET/CT was 94.3% compared to 78.1% with bone scanning and the specificity was, respectively, 98.8% and 97.4%. Among the 346 bone metastases detected by PET/CT, 55 were in the thoracic spine, 28 in the scapula or clavicles (fig. 4), 12 in the sternum and 56 in the ribs (fig. 5), *i.e.* 44% of the foci were in the chest. The main problem of PET is poor anatomical resolution (fig. 6).

MRI is the best imaging procedure whenever spinal cord compression is suspected.

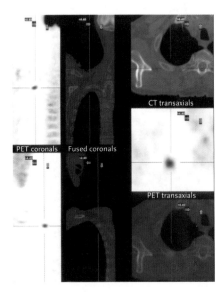

Figure 6. Rib metastasis in a patient with a left hilar relapse of a lung adenocarcinoma without CT finding.

Conclusions

The chest is a frequent site of metastasis, especially for lung, breast, kidney, prostate, colon and ovary carcinomas. The prognosis of these metastases is more related to the possibilities of control of the underlying neoplasm than to their possible immediate complications (*e.g.* tamponade). However, some of metastases may alter quality of life, such as bone metastases, with a special attention to be paid to the spine because of the risk of cord compression.

Further reading

- Anderson CB, *et al.* (1974). The treatment of malignant pleural effusion. *Cancer*, 33: 916–922.
- Chatkin JM, *et al.* (2007). Microscopic pulmonary neoplastic emboli: report of a case with respiratory failure but normal imaging. *Prim Care Respir*, 16: 115–117.
- Costelloe CM, *et al.* (2009). Imaging bone metastases in breast cancer: techniques and recommendations for diagnosis. *Lancet Oncol*, 10: 606–614.
- Dequanter D, *et al.* (2008). Severe pericardial effusion in patients with concurrent malignancy: a retrospective analysis of prognostic factors influencing survival. *Ann Surg Oncol*, 15: 3268–3271.
- Dizon DS, *et al.* (2008). The differential diagnosis of dyspnea in a woman with metastatic breast cancer—consideration beyond pulmonary embolism. *Breast J*, 14: 90–91.
- Kreisman H, *et al.* (1983). Breast cancer and thoracic metastases: review of 119 patients. *Thorax*, 38: 175–179.
- Milleron B, *et al.* (1986). Endobronchial metastases of cancer. A propos of 29 cases. *Rev Pneumol Clin*, 42: 231–234.
- Ou SH, *et al.* (2008). Validation study of the proposed IASLC staging revisions of the T4 and M non-small cell lung cancer descriptors using data from 23583 patients in the California Cancer registry. *J Thorac Oncol*, 3: 216–227.
- Park CM, *et al.* (2004). Endobronchial metastasis from renal cell carcinoma: CT findings in four patients. *Eur J Radiol*, 51: 155–159.

- Riquet M, *et al.* (2009). Intrathoracic lymph node metastases from extrathoracic carcinoma: the place of surgery. *Ann Thorac Surg*; 88: 200–205.
- Seo JB, *et al.* (2001). Atypical pulmonary metastases: spectrum of radiologic findings. *Radiographics*; 21: 403–417.
- Shie P, *et al.* (2008). Meta-analysis: comparison of F-18 fluorodeoxyglucose-positron emission tomography and bone scintigraphy in the detection of bone metastases in patients with breast cancer. *Clin Nucl Med*; 33: 97–101.
- Song JW, *et al.* (2009). Efficacy comparison between 18-FDG PET/CT and bone scintigraphy in detecting bony metastases of non-small cell lung cancer. *Lung Cancer*; 65: 333–338.
- Sorensen B (2004). Endobronchial metastases from extrapulmonary solid tumors. *Acta Oncologica*; 43: 73–79.
- Thomas JM, *et al.* (1979). The spread of breast cancer: importance of the intrathoracic lymphatic route and its relevance to treatment. *Br J Cancer*; 40: 540–547.

Pleural and chest wall tumours

Arnaud Scherpereel

Pleural and chest wall malignancies are quite common diseases in our practice. Malignant pleural effusions (MPEs) and pleural metastases are much more frequent than primary tumours of these tissues (mesothelioma, sarcoma, lymphoma, *etc.*). Primary chest wall tumours are a heterogeneous group of rare tumours (<2% of all primary tumours; 60% of them are malignant) developing in the bones and soft tissues of the thoracic cage, but having similar diagnostic and therapeutic issues.

Epidemiology and pathogenesis

Malignant pleural mesothelioma (MPM), a highly aggressive tumour involving the pleura in 90% of cases, is a rare tumour but with increasing incidence. MPM may occur in subjects up to 40 years of age after occupational asbestos exposure (found in

>80% of male cases but <40% of females), the main factor involved in MPM pathogenesis.

Pleural metastases and MPEs Pleural tumour involvement may result from a direct invasion from adjacent structures (lung, chest wall, *etc.*), blood dissemination or, more often, from tumour emboli to the visceral pleura with secondary seeding to the parietal pleura (lung cancer). Effusion may be due to the pleural tumour lesions or to a lymphatic blockade at the mediastinal level. MPEs also depend on interactions between tumour cells and mesothelial cells through growth factors such as vascular endothelial growth factor that increase vascular permeability and angiogenesis.

A MPE is found in up to 6% of patients with malignancy. In half of these cases, MPE may reveal the cancer. Neoplasias responsible for pleural metastases and/or MPE are mostly lung cancer (~30% of cases) or breast cancer (10–15%), but other cancers include carcinomas (ovary, stomach, *etc.*) or noncarcinoma proliferations such as lymphoma, sarcoma, melanoma, seminoma or thymoma.

Pleural effusion is the main clinical element but it is not found in all pleural malignancies. Moreover, pleurisy is not systematically synonymous with MPE in cancer patients because it may be induced by other mechanisms, such as pneumonia and/or atelectasis due to bronchial obstruction, transudate induced by severe denutrition or cardiac failure, or even drug- or radiotherapy-induced effusion. Therefore, the diagnostic strategy may differ depending on whether the patient has a cancer

---

Key points

- MPEs are much more frequent than primary pleural or chest wall tumours.

- Diagnostic strategy includes pleural cytology, but a firm and reliable diagnosis of cancer is based on histology, usually best obtained by biopsies during thoracoscopy.

- Talc pleurodesis by thoracoscopy is the best local treatment of recurrent or massive MPE, but indwelling pleural catheters represent an interesting alternative.

- Figures 1 and 2 summarise a proposal for MPE and MPM management.

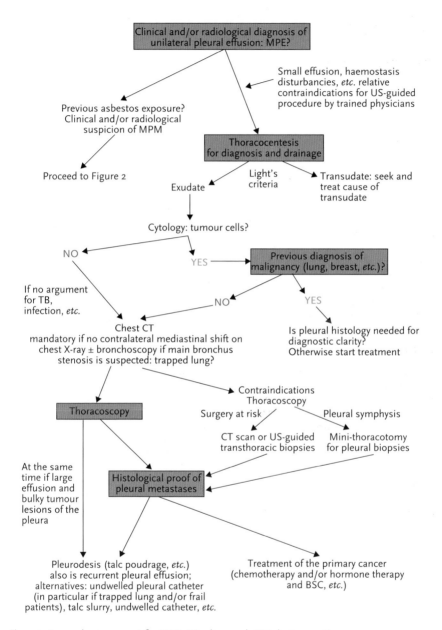

Figure 1. Proposed management for MPE. US: ultrasound; BSC: best supportive care.

background or not but should always rely on cytology or, better still, on histology.

Lymphoma and chest wall sarcoma Initial thoracic involvement of lymphoma is common but mostly involves the mediastinum. Lung parenchyma and/or pleural localisations are less frequent and need to be histologically proven because they modify the staging and prognosis of the

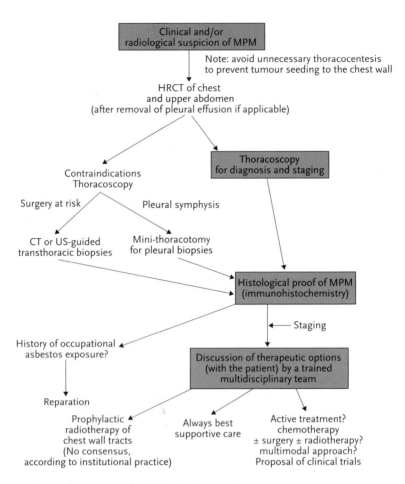

Figure 2. *Proposed management for MPM. US: ultrasound.*

tumour. Primary soft-tissue sarcoma of the chest wall is a rare disease (<10% of the 8000 new cases per year of soft-tissue sarcomas in the USA). The most common sarcomas of the chest wall are chondrosarcoma, osteosarcoma, Ewing's sarcoma/primitive neuroectodermal tumour, malignant fibrous histiocytoma and fibrosarcoma. Primary pleural and pulmonary sarcomas are rare.

Prognosis

The prognosis of patients with pleural metastases or MPM is poor (median survival <12 months). However, survival may vary according to the primary cancer

(better outcome for breast cancer or lymphoma) and/or presence of favourable markers (*EGFR* mutation or *ALK* amplification in non-small cell lung cancer, *etc.*). Sarcomas have a variable prognosis, with a reported 5-year survival from 15% to 90%, depending mostly on the localisation, grade and differentiation the tumour, and the possibility of achieving an early wide resection of the sarcoma.

Diagnosis

Clinical signs Dyspnoea on exertion and dry cough are the most common signs of MPE. Dyspnoea is usually progressive and more marked as the effusion becomes larger but it may be also modulated by other factors, *i.e.* bronchus obstruction, carcinomatous lymphangitis or associated (pulmonary or cardiac) comorbidities. Chest pain suggests chest wall involvement. Other signs may include weight loss, anorexia, asthenia, haemoptysis (lung cancer), adenopathy, peritoneal effusion, *etc.* However, MPE or MPM may be diagnosed in asymptomatic patients by routine chest imaging. A diagnosis of MPM should not be based on unspecific and usually late clinical signs. However, the association of chest pain, thoracic 'shrinkage', and/or a unilateral pleural effusion or thoracic mass in asbestos-exposed patients may suggest this diagnosis.

There are no reliable clinical features for distinguishing benign from malignant chest wall tumours. A palpable mass and pain are common in both groups of tumours. The final diagnosis is often obtained only after surgery.

Imaging Pleural metastases usually exhibit a moderate-to-large, nonloculated and unilateral pleural effusion. MPE may be associated with an irregular pleural thickening. Typically, this large pleural effusion induces a contralateral mediastinal shift. If not, one should suspect an obstruction of a main bronchus by lung cancer or metastasis, a fixed mediastinum caused by the cancer and/or lymph nodes, an extensive tumour infiltration of the ipsilateral lung mimicking a large effusion, or MPM.

In MPM patients, chest radiography or, better, CT typically shows an unspecific, unilateral (95% of cases) pleural effusion with or without mediastinal shift. More rarely, pleural thickening or mass, without pleurisy, may be observed. Pleural plugs are very common (70% of cases); about 20% of patients exhibit the association of asbestos-induced pulmonary interstitial fibrosis. Definitive diagnosis of MPM is not possible by CT but this is recommended for diagnosis and staging (after removal of pleural effusion if applicable). MRI is mostly useful to assess the tumour extent into the diaphragm and chest wall.

^{18}F-fluorodeoxyglucose positron emission tomography (PET) usually shows hypermetabolism of pleural mesothelioma, metastatic adenopathy and metastasis, but should not currently be performed for the diagnosis of MPM. Pleural hypermetabolism is also found after talc pleurodesis. PET may be helpful for the staging of pleural malignancies or in the search of primary cancer.

Although histological analysis is almost always required for accurate diagnosis, imaging is important for staging of chest wall sarcomas, and several of these tumours have distinctive radiological features, allowing the radiologist to narrow the differential diagnosis.

Pathology and diagnostic procedures In patients suspected of having MPE, a thoracocentesis is the first diagnostic step (American Thoracic Society/European Respiratory Society (ERS) guidelines). Pleural fluid analysis usually finds an exudate according to Light's criteria but a transudate due to major hypoproteinaemia with cachexia or to malignant pericardial effusion does not eliminate the diagnosis of MPE. Assessment of the pleural level of adenosine deaminase can yield false-positive results in some cases of MPM or lymphoma but may be helpful in countries with medium-to-high prevalence of TB. The diagnostic sensitivity of pleural cytology in MPE may vary depending on the extension of the pleural lesions and the primary cancer, from 62% to 90% in case series. Thus, in a patient with a history of cancer, cytology may be enough for the diagnosis of pleural metastases. A diagnosis of MPM should not be based on cytology alone because of its poor sensitivity (30%) and specificity (potential confusion with reactive mesothelial cells or adenocarcinoma cells).

Closed, percutaneous needle (*e.g.* Abrams) pleural biopsies are quite easy to perform with local anaesthesia on an outpatient basis. However, due to the potentially scarce and irregular distribution of the tumour lesions in the pleural cavity, the positive yield of blind biopsies is low (30–40%), adding little to a negative cytology, except in countries with a high incidence of TB.

CT- or ultrasound-guided biopsies have a better diagnostic sensitivity than blind biopsies in series of MPEs (70–80% sensitivity), but lower than that of thoracoscopy. They are not recommended for MPM diagnosis except in patients for whom thoracoscopy (or mini-thoracotomy with pleural symphysis) is contraindicated or rejected by the patient. If MPM is not clearly suspected, closed needle biopsies may first be proposed in young patients with pleural lesions and exudative, cytology-negative pleural effusion from countries with a relatively high prevalence of TB.

Medical (pleuroscopy) or surgical (video-assisted thoracoscopic surgery) thoracoscopy with multiple pleural biopsies is the 'gold standard' for obtaining a diagnosis of MPM or pleural metastasis. Diagnostic accuracy is >90% and complications occur in <10% of cases. MPM or pleural metastasis will usually appear as nodules or masses of various diameters. Thoracoscopy is also useful for the staging of MPM and may permit talc pleurodesis in case of massive and/or recurrent MPE. However, access to thoracoscopy may be limited in many places worldwide, as significant resources and expertise are required.

Immunohistochemistry is helpful in the search for the primary cancer for pleural metastases or to obtain an accurate diagnosis of mesothelioma, referring to the international classification of pleural tumours (World Health Organization, 2004). The epithelioid subtype is the most frequent mesothelioma subtype.

Soluble biomarkers have been searched to obtain an early and reliable diagnosis of pleural malignancies but none was considered as valuable in routine practice. Soluble mesothelin (or soluble mesothelin-related peptides (SMRPs)) levels were increased in the serum and pleural fluid of patients with MPM compared with healthy asbestos-exposed subjects or patients with benign pleural lesions or pleural metastasis.

SMRPs showed interesting sensitivity (70–80%) and specificity (80–100%) as diagnostic markers for MPM. However, SMRPs do not capture sarcomatoid (and some mixed) mesothelioma subtypes, and should not be used for MPM screening.

Staging and pre-therapeutic assessment of MPM

It is recommended to use the Union Internationale Contre le Cancer/International Mesothelioma Interest Group 1995 TNM staging system, even if it is inaccurate in describing tumour and node extent by current imaging procedures. Only a patient's performance status and histological subtype are recognised as prognostic factors for the management of MPM in routine.

The 2010 ERS/European Society of Thoracic Surgeons (ESTS) guidelines on MPM management proposed a simple and sequential three-step pretreatment assessment (Scherpereel et al., 2010).

Treatment

Treatment includes palliative local therapies, mostly to improve the patient's symptoms, and treatment of the primary cancer depending of the nature of the malignancy, and the clinical status and the wishes of the patient.

Treatment of primary cancer MPM treatment, summarised by the 2010 ERS/ESTS guidelines, relies mostly on best supportive care (BSC) (oxygen, pain relief, nutrition, etc.) associated with chemotherapy.

There is limited evidence for the efficacy of radical surgery for mesothelioma, except parietal pleurectomy in very early and rare stage Ia disease. Debulking surgery (radical pleurectomy or pleurectomy/decortication (P/D)) is now preferred to extrapleural pneumonectomy because of the lower morbidity/mortality and better outcome when combined with chemotherapy or radiotherapy. Both surgical procedures should be performed only in clinical trials, in specialised centres and as a part of multimodal treatment. P/D can also be considered to achieve symptom control, especially in symptomatic patients with entrapped lung syndrome who cannot benefit from chemical pleurodesis.

Palliative radiotherapy aimed at pain relief may be considered in the case of painful chest wall infiltration or nodules. The value of prophylactic radiotherapy to prevent subcutaneous metastasis developing along drainage channels or thoracocentesis tracts is questionable based on recent studies and does not permit any recommendation.

When a decision is made to treat patients with chemotherapy, subjects with a good performance status should be treated with first-line chemotherapy combining platinum and an antimetabolite (pemetrexed), or could be included in clinical trials. No drug has been validated in second-line chemotherapy, and patients with a good performance status should be proposed to enter into clinical trials. Patients demonstrating prolonged symptomatic and objective response with first-line chemotherapy may be treated again with the same regimen in the event of relapse. For tumour assessment and follow-up of MPM, only chest CT is recommended. PET and biological markers (SMRP) are promising tools but still under investigation. The modified Response Evaluation Criteria In Solid Tumors (RECIST) criteria are the preferred method of measuring response to treatment.

Pleural metastases Treatment of metastatic cancer relies on chemotherapy and/or hormone therapy, and BSC. The choice of cytotoxic drugs depends on the nature of the primary cancer. Mediastinal radiotherapy may be combined with chemotherapy for lymphoma.

Chest wall sarcomas The treatment of choice is an early adequate and wide resection of the sarcoma. Adjuvant radio- and/or chemotherapy are considered for high-grade sarcomas.

Local treatment Pleurodesis is useful in treating a patient's symptoms and preventing recurrent effusions. Sterile talc is the most effective agent available for pleurodesis and may be administered in the pleural space through a chest drain ('talc slurry') or, better, during thoracoscopy ('talc poudrage'). Pleurodesis is most effective when performed early in the disease process before effusions have become loculated and/or the lung has become fixed and is unable to expand fully, but it should not be performed before sufficient tissue for diagnosis has been obtained. Criteria for talc pleurodesis are a sufficient World Health Organization performance status (WHO PS) <2, an estimated survival >3 months, an established diagnosis of the tumour and no arguments for either a trapped lung (suspected if a pneumothorax persists after thoracocentesis) or an endobronchial tumour (massive pleural effusion without a contralateral mediastinal shift). This may justify a bronchoscopy or a pleural manometry before pleurodesis. To decrease the risk of pleurodesis failure in MPE, it is recommended to use 4 g of talc after complete aspiration of pleural effusion. In a phase III multicentric randomised study, success rates in talc poudrage *versus* slurry in patients with MPE were, respectively, 67% *versus* 56% (p=0.045), and 82% *versus* 67% in the subgroup of lung or breast cancers (p=0.022). Benign usual side-effects of talc (fever and chest pain) were observed with both methods, but no acute respiratory distress syndrome and death.

Alternatives to talc pleurodesis are repeated pleural punctures or better indwelling/tunnelled pleural catheters (TPCs). In fact, current guidelines consider TPCs an effective and ambulatory procedure for symptomatic, recurrent MPE. Their use as a first-line treatment is feasible; TPCs should be preferred for patients with trapped lung or those who are not considered good candidates for chemical pleurodesis because of short life expectancy, rather than a second talc pleurodesis, a pleuroperitoneal shunt with a high risk of complications, or parietal pleurectomy. Spontaneous pleurodesis may be obtained by TPC without mortality or major morbidity in nearly half of the cases when pleural drainage is performed *via* the catheter every other day, or even up to 70% in MPE patients fit for pleurodesis.

Further reading

- Antony VB, et al. (2001). Management of malignant pleural effusions. *Eur Respir J*; 18: 402–419.
- Chee A, et al. (2011). The use of tunneled pleural catheters in the treatment of pleural effusions. *Curr Opin Pulm Med*; 17: 237–241.
- Foran P, et al. (2011). Imaging of thoracic sarcomas of the chest wall, pleura, and lung. *Semin Ultrasound CT MR*; 32: 365–376.
- Gross JL, et al. (2005). Soft-tissue sarcomas of the chest wall: prognostic factors. *Chest*; 127: 902–908.
- Janssen JP, et al. (2007). Safety of pleurodesis with talc poudrage in malignant pleural effusion: a prospective cohort study. *Lancet*; 369: 1535–1539.
- Maskell NA, et al. (2003). Standard pleural biopsy *versus* CT-guided cutting-needle biopsy for diagnosis of malignant disease in pleural effusions: a randomised controlled trial. *Lancet*; 361: 1326–1330.
- Rodriguez-Panadero F. Effusions from malignancy. *In:* Light RW, et al., eds. Textbook of Pleural Diseases. 2nd Edn. London, Hodder Arnold, 2008; pp. 323–333.
- Sahn SA. Malignant pleural effusions. *In:* Bouros D, ed. Pleural Disease. Vol. 186. New York, Marcel Dekker, 2004: pp. 411–438.
- Scherpereel A, et al. (2010). Guidelines of the European Respiratory Society and the European Society of Thoracic Surgeons for management of malignant pleural mesothelioma. *Eur Respir J*; 35: 479–495.
- Travis WD, et al., eds. World Health Organization Classification of Tumors. Tumors of the Lung, Pleura, Thymus and Heart. Lyon, IARC, 2004.
- van der Bij S, et al. (2011). Markers for the non-invasive diagnosis of mesothelioma: a systematic review. *Br J Cancer*; 104: 1325–1333.

Mediastinal tumours

Paul E. Van Schil, Patrick Lauwers and Jeroen M. Hendriks

Variety of compartments and organs

Although no universal agreement exists, the mediastinum is commonly divided into a superior compartment above a straight line from the sternal angle of Louis to the vertebral column, and an inferior part below this imaginary line. The latter is composed of an anterior compartment in front of the heart, a middle compartment at the level of the heart, and a posterior part lying behind the heart. Each compartment contains different organs and structures, varying from the heart and great vessels to lymphatic tissue and pluripotent cells.

Variety of histological types and tumours

In both young and old patients, a range of primary tumours and cysts is encountered in the mediastinum; these are summarised in table 1. Metastases may also occur in the mediastinum.

Variety of symptoms

Mediastinal tumours can grow to a large size before symptoms appear. Pressure on surrounding structures may result in hoarseness, dyspnoea, dysphagia and superior vena cava syndrome. Various paraneoplastic syndromes have been described, such as myasthenia gravis and pure red cell aplasia in case of thymoma (fig. 1).

Variety of diagnostic means

Chest CT, MRI and positron emission tomography provide exact anatomical delineation of a tumour and may suggest a specific entity. To obtain a precise histological diagnosis, CT-guided puncture, endoscopic or endobronchial ultrasound, mediastinoscopy, mediastinotomy, and video-assisted thoracic surgery are used. In the case of suspicion of lymphoma, germ

---

Key points

- Mediastinal tumours are characterised by a wide variation in clinical presentation, histological features and treatment options.

- A multidisciplinary approach is necessary to determine optimal treatment.

- Surgical treatment should aim at complete resection.

- The mediastinum, which is defined as the anatomical compartment between both lungs, is a fascinating region due to its surprising complexity and variety.

Table 1. *Primary tumours and cysts encountered in the mediastinum*

Superior mediastinum	Substernal goitre
	Ectopic thyroid
Inferior mediastinum	
Anterior	Thymoma
	Thymic cyst
	Germ cell tumours
	Pleuropericardial cysts
Middle	Lymphoma
	Bronchogenic cyst
Posterior	Neurogenic tumours
	Enterogenic cysts

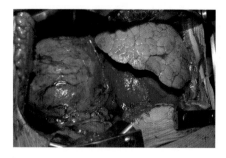

Figure 1. A large thymoma in the right hemithorax presenting with myasthenia gravis. The tumour was resected by a bilateral anterior thoracotomy (clam-shell incision).

cell tumour or thymoma, large biopsies are required. Well-circumscribed tumours in young patients should be excised at once so as not to breach the surrounding capsule.

Variety of therapeutic strategies

Operable lesions are treated by surgical excision. Minimally invasive and even robotic techniques can be applied if a complete resection can be obtained by this approach. In the case of incomplete resection or transcapsular invasion, adjuvant radio- or chemotherapy may be indicated. Inoperable lesions and lymphomas are treated by a combination of chemo- and radiotherapy. In selected cases, induction therapy may be a valid approach to downstage a locally aggressive tumour. Salvage surgery may be attempted in tumours that are no longer responsive to chemo- or radiotherapy. Long-term survival depends on histological type and completeness of resection.

Further reading

- Date H (2009). Diagnostic strategies for mediastinal tumors and cysts. *Thorac Surg Clin*; 19: 29–35.
- Hoffman R, *et al.*, eds. Hematology: Basic Principles and Practice. 5th Edn. Philadelphia, Churchill Livingstone Elsevier, 2009.
- Spaggiari L, *et al.* (2012). Multi-disciplinary treatment of malignant thymoma. *Curr Opin Oncol*; 24: 117–122.

Obstructive sleep apnoea/hypopnoea syndrome

Wilfried De Backer

Obstructive sleep apnoea/hypopnoea syndrome (OSAHS) is characterised by recurrent episodes of partial or complete upper airway collapse during sleep. The collapse is highlighted by a reduction in, or complete cessation of, airflow despite ongoing inspiratory efforts. Due to the lack of adequate alveolar ventilation that results from the upper airway narrowing, oxygen saturation may drop and carbon dioxide tension may occasionally increase. The events are mostly terminated by arousals. Clinical consequences are excessive daytime sleepiness related to the sleep disruption. Minimal diagnostic criteria have been defined for OSAHS. Patients should have excessive daytime sleepiness that cannot be better explained by other factors, or experience two or more of the following symptoms, again that are not better explained by other factors:

- choking or gasping during sleep
- recurrent awakenings from sleep
- unrefreshing sleep
- daytime fatigue
- impaired concentration

> **Key points**
>
> - OSAHS is characterised by recurrent episodes of partial or complete upper airway collapse during sleep.
>
> - Minimal diagnostic criteria exist for OSAHS.
>
> - Overnight polysomnography is the gold standard for OSAHS diagnosis.

All patients should have more than five obstructed breathing events per hour during sleep. An obstructive apnoea or hypopnoea can be defined as an event that lasts for $\geqslant 10$ s and is characterised by an absence or a decrease from baseline in the amplitude of a valid measure of breathing during sleep that either reaches >50% with an oxygen desaturation of 3% or an arousal (alternatively a 30% reduction with 4% desaturation). These definitions are recommended by the American Academy of Sleep Medicine (AASM). The AASM Task Force also states that there are common pathogenic mechanisms for obstructive apnoea syndrome, central apnoea syndrome, sleep hypoventilation syndrome and Cheyne–Stokes breathing. It was more preferable to discuss each of these separately, although they could be placed under the common denominator of 'sleep-disordered breathing syndrome'. The definition of OSAHS using two components, daytime symptoms and breathing pattern disturbances during sleep, may suggest that there is a tight correlation between the two. However, unfortunately, this is not the case. The breathing pattern abnormalities, mostly described by an AHI, only weakly correlate with quantified measures of sleepiness, such as the Epworth Sleepiness Scale (ESS). This probably means that interindividual sensitivity, with some individuals coping better with sleep fragmentation than others, does compromise the relationship between the AHI and daytime sleepiness scores. In addition, epidemiological studies show a broad range of sleepiness in the general population. Obviously, epidemiological studies investigating the prevalence of OSAHS are all biased by the lack of a uniform definition. The prevalence of an AHI of >5 events·h^{-1} in a general population (without taking into account symptoms of sleepiness) has previously been estimated to be 24% in a male population. When symptoms of sleepiness were also taken into account, the prevalence decreased to 4% in males and 2% in females.

Assessment of OSAHS

The most widely used gold standard for diagnosis is overnight polysomnography including nasal and/or oral airflow, thoracoabdominal movement, snoring, electroencephalography, electro-oculography, electromyography and oxygen saturation. Cardiorespiratory monitoring alone can be considered as highly sensitive (78–100%) and specific (67–100%). Sleepiness is often evaluated using the ESS, which assesses the global level of sleepiness and is independent of short-term variations in sleepiness. The ESS discriminates between normal and pathological sleepiness.

Pathophysiology

Structural narrowing of the upper airway at one specific location is unlikely to be a major cause. Studies have shown that the upper airway collapse is not restricted to one place but is rather a dynamic phenomenon, starting at a certain level and spreading caudally. Upper airway obstruction involves more than one specific site of the upper airway in the majority of sleep apnoea patients. The upper airway can collapse when insufficient load compensation is generated when an imbalance between the activation of the upper airway dilator muscles and the diaphragm occurs. When this occurs, the airway will collapse during inspiration or at least narrow with the development of flow limitation. However, there is increasing evidence that the collapse of the upper airway occurs during expiration. Furthermore, it has been convincingly shown that the upper airway behaves like a Starling resistor, making the collapse independent of the suction force brought about by the diaphragm but dependent on the balance between the upper airway

pressure and the tissue pressure at the collapsible site. The airway remains patent, regardless of the excessive pressure applied, as long as the critical pressure of positive end-expiratory pressure (P_{crit}) remains low relative to the pressure upstream to the collapsible segment (P_u). Closure of the upper airway occurs when P_u falls below the surrounding tissue pressure (P_{crit}). In the model of the Starling resistor, maximal flow (V'_{max}) becomes a function of the pressure gradient and the resistance in the segment upstream to the collapsible segment (R_u):

$$V'_{max} = (P_u - P_{crit})/R_u \qquad (1)$$

The collapse of the upper airway then finally occurs during expiration when, due to the absence of dilator muscle, P_{crit} exceeds the upstream pressures. Prolonged expiratory time, as occurs during central apnoeas, therefore predisposes to collapse, but other factors may contribute and can be considered as risk factors (table 1).

Central and obstructive events are closely linked. Sometimes a central event with an already partially collapsed upper airway can transit towards an obstructive event with ongoing occlusion of the upper airway despite the resumption of effort. Often, however, with resumption of effort at the end of the central apnoea, the obstruction of the upper airway disappears, presumably due to reactivation of the upper airway dilator muscles. However, the mechanisms remain unclear and more research is needed to understand why central apnoeas are sometimes followed by obstructive apnoeas and, in some cases, followed by reopening of the airways. In any case, since central apnoeas can trigger classical obstructive apnoeas, the mechanisms leading to unstable breathing (and thus central apnoeas) are also important in the genesis of obstructive apnoeas.

Consequences

Cardiovascular Obstructed airways may generate negative intrathoracic pressure that increases left ventricular transmural pressure and left ventricular afterload. The negative pressure also draws more blood into the thorax and increases right ventricular

TABLE 1. Risk factors for OSA: factors promoting upper airway collapse

Abnormal anatomy of the upper airway
Skeletal factors
Maxillary and/or mandibular hypoplasia or retroposition
Hyoid position (inferior displacement)
Soft tissue factors
Increased volume of soft tissues
Adenotonsillar hypertrophy
Macroglossia
Thickened lateral pharyngeal walls
Increased fat deposition
Pharyngeal inflammation and/or oedema
Increased vascular volume
Increased muscle volume
Pharyngeal muscle factors
Insufficient reflex activation of upper airway dilator muscles
Impaired strength and endurance of pharyngeal dilators
Pharyngeal compliance
Increased upper airway collapsibility
Sensory function
Impaired pharyngeal dilator reflexes
Impaired mechanoreceptor sensitivity
Lung volume dependence of upper airway cross-sectional area
Increased below functional residual capacity
Ventilatory control system factors
Unstable ventilatory control
Increased ventilatory responses and loop gains
Sex factors
Male influences
Centripetal pattern of obesity
Absence of progesterone
Presence of testosterone
Weight
Obesity causing peripharyngeal fat accumulation

Reproduced from Verbraecken et al. (2009) with permission from the publisher.

preload. Intermittent hypoxia related to OSA will also impair cardiac contractility and diastolic relaxation (fig. 1).

OSA patients also have attenuated endothelium-dependent vasodilation and decreased circulating markers of nitric oxide. These effects, together with increased sympathetic vasoconstrictor activity and inflammation, will predispose to hypertension and atherosclerosis. In addition, platelet activation and aggregability are increased and predispose to thrombotic disease. Epidemiological studies indicate that OSA can initiate or promote cardiovascular disease, such as hypertension, coronary heart disease, heart failure, cardiac arrhythmias (bradyarrhythmias, atrial fibrillation and ventricular ectopy) and cerebrovascular disease.

Metabolic OSA is associated with several components of the metabolic syndrome, mainly insulin resistance and abnormal lipid metabolism. Sleep restriction causes insulin resistance by inducing a pro-inflammatory state (increased release of interleukin (IL)-6 and tumour necrosis factor (TNF)-α). Epidemiological studies have shown that sleep-related hypoxaemia is associated with glucose intolerance independent of age, sex, BMI and waist circumference. Metabolic syndrome can be triggered by both intermittent hypoxia and sleep fragmentation/deprivation. The mechanisms are shown in figure 2.

Metabolic syndrome can be due to the release of free fatty acids, angiotensin II and adipokines by adipose tissue, which may damage the pancreas, leading to insufficient insulin release and apparent insulin resistance.

Mean and nadir Sa,O_2 during sleep is an independent predictor of metabolic syndrome in overweight children and adolescents.

CPAP treatment

Therapy with nasal CPAP nCPAP is perceived by most physicians as a very effective treatment for sleep apnoea and has been shown to be effective in controlled studies.

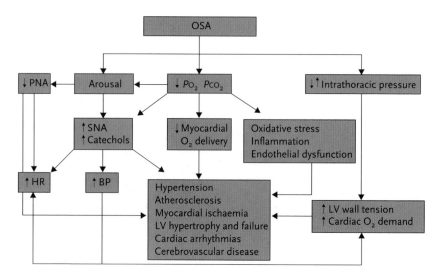

Figure 1. *Cardiovascular consequences of OSA. PNA: parasympathetic nerve activity; PO₂: oxygen tension; PCO₂: carbon dioxide tension; SNA: sympathetic nerve activity; HR: heart rate; BP: blood pressure; LV: left ventricle. Reproduced and modified from Bradley et al. (2009) with permission from the publisher.*

nCPAP results in better sleep quality with a lower arousal index, and less stage 1 and more stage 3 and 4 sleep in a placebo-controlled (using placebo capsules) study. In addition, in milder forms of sleep apnoea, nCPAP improved self-reported symptoms of OSA, including snoring, restless sleep, daytime sleepiness and irritability. Neuropsychological tests also improved after nCPAP compared with ineffective nCPAP. Blood pressure can also be reduced with nCPAP when compared with an oral placebo, especially in patients using nCPAP for ≥3.5 h·night⁻¹ and in those with >20 desaturations of 4% per hour.

nCPAP and the upper airway Occlusion of the upper airway can be prevented when either the resistance of the upper airway upstream, R_U or P_{crit} can be lowered. Regardless of the severity of the changes in P_{crit} and P_U, nCPAP can effectively increase (or restore) flow, largely through its effect on P_U (equation 1). Appropriate titration of the CPAP restores flow. nCPAP can increase P_U much more than local interventions, such as uvulopalatopharyngoplasty. Therefore, it also explains why overall nCPAP is much

more clinically effective than was shown in previous controlled studies.

nCPAP and control of breathing As mentioned previously, some clinical observations initially indicated that unstable breathing is part of OSAS, while more recent systematic analysis confirmed the increased loop gain and instability in the breathing pattern in OSA patients. It can be questioned, therefore, whether nCPAP can influence control of breathing in (obstructive) sleep apnoea patients. One could demonstrate that prolonged treatment with nCPAP significantly decreases the slope of the hypercapnic ventilatory response curve when measured during wakefulness, together with an increase in P_{aO_2} and a decrease in the arterial–alveolar oxygen tension difference. It is clear that all of these changes may contribute to lowering of the gain in the system and promote a more stable breathing pattern. Changes in lung volume, although mostly small, can also be observed during nCPAP therapy.

nCPAP has also been demonstrated to be effective in central sleep apnoea (CSA). nCPAP can increase carbon dioxide tension

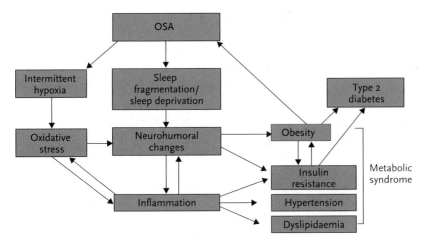

Figure 2. Mechanisms linking OSA and the metabolic syndrome. Reproduced and modified from Tasali et al. (2008) with permission from the publisher.

above the apnoeic threshold and, therefore, eliminate central apnoeas. However, central apnoeas are often also characterised by (near) occlusion of the upper airway; as highlighted earlier, nCPAP can also presumably be effective in preventing this collapse and its associated local reflexes.

nCPAP and the heart nCPAP can effectively be used to treat acute cardiogenic pulmonary oedema with shifting volume from intra- to extrathoracic compartments.

nCPAP may relieve CSA in chronic heart failure patients by increasing the $P_{a}CO_2$ above the apnoeic threshold. nCPAP may reduce ventilation by redistributing excess lung water to extrathoracic compartments, thereby reducing stimulation of pulmonary vagal irritant receptors. nCPAP may also unload the inspiratory muscles by increasing lung compliance, again due to extrathoracic redistribution of lung water.

nCPAP may significantly reduce left ventricular afterload by lowering the transmural pressure in patients with compromised cardiac function and, thus, overcome the burden of OSA on the cardiovascular system, as shown in figure 1. In the normal heart, where cardiac output is largely preload dependent, CPAP decreases

cardiac output by reducing left ventricular preload. In contrast, the failing heart is relatively insensitive to changes in preload but very sensitive to reductions in afterload. CPAP-induced reductions in left ventricular transmural pressure (and afterload) can augment cardiac output.

nCPAP may also attenuate sympathetic nervous activity and increase cardiac vagal modulation of the heart with favourable effects on blood pressure regulation.

In a large prospective study, severe untreated OSA patients had more fatal and nonfatal cardiovascular events; this difference disappeared with nCPAP treatment.

nCPAP and metabolic/systemic effects of OSA nCPAP may improve metabolic syndrome, although it is not always certain that nCPAP has an independent effect. nCPAP also lowers TNF-α, IL-6 and C-reactive protein levels.

Non-CPAP treatment

Mandibular advancement devices (MADs) are the most common oral appliances used for the treatment of OSA and/or snoring. They have either a one-piece (monobloc) or two-piece (duobloc) configuration. Customised devices have a better retention, tolerance and efficacy. MADs are effective if they increase the volume of the upper airway, which may enlarge at some sites and also narrow at other sites. Therefore, the overall efficacy is sometimes suboptimal; 65% of patients achieve a 50% reduction in AHI. In addition, snoring, excessive daytime sleepiness, neuropsychological function and cardiovascular risk may decrease. It is important to try to predict the outcome. Imaging and modelling studies can be of help for this purpose. Overall, these oral appliances are recommended for patients with mild-to-moderate OSA and for those with more severe disease when they do not tolerate CPAP. Side-effects, such as pain in the teeth and jaws, are mostly mild. Short-term compliance seems to be very high while long-term compliance (after >2 years) is ~50%.

Surgical treatment Several techniques have been performed, all with the aim of enlarging the volume of the upper airway and reducing the closing pressure. Uvulopalatopharyngoplasty reduces upper airway obstruction by shortening the uvula, trimming the soft plate, and suturing back the anterior and posterior pharyngeal pillars. Tonsillectomy is performed at the same time if the tonsils are found to be enlarged. Maxillomandibular advancement osteotomy advances the maxilla and mandible to enlarge the retrolingual and retropalatal spaces. This technique is not yet often used but additional studies are needed to establish its place, presumably in the more severe OSA patients who do not tolerate nCPAP and where an adequate therapy is needed to improve daytime sleepiness and prevent cardiovascular and metabolic consequences. Adenotonsillectomy is the first-line treatment in children. Electrical stimulation of the genioglossus with an implanted pacemaker has recently been tested and found to be efficient in selected patients, although more clinical studies are needed in order to learn which patients will benefit most. Overall, the results of upper airway surgery are poor when patients are unselected. Therefore, one must try to identify the site of the upper airway collapse and correct the anatomical abnormalities at

that site. Sleep endoscopy has been most widely used to identify the site of collapse, although pressure catheters with multiple sensors have also been used to identify the site of collapse; in addition, functional imaging of the upper airway maybe a promising tool.

Bariatric surgery

Several techniques have been used to perform bariatric surgery including gastric banding, use of a gastric balloon, gastric sleeve resection and gastric bypass. Bariatric surgery is used in morbidly obese patients with a BMI $\geqslant 40$ kg·m^{-2}. Almost half of patients improve after these interventions but, therefore, a substantial number of patients has still to continue with nCPAP.

Drug treatment

Several drugs have been tried, such as protriptyline (a tricyclic antidepressant), paroxetine (a serotonin reuptake inhibitor) and mirtazapine (a serotonin receptor agonist). None of these has given convincing results. Acetazolamide, although quite efficient in the treatment of central apnoeas, has also no effect on obstructive apnoeas.

Further reading

- Bradley TD, et al. (2009). Obstructive sleep apnoea and its cardiovascular consequences. *Lancet*; 373: 82–93.
- Chan AS, et al. (2008). Non-positive airway pressure modalities: mandibular advancement devices/positional therapy. *Proc Am Thorac Soc*; 5: 179–184.
- De Backer WJ, et al. (2008). Novel imaging techniques using computer methods for the evaluation of the upper airway in patients with sleep-disordered breathing: a comprehensive review. *Sleep Med Rev*; 12: 437–447.
- Jennum P, et al. (2009). Epidemiology of sleep apnoea/hypopnoea syndrome and sleep-disordered breathing. *Eur Respir J*; 33: 907–914.
- Levy P, et al. (2009). Sleep, sleep-disordered breathing and metabolic consequences. *Eur Respir J*; 34: 243–260.

- Marin JM, *et al.* (2005). Long-term cardiovascular outcomes in men with obstructive sleep apnoea-hypopnoea with or without treatment with continuous positive airway pressure: an observational study. *Lancet*; 365: 1046–1053.
- Marklund M, *et al.* (2012). Non-CPAP therapies in obstructive sleep apnoea: mandibular advancement device therapy. *Eur Respir J*; 39: 1241–1247.
- McArdle N, *et al.* (2001). Effect of continuous positive airway pressure on sleep architecture in the sleep apnea-hypopnea syndrome: a randomized controlled trial. *Am J Respir Crit Care Med*; 164: 1459–1463.
- Randerath WJ, *et al.* (2011). Non-CPAP therapies in obstructive sleep apnoea. *Eur Respir J*; 37: 1000–1028.
- Sleep-related breathing disorders in adults: recommendations for syndrome definition and measurement techniques in clinical research. The Report of an American Academy of Sleep Medicine Task Force. *Sleep*; 22: 667–689.

- Tasali E, *et al.* (2008). Obstructive sleep apnea and metabolic syndrome: alterations in glucose metabolism and inflammation. *Proc Am Thorac Soc*; 5: 207–217.
- Verbraecken JA, *et al.* (2009). Upper airway mechanics. *Respiration*; 78: 121–133.
- Verhulst SL, *et al.* (2007). Sleep-disordered breathing and the metabolic syndrome in overweight and obese children and adolescents. *J Pediatr*; 150: 608–612.
- Won CH, *et al.* (2008). Surgical treatment of obstructive sleep apnea: upper airway and maxillomandibular surgery. *Proc Am Thorac Soc*; 5: 193–199.
- Young TM, *et al.* (1993). The occurrence of sleep-disordered breathing among middle-aged adults. *N Engl J Med*; 328: 1230–1235.
- Younes M, *et al.* (2007). Mechanisms of breathing instability in patients with obstructive sleep apnea. *J Appl Physiol*; 103: 1929–1941.

Central sleep apnoea

Konrad E. Bloch and Thomas Brack

Central sleep apnoea/hypopnoea refers to the cessation or reduction of ventilation lasting for $\geqslant$10 s (in adults) due to a transient loss of neural output to the respiratory muscles. Many patients with central sleep apnoea (CSA) have mild hypocapnia or normocapnia but hypercapnia is less common, although hypoventilation may also accompany CSA. A periodic pattern of waxing and waning of ventilation with periods of hyperventilation alternating with central apnoea/hypopnoea is termed Cheyne–Stokes respiration (CSR).

Prevalence, aetiology and pathophysiology

The prevalence of CSA in the general population is not known. However, it seems

Key points

- CSA signifies the loss or reduction in ventilation due to a transient loss of neural output to the respiratory muscles.

- A high prevalence of CSA is observed in association with conditions such as CHF, pulmonary hypertension, cerebral stroke, neuromuscular disease, obesity hypoventilation syndrome and opioid use.

- Risk factors for CSA/CSR are age >60 years, male sex, severe heart failure, hypocapnia and atrial fibrillation.

- Treatment includes oxygen, acetazolamide and positive pressure ventilation, in particular adaptive servoventilation.

to be significantly less common than OSA, as <5% of patients referred to a sleep laboratory revealed predominant CSA. In contrast, a relatively high prevalence of CSA is observed in association with various conditions including CHF, pulmonary hypertension, ischaemic stroke, neuromuscular disease, obesity hypoventilation syndrome and narcotic use, or during initiation of CPAP therapy in certain patients with OSA. In healthy subjects, CSA may occur during hypoxia at altitude. Idiopathic CSA, by definition, is not associated with any comorbid condition.

Pathophysiological mechanisms underlying CSA include:

- respiratory control instability, due to an increased chemical drive, so that the prevailing $P\text{a}CO_2$ approaches the apnoea threshold
- a prolonged circulation time
- altered respiratory mechanics

Subsequently, different forms of CSA will be discussed.

CSR/CSA syndrome in CHF patients

Left-heart failure that increases pulmonary venous pressure is regarded as a source of CSR, as pulmonary congestion stimulates stretch receptors that sensitise the peripheral chemoreceptors to carbon dioxide through vagal afferents. The increased ventilatory sensitivity to carbon dioxide drives the $P\text{a}CO_2$ closer to the apnoea threshold, thereby promoting the susceptibility to central apnoea. Moreover, hypoxia that follows apnoea/hypopnea enhances post-apnoeic hyperventilation. If chemical control prevails over cortical influences on the respiratory controller, as typically occurs during sleep, patients develop an oscillatory breathing pattern that causes sympathetic overstimulation in patients who are already sympathetically stimulated through their heart failure.

Among patients with moderate to severe heart failure (left ventricular ejection fraction (LVEF) ≤55%) the prevalence of sleep apnoea (both obstructive and central) is very high irrespective of the clinical suspicion (fig. 1).

Criteria for CSR/CSA have not been uniformly accepted. According to the American Academy of Sleep Medicine, CSR should be scored if at least three successive cycles of cyclic crescendo–decrescendo changes in breathing amplitude are present for at least 10 consecutive minutes or when a central AHI >5 events·h^{-1} arises. In the Canadian Continuous Positive Airway Pressure for Patients with Central Sleep Apnea and Heart Failure (CANPAP) trial, a large multicentre study that evaluated the effectiveness of CPAP therapy in patients with heart failure and CSA, inclusion criteria required ≥15 apnoeas/hypopnoeas per hour

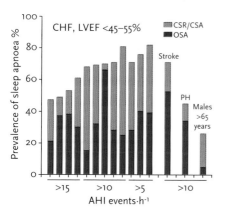

Figure 1. The prevalence of OSA and CSR/CSA in patients with CHF is very high (47–82%), depending on the severity of heart failure and on the cut-off level of the AHI. Sleep apnoea is also common in patients with stroke or pulmonary hypertension (PH). For comparison, data from a community sample of males aged >65 years are also shown. Reproduced and modified from Brack et al. (2012) with permission from the publisher.

with >50% central events and a LVEF <40%. Obviously, the AHI threshold used to define the presence of CSR has a major impact on prevalence estimates (fig. 1).

In some patients, CSR/CSA and OSA may coexist and alternate over the course of a night. Symptoms attributable to CSR/CSA are not well defined and may include paroxysmal nocturnal dyspnoea, poor sleep quality, excessive daytime sleepiness, fatigue and poor exercise tolerance.

CSR/CSA in heart failure patients is associated with poor prognosis. Several studies have found an increased mortality in patients with CSR/CSA even after controlling for the severity of heart failure, age, sex and other potential confounders. Mortality was particularly high in patients presenting with daytime CSR during physical activity (fig. 2).

Sleep-related breathing disturbances should be suspected in all patients with heart failure who suffer from nocturnal dyspnoea, unrefreshing sleep or daytime sleepiness. Particular risk factors for CSA/CSR include:

- severe heart failure
- older age (≥60 years)
- male sex
- hypocapnia
- atrial fibrillation
- CSR observed during the day

The diagnosis should be evaluated by polysomnography or a cardiorespiratory sleep study, as pulse oximetry cannot make the important distinction between CSA and OSA.

Optimised medical therapy of heart failure is the first step in the treatment of CSR/CSA. Cardiac resynchronisation by biventricular pacing and heart transplantation may also alleviate CSR/CSA. If medical therapy alone is ineffective, NIV may also be required. Nocturnal CPAP has been shown to improve nocturnal CSR/CSA, oxygen saturation, LVEF, sympathetic nervous system activity and 6-min walking distance. These effects are thought to be mediated by the increase in intrathoracic pressure induced by CPAP, which reduces both afterload and preload by decreasing transmural ventricular pressure and venous return so that cardiac function

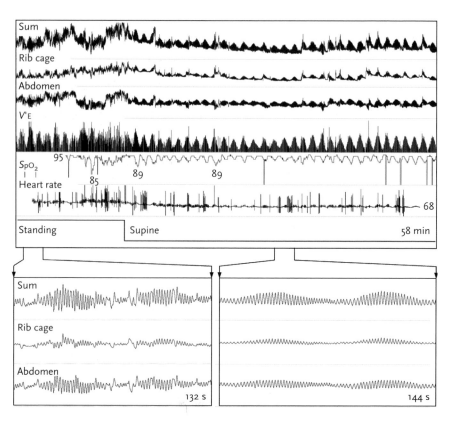

Figure 2. CSR in a patient with CHF. Inductive plethysmographic signals from rib cage and abdominal sensors showing regular waxing and waning of ventilation with central hypopnoeas and corresponding oscillations of oxygen saturation. The upper panel represents a 58-min daytime recording, the lower panels show enlarged portions obtained while standing (left) and in the supine position (right). Reproduced and modified from Brack et al. (2007) with permission from the publisher.

improves in patients with increased filling pressures. Additionally, CPAP stabilises CSR by raising the end-expiratory lung volume. Despite its positive effects on several outcomes described above, CPAP did not prolong survival without heart transplantation during a 2-year follow-up in a large trial (CANPAP). Yet, a *post hoc* analysis suggested a survival benefit in a subgroup of patients in whom CPAP sufficiently suppressed CSR/CSA. Adaptive servoventilation is a mode of bilevel positive airway pressure ventilation that continuously adjusts pressure support according to the breathing pattern of the patient in order to stabilise periodic breathing (fig. 3). It is a promising treatment option for CSR/CSA as it has been shown to improve nocturnal breathing pattern, daytime vigilance and quality of life after treatment for several weeks. Studies in larger patient cohorts over longer time periods are needed to confirm these effects and to evaluate a potentially improved survival. Acetazolamide and theophylline both have reduced CSR/CSA in some studies but these drugs are currently not generally recommended because of limited data on their effectiveness and potential adverse effects. Supplemental nocturnal oxygen has provided inconsistent results with some studies showing a reduction in CSR/CSA, along with improvements in physical performance or quality of life while others failed to reproduce these benefits. Further studies are required to better define the role of these adjuncts for the treatment of heart failure in patients with CSR/CSA.

Complex sleep apnoea syndrome

In some patients diagnosed with OSA, a CSR/CSA breathing pattern may emerge during initial CPAP therapy. The clinical relevance of this phenomenon, referred to as complex sleep apnoea, is still a matter of debate, as studies suggest that CSA disappears in the majority of OSA patients during prolonged CPAP therapy. However, persistent residual CSA may disturb sleep quality, prevent complete symptomatic improvement and may lead to CPAP intolerance in OSA patients. In this setting, adaptive servoventilation has been successfully used to normalise the breathing pattern and improve sleep quality.

Idiopathic CSA syndrome

Idiopathic CSA syndrome (fig. 4) is, by definition, not associated with any underlying disease. CSA causes sleep fragmentation, which may be perceived as unrefreshing sleep and result in daytime sleepiness. Idiopathic CSA is thought to be much less common than OSA, although no systematic epidemiological studies have been performed. Treatment options include acetazolamide, theophylline, CPAP and adaptive servo-ventilation.

CSA in various conditions

CSA and ataxic breathing have been observed in patients on chronic opioid medication and can be successfully treated with adaptive servoventilation, although the relevance of the breathing disturbances requires further study. Patients with stroke and neuromuscular disease, such as post-polio syndrome, motor neuron disease or multiple system atrophy, or with idiopathic central hypoventilation may exhibit CSA with or without associated OSA and/or hypoventilation. Depending on the prevailing breathing disturbance, bilevel positive pressure ventilation, CPAP or adaptive servoventilation may improve breathing and alleviate symptoms.

High-altitude periodic breathing

In healthy subjects, hypobaric hypoxia at altitudes of >1600 m may induce periodic breathing with central apnoea/hypopnoea. Breathing instability is related to an

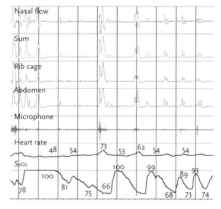

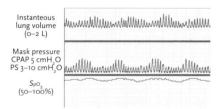

Figure 3. Recordings of instantaneous lung volume by respiratory inductive plethysmography and mask pressure during adaptive servoventilation in a patient with severe heart failure. In this mode of pressure support ventilation, the inspiratory pressure support is increased during hypopnoeic or apnoeic phases of CSR whereas pressure support is reduced to a minimal level during hyperpnoeic phases. PS: pressure support.

Figure 4. Idiopathic CSA in a 56-year-old male suffering from unrefreshing sleep. The 5-min recording shows repetitive central apnoeas of variable duration (20–90 s) associated with severe oxygen desaturation (minimal value of 66%). The absence of excursions in the inductive plethysmographic rib cage and abdominal signals during cessation of airflow indicates that apnoeas are due to intermittent loss of respiratory muscle activity.

enhanced chemosensitivity (high controller gain) causing a tendency for a ventilatory overshoot and hyperventilation with a reduced carbon dioxide reserve, *i.e.* the eupnoeic carbon dioxide tension approaches the apnoeic threshold, which promotes apnoea during minor ventilatory alterations. Symptoms may include paroxysmal dyspnoea and poor sleep quality. In some subjects, high-altitude periodic breathing is associated with acute mountain sickness, a syndrome characterised by headaches, insomnia, poor appetite, fatigue and, in more severe forms, ataxia and altered consciousness. The diagnosis of high-altitude periodic breathing is based on clinical observations in the appropriate context combined with pulse oximetry or more sophisticated sleep studies. Treatment is often not required but can be performed by altitude descent or the administration of supplemental oxygen or acetazolamide, which is also effective against acute mountain sickness.

Conclusions

In conclusion, CSA/CSR is less common than OSA. However, in certain conditions, including CHF, neuromuscular disorders, opioid use and high altitude, the prevalence of CSA is high. Treatment for CSA is not as well established as that for OSA, and it may include oxygen, acetazolamide and positive pressure ventilation, in particular adaptive servoventilation.

Further reading

- Aurora N, *et al.* (2012). The treatment of central sleep apnoea syndromes in adults: practice parameters with an evidence-based literature review and meta-analyses. *Sleep*; 35: 17–40.
- Brack T, *et al.* (2007). Daytime Cheyne–Stokes respiration in ambulatory patients with severe congestive heart failure is associated with increased mortality. *Chest*; 132: 1463–1471.
- Brack T, *et al.* (2012). Cheyne–Stokes respiration in patients with heart failure: prevalence, causes, consequences and treatments. *Respiration*; 83: 165–176.
- Bradley DT, *et al.* (2005). Continuous positive airway pressure for central sleep apnea and heart failure. *N Engl J Med*; 353: 2025–2033.
- Dai Y, *et al.* (2008). Central sleep apnea and Cheyne–Stokes respiration. *Proc Am Thorac Soc*; 5: 226–236.
- Eckert DJ, *et al.* (2007). Central sleep apnea. *Chest*; 131: 595–607.
- Javaheri S, *et al.* (2009). The prevalence and natural history of complex sleep apnea. *J Clin Sleep Med*; 5: 205–211.
- Schmidt-Nowara W. Patient information: Sleep apnea in adults (Beyond the Basics). www.uptodate.com/contents/sleep-apnea-in-adults-beyond-the-basics?.
- Walker JM, *et al.* (2007). Chronic opioid use is a risk factor for the development of central sleep apnea and ataxic breathing. *J Clin Sleep Med*; 3: 455–461.

Hypoventilation syndromes

Jean-François Muir

Sleep-related hypoventilation syndromes, together with central and obstructive sleep apnoea syndromes, are a part of so-called sleep-related breathing disorders (table 1).

Key points

- Sleep-induced hypoventilation is characterised by increased $PaCO_2$ levels of >45 mmHg.

- Nocturnal hypoventilation is associated with decreased ventilatory drive, respiratory iatrogenic depression, alteration of respiratory nerve conductance, muscular disease, chest wall deformities or severe obesity.

- OHS is the association of obesity and sleep-disordered breathing with daytime hypersomnolence and hypercapnia in the absence of other respiratory diseases.

- OHS is nowadays the most common sleep-related hypoventilation syndrome.

- Nocturnal polygraphy evaluation is needed in order to diagnose OHS.

- In OHS, NIV is used as the first-line treatment with supplementary oxygen when $PaCO_2$ ⩾50 mmHg; if $PaCO_2$ <50 mmHg, nasal CPAP (nCPAP) plus oxygen may be discussed as a first-line treatment after a night trial of nCPAP plus oxygen.

Sleep-induced hypoventilation is characterised by elevated levels of $PaCO_2$ of >45 mmHg while asleep or disproportionately increased relative to levels during wakefulness.

Pathophysiology

Nocturnal hypoventilation can be attributed to respiratory pump failure in relation with decreased ventilatory drive (won't breathe), which may be due to respiratory dysfunction secondary to polio sequelae, central hypoventilation, amyotrophic lateral sclerosis, Arnold–Chiari malformation, or the following: respiratory centres depression (hypnotics); alteration of respiratory nerve conduction (Guillain–Barré syndrome), transmission to the respiratory muscles (myasthenia) or worsening mechanics (can't breathe) with respiratory muscle alteration (muscular dystrophy), chest wall deformities or severe obesity. In the latter situations, lungs are normal, and associated hypoxaemia is due to the displacement of oxygen in the alveoli from increasing carbon dioxide levels, as predicted by the alveolar air equation. If the lungs are abnormal (COPD, tuberculous sequelae, CF or diffuse bronchiectasis), hypercapnia is mainly due to worsening mechanics and ventilation–perfusion inequalities.

During the night, ventilatory response to hypoxaemia and hypercapnia is largely reduced during rapid eye movement (REM) sleep with dysrhythmic breathing and less reduced during non-REM sleep. The result is a reduction of alveolar ventilation by altering $V'E$ and/or dead space volume/tidal volume (fig. 1).

Table 1. *Sleep-related breathing disorders*

Presence of an extra-/intraspulmonary restrictive disorder

OHS

Neuromuscular diseases

Duchenne muscular dystrophy, Steinert myotony, polio sequelae, amyotrophic lateral sclerosis, high spinal injuries with tetraplegia and respiratory paralysis (less frequent: acid maltase deficiency and spinal muscular atrophy)

Chest wall diseases

Kyphoscoliosis and/or tuberculosis sequelae

Other conditions

Respiratory centers depressant drugs

Neurologic conditions

Arnold-Chiari malformations, brainstem tumors, space occupying lesions, vascular malformations, central nervous system infection, stroke and neurosurgical procedure which may be associated with central hypoventilation

Congenital central hypoventilation

Presence of an obstructive disorder

COPD, diffuse bronchiectasis and CF are the most frequent conditions

Respiratory mechanics change during sleep and thereby worsen gas exchange, particularly in neuromuscular diseases and obstructive airways diseases. REM sleep induces skeletal muscle hypotonia sparing the diaphragm and not the accessory respiratory muscles, with deleterious effects in conditions for which these muscles are

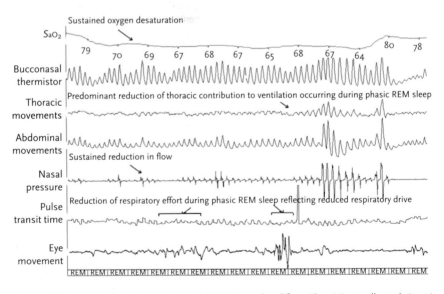

Figure 1. *REM hypoventilation in a patient with OHS. Reproduced from Chouri Pontarollo et al. (2007).*

necessary to maintain normal ventilation. REM sleep also alters upper airways patency and reduces chronic respiratory failure.

Clinical features

Hypoventilation *per se* generates a clinical syndrome associated with, in typical cases, dyspnoea during activities of daily living in the absence of paralysis, poor sleep quality, excessive daytime fatigue and sleepiness, nocturnal or early morning headache, cyanosis and evidence of right heart failure.

Diagnosis

The presence of such symptoms highlights the need to perform a physical examination, pulmonary function tests, a chest radiograph as well as measurement of arterial blood gases in the awake and asleep patient, *i.e.* SaO_2 and transcutaneous carbon dioxide tension. The results of this initial investigation are concluded by full night ventilatory polygraphy (respiratory signals only) or polysomnography (respiratory and neurological signals; electroencephalography (EEG), electrooculography (EOG), electromyography (EMG)). Chronic daytime hypercapnia is associated with and preceded by sleep-related hypoventilation.

Aetiology

Presence of an extra-/intrapulmonary restrictive disorder If obesity is present the most frequent diagnosis is obesity hypoventilation syndrome. Previously called the 'Pickwickian syndrome', obesity hypoventilation syndrome (OHS) is defined as the association of obesity (BMI >30 kg·m^{-2}) and sleep-disordered breathing with daytime hypersomnolence and hypercapnia ($PaCO_2$ >45 mmHg) in the absence of any other respiratory disease. The prevalence of OHS is 36% in patients with a BMI of 35–40 kg·m^{-2} and 48% if BMI is ⩾50 kg·m^{-2}.

The pathogenesis of OHS involves abnormal pulmonary mechanics with an excessive work of breathing and altered hypoxic and hypercapnic ventilatory responses, linked, in part, to chronic hypoxaemia and poor sleep quality, upper airway obstruction and, possibly, the influence of leptin.

Without adequate treatment, patients with OHS develop cor pulmonale, recurrent episodes of hypercapnic respiratory failure and loss of survival. OHS is one of the many aetiologies of chronic respiratory failure and has become a growing indication to initiate acute and/or long-term mechanical NIV. Mechanisms of action include resting of the respiratory muscles, an increase in thoracic compliance and resetting of the respiratory centres. In OHS, nocturnal mechanical NIV has been shown to be clinically effective because of a rapid and sustained improvement of daytime arterial blood gas levels and a net reduction of daytime sleepiness.

In order to establish a diagnosis of OHS, polysomnographic evaluation is needed and the ventilatory treatment needs to be adapted. The sleep respiratory pattern can present as obstructive apnoeas and hypopnoeas (90% of cases), obstructive hypoventilation due to increased upper airway resistance and/or central hypoventilation (10% of cases) (fig. 2). Data from a large cohort of OHS patients who had been treated with mechanical NIV showed a very significant decrease in the number of hospital stays for cardiac and/or respiratory illness for the 3 years following the initiation of mechanical NIV, compared with the year prior to the start of treatment. A dramatic improvement in arterial blood gases was observed and a good compliance suggests that this treatment is cost-effective and improves morbidity and mortality in such patients. Recent studies discussed the necessity to begin with mechanical NIV as first-line treatment *versus* nasal CPAP (nCPAP) with supplemental oxygen; in patients with low levels of hypercapnia, a trial of night CPAP is useful to detect patients without severe nocturnal hypoxemia who could be proposed to nCPAP plus oxygen as a first line treatment. In patients who demonstrate a severe nocturnal hypercapnia, mechanical NIV is chosen; expiratory positive airway pressure (EPAP) is titrated to control hypopnoeas and apnoeas and inspiratory positive airway pressure (IPAP) is added to control P_{aCO_2}. If pressure pre-set NIV fails, target-volume ventilation or, in some cases, nasal volume pre-set ventilation may be used. In patients with OHS and predominant OSA, once hypercapnia has improved using mechanical NIV (which may take several weeks or months), mechanical NIV may be changed to nCPAP (fig. 3). Mechanical NIV has also largely improved the immediate vital prognosis of OHS and acute respiratory failure.

Medical management is mainly orientated towards weight loss. A reduction of 5–10% of body weight can result in a significant decrease in P_{aCO_2}. Unfortunately, weight loss by diet alone is difficult to achieve and sustain; thus, bariatric surgery may be proposed in the youngest patients. After significant weight-reduction surgery, patients with OHS experience long-term improvement of arterial blood gases and dyspnoea, which may lead, after night ventilator polygraphy monitoring showing disappearance of sleep-disordered breathing, to discontinuation of the ventilator treatment.

If obesity is absent or not predominant, the most frequent conditions are: neuromuscular diseases with Duchenne muscular dystrophy; Steinert myotony; polio sequelae; amyotrophic lateral sclerosis; and high spinal injuries with tetraplegia and respiratory paralysis (less frequent are acid maltase deficiency and spinal muscular atrophy), and chest wall diseases with kyphoscoliosis and/or TB sequelae.

These diseases represent the best indication for the application of acute and chronic mechanical ventilation (mainly with NIV) and, in some severe situations or after failure of NIV, with invasive mechanical ventilation and tracheostomy.

Other conditions of sleep-related hypoventilation There are less frequent conditions including neurological conditions such as Arnold–Chiari malformations, brainstem tumours, space occupying lesions, vascular malformations, central nervous system infection, stroke, or neurosurgical procedure which may be associated with central hypoventilation.

Congenital central hypoventilation syndrome is a rare disorder of ventilatory control that typically presents in newborns and mainly results from a polyalanine repeat expansion mutation in the *PHOX2B* gene. It results in the failure of automatic central

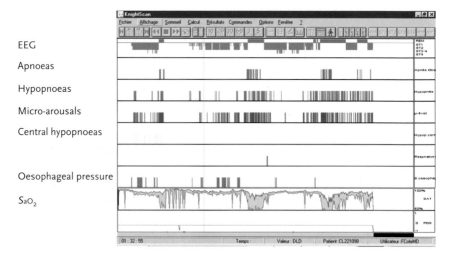

Figure 2. A ventilator polygraphy from a patient with severe OHS (J.L. Pepin, personal communication, with permission).

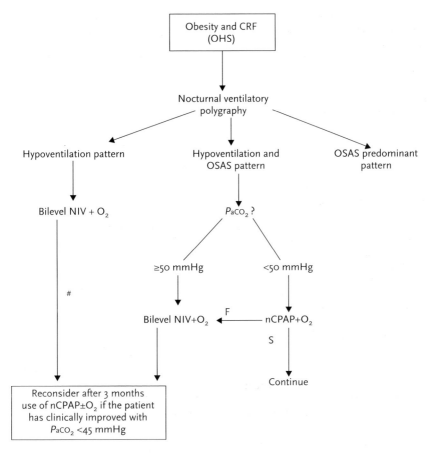

Figure 3. A ventilator management algorithm in a patient with severe OHS presenting with chronic respiratory failure (CRF). F: failure; S: success. #: an alternative is assisted control ventilation.

control of breathing in infants who do not breathe spontaneously or who breathe shallowly and erratically. Sufferers are generally treated by mechanical ventilation with tracheostomy and, in less severe situations, by mechanical NIV. Electrostimulation of the phrenic nerves and/or the diaphragm is currently being tested as a new therapeutic option.

Some rare conditions of proven sleep-related hypoventilation for which all the previous aetiologies have been ruled out are considered as idiopathic; it is always important to review the medications of such patient in order to detect intake of respiratory centres depressors (morphine, antitussive drugs, hypnotic and sedatives compounds) which are often used by elderly people.

Presence of an obstructive disorder

COPD, diffuse bronchiectasis and CF are the most frequent conditions. During sleep there is a worsening of awake hypoxaemia and hypercapnia, especially during REM sleep. Mechanical NIV is generally proposed after failure of long-term oxygen therapy in hypercapnic COPD when frequent episodes of acute respiratory decompensation occur and/or when baseline $P_{a}CO_2$ progressively worsens. COPD patients with obesity must be investigated for possible overlap syndrome, which is associated with obstructive sleep apnoea and COPD and is frequently a good responder to mechanical NIV.

Further reading

- Bannerjee D, et al. (2007). Obesity hypoventilation syndrome: hypoxemia during CPAP. Chest; 131: 1678–1684.
- Casey KR, et al. (2007). Sleep related hypoventilation/hypoxemic syndromes. Chest; 131: 1936–1948.
- Chouri-Pontarollo N, et al. (2007). Impaired objective daytime vigilance in obesity-hypoventilation syndrome: impact of noninvasive ventilation. Chest; 131: 148–155.
- Cuvelier A, et al. (2007). Obesity hypoventilation syndrome. New insights in the Pickwick papers. Chest; 131: 7–8.
- de Lucas-Ramos P, et al. (2004). Benefits at 1 year of nocturnal intermittent positive pressure ventilation in patients with obesity-hypoventilation syndrome. Respir Med; 98: 961–967.
- Guo YF, et al. (2007). Respiratory patterns during sleep in OHS patients treated with nocturnal pressure support. Chest; 131: 1090–1099.
- Kessler, R, et al. (2001). The obesity-hypoventilation syndrome revisited: a prospective study of 34 consecutive cases. Chest; 120: 369–376.
- Mokhlesi B (2007). Positive airway pressure titration in obesity hypoventilation syndrome. CPAP or bi-level AP? Chest; 131: 1624–1626.
- Mokhlesi B (2010). Obesity hypoventilation syndrome. A state of the art review. Respir Care; 55: 1347–1365.
- Muir JF, et al. Management of chronic respiratory failure and obesity. In: Ambrosino N, eds. Ventilatory Support for Chronic Respiratory Failure. Vol. 1. New York, Informa Healthcare, 2008; pp. 433–444.
- Piper AJ, et al. (2011). Obesity hypoventilation syndrome: mechanism and management. Am J Respir Crit Care Med; 183: 292–298.

Pulmonary diseases in primary immunodeficiency syndromes

Federica Pulvirenti, Cinzia Milito, Maria Anna Digiulio and Isabella Quinti

Almost all patients with primary antibody deficiencies suffer from upper and lower respiratory tract bacterial infections. Severe and recurrent infections with capsulated bacteria, asthma, and bronchiectasis represent the most important morbidity and mortality factors. The pathogens commonly isolated from the sputum are *Haemophilus influenzae*, *Streptococcus pneumoniae* and *Streptococcus pyogenes*, with *Pseudomonas aeruginosa* and *Moraxella catarrhalis* occurring less frequently (table 1).

Key points

- PIDs include multiple genetic defects that belong to the group of rare diseases. The World Health Organization recognises >70 diseases classified as PID.

- The risk and type of infections change according to the main defect of the immune system: they are classified as antibody deficiencies, combined immunodeficiencies, phagocytic disorders and innate immunity disorders.

- In pulmonology, a PID diagnosis should be considered in patients presenting with: 1) severe and recurrent respiratory infections; 2) granulomatous diseases; and 3) life-threatening invasive pulmonary infections. In some cases, there are unique features of lung abnormalities in specific defects.

Pneumonia is a common acute infection in primary antibody deficiency (PAD). Studies of PAD patients have revealed that at least two-thirds of patients have one or more episodes of pneumonia prior to diagnosis. Patients are prone to pneumonia-associated complications that require hospitalisation. Respiratory infections lead over time to permanent lung damage.

Chronic lung disease (CLD) represents the principal morbidity factor. As already demonstrated in patients with CF, dyspnoea and sputum production are conditioning factors of increased morbidity. Accumulated mucus in the airways is the prominent feature of bronchiectasis, leading to airway obstruction, bacterial colonisation and recurrent infections.

The events that define the pathogenesis of an infection depend on a large range of variables, including the specific infecting organism, its virulence and the overall immunological state of the host. IgG antibodies are only one player in the complex network of cells and mediators required to protect the respiratory tract against various insults, including infections. In support of this, data indicate the role of a very low IgA level as a major independent risk factor for all the main primary immunodeficiency (PID)-associated clinical conditions (pneumonia, CLD, and acute and chronic sinusitis), underlining the well-known role of IgA in immune defence against a variety of potentially pathogenic organisms when they are encountered in the respiratory and intestinal tracts. The generation of secretory IgA has a basic impact on the epithelial barrier, a function lacking in the majority of PID patients. Moreover, low IgA levels reflect a severely impaired

Table 1. Microorganisms in PID

	Antibody deficiencies	Combined immunodeficiencies	Phagocytic defects
Viruses	Enteroviruses	CMV Respiratory syncytial virus EBV Parainfluenza virus type 3	No
Bacteria	*Streptococcus pneumoniae* *Haemophilus influenzae* *Moraxella catarrhalis* *Pseudomonas aeruginosa* *Staphylococcus aureus* *Neisseria meningitidis* *Mycoplasma* *pneumoniae* *Campylobacter*	As for antibody deficiencies, plus: *Salmonella typhi* *Listeria monocytogenes*	*Staphylococcus* *aureus* *Pneumoniae* *aeruginosa* *Nocardia asteroides* *Salmonella typhi*
Mycobacteria	No	Nontuberculous, including BCG	Nontubercolous, BCG
Fungi	No	*Candida* *Pneumocystis jirovecii*	*Aspergillus*

CMV: cytomegalovirus; EBV: Epstein–Barr virus; BCG: bacille Calmette–Guérin. Reproduced and modified from Notarangelo (2010) with permission from the publisher.

isotype-switching process. Thus, the loss of function of memory B-cells seems to represent the major cause of PID-associated clinical conditions, as demonstrated in common variable immunodeficiency (CVID) patients with bronchiectasis: patients with decreased frequencies of memory B-cells have low levels of IgG/IgM, and high rates of autoimmune disease and bronchiectasis. Thus, assessment of memory B-cells could be considered a prognostic factor in CVID patients.

In patients with cellular and combined immunodeficiencies and in patients with PID who have undergone a haematopoietic stem cell transplant, respiratory viral infections are major causes of morbidity and mortality. Any virus may be detected and all worsen the clinical outcome. Herpes viruses, paramyxoviruses and adenoviruses are common significant pathogens in these patients. Aggressive antiviral treatments may reduce viral replication and lung damage. Fungal infections can result in significant morbidity and potentially fatal outcomes if misdiagnosed or not correctly treated.

Noninfectious associated respiratory diseases might also occur in PID patients and should be taken into consideration in the differential diagnosis: nonspecific interstitial pneumonia, granulomatous lymphocytic interstitial pneumonia, cryptogenic organising pneumonia and lymphocyte interstitial pneumonia.

Medical imaging, especially HRCT, plays a crucial role in the initial detection and characterisation of changes, and in monitoring the response to therapy. The spectrum of abnormalities seen in thoracic imaging includes noninfectious airway disorders, infections, CLD, chronic inflammatory conditions, and benign and malignant neoplasm. Bronchial wall thickening and bronchiectasis are the most common pulmonary changes observed in patients with primary humoral immunodeficiencies: their presence is indicative of a poor prognosis and is suggestive of the evolution of the disease process to an irreversible stage (e.g. lung fibrosis). Small airway involvement leads to ventilation abnormalities and chronic obstructive disease, which are found in 33–43% of patients with PAD and are almost always irreversible. In addition, air trapping, emphysema, bullae, ground-glass nodules and parenchymal abnormalities are common.

Granulomatous-lymphocytic interstitial lung disease (GLILD) is a 'sarcoid-like' inflammatory process with nodular lymphocytic infiltrates, bronchus-associated lymphoid tissue (BALT) hyperplasia and peribronchiolar lymphocytic infiltrates, perivascular granuloma, and lymphocytic interstitial pneumonia. It is present in as many as 8% of patients with PAD. The presence of sarcoid-like granulomatosis is indicative of a dismal prognosis, with terminal respiratory insufficiency developing in ~24% of cases. By HRCT, interstitial nonspecific pneumonia findings include ground-glass opacities (in one-third of cases, these are the only abnormalities), lobe volume loss, a reticular pattern, traction bronchiectasis, and areas of fibrosis predominantly at the basal level with a subpleural, peribronchovascular distribution.

Lung alterations in patient with PID might be evaluated also by MRI, a radiation-free alternative to CT. Lung function tests are also useful: they show ventilatory disturbance, an obstructive pattern or pattern mix.

Treatment

In PID where the defect is an inability to produce an effective antibody response to pathogens, IgG can be replaced. However, despite IgG replacement, the percentage of patients with CLD and bronchiectasis increases over time (>50% in adults and 30–40% in children). The overall probability of developing CLD reaches ~80% after 17 years of follow-up. In fact, substitutive therapy with IgG reduces the risk of acute respiratory infections, particularly of pneumonia, but has a low efficacy in the reduction of chronic lung complications, infective exacerbations and asthma promoted by vicious circle infection–inflammation (protease release from polymorphonucleates, epithelial damage, epithelial cuboidalisation, mucus accumulation predisposing to recurrent infections and chronic inflammatory phenomena favouring remodelling).

Treatment strategies for progressive GLILD in CVID include corticosteroids, methotrexate, azathioprine, leflunomide or mofetil mycophenolate. Biological therapies have been used in single patients or in small trials. Aside from immunoglobulin replacement, a strategy to reduce lung

Table 2. Clinical presentation and clinical respiratory diagnosis in primary antibody deficiencies

Symptoms and signs	Respiratory clinical diagnosis
Recurrent chest infection	Bronchiectasis
Productive cough	Recurrent chest infection/pneumonia
Wheeze	Asthma
Weight loss	Granulomatous lung disease
Rhinosinusitis	Emphysema
Otitis media	Previous TB
Progressive dyspnoea	Cavitating lung lesion
Hypoxaemia	Rhinosinusitis
T_{LCO} alteration	
Polycythaemia	
Cyanosis	

damage should be approached. Prophylactic antibiotics, macrolides as anti-inflammatory agents, inhaled corticosteroids, bronchodilators, mucolytic agents, or mechanical or rehabilitative respiratory methods need to be considered.

In conclusion, a PID diagnosis should be considered in patients presenting with severe and recurrent respiratory infections, with granulomatous diseases or with life-threatening invasive pulmonary infections (table 2).

Further reading

- Alachkar H, et al. (2006). Memory switched B cell percentage and not serum immunoglobulin concentration is associated with clinical complications in children and adults with specific antibody deficiency and common variable immunodeficiency. Clin Immunol; 120: 310–318.
- Associazione Italiana Ematologia Oncolgia Pediatrica. www.aeiop.org
- Carsetti R, et al. (2005). The loss of IgM memory B cells correlates with clinical disease in common variable immunodeficiency. J Allergy Clin Immunol; 115: 412–417.
- Costa-Carvalho BT, et al. (2011). Pulmonary complications in patient with antibody deficiency. Allergol Immunopathol (Madr); 39: 128–132.
- Crooks BN, et al. (2000). Respiratory viral infections in primary immune deficiencies: significance and relevance to clinical outcome in a single BMT unit. Bone Marrow Transplant; 26: 1097–1102.
- Guillaume B, et al. (2009). Thoracic manifestations of primary humoral immunodeficiency: a comprehensive review. RadioGraphics; 29: 1909–1920.
- Notarangelo LD (2010). Primary immunodeficiencies. J Allergy Clin Immunol; 125: Suppl. 2, S182–S194.
- Pilette C, et al. (2001). Lung mucosal immunity: immunoglobulin-A revisited. Eur Respir J; 18: 571–588.
- Plebani A, et al. (2002). Clinical, immunological, and molecular analysis in a large cohort of patients with X-linked agammaglobulinemia: an Italian multicenter study. Clin Immunol; 104: 221–230.
- Primary immunodeficiency diseases. Report of an IUIS Scientific Committee. International Union of Immunological Societies. Clin Exp Immunol; 118: Suppl. 1, 1–28.
- Quinti I, et al. (2007). Long-term follow-up and outcome of a large cohort of patients with common variable immunodeficiency. J Clin Immunol; 27: 308–316.
- Quinti I, et al. (2011). Effectiveness of immunoglobulin replacement therapy on clinical outcome in patients with primary antibody deficiencies: results from a multicenter prospective cohort study. J Clin Immunol; 31: 315–322.
- Sanchez-Ramon S, et al. (2008). Memory B cells in common variable immunodeficiency: clinical associations and sex differences. Clin Immunol; 128: 314–321.
- Serra G, et al. (2011). Lung MRI as a possible alternative to CT scan for patients with primary immune deficiencies and increased radiosensitivity. Chest; 140: 1581–1589.
- Thickett KM, et al. (2002). Common variable immune deficiency: respiratory manifestations, pulmonary function and high-resolution CT scan findings. QJM; 95: 655–662.
- Vodjgani M, et al. (2007). Analysis of class-switched memory b cells in patients with common variable immunodeficiency and its clinical implications. J Investig Allergol Clin Immunol; 17: 321–328.
- Wood P, et al. (2007). Recognition, clinical diagnosis and management of patients with primary antibody deficiencies: a systematic review. Clin Exp Immunol; 149: 410–423.

HIV-related disease

Marc C.I. Lipman and Rob F. Miller

Key points

- In populations with access to antiretroviral therapy, use of combination antiretroviral therapy (CART) has led to a marked reduction in the incidence of many HIV-associated pulmonary diseases and improved overall outcome following a severe respiratory event.

- Despite CART, bacterial infections remain more common in HIV-infected people than in the general population.

- In response to starting CART, there may be an overexuberant and uncontrolled immune response to exogenous antigen. This phenomenon of immune reconstitution disease can mimic a variety of other conditions and may be life threatening.

- TB may occur at any stage of HIV infection. Cases should be managed in line with appropriate public health and infection control guidance.

- Noninfectious respiratory complications of HIV are increasingly recognised in an ageing population. Many of these, such as COPD and lung cancer, are linked to smoking, and can run an accelerated course compared with the general population.

- Quitting smoking is an important component of long-term respiratory health maintenance.

Most HIV-infected people experience at least one significant episode of respiratory disease during their lifetime. Although the widespread use of effective combination antiretroviral therapy (CART) has led to a 50–90% fall in the incidence of many HIV-associated opportunistic infections and some malignancies, the associated reduction in short-term mortality means that people with HIV infection are now living longer, and so are developing (often at an increased frequency) noninfectious pulmonary conditions usually present in older age. Thus, HIV patients with respiratory symptoms require careful, systematic investigation to exclude a wide variety of illnesses and pathogens.

This chapter will focus upon common causes of HIV-related respiratory disease (table 1). For an individual, the scope and scale of the problem depends on a number of factors including their risk of exposure to pathogens (*e.g.* through geography or lifestyle, such as injecting drug use; their ability to obtain and consistently use CART successfully; the use of specific preventive therapies such as co-trimoxazole; and co-factors such as cigarette smoking). Unfortunately, there are still a large number of people who present with severe respiratory disease and undiagnosed HIV infection. This is avoidable and should be regarded as a failure of societal medical care.

In the following sections we use blood absolute CD4 counts to categorise the stages of HIV infection. This is a reasonably accurate measure of systemic and local immunity (in HIV-uninfected individuals, the CD4 count is typically >500 cells·μL^{-1}). In HIV-infected subjects with preserved immunity, typical community-acquired

Table 1. Common causes of HIV-associated respiratory disease

Infectious conditions	Non-infectious conditions
Upper respiratory tract infection	**Malignancy**
Acute sinusitis	Kaposi sarcoma
Chronic sinusitis	Lymphoma
Acute bronchitis	Bronchial carcinoma
Bronchiectasis	**Nonmalignant conditions**
Bacterial pneumonia	COPD
Streptococcus pneumoniae	HIV-associated pneumonitis *e.g.* NSIP and LIP
Haemophilus influenzae	Pulmonary arterial hypertension
Viral infection	Pneumothorax
Influenza A	HIV therapy causing respiratory symptoms *e.g.* IRD
TB	
Fungal infection	
Pneumocystis pneumonia	
Histoplasma capsulatum	
Cryptococcus neoformans	

NSIP: nonspecific interstitial pneumonitis; LIP: lymphocytic interstitial pneumonitis; IRD: immune reconstitution disease

infections occur but at a greater frequency than in the general population. With advancing HIV-induced immuno-suppression (CD4 counts $<$200 cells·µL^{-1}), the risk of opportunistic infections and malignancy rapidly increases.

Infections

Bacterial infection Upper respiratory tract infections, acute bronchitis, and acute and symptomatic chronic sinusitis occur more frequently in HIV-infected patients than in the general population.

Bronchiectasis is increasingly recognised in patients with advanced HIV disease. It probably arises as a consequence of recurrent *Pneumocystis jiroveci* pneumonia or bacterial infection.

Compared with HIV-negative populations, bacterial pneumonia is six to 10 times more frequent in HIV-infected subjects not using CART. Injecting drug users are particularly vulnerable (with a risk approximately double that of other HIV-infected people). The presentation of HIV-associated community-acquired bacterial pneumonia is similar to that in HIV-negative subjects. However, the chest radiograph may be atypical, and mimic *P. jiroveci* pneumonia in up to half of cases. The usual pathogens isolated are

Streptococcus pneumoniae and *Haemophilus influenzae*. Infection with *Staphylococcus aureus* and Gram-negative organisms may occur in advanced HIV disease. *Mycoplasma*, *Legionella* and *Chlamydia* species are probably no more frequent.

Bacteraemia is reported to be up to 100 times more common in HIV-infected patients with bacterial pneumonia, irrespective of blood CD4 count. These data come from studies performed prior to CART. Even so, it highlights the importance of undertaking a full set of investigations (including blood cultures) in HIV-infected individuals presenting with community-acquired pneumonia.

Complications of bacterial infection include intrapulmonary cavitation, abscess formation and empyema. There is a high relapse rate, despite appropriate antibiotic therapy.

Immunisation with pneumococcal vaccine is recommended in all adults and adolescents (at diagnosis of HIV infection and after 5 years). Conjugate vaccines appear to offer better protection than polysaccharide vaccines. Humoral responses and clinical efficacy are probably impaired in those with CD4 counts $<$200 cells·µL^{-1}, although vaccination can be successfully re-administered to subjects on CART who have not developed protective immunity from prior vaccination when not using CART.

Viral infection The recent influenza A H1N1 pandemic has served as a reminder that opportunistic viral infections, such as *Cytomegalovirus* pneumonitis, are, for many HIV-infected individuals, much less of an issue than common viral pathogens. H1N1 appears to have a similar presentation and outcome when associated with HIV co-infection. CART probably offers little specific protection and annual influenza immunisation is recommended.

Fungal infection P. *jiroveci*, formerly P. *carinii*, is the cause of *Pneumocystis* pneumonia (PCP). It remains a common problem in individuals unaware of their HIV serostatus and also among HIV-infected patients intolerant of, or nonadherent with, PCP prophylaxis and/or CART.

Patients present with nonproductive cough and progressive exertional breathlessness of several days' to weeks' duration, with or without fever. On auscultation, the chest is usually clear; occasionally, end-inspiratory crackles are audible. In early PCP, the chest radiograph may be normal ($\sim$10% of cases). The most common abnormality is bilateral perihilar, interstitial infiltrates, which may progress to diffuse alveolar shadowing over a period of days. Atypical radiographic appearances include upper zone infiltrates resembling TB, hilar/mediastinal lymph-adenopathy, intrapulmonary nodules and lobar consolidation (present in up to 20% of cases).

Treatment is usually started empirically in patients with typical clinical and radiological features and a CD4 count of <200 cells·μL^{-1}, pending diagnosis by cytological analysis of bronchoalveolar lavage (BAL) fluid or induced sputum samples.

Several factors present at, or soon after, hospitalisation predict poor outcome from PCP. These include increasing patient age, a second or third episode of PCP, hypoxaemia, low haemoglobin, co-existent pulmonary Kaposi sarcoma and medical comorbidity.

Once hospitalised, development of pneumothorax, admission to the intensive care unit and the need for mechanical ventilation are associated with a worse outcome.

PCP can be stratified clinically as mild (PaO$_2$ >11.0 kPa, SaO$_2$ >96% breathing air at rest), moderate (PaO$_2$ 8.0–11.0 kPa, SaO$_2$ 91–96%) or severe (PaO$_2$ <8.0 kPa, SaO$_2$ <91%). This categorisation is helpful, as oral therapy may be given to those with mild disease. The first-choice treatment for PCP of all severity is high-dose co-trimoxazole (sulphamethoxazole 100 mg·kg^{-1}·day^{-1} with trimethoprim 20 mg·kg^{-1}·day^{-1}) in two to four divided doses orally or intravenously for 21 days. Approximately two-thirds of patients will successfully complete this regimen. Treatment-limiting drug toxicity (*e.g.* intense gastro-intestinal upset, rash, bone marrow suppression, or renal or liver dysfunction) is common, while <10% who tolerate therapy do not respond to treatment (defined by deterioration ⩾5 days after initiation).

In patients with drug toxicity or poor response to co-trimoxazole, alternative therapy in mild/moderate disease includes clindamycin (450–600 mg four times daily orally or *i.v.*) plus oral primaquine (15 mg daily), oral dapsone (100 mg daily) with trimethoprim (20 mg·kg^{-1}·day^{-1}), or oral atovaquone suspension (750 mg twice daily). In severe disease, alternative therapy is clindamycin with primaquine or *i.v.* pentamidine (4 mg·kg^{-1} daily).

Patients with an admission PaO$_2$ ⩽9.3 kPa should also receive adjunctive gluco-corticoids within 72 h of starting specific anti-PCP treatment. A frequently used regimen is prednisolone, 40 mg twice daily for 5 days, then 40 mg daily on days 6–10, and 20 mg daily on days 11–21. This has been shown to reduce mortality. Patients should be monitored carefully for steroid-related adverse events, including hyper-tension, hyperglycaemia, and local and systemic viral reactivation.

Co-trimoxazole, dapsone and primaquine should be avoided in patients with glucose-6-phosphate dehydrogenase deficiency, and testing for the enzyme deficiency is recommended as standard practice.

Patients are at increased risk of PCP as their blood CD4 count decreases.

Regimens for PCP prophylaxis are listed in table 2.

Indications for primary prophylaxis are:

- blood absolute CD4 count <200 cells·µL^{-1}
- blood CD4 count <14% of total lymphocyte count
- unexplained fever (>3 weeks' duration)
- persistent or recurrent oral/pharyngeal *Candida*
- history of another AIDS-defining diagnosis, *e.g.* Kaposi sarcoma

The indication for secondary prophylaxis is:

- all patients who have had a previous episode of PCP

Indications for discontinuing secondary prophylaxis are:

- patients on CART with a sustained increase in blood CD4 count

(>200 cells·µL^{-1}) and undetectable plasma HIV RNA for ≥3 months (note that if CD4 count subsequently falls below 200 cells·µL^{-1} and/or the HIV RNA load increases, prophylaxis should be re-instituted)

- based on the rates of recurrent PCP noted within observational cohorts, some clinicians will discontinue treatment if the HIV load is undetectable and blood CD4 is >100 cells·µL^{-1}

It is recommended that, if possible, all patients with an episode of PCP start CART within 2 weeks of completing their anti-*Pneumocystis* treatment.

Tuberculosis All patients with TB and unknown HIV status should be offered an HIV test. Active TB is estimated to occur between 20 and 40 times more frequently in HIV-infected subjects. Worldwide, almost 15% of new TB cases occur in HIV-infected subjects. TB accounts for ~25% of all HIV-related deaths. TB is also covered in other chapters, so here the focus is on issues of particular relevance in HIV infection.

More than two-thirds of patients with TB and HIV co-infection present with

Table 2. Recommended PCP prophylaxis regimens

	Drug	Dosage	Notes
First choice	Co-trimoxazole (sulphamethoxazole + trimethoprim 5:1)	960 mg once daily[#] 480 mg once daily 960 mg thrice weekly	Protects against certain bacterial infections and reactivation of toxoplasmosis Adverse effects include nausea (40%), rash (up to 20%), bone marrow suppression (20%)
Second choice	Aerosolised pentamidine	300 mg once per month *via* jet nebuliser	Use once per fortnight if CD4 count <50 cells·µL^{-1}
	Dapsone	100 mg once daily	Plus oral pyrimethamine 25 mg once per week against reactivation of toxoplasmosis
Third choice	Atovaquone	Suspension 750 mg twice daily	
	Azithromycin	1250 mg once per week	

[#]: the use of lower doses of co-trimoxazole may be associated with fewer adverse events.

pulmonary disease. When blood CD4 counts are normal or only slightly reduced (e.g. >350 cells·µL⁻¹), clinical features are similar to adult post-primary disease. Chest radiography often shows upper lobe infiltrates and cavitary changes. Sputum and BAL fluid are often smear positive.

In advanced HIV disease, and/or with a low blood CD4 count (<200 cells·µL⁻¹), the presentation is often with nonspecific malaise, fatigue, weight loss and fever. Chest radiographic abnormalities may not be specific for TB and include diffuse or miliary-type shadowing, mediastinal/hilar lymphadenopathy and pleural effusions; cavitation is uncommon. Sputum or BAL fluid is often smear negative though culture positive. Extrapulmonary TB is common in patients with CD4 counts <100 cells·µL⁻¹. Local or disseminated infection may involve lymph nodes and bone marrow, blood cultures may be positive and it is worth obtaining specimens from as many body sites or fluids as clinically practical. For example, the yield from early-morning urine cultures is reasonable.

If smears or unspeciated mycobacterial cultures are positive, treatment should initially include a four-drug anti-TB regimen with a rifamycin (either rifampicin or rifabutin) plus isoniazid, pyrazinamide and ethambutol, until mycobacterial identification and drug sensitivities are known. TB diagnosis using rapid nucleic acid amplification tests are increasingly sensitive in HIV infected individuals, although, generally, this remains less than in HIV-negative TB patients. The molecular probes can distinguish Mycobacterium tuberculosis from opportunistic mycobacteria and identify common mutations in the rpoB gene associated with rifampicin resistance, as well as isoniazid (katG and inhA genes) and mutations associated with resistance to other anti-TB drugs, depending on the test kit used.

Rapid molecular diagnostic assays, such as the Xpert MTB/RIF (Cepheid, Sunnyvale, CA, USA), are increasingly simple to use in a field setting. They enable often scarce resources to be allocated effectively; for example, if a patient is shown to have rifampicin resistance using the probe, then an early decision can be made to treat for multidrug-resistant TB in the first instance and appropriate samples set up for mycobacterial culture and sensitivity testing, which may not be a part of local, routine care.

Point-of-care rapid antigen assays using relatively easily obtained body fluids (e.g. the mycobacterial cell wall antigen lipoarabinomannan tested in urine) may be of more value in HIV-infected than -uninfected individuals with suspected active TB. However, despite good specificity, their sensitivity appears generally low other than in patients with TB and advanced HIV infection (presumably due to such individuals having a greater mycobacterial load).

The wider use of rapid mycobacterial detection systems has led to the discovery that 'subclinical' TB is common in HIV-infected subjects from TB endemic areas. Here, patients are generally well but have viable bacilli isolated from, for example, sputum and, hence, require treatment for TB. This has been reported in up to 20% of patients being screened for active TB prior to starting CART. In lower TB prevalence areas, it is less common and probably occurs in, at most, 5% of such individuals.

Short- and long-term response to treatment with a 6-month four-drug regimen is generally good, although patients with disseminated disease are often treated for 9–12 months. Given the reported increased risk of developing drug-resistant disease, it is recommended that HIV patients with high mycobacterial loads (e.g. disseminated disease, as is often present in patients with low blood CD4 counts) receive daily and not higher-dose (twice- or thrice-weekly) intermittent therapy. Compared with non-HIV-infected individuals, there is possibly a greater incidence of adverse reactions to anti-TB drugs and an increased risk of death.

CART reduces short- and long-term mortality in co-infected patients and should be started as soon as possible in subjects receiving treatment for active TB. Generally, the lower the blood CD4 count, the more pressing is the clinical need to start CART (e.g. if blood CD4 <200 cells·μL⁻¹, then commence within 2–4 weeks of start of anti-TB treatment).

Issues with early use of CART in TB patients include:

- high pill burden
- overlapping toxicities, e.g. neuropathy
- drug–drug interactions, e.g. CART and rifamycins
- poor adherence to complex regimens
- increased risk of immune reconstitution disease (IRD) (see later, and of particular relevance when starting CART within days of anti-TB treatment in cerebral TB)

Multidrug- and extensively drug-resistant TB have been associated epidemiologically with HIV infection. This is probably due to the rapid development of active (and, hence, infectious) TB in the HIV co-infected population exposed to drug-resistant cases and, hence, reflects general susceptibility to developing mycobacterial disease rather than to infection with specific drug-resistant strains.

Given the high risk of latent TB infection (LTBI) progressing to active disease, the World Health Organization recommends that HIV-infected patients with LTBI should receive preventive treatment. As, by definition, LTBI diagnosis requires a positive immune response (e.g. tuberculin skin test or blood interferon-γ release assay) in an asymptomatic individual, these assessments can be affected by the immune dysregulation present in HIV co-infected subjects.

Malignant conditions

Kaposi sarcoma Kaposi sarcoma is the most common HIV-associated malignancy. Before the advent of CART, 15–20% of AIDS diagnoses were due to Kaposi sarcoma. It is associated with human herpes virus-8 (also called Kaposi sarcoma-associated virus) co-infection. Pulmonary Kaposi sarcoma is almost always accompanied by cutaneous or lymphadenopathic Kaposi sarcoma (palatal disease strongly predicts the presence of pulmonary lesions). Presentation is with nonspecific cough and progressive dyspnoea; haemoptysis is uncommon.

As Kaposi sarcoma may involve both the airways and lung parenchyma; radiological findings include interstitial or nodular infiltrates and alveolar consolidation. Hilar/mediastinal lymphadenopathy occurs in ~25% of patients and up to 40% have a pleural effusion.

Diagnosis is confirmed at bronchoscopy in >50% cases by the appearance of multiple, raised or flat, red or purple endotracheal and endobronchial lesions. Biopsy is rarely performed since cutaneous Kaposi sarcoma is usually present and diagnostic yield from biopsy is <20%. CART may induce remission of lesions and is used in addition to chemotherapy.

Lymphoma High-grade B-cell non-Hodgkin lymphoma is the most common HIV-associated thoracic lymphoma and is usually found in association with disease elsewhere. Presenting symptoms are nonspecific. Chest radiographic abnormalities include mediastinal lymphadenopathy, pleural masses or effusions. The prognosis is considerably better if patients treated with chemotherapy also receive CART.

Bronchial carcinoma Lung cancer appears to be around twice as common in HIV-infected compared with HIV-negative smokers. It is now more frequently diagnosed than in the pre-CART era and probably reflects the protection CART offers from other conditions that otherwise would have occurred. The clinical presentation is often late and, despite specific treatment, plus the use of CART if not already prescribed, the prognosis is, therefore, generally poor.

Nonmalignant, noninfectious conditions

Chronic obstructive pulmonary disease HIV-infected smokers are at increased risk (approximately 20–30%) of developing COPD. Although this does not approach the relative risk associated with many respiratory infections, in a similar manner to lung cancer, the onset of symptoms appears to be at a younger age. Some studies suggest that such individuals have a greater degree of breathlessness and functional disability compared with HIV-negative COPD patients with equivalent lung function.

The large number of HIV-positive ageing smokers together with the synergistic effects of smoking, recurrent bacterial and opportunistic infections, injecting drug use, and possibly the direct effect of HIV in the lung (plus also the inflammatory response generated by use of CART), argue strongly for scaling up smoking cessation services. This is important as in many developed-world settings, smoking rates in HIV-infected populations are higher than national averages. Smoking cessation will also impact on other smoking-related illnesses such as cardiovascular disease, which are increasingly prevalent in HIV-infected communities.

HIV-associated pneumonitis Nonspecific pneumonitis mimics PCP but often occurs at higher blood CD4 counts. Diagnosis requires transbronchial, video-assisted thoracoscopic or open-lung biopsy. Most episodes are self limiting, but prednisolone may be beneficial.

Lymphocytic interstitial pneumonitis is generally seen in HIV-infected children and clinically resembles idiopathic pulmonary fibrosis. Diagnosis requires biopsy. Treatment with CART is often effective.

Pulmonary arterial hypertension Pulmonary arterial hypertension is reported to be six to 12 times more common in HIV-infected populations. The presentation and management are similar to immunocompetent individuals, although CART is associated with improved haemodynamics and survival.

Pneumothorax occurs more frequently in HIV-infected patients than in the age-matched general medical population. Cigarette smoking and receipt of nebulised pentamidine are risk factors. PCP should be excluded in any patient presenting with a pneumothorax.

HIV therapy causing respiratory symptoms
The clear beneficial impact of antiretroviral therapy on long-term morbidity and mortality

means that CART is now a global standard of care for most HIV-infected people. The changes in immunity that occur when it is first started can be intense. In up to 30% subjects who have documented or subclinical co-infection, the immune response may be overexuberant and manifest as a clinical deterioration in health status. This has been given several names including immune reconstitution inflammatory syndrome and IRD. It has been reported to occur with a number of conditions, but particularly mycobacterial disease and chronic fungal and viral infections.

The underlying mechanism is not completely understood, and its clinical features represent both innate and acquired host responses to exogenous antigen. The 'paradoxical' type of IRD is similar to that seen in non-HIV-infected patients being treated for TB but is generally more intense. Here, subjects with known TB improving on treatment start CART and within a median of 2–3 weeks develop new clinical manifestations, e.g. peripheral lymph-adenopathy, pleural or pericardial effusions or cerebral disease. There is no specific diagnostic test and so drug resistance, patient nonadherence to treatment and other disease processes must be actively excluded. It is more likely in people with low baseline CD4 counts ($<$100 cells·μL^{-1}), faster suppression of HIV viral load and shorter time between starting anti-TB therapy and CART. IRD can be severe, though is rarely fatal. When this does happen it is generally due to the pressure effects associated with a rapid increase in size of the inflammatory lesions. Hence, care must be taken with IRD associated with cerebral, pericardial and, sometimes, mediastinal disease. Treatment is largely symptomatic and may involve oral glucocorticoid therapy.

A second form of IRD is the 'unmasking' of TB. Here, a patient with latent, asymptomatic infection will rapidly develop highly inflammatory active TB a median of 3–6 weeks after starting CART. Treatment is generally directed at the underlying mycobacterial infection. In TB-endemic areas, such as sub-Saharan Africa and South-East Asia, screening subjects for subclinical TB prior to CART initiation is important. Studies have indicated that up to one in five of individuals who are minimally symptomatic will have sputum culture-positive TB and, hence, require treatment. The use of rapid molecular and mycobacterial diagnostic tests (described earlier in this chapter) are a useful and effective means of excluding TB in people who need to start CART.

The antiretroviral nucleoside analogue abacavir can cause a hypersensitivity reaction (in up to 3% of subjects) with fever, rash and pulmonary symptoms. In these cases, recovery occurs if the drug is withdrawn. It should not be given again.

Further reading

- Benfield T. Noninfectious conditions in patients with human immunodeficiency virus infection. *In:* Spiro SG, *et al.*, eds. Clinical Respiratory Medicine. 4th Edn. Philadelphia, Elsevier Saunders, 2012.
- Benfield T, *et al.* (2008). Second-line salvage treatment of AIDS-associated *Pneumocystis jirovecii* pneumonia: a case series and systematic review. *J Acquir Immune Defic Syndr;* 48: 63–67.
- Crothers K, *et al.* (2011). Longitudinal studies of HIV-associated lung infections and complications in the era of anti-retroviral therapy. *Proc Am Thorac Soc;* 8: 275–281.
- Dockrell DH, *et al.* (2011). British HIV Association guidelines for the treatment of opportunistic infection in HIV-positive individuals 2010: pulmonary opportunistic infections. *HIV Med;* 12: Suppl. 2, 1–140.
- Kaplan JE, *et al.* (2009). Guidelines for prevention and treatment of opportunistic infections in HIV-infected adults and adolescents: recommendations from CDC, the National Institutes of Health, and the HIV Medicine Association of the Infectious Diseases Society of America. *MMWR Recomm Rep;* 58: 1–207.
- Lipman MCI, *et al.* An Atlas of Differential Diagnosis in HIV Disease. 2nd Edn. London, Parthenon Publishing, 2004.
- Miller RF, *et al.* Pulmonary infections in patients with human immunodeficiency virus disease. *In:* Spiro SG, *et al.*, eds. Clinical Respiratory Medicine. 4th Edn. Philadelphia, Elsevier Saunders, 2012.
- Pozniak AL, *et al.* (2011). British HIV Association guidelines for the treatment of TB/HIV coinfection 2010. *HIV Med;* 12: 517–524.

Graft *versus* host disease

Federica Pulvirenti, Cinzia Milito, Maria Anna Digiulio and Isabella Quinti

Pathogenesis

Graft *versus* host disease (GVHD) is the principal complication of allogeneic haematopoietic stem cell transplantation (HSCT): it limits HSCT success and is fatal to ~15% of transplant recipients. The number of patients at high risk for GVHD is increasing, as more HSCTs are performed from unrelated donors, mainly in older patients. GVHD results from immunological attack on target recipient organs or tissues (such as the skin, liver and gut) by donor allogeneic T-cells that are transferred along with the allograft. The development and severity of GVHD in transplant recipients depends on many factors, such as recipient age, toxicity of the conditioning regimen, haematopoietic graft source and GVHD prophylaxis approaches.

GVHD is divided into acute and chronic forms. Acute GVHD and chronic GVHD involve distinct pathological processes: acute GVHD has strong inflammatory components, whereas chronic GVHD displays more autoimmune and fibrotic features.

Chronic GVHD is defined as occurring after the first 100 days post-HSCT and has a characteristic clinical presentation, which resembles autoimmune vascular diseases and is distinct from that observed in acute GVHD. Chronic GVHD occurs in 30–65% of allogeneic HSCT recipients, can be highly debilitating in its extensive form and has a 5-year mortality rate of 30–50%, mainly due to immune dysregulation and opportunistic infections.

Acute GVHD was thought to be a process driven mainly by T-helper (Th)1- and Th17-type immune responses, whereas chronic GVHD was thought to be predominately medi-ated by Th2-type responses. Vascular endothelial damage and increased secretion of

> **Key points**
>
> - Graft *versus* host disease (GVHD) is the principal complication of allogeneic HSCT.
>
> - Vascular endothelial damage and increased secretion of pro-inflammatory cytokines are involved in the pathogenesis of lung disorders.
>
> - Acute and subacute patterns of lung injury include: idiopathic interstitial pneumonia, bronchiolitis obliterans syndrome, organising pneumonia, alveolar haemorrhage, capillaritis, post-transplant lymphoproliferative disorders.
>
> - CMV infection is the most frequent viral complication in patients undergoing HSCT and acute GVHD significantly affects active CMV infection recurrence.
>
> - GVHD has beneficial effect of on the incidence of leukaemia relapse and increase the overall survival of patients with leukaemia: this phenomenon is known as the graft-versus-tumour effect.
>
> - New insights from basic immunology, preclinical models and clinical studies have led to novel approaches for prevention and treatment.

pro-inflammatory cytokines are involved in systemic disorders post-HSCT, including GVHD and cytomegalovirus (CMV) infection. The pathology of acute GVHD can be considered in a framework of sequential phases. Initially, the recipient-conditioning regimen damages host tissues and causes release of pro-inflammatory cytokines; host antigen-presenting cells mature, acquire adhesion and co-stimulatory molecules that activate mature donor T-cells; these cells proliferate and produce additional cytokines inducing inflammatory and cellular effectors that amplify the inflammatory responses that cause tissue damage.

The pivotal role of T-cells in acute GVHD is supported by the complete abrogation of GVHD following T-cell depletion from the graft, an approach that remains the most effective in preventing acute GVHD.

Tissue damage caused by the cytotoxic T-cells leads to the recruitment of other effector cells (including natural killer (NK) cells and neutrophils), which further increase tissue injury and result in a self-perpetuating state of GVHD that is difficult to control once it is fully initiated

Current data implicate the innate immune response as being responsible for initiating or amplify-ing acute GVHD. Molecules such as bacterial lipopoly-saccharide (LPS), released from the injured gut during the conditioning regimen, activate innate immune receptors, including Toll-like receptors (TLRs), and cause a cytokine storm, which favours the devel-opment of acute GVHD. Commensal microflora may modulate innate response and reduce the severity of GVHD by stimulating other TLRs (TLR): to re-address the gut flora to make it less GVHD favourable might be a way to ameliorate GVHD, as suggested by the decreased severity of GVHD and improved survival of animals following the administration of probiotic bacteria.

Great progresses have been recently achieved in discerning the role of antigen presenting cells (APCs) in GVHD: MHC class II-bearing host haematopoietic APCs were previously thought to be essential for the induction of CD4$^+$ T-cell-dependent acute GVHD. Recent studies have shown that host haematopoietic professional APCs in lymphoid organs may have only a limited capacity to induce GVHD, and host dendritic cells (DCs) may not be required. Parenchymal tissue cells can acquire APCs functions and they have been shown to promote a marked expansion of allo-reactive donor T-cell populations in the gastrointestinal tract. In the absence of functional host haematopoietic APCs, the presentation of minor histocompatibility antigens by donor haematopoietic APCs or host non-haematopoietic APCs is sufficient for GVHD induction.

The graft *versus* tumour effect

Obstacles to the improvement of HSCT treatment include the linkage between GVHD toxicity and the beneficial graft *versus* leukaemia effect, as well as the impairment of immune reconstitution leading to life-threatening infections.

The long-known beneficial effect of GVHD on the incidence of leukaemia relapse and the overall survival of patients with leukaemia is known as the graft *versus* tumour (GVT) effect.

The role of T-cells in both GVHD and the GVT effect was supported by the finding that T-cell depletion from the graft eliminates GVHD but at the expense of an increased leukaemia relapse rate. The major GVT effectors are cytotoxic T-cells that recognize allogeneic histocompatibility antigens and unique tumour antigens. In addition, NK cells and NK T-cells can directly recognize MHC class-I molecules and stress-induced peptides and mount anti-tumour responses.

Current strategies to improve GVT effects are based on selectively targeting tumour-specific killing and inhibiting immune escape mechanisms commonly used by tumours. These immune escape mechanisms include the loss of tumour-specific molecules on presented peptides, the downregulation or loss of MHC class-I or co-stimulatory molecules expression by tumour cells, the induction of functional defects in T-cells or NK cells, the production of soluble inhibitors of NK cell function, the expression of death receptor ligands such as CD95 ligand by tumour cells, and tumour cell resistance to apoptosis.

Treatment

Systemic corticosteroid therapy, despite its major shortcomings, remains the standard primary therapy for GVHD. Patients with steroid-refractory acute GVHD have a dismal outcome, with long-term mortality rates that can reach 90%.

New and improved therapies are therefore des-perately needed, particularly in cases of steroid-refractory chronic GVHD. Most of the current therapeutic approaches that are routinely used for GVHD (like corticosteroid and the calcineurin inhibitors) are broad-spectrum approaches that target T-cells and are therefore likely have a negative impact on GVT responses as well as immune reconstitution.

Novel approaches to prevent or treat GVHD are linked to the generation of new monoclonal antibodies, immunomodulatory therapy, innovative strategies that target both soluble and cellular effectors.

Because of donor $CD4^+$ and donor $CD8^+$, T-cells have a crucial role in the pathogenesis of GVHD, the most effective approaches for GVHD prevention and therapy focus on the depletion, tolerisation or func-tional incapacitation of donor T-cells. Recently the role of TH17 cells has been highlighted. The TH17 cells are a T-lymphocyte helper subset characterised by the production of interleukin (IL)-17A, IL-17F, IL-21 and IL-2; they have been shown to have a direct role in GVHD pathogenesis and they may yet prove to be a viable target for neutralisation in patients with GVHD in the gut. The TH17-type cytokine, IL-21, is another potential neutralisation target, given its role in promoting the activation, differentiation, maturation or expansion of NK cell, B-cell, T-cell and APC populations. Inhibition of IL-21 receptor signaling *in vivo* reduced acute GVHD activity in the gut, and this effect was associated with decreased TH1 cell and increased regulatory T-cell (Treg) numbers in the gut mucosa. An alternative approach to manipulating the TH17 cell response is to target the cytokines that are involved in the induction of TH17 cells, such as IL-6. Together with transforming growth factor (TGF)-β, IL-6 promotes the differentiation of naïve T-cells into TH17 cells. Infusion of an IL-6 receptor-specific monoclonal anti-body in a model of acute GVHD led to increased Treg numbers and a reduction in GVHD-induced pathological damage, particularly in the gut. The neutralisation of IL-6 may result in a direct anti-tumour response, particularly in multiple myeloma.

Because of the key role for pro-inflammatory cytokines in acute GVHD, inhibition of cytokine-induced signal transduction is an appealing approach for GVHD treatment. Janus kinases (JAKs) are cyto-plasmic protein tyrosine kinases that initiate cytokine-triggered signaling events by activating the cyto-plasmic latent forms of STAT proteins. In preclini-cal models, a small-molecule inhibitor of JAK3 has shown great promise in reducing lethality from GVHD without impeding GVT effects. Small-molecule inhibitors of JAK2 or JAK3 may therefore prove to be useful in inducing donor cell tolerance towards the host.

Other tyrosine kinase inhibitors, such as imatinib, which is commonly used to treat chronic myeloid leukaemia, have been shown to have marked anti-GVHD effects, especially in patients with chronic GVHD. Although the exact mechanism of action of imatinib in GVHD seems to be independent of its capacity to inhibit the platelet-derived growth factor receptor (PDGFR), imatinib represents an attractive agent for suppressing chronic GVHD and preserving GVT responses.

Proteasome inhibitors, such as bortezomib, prevent or treat GVHD in mice because they have inhibitory effects on cytokine signaling and nuclear factor (NF)-κB acti-vation. Bortezomib, even at very low doses, can specifically deplete alloreactive T-cells, allow T-Reg cell survival and attenuate IL-6-mediated T-cell differentia-tion; it can also inhibit APCs by targeting TLR4-mediated activation. Bortezomib and possibly other proteasome inhibitors are attractive therapeutic agents and worth testing in various clinical HSCT settings.

Modulating the trafficking patterns of alloreactive T-cells could be an efficacious mean of ameliorating GVHD. Inhibition of T-cell homing to inflamed tissues can be accom-plished by interrupting one of four key stages of T-cell migration: 1) tethering and rolling on the endothelium; 2) chemokine ligand–receptor interactions; 3) adhesion to the endothelium; and 4) migration in response to sphingosine-1-phosphate.

Other approaches include NK cell infusion and the *in vivo* activation of NK cells to promote the deletion of alloreactive T-cells; infusion of mesenchymal stem cells (MSCs), transfer of donor-derived Treg populations, infusion of myeloid-derived suppressor cell (MDSC) populations expanded *ex vivo* using granulocyte colony-stimulating factor (G-CSF) and granulocyte–macrophage colony-stimulating factor (GM-CSF), sirolimus, anti-tumour necrosis factor and anti-lymphocyte function-associated (anti-LFA)-3 antibodies, extracorporeal photopheresis.

Non-infectious pulmonary-associated complications

Common pulmonary complications occur in 25–50% of HSCT recipients and are responsible for 50% of transplant related deaths (table 1). Acute and subacute patterns of lung injury have been recognised. Idiopathic pneumonia syndrome occurs within the first 120 days after HSCT with a rapidly progressing fulminant course resulting in death in 60–80% of patients. By contrast, subacute noninfectious lung injury (alloimmune lung syndromes), including idiopathic pneumonia syndrome, bronchiolitis obliterans syndrome and bronchiolitis obliterans with organising pneumonia, can occur in the early post-transplant period or in the months post-HSCT. Although long-term disease-free survival after HSCT could exceed 60%, pulmonary infiltrates, due to either inflammatory or infectious pneumonitis, occur in 40–60% of HSCT recipients causing the 80% of transplant-related deaths. In children undergoing HSCT, the incidence of pulmonary complications varies from 10% to 25%. Open lung biopsy has been recommended to make a definitive diagnosis and the appropriate treatment. Idiopathic interstitial pneumonitis and CMV pneumonitis are the most common causes and should be suspected in patients with diffuse interstitial infiltrates. Epidemiological data suggest that, although GVHD reactions may play an aetiological role, the major contributing

Table 1. Frequency and mortality due to pulmonary complications after bone marrow transplantation.

	Frequency	Mortality
Infectious aetiology	34.3	50
CMV pneumonitis		71.4
Tuberculosis		33.4
PCP		0
Aspergillosis		0
Non infectious aetiology	65.7	30.4
Idiopathic interstitial pneumonitis		14.3
Organising pneumonia		20
Alveolar haemorrhage		100
Capillaritis		100
Post-transplant lymphoproliferative disorders		100

Data are presented as %. CMV: cytomegalovirus; PCP: *Pneumocystis jiroveci* pneumonia. Adapted from Wang *et al.* (2004)

factor is a conditioning-related toxicity. Moreover, engraftment syndrome, diffuse alveolar haemorrhage and pulmonary veno-occlusive disease are also possible complications.

Infectious pulmonary-associated complications

Respiratory virus infections in HSCT patients are observed in 1–56% of patients. CMV infection is the most frequent viral complication in patients undergoing HSCT. Despite advanced diagnostic methods and pre-emptive antiviral therapy, CMV disease continues to be a life-threatening complication. Clinical manifestations could vary from an asymptomatic infection, defined as active CMV replication in the blood in the absence of clinical manifestations, or organ failure abnormalities characterised by CMV infection with clinical symptoms or organ function abnormalities. Active CMV infection interacts significantly in several ways with GVHD. Acute GVHD increases the chances of a poor outcome. CMV prophylaxis or pre-emptive therapy adopted during the last few years in allogeneic HSCT recipients has changed the natural history of the disease. As prophylaxis, antiviral drugs are administered before any evidence of the virus, and in pre-emptive therapy antiviral drugs are administered when there is laboratory evidence of an active but asymptomatic infection. Acute GVHD significantly affects active CMV infection recurrence. CMV infection recurrence is more frequent with short courses of antiviral therapy. The poor bioavailability of oral ganciclovir may account for this; drug resistance may also be a

supplementary factor. Knowledge of these complications is now a part of the contemporary practice of pulmonary medicine and no longer isolated to the transplant pulmonologists.

Further reading

- Blazar BR, et al. (2012). Advances in graft-versus-host disease biology and therapy. Nat Rev Immunol; 12: 443–458.
- Castagnola E, et al. (2004). Cytomegalovirus infection after bone marrow transplantation in children. Human Immunol; 65: 416–422.
- Paczesny S, et al. (2009). Acute graft-versus-host disease: new treatment strategies. Curr Opin Hematol; 16: 427–436.
- Takatsuka H, et al. (2000). Complications after bone marrow transplantation are manifestations of systemic inflammatory response syndrome. Bone Marrow Transplant; 26: 419–426.
- Versluys AB, et al. (2010). Strong association between respiratory viral infection early after hematopoietic stem cell transplantation and the development of life-threatening acute and chronic alloimmune lung syndromes. Biol Blood Marrow Transplant; 16: 782–791.
- Wang JY, et al. (2004). Diffuse pulmonary infiltrates after bone marrow transplantation: the role of open lung biopsy. Ann Thorac Surg; 78: 267–272.
- Yoshihara S, et al. (2007). Bronchiolitis obliterans syndrome (BOS), bronchiolitis obliterans organizing pneumonia (BOOP) and other late-onset noninfectious pulmonary complications following allogeneic hematopoietic stem cell transplantation. Biol Blood Marrow Transplant; 13: 749–759.

Amyloidosis

Helen J. Lachmann

Amyloidosis is a group of diseases caused by accumulation of protein as insoluble fibrillar deposits within the extracellular space. These progressively disrupt the structure and function of affected tissues. Amyloidosis may be either acquired or inherited and $\geqslant 26$ different proteins can form amyloid fibrils *in vivo* in humans. The ultrastructural morphology and histochemical properties of all amyloid fibrils, regardless of the precursor protein type, are remarkably similar. Diffraction studies of amyloid fibrils have demonstrated a shared common core structure consisting of antiparallel β-strands lying perpendicular to the long axis of the fibril. This extremely abnormal, highly ordered conformation underlies the distinctive physicochemical properties of amyloid fibrils: they are relatively stable and are resistant to proteolysis, and they all bind molecules of the dye Congo red in a spatially organised manner, which results in the pathognomonic apple-green birefringence when viewed under cross-polarised light. Amyloid deposits also always contain the normal plasma glycoprotein, serum amyloid P component (SAP) as a nonfibrillar constituent. The universal presence of SAP in amyloid deposits reflects its specific binding to an, as yet, uncharacterised ligand common to all amyloid fibrils, which forms the basis for diagnostic scintigraphic imaging of amyloid with radiolabelled SAP.

Untreated amyloidosis progresses relentlessly and systemic forms of the disease are generally fatal, but deposits can regress if the supply of fibril precursors is reduced.

Amyloidosis can present to respiratory physicians in a number of ways:

- chronic lung conditions may give rise to systemic amyloidosis
- systemic amyloidosis may present with respiratory symptoms
- localised pulmonary and respiratory tract amyloid deposits may present either symptomatically or as an incidental finding on imaging

Systemic amyloidosis complicating respiratory diseases

AA amyloidosis is a potential complication of any sustained inflammatory condition, which usually presents as proteinuric renal impairment. The amyloid fibrils are derived from the acute-phase reactant serum amyloid A protein (SAA). The major respiratory disease underlying AA amyloidosis in the industrialised world is

> **Key points**
>
> - Amyloidosis is a protein deposition disease.
>
> - Diagnosis is by biopsy and Congo red staining.
>
> - Systemic amyloidosis is a life threatening condition that usually affects several organs.
>
> - Localised amyloidosis can present with obstructive symptoms, haemoptysis or as an incidental finding on imaging.
>
> - Treatment depends on the type and distribution of amyloid deposits.

longstanding bronchiectasis, which underlies 5% of cases. Previously, tuberculosis was common, and other associations include lung neoplasia (Castleman's tumours, lymphoma and adenocarcinoma; accounting for 3% of AA amyloidosis cases), CF, sarcoidosis and Kartagener's syndrome. The prognosis of AA amyloidosis depends on the degree of renal damage and whether the underlying inflammatory disease can be completely controlled. Treatment depends on the underlying disease and may involve surgery, antimicrobials or immuno-suppression.

Systemic, amyloid light chain (AL) amyloidosis is the commonest type, accounting for 60% of cases, and may occur in association with any B-cell dyscrasia, as the amyloid fibrils are derived from mono-clonal immunoglobulin light chains. A number of chest-localised conditions can underlie systemic AL amyloidosis, including Sjögren's syndrome, plasmacytomas and Castleman's tumours.

Respiratory system symptoms arising from systemic AL amyloidosis

Although lung deposits are universal on *post mortem* examination, symptoms are rare and dyspnoea generally reflects amyloid cardiomyopathy. Chest radiographs are usually normal but can demonstrate diffuse reticulonodular infiltration. Lung function tests may be restrictive and extensive alveolar deposits can reduce gas transfer. Persistent pleural effusions are usually due to cardiac infiltration by amyloid but can rarely be caused by amyloidotic disruption of the pleura and may require recurrent drainage or pleurodesis. Treatment of systemic AL amyloidosis is chemotherapy directed against the underlying B-cell clone. Serious pulmonary side-effects from treatment are rare but fever and asthma-like symptoms and progression to respiratory failure with pulmonary infiltrates have been reported following treatment with the proteasome inhibitor bortezomib. There have also been descriptions of lung toxicity following the use of thalidomide and lenalidomide with toxic granulomatous

interstitial pulmonary disease, which may be steroid responsive.

Amyloidosis localised to the respiratory tract

This results either from local production of fibril precursors or from properties inherent to a particular microenvironment, which favour fibril formation of a widely distributed precursor protein. The majority of deposits are AL-associated with monoclonal B-cells confined to the affected site. Apparently localised amyloid deposits can be manifestations of systemic disease and should always be fully investigated to exclude systemic amyloidosis.

Laryngeal amyloidosis

Amyloidosis represents 0.5–1% of benign laryngeal disease and the incidence increases with age. It usually presents as hoarseness and is relatively benign but can be progressive or recur after treatment. Fatal haemorrhage has been reported. Endoscopic or laser excision is the treatment of choice, aiming to preserve voice quality and airway patency. Very rarely, apparently localised laryngeal amyloid deposits can be a feature of hereditary apolipoprotein AL amyloidosis.

Tracheobronchial amyloidosis

This typically presents in the fifth or sixth decades with dyspnoea, cough and haemoptysis. Airway narrowing may cause pneumonia or lobar collapse and solitary nodules can mimic endobronchial neoplasia. There is no proven therapy although chemotherapy has been tried in patients with progressive disease. Management is dictated by symptoms and includes resection, stenting or laser ablation. Survival is <45% at 6 years.

Parenchymal pulmonary amyloidosis

This is typically an incidental finding on chest radiography of solitary/multiple nodules or a diffuse alveolar–septal pattern. Although the lesions must be differentiated from neoplasia, the prognosis is usually excellent and no treatment is required.

Pulmonary amyloidosis associated with Sjögren's syndrome

This chronic, organ-specific autoimmune disease predominantly affects females and carries a 44-fold increase in lymphoproliferative disorders. Pulmonary AL amyloidosis is a rare but well recognised complication, resulting in cough and dyspnoea.

Mediastinal and hilar amyloid lymphadenopathy

The lymphadenopathy may be massive and typically complicates a low-grade lymphoma. Disease progression is slow and calcification frequent. Tracheal compression or superior vena cava obstruction occasionally result.

Conclusion

Amyloidosis can both complicate long-standing pulmonary disease and be deposited within the respiratory system. The presentation and prognosis of amyloid deposits depend on their aetiology and distribution, and can be benign or life threatening. In most cases of localised disease, management is essentially supportive or involves resection of symptomatic deposits. In contrast, systemic treatment can be extremely effective in patients with generalised AA and AL amyloidosis.

Further reading

- Berk JL, et al. (2002). Pulmonary and tracheobronchial amyloidosis. *Semin Respir Crit Care Med*; 23: 155–165.
- Gilad R, et al. (2007). Severe diffuse systemic amyloidosis with involvement of the pharynx, larynx, and trachea: CT and MR findings. *Am J Neuroradiol*; 28: 1557–1558.
- Lachmann HJ, et al. (2006). Amyloidosis and the lung. *Chron Respir Dis*; 3: 203–214.
- Ma L, et al. (2005). Primary localized laryngeal amyloidosis: report of 3 cases with long-term follow-up and review of the literature. *Arch Pathol Lab Med*; 129: 215–218.
- O'Regan A, et al. (2000). Tracheobronchial amyloidosis. The Boston University experience from 1984 to 1999. *Medicine (Baltimore)*; 79: 69–79.
- Pepys MB, et al. Amyloidosis. *In:* Warrell DA, et al., eds. Oxford Textbook of Medicine. 5th Edn. Oxford, Oxford University Press, 2010; pp. 1766–1779.
- Rajagopala S, et al. (2010). Pulmonary amyloidosis in Sjogren's syndrome: a case report and systematic review of the literature. *Respirology*; 15: 860–866.
- Shah P, et al. (2002). The importance of complete screening for amyloid fibril type and systemic disease in patients with amyloidosis in the respiratory tract. *Sarcoidosis Vasc Diffuse Lung Dis*; 19: 134–142.
- Travis WD, et al. Non-neoplastic disorders of the lower respiratory tract. *In:* Travis WD, et al., eds. Atlas of Nontumor Pathology. Washington DC, American Registry of Pathology, 2002; pp. 873–881.
- Turner CA, et al. (2007). CT appearances of amyloid lymphadenopathy in a patient with non-Hodgkin's lymphoma. *Br J Radiol*; 80: e250–e252.

Pulmonary alveolar proteinosis

Maurizio Luisetti

Pulmonary alveolar proteinosis (PAP) is a rare syndrome occurring worldwide with an estimated prevalence of 0.1 cases per 100 000 individuals. PAP is characterised by accumulation of surfactant within alveolar macrophages in the alveoli and terminal airspaces, with impairment of gas transfer, and by a variable clinical course, ranging from spontaneous resolution to progressive respiratory failure.

Surfactant clearance impairment is the likely common pathophysiology of PAP, which can be classified as follows.

- Primary PAP is due to disruption of granulocyte–macrophage colony-stimulating factor (GM-CSF) signalling, either by the presence in plasma and lungs of high levels of neutralising anti-GM-CSF autoantibodies (GMAb) (autoimmune PAP, formerly known as idiopathic PAP) or by mutations in the GM-CSF receptor α or β chains. Passive transfer of PAP features in monkeys inoculated with human GMAb strongly supports the concept that GMAb are the causative factor of autoimmune PAP.
- Secondary PAP occurs as a consequence of the presence of several underlying diseases associated with PAP, such as haematological disorders (mostly myelodysplastic syndrome), immunodeficiency, dust inhalation or lysinuric protein intolerance.
- A third group (PAP-like diseases) is characterised by surfactant production impairment and includes genetic disorders due to mutations in the genes encoding surfactant protein (SP)-B and SP-C genes, as well as in the *ABCA3* (ATP-binding cassette subfamily A member 3) gene.

Key points

- PAP is a rare syndrome caused by surfactant clearance impairment.
- >90% of PAP cases are associated with the presence of neutralising autoantibodies against GM-CSF (GMAb; primary autoimmune PAP).
- Diagnosis of primary autoimmune PAP is based on the following triad: 1) crazy paving pattern on HRCT; 2) milky appearance and cytology of BAL fluid; and 3) elevated serum level of GMAb.
- WLL is the current standard of care of PAP but alternative therapies (especially GM-CSF administration) are under active investigation.

According to a recently published meta-analysis and large cohort report, >90% of immune PAP patients are middle-aged adults, complaining of progressive exertional dyspnoea and cough; interestingly, about one-third of a large Japanese PAP series was asymptomatic. Physical examination of PAP patients is often unremarkable. Pulmonary function tests may be normal but, usually, the first abnormality is represented by a decrease in lung diffusing capacity and increased exertional alveolar–arterial oxygen tension gradient. The classic chest radiographic presentation is a diffuse bilateral infiltrate with a distribution that is sometimes similar to that of pulmonary oedema (fig. 1a). More typical is the HRCT presentation defined as 'crazy paving' (thickening of interlobular and intralobular septa and ground-glass opacities, with a patchy distribution) (fig. 1b). Although surgical biopsy is traditionally considered mandatory to establish the diagnosis of PAP, more recently, the triad represented by:

1) typical crazy paving pattern on HRCT

2) macroscopic appearance of milky fluid and cytology of bronchoalveolar lavage (BAL) fluid

3) elevated serum level of GMAb (whose sensitivity and specificity for diagnosing PAP is ~100%)

is now considered sufficient to establish the diagnosis of autoimmune PAP. Lung biopsy should be considered when one or more of the previous findings are unclear. Histopathology usually shows well preserved alveolar wall architecture, and alveolar spaces filled with lipoproteinaceous, eosinophilic, Periodic Acid–Schiff-positive material and foamy macrophages.

The natural history of the PAP has been greatly influenced by the treatment. In the pre-whole-lung lavage (WLL) era, progressive deterioration occurred in ~30% of PAP patients. Death occurred mostly because of irreversible respiratory failure and, to a lesser extent, respiratory infection. The latter is a typical complication of the clinical course of PAP: pulmonary and systemic infections due to opportunistic organisms such as *Nocardia*, mycobacteria and *Cryptococcus* are often reported. Increased susceptibility to lung infections is traditionally attributed to the impairment of alveolar macrophages engulfed by surfactant but systemic infections have been ascribed more recently to GM-CSF signalling impairment.

The adoption of WLL, first described in the mid-1960s, has changed the natural history of PAP by dramatically reducing the death rate. It is considered the standard of care for PAP and 95% of PAP patients respond positively to the procedure, although a considerable fraction of patients may show relapses or incomplete resolution. GM-CSF administration, based on

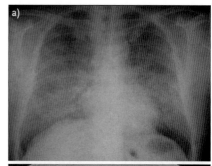

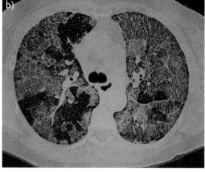

Figure 1. a) Radiographic and b) HRCT 'crazy paving' presentation of PAP.

the pathophysiology of the disorder, is considered an attractive alternative to WLL. Unfortunately, limited experience and, more importantly, difficult access to the drug have so far precluded diffusion of this therapeutic option. Possible alternatives are plasma-pheresis or immunosuppressive agents such as rituximab, but data are so far insufficient. Lung transplantation is considered in end-stage disease but PAP may recur.

Further reading

- Beccaria M, *et al.* (2004). Long-term durable benefit after whole lung lavage in pulmonary alveolar proteinosis. *Eur Respir J*; 23: 526–531.
- Inoue Y, *et al.* (2008). Characteristics of a large cohort of patients with auto-immune pulmonary alveolar proteinosis in Japan. *Am J Respir Crit Care Med*; 177: 752–762.

- Luisetti M, *et al.* Pulmonary alveolar proteinosis. *In:* Schwarz MI, *et al.*, eds. Interstitial Lung Disease, 5th Edn. Maidenhead, McGraw-Hill, 2010.
- Orphanet. 2009 Activity Report. www.orpha.net/orphacom/cahiers/docs/GB/ActivityReport2009.pdf
- Ramirez J, *et al.* (1963). Pulmonary alveolar proteinosis: a new technique and rationale for treatment. *Arch Int Med*; 112: 419–431.
- Sakagami T, *et al.* (2009). Human GM-CSF autoantibodies and reproduction of pulmonary alveolar proteinosis. *N Engl J Med*; 361: 2679–2681.
- Seymour JF, *et al.* (2002). Pulmonary alveolar proteinosis: progress in the first 44 years. *Am J Respir Crit Care Med*; 166: 215–235.
- Suzuki T, *et al.* (2010). Hereditary pulmonary alveolar proteinosis: pathogenesis, presentation, diagnosis, and therapy. *Am J Respir Crit Care Med*; 182: 1292–1304.
- Trapnell BC, *et al.* (2003). Pulmonary alveolar proteinosis. *N Engl J Med*; 349: 2527–2539.
- Uchida K, *et al.* (2007). GM-CSF auto-antibodies and neutrophil dysfunction in pulmonary alveolar proteinosis. *N Engl J Med*; 356: 567–579.

Adult pulmonary Langerhans' cell histiocytosis

Vincent Cottin, Romain Lazor and Jean-François Cordier

Langerhans' cells are bone marrow-derived dendritic cells, the physiological function of which is to process and present antigens to lymphocytes. Langerhans' cell histiocytosis (LCH) is a rare systemic disorder characterised by aberrant accumulation of Langerhans' cells in various organs, usually in the form of granulomas. LCH is part of a spectrum of other histiocytic disorders that includes include LCH, non-Langerhans' histiocytosis such as Erdheim–Chester disease and Rosai–Dorfman disease, and malignant histiocytic disorders. LCH in adults may especially involve the lung, bones, skin and pituitary gland. The presentation in childhood is different, with acute disseminated disease and a poor prognosis, and, in older children and adolescents, with multifocal involvement including the bone. However, single-system involvement of LCH is possible. Pulmonary LCH is characterised by polyclonal accumulation of Langerhans' cells and other inflammatory cells in the small airways, resulting in nodular inflammatory lesions that may evolve into extensive cavitating

destruction of the lung parenchyma and respiratory insufficiency.

Epidemiology

Pulmonary LCH in adults is a rare disease with an estimated prevalence of less than one case in 200 000. It occurs almost exclusively in smokers, with no sex predominance, between the ages of 20 and 40 years, and is more common in the white population.

Pathologic features

Pulmonary LCH is characterised by granulomatous bronchiolocentric organisation of Langerhans' cells associated with inflammatory cells including eosinophils. Langerhans' cells do not differ from their normal counterpart in tissues, exhibiting convoluted irregular nuclei with characteristic Birbeck granules visible by electron microscopy. These cells stain positive with anti-CD1a and anti-CD207 (langerin) antibodies. Some features of alveolar macrophage pneumonitis (desquamative interstitial pneumonia) or respiratory bronchiolitis with interstitial lung disease are often associated with LCH. Progression of the bronchiolocentric granulomatous lesions results in fibrosis with end-stage stellar fibrotic scars and adjacent cystic cavities.

Clinical features

The respiratory manifestations are not specific, with cough (often overlooked in patients who are smokers) and gradually progressive dyspnoea on exercise. Spontaneous pneumothorax is the first manifestation leading to diagnosis in about

---

Key points

- Pulmonary LCH is characterised by cough, dyspnoea on exercise, and diffuse pulmonary nodules and cysts on chest imaging in smokers that may evolve into respiratory failure.

- Smoking cessation should be attained. No medical therapy has demonstrated efficacy.

10–20% of patients. A number of patients have almost no reported symptoms and the disease is discovered incidentally on routine chest X-ray or CT. Pulmonary LCH is solitary in a large majority of patients; however, involvement of other systems may be the first manifestation of the disease. These include bone lesions (which are often characteristic, well demarcated and osteolytic on imaging; rib involvement with possible chest pain), hypothalamic–pituitary involvement resulting in diabetes insipidus (polyuria and polydipsia) and skin lesions.

Imaging

The chest X-ray is usually abnormal, with micronodular and reticular opacities, typically sparing the lower lobes. In advanced disease, nodules are absent and the chest X-ray may suggest emphysema.

HRCT of the chest usually shows characteristic features in early disease with disseminated infracentimetric nodules, which may show cavitation and may spontaneously disappear. The cavitated nodules may evolve to thick- then thin-walled cysts (fig. 1). The cysts may then enlarge and become confluent, with HRCT features resembling emphysema.

The differential diagnosis includes other multiple cystic lung diseases on imaging, especially Birt–Hogg–Dubé syndrome and spontaneous familial pneumothorax related to FLCN mutations, lymphangio-leiomyomatosis, Sjögren's syndrome, and nonamyloid immunoglobulin deposition

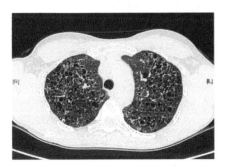

Figure 1. HRCT of the chest demonstrating numerous thin-walled cysts in a patient with LCH.

disease. Pleural effusion and mediastinal lymphadenopathy are exceptional. Pulmonary artery enlargement is present in patients with pulmonary hypertension.

Lung function tests

Lung function tests may be normal or only mildly impaired in patients with nodular involvement. However, TLCO is usually decreased, including in patients with relatively few lesions on imaging. About one-third of patients develop airflow obstruction with hyperinflation, which may progress to severe obstructive respiratory insufficiency.

Diagnosis

The gold standard for diagnosis of LCH is lung biopsy showing the characteristic features described above. Surgical biopsy is often obtained during pleurodesis for recurrent pneumothorax. Because of the plurifocal distribution of the lesions in the lung, the yield of transbronchial lung biopsy is usually limited. Bronchoalveolar lavage (BAL) is currently considered of little (if any) value. It shows an increase in total cell counts with a large predominance of macrophages with possible slight increase in eosinophils. The CD4$^+$/CD8$^+$ lymphocyte ratio is decreased. The identification of Langerhans' cells in BAL with antibodies against CD1a has only poor sensitivity and specificity, and their proportion is usually similar to that in smokers without LCH. Common laboratory tests do not contribute to the diagnosis of LCH.

A presumptive diagnosis of pulmonary LCH may be accepted in patients with characteristic HRCT features, and limited symptoms and impaired lung function. Lung biopsy is indicated in those patients with significant symptoms and deteriorated or deteriorating lung function who are considered for treatment. In patients with diffuse cystic lesions on HRCT with irreversible lung function impairment, lung biopsy is of limited benefit, especially as it may not show characteristic granulomatous lesions.

Evolution

About half of the patients improve spontaneously or with corticosteroid treatment (which has, however, not been rigorously evaluated). Poor outcome with respiratory failure may occur, especially in older patients with systemic involvement and deteriorating lung function tests. Pulmonary hypertension often severe is common in advanced disease. Lung cancer may develop resulting from smoking habits.

Treatment of pulmonary LCH

Given the possibility of spontaneous recovery in a number of patients and the absence of controlled therapeutic trials, there is currently no evidence of efficacy of any treatment.

The strong association between pulmonary LCH and tobacco smoking suggests a causal relationship, and numerous observations have reported improvement of the disease following smoking cessation. However, worsening or relapse despite smoking cessation has also been described. In any case, smoking cessation is an essential component of management in pulmonary LCH, at least to prevent further development of COPD and/or lung cancer.

Although without evidence of efficacy, corticosteroid treatment is often used in patients with symptomatic disease and worsening lung function, starting with prednisone $0.5-1$ mg·kg^{-1} then tapering over 6–12 months. Whether improvement, when occurring, results from treatment efficacy or from spontaneous improvement cannot be established.

Cytotoxic agents (especially vinblastine) have been occasionally used with no conclusive efficacy. 2-chloro-deoxyadenosine (cladribine) has consistently been shown to be efficient in isolated cases. However, cladribine may induce profound myelo- and immunosuppression, and should be administered only in expert centres.

Pulmonary hypertension, when present, may be improved by pulmonary arterial hypertension treatment in some patients.

Lung transplantation (single or double lung, or heart–lung) may be considered in patients with end stage disease. The majority of them present with moderate-to-severe pulmonary hypertension. Post-transplant survival is rather good, with 10-year survival >50%. However, pulmonary LCH may recur in about one-fifth of patients.

Further reading

- Allen TC (2008). Pulmonary Langerhans cell histiocytosis and other pulmonary histiocytic diseases. *Arch Pathol Lab Med*; 132: 1171–1781.
- Caminati A, et al. (2006). Smoking-related interstitial pneumonias and pulmonary Langerhans cell histiocytosis. *Proc Am Thorac Soc*; 3: 299–306.
- Dauriat G, et al. (2006). Lung transplantation for pulmonary Langerhans' cell histiocytosis: a multicenter analysis. *Transplantation*; 81: 746–750.
- Fartoukh M, et al. (2000). Severe pulmonary hypertension in histiocytosis X. *Am J Respir Crit Care Med*; 161: 216–223.
- Kiakouama L, et al. (2010). Severe pulmonary hypertension in histiocytosis X: long-term improvement with bosentan. *Eur Respir J*; 36: 1–3.
- Lazor R, et al. (2009). Progressive diffuse pulmonary Langerhans cell histiocytosis improved by cladribine chemotherapy. *Thorax*; 64: 274–275.
- Le Pavec J, et al. (2012). Pulmonary Langerhans cell histiocytosis-associated pulmonary hypertension: clinical characteristics and impact of pulmonary arterial hypertension therapies. *Chest*; 142: 1150–1157.
- Lorillon G, et al. (2012). Cladribine is effective against cystic pulmonary Langerhans cell histiocytosis. *Am J Respir Crit Care Med*; 186: 930–932.
- Mendez JL, et al. (2004). Pneumothorax in pulmonary Langerhans cell histiocytosis. *Chest*; 125: 1028–1032.
- Tazi A (2006). Adult pulmonary Langerhans' cell histiocytosis. *Eur Respir J*; 27: 1272–1285.
- Vassallo R, et al. (2000). Pulmonary Langerhans' cell histiocytosis. *N Engl J Med*; 342: 1969–1978.

Lymphangioleiomyomatosis

Vincent Cottin, Romain Lazor and Jean-François Cordier

Epidemiology and genetics

Lymphangioleiomyomatosis (LAM) is a rare (so-called orphan) lung disease affecting about 3.4–7.8 per million adult females (usually of childbearing age). It may be sporadic, or associated with tuberous sclerosis complex (TSC), where it affects 30–40% of adult women and exceptionally men.

TSC is associated with inherited mutations of the *TSC1* and *TSC2* genes, while acquired somatic mutations of *TSC2* are associated with sporadic LAM, resulting in constitutive activation of the kinase mammalian target of rapamycin (mTOR) signalling pathway in affected cells (LAM cells).

Lung pathology

In LAM, the lung parenchyma is progressively replaced by cysts associated with a proliferation of immature smooth muscle cells and perivascular epithelioid cells (LAM cells). LAM cell proliferation usually develops around lymphatic vessels in the lung and, possibly, the axial lymphatics and the thoracic duct. LAM cells stain with antibodies against smooth muscle actin, desmin and HMB-45 (detecting characteristic pre-melanocyte proteins). As LAM cells have been shown to invade the lymphatic vessels and spread to selected distant sites such as the lung and kidney, LAM is increasingly considered a low-grade metastatic tumour. The source and physiological counterpart of LAM cells are currently unknown. LAM cell clusters have recently been found in the uterus of 90% patients with LAM, suggesting that these cells could originate from this organ.

Clinical manifestations and lung function tests

Dyspnoea on exertion is the most common symptom and pneumothorax the most common mode of presentation (often relapsing and maybe bilateral). Chylous effusion (chylothorax and chylous ascites) may be present.

Lung function tests are characterised by airflow obstruction and impaired gas transfer with a decrease in T_{LCO}. Exercise performance and maximal oxygen uptake are impaired. Hypoxaemia is present in advanced disease.

Imaging

Chest X-ray shows reticular opacities, cysts, pleural effusion or pneumothorax.

HRCT of the chest plays a major role in diagnosis. It shows characteristic multiple round, thin-walled cysts evenly distributed

---

Key points

- LAM is a rare disease occurring in women of child-bearing age, characterised by dyspnoea on exertion, relapsing pneumothorax and numerous thin-walled cysts on chest imaging.

- Diagnostic criteria have been proposed recently.

- The disease may slowly progress to respiratory insufficiency.

- No effective therapy is available.

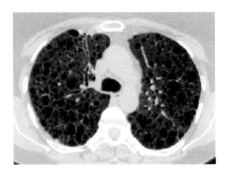

Figure 1. HRCT of the chest demonstrating numerous thin-walled cysts in a patient with LAM.

throughout the lung parenchyma; these cysts may progressively become confluent (fig. 1).

Cysts may be associated with small nodules in TSC (corresponding to multifocal micronodular pneumocyte hyperplasia), pleural effusion and pneumothorax. The axial lymphatics of the thorax and retroperitoneum may be dilated with lymphadenopathy and abdominal cystic lymphatic collections called lymphangiomas (in up to 20% of patients) that may result in abdominal discomfort or compression.

Angiomyolipoma

Angiomyolipomas (AMLs) of the kidney are benign tumours composed of blood vessels, smooth muscle and adipose tissue that are easily identified by HRCT. AMLs are found in ~50% of patients with sporadic LAM and 80% of patients with TSC, in whom they are more often bilateral and larger. AMLs may slowly enlarge with time and become prone to bleeding, especially when >4 cm or rich in microaneurysms (percutaneous embolisation or, rarely, nephron-sparing nephrectomy is therefore indicated). Regular screening for AML is recommended in patients with LAM.

Diagnostic criteria

Diagnostic criteria for LAM have recently been proposed by a European Respiratory Society Task Force (table 1). The gold standard for diagnosis of LAM is lung biopsy fitting the pathological criteria.

However, the combination of characteristic HRCT features with AML or other characteristic features of LAM may obviate the need for biopsy. The differential diagnosis comprises other multiple-cystic lung diseases associated with mutations of the folliculin gene (*FLCN*), especially Birt–Hogg–Dubé syndrome and familial isolated primary spontaneous pneumothorax, Langerhans' cell histiocytosis, cysts associated with lymphoid interstitial pneumonia, nonamyloid immunoglobulin deposition disease, *etc*. A diagnostic work-up for alternative causes of multiple-cystic lung disease is mandatory in patients with probable and especially possible LAM. Levels of vascular endothelial growth factor (VEGF)-D, a major angiogenic growth factor produced by tumour cells that promotes formation of lymphatic vessels and spread of tumour cells to lymph nodes, are increased in the serum of patients with LAM, as compared with other cystic lung diseases and healthy controls. Serum VEGF-D level contributes to the noninvasive diagnosis of LAM if elevated (high positive predictive value if >800 pg·mL^{-1}) but does not rule out the disease if normal.

Evolution and prognosis

Disease progression is variable, with some patients remaining relatively stable for a long time but others deteriorate rapidly with ensuing respiratory insufficiency. Median annual FEV1 decline is around 100 mL·year^{-1}. Repeated measurement of FEV1 and TLCO is used to assess disease progression with arterial oxygen measurement in advanced disease. Pulmonary hypertension, usually mild, may develop.

The 10-year survival was about 70–90% in recent large series.

Management

As LAM occurs in women of childbearing age, oestrogens have been suspected to enhance and progesterone to prevent the development of LAM. However, hormonal interventions have not demonstrated significant advantages. Nevertheless, oestrogens (the contraceptive pill or hormone replacement) should be avoided.

Table 1. *European Respiratory Society diagnostic criteria for LAM*

Definite LAM
1. Characteristic[#] or compatible[¶] lung HRCT and lung biopsy fitting the pathological criteria for LAM[#,¶] or
2. Characteristic[#] lung HRCT and any of the following
AML (kidney)[+]
Thoracic or abdominal chylous effusion[§]
Lymphangioleiomyoma[f] or lymph node involvement of LAM[f]
Definite or probable TSC
Probable LAM
1. Characteristic[#] lung HRCT and compatible clinical history[##] or
2. Compatible[¶] lung HRCT and any of the following
AML (kidney)[+]
Thoracic or abdominal chylous effusion[§]
Possible LAM
Characteristic[#] or compatible[¶] lung HRCT
[#]: multiple thin-walled, round, well-defined, air-filled cysts; [¶]: only a few (more than two but ⩽10) cysts, <30 mm in diameter; [+]: diagnosed by characteristic CT features and/or on pathological examination; [§]: based on visual and/or biochemical characteristics of the effusion; [f]: based on pathological examination; [##]: compatible clinical features include pneumothorax (especially multiple and/or bilateral) and/or altered lung function tests as in LAM.

The mTOR inhibitor and immunosuppressive agent sirolimus has recently been shown to stabilise lung function in patients with LAM compared with placebo. However, significant side-effects occurred (mouth ulcers, diarrhoea, nausea, increased blood cholesterol levels, skin rash and swelling of the extremities) and disease progression resumed when sirolimus was stopped. Sirolimus and everolimus also appeared effective on chylous effusion in small observational studies, and in AML not amenable to embolisation therapy. As mTOR inhibitors are not currently approved for LAM, their compassionate use should be restricted to expert centres.

There is a greater risk of pneumothorax and chylous effusion during pregnancy. Whether or not to become pregnant is the patients' decision; however, pregnancy may be discouraged in patients with severe disease.

Influenza and pneumococcal vaccination should be offered to patients with LAM.

Inhaled bronchodilators should be prescribed to patients with airflow obstruction and continued if a response is observed.

In patients with end-stage LAM, lung transplantation (single or bilateral) is an efficient procedure, with results comparing favourably with transplantation for other pulmonary diseases. As many LAM patients are rather young, lung transplantation may be proposed in the most severe cases with poor prognosis. Recurrence of LAM on transplant is possible but does not affect survival.

Further reading

- Avila NA, et al. (2000a). Pulmonary lymphangioleiomyomatosis: correlation of ventilation-perfusion scintigraphy, chest radiography, and CT with pulmonary function tests. *Radiology*; 214: 441–446.

- Avila NA, *et al.* (2000b). Lymphangioleiomyomatosis: abdomino-pelvic CT and US findings. *Radiology*; 216: 147–153.
- Benden C, *et al.* (2009). Lung transplantation for lymphangioleiomyomatosis: the European experience. *J Heart Lung Transplant*; 28: 1–7.
- Bissler JJ, *et al.* (2008). Sirolimus for angiomyolipoma in tuberous sclerosis complex or lymphangioleiomyomatosis. *N Engl J Med*; 358: 140–151.
- Chang WY, *et al.* (2012). Clinical utility of diagnostic guidelines and putative biomarkers in lymphangioleiomyomatosis. *Respir Res*; 13: 34.
- Cottin V, *et al.* (2012). Pulmonary hypertension in lymphangioleiomyomatosis: characteristics in 20 patients. *Eur Respir J*; 40: 630–640.
- Harknett EC, *et al.* (2011). Use of variability in national and regional data to estimate the prevalence of lymphangioleiomyomatosis. *Q J Med*; 104: 971–979.
- Hayashi T, *et al.* (2011). Prevalence of uterine and adnexal involvement in pulmonary lymphangioleiomyomatosis: a clinicopathologic study of 10 patients. *Am J Surg Pathol*; 35: 1776–1785.
- Johnson SR, *et al.* (2000). Clinical experience of lymphangioleiomyomatosis in the UK. *Thorax*; 55: 1052–1057.
- Johnson SR, *et al.* (2010). European Respiratory Society guidelines for the diagnosis and management of lymphangioleiomyomatosis. *Eur Respir J*; 35: 14–26.
- Lazor R, *et al.* (2004). Low initial K_{CO} predicts rapid FEV_1 decline in pulmonary lymphangioleiomyomatosis. Groupe d'Etudes et de Recherche sur les Maladies "Orphelines" Pulmonaires (GERM"O" P). *Respir Med*; 98: 536–541.
- McCormac FX, *et al.* (2011). Efficacy and safety of sirolimus in lymphangioleiomyomatosis. *New Engl J Med*; 364: 1595–1606.
- McCormack FX, *et al.* (2012). Lymphangioleiomyomatosis. Calling it what it is: a low-grade, destructive, metastasizing neoplasm. *Am J Respir Crit Care Med*; 186: 1210–1212.
- Moss J, *et al.* (2001). Prevalence and clinical characteristics of lymphangioleiomyomatosis (LAM) in patients with tuberous sclerosis complex. *Am J Respir Crit Care Med*; 164: 669–671.
- Ryu JH, *et al.* (2006). The NHLBI Lymphangioleiomyomatosis Registry: characteristics of 230 patients at enrollment. *Am J Respir Crit Care Med*; 173: 105–111.
- Taveira-DaSilva AM, *et al.* (2011). Changes in lung function and chylous effusions in patients with lymphangioleiomyomatosis treated with sirolimus. *Ann Intern Med*; 154: 797–805.
- Urban T, *et al.* (1999). Pulmonary lymphangioleiomyomatosis. A study of 69 patients. Groupe d'Etudes et de Recherche sur les Maladies "Orphelines" Pulmonaires (GERM"O"P). *Medicine (Baltimore)*; 78: 321–337.
- Young LR, *et al.* (2010). Serum vascular endothelial growth factor-D prospectively distinguishes lymphangioleiomyomatosis from other diseases. *Chest*; 138: 674–681.

Respiratory physiotherapy

Julia Bott

Respiratory physiotherapy spans a broad range of services, advice and nonpharmacological interventions, used to help patients with a variety of respiratory conditions. Its use has been documented for over a century: postural drainage was reported for secretion removal in bronchiectasis in 1901, and in 1915, breathing exercises and physical exercise for chest injuries.

General principles of physiotherapy

Physiotherapy is aimed at treating or alleviating problems rather than diseases. Strategies are used to restore, improve or maintain movement and/or function, and maximise participation in everyday life. Physiotherapists are thus vital to the delivery of effective pulmonary rehabilitation.

Key points

Physiotherapy is indicated in most respiratory conditions, both for groups and individuals, for:

- self-management advice and education on lifestyle modifications,

- breathlessness management,

- improvement or maintenance of mobility and function,

- airway clearance in well-defined cases,

- prescription of exercise and exercise training,

- prescription of walking aids.

Physiotherapy is provided across all healthcare settings, from the patient's own home to the critical care unit. Physiotherapists are well qualified to provide assessment and monitoring of, for example, ventilatory function and cough effectiveness or exercise tolerance, including for ambulatory oxygen assessment. Interestingly, there is wide variance in tasks undertaken by physiotherapists across countries; for example, in some, assisting in delivery of pharmacotherapy, oxygen therapy and NIV is the role of the respiratory physiotherapist, while in others, these roles may be provided by other healthcare professionals.

Airway clearance

To help the patient better manage their secretions, a range of airway clearance techniques are available, including:

- independent techniques
- mechanical or other devices
- postural drainage
- nebulised substances (e.g. hypertonic saline)
- techniques for cough enhancement or support

Physiotherapists' physiological knowledge and practical skills means they are well placed to assist in the delivery of pharmacotherapy (inhalers) and their timing with respect to the physiotherapy intervention. Physiotherapists can also help in the delivery and correct application of oxygen therapy, including ambulatory oxygen, as well as in offering improvement of poor ventilatory function, including in the sedated and paralysed patient.

Enhancing ventilation and gas exchange

Strategies to enhance ventilation and gas exchange include:

- Positioning
- Breathing techniques
- Manual hyperinflation
- Intermittent positive pressure breathing (IPPB)
- CPAP
- NIV

Physiotherapists are considered by many to be invaluable in the delivery of an effective NIV service.

Physiotherapy is commonly helpful for postural problems and/or musculoskeletal dysfunction and pain, as well as for improving continence. With an increased prevalence compared to that of nonrespiratory populations, this is especially warranted during coughing and forced expiratory manoeuvres.

Disease-specific physiotherapy

Chronic obstructive pulmonary disease Taking account of the altered mechanics of breathing in those with COPD is essential for effective breathlessness management and advice.

Breathlessness management includes:

- positioning to fix the shoulder girdle passively
- forward-leaning postures to improve the length/tension ratio of the diaphragm
- breathing techniques help the patient better control dyspnoea and panic, both at rest and during exertion

Physical activity and exercise should be encouraged throughout the course of the disease, including during hospital admission where possible and appropriate. When supervised and carried out at appropriate intensity these exercises are more effective. Exercise training programs are indicated for patients who have symptoms and impaired physical activities in daily life. Selected patients may benefit from inspiratory muscle training.

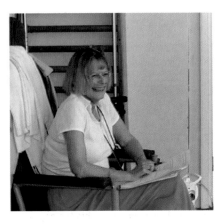

'Thank you for giving me my life back.'

In both the acute and domiciliary settings:

- wheeled walking aids (rollator frame) reduce the ventilatory requirements of ambulation
- wheeled walking aids are especially useful for those who are more disabled by breathlessness and those using ambulatory oxygen
- patients severely disabled by breathlessness may find using a high-gutter rollator frame allows some mobility
- along with occupational therapists, physiotherapists may promote energy conservation strategies to minimise the work of the activities of daily living

Airway clearance techniques should be used where indicated and IPPB may be considered in acute exacerbations of COPD for patients with retained secretions who are too weak or tired to generate an effective cough. NIV is now the first-line therapy for hypercapnic respiratory failure, and both NIV and oxygen therapy should be delivered as per current guidance.

Asthma Some form of breathing retraining, using reduced volume and/or frequency with relaxation, is indicated to reduce symptoms and improve quality of life, along with prescribed medication. Several schools advocate specific techniques, but it is important to stress that these techniques are adjunctive to medication and not a replacement therapy.

Routine or regular airway clearance is rarely indicated in the asthmatic patient

Disordered breathing (hyperventilation syndrome) Breathing exercises, with an emphasis on nasal breathing and either a smaller tidal volume or lower respiratory rate, or both, to reduce $V'E$, combined with relaxation (technique as for asthma), is an effective strategy to reduce symptoms once the diagnosis is confirmed.

CF and non-CF bronchiectasis Physiotherapy is integral to the management of patients with bronchiectasis from any cause, including CF, with airway clearance and exercise being central to this therapy. The acceptability of techniques and regimes, to enhance concordance with treatment, is vital to the success of therapy.

A variety of airway clearance techniques, including those with and without mechanical assistance if necessary, should be offered to find one that is both acceptable and effective. The simplest technique that impinges the least on the patient's life is a good starting point.

Effective treatment might need to be supported by inhaled therapies (*e.g.* bronchodilators or hypertonic saline, oxygen and NIV or IPPB). These supportive therapies and postural drainage to enhance airway clearance or exercise tolerance should be assessed for benefit on an individual basis. Regular review is advised to ensure continuing effectiveness and concordance with therapy; appropriate adjustment of treatment can be made if necessary.

- Physiotherapy for patients with CF should include assessment and treatment for musculoskeletal and postural disorders
- Physiotherapists need to be scrupulous about hygiene for infection control in this population
- For those with either CF or bronchiectasis, continence problems should be identified and treated
- For patients with bronchiectasis, pulmonary rehabilitation is indicated when dyspnoea is impacting on exercise tolerance or functional activities
- Exercise for the patient with CF must be undertaken individually to reduce risk of cross-infection

Interstitial lung diseases There is little published evidence on physiotherapy for interstitial lung diseases. Studies on the effectiveness of engaging in exercise training are emerging and patients with interstitial lung diseases can gain benefit from pulmonary rehabilitation providing they are referred early in the disease process. Patients at a later stage of disease may benefit from wheeled walking aids, ambulatory oxygen, breathlessness management and energy conservation strategies.

Community-acquired pneumonia Traditional airway clearance techniques are rarely indicated.

For patients admitted to hospital with uncomplicated community-acquired pneumonia (CAP):

- Regular use of positive expiratory pressure may reduce length of stay
- Medical condition permitting, early mobilisation is indicated
- Patients should be encouraged to sit out of bed for $\geqslant 20$ min on the first day, increasing the time and general mobility each subsequent day

CPAP may be helpful for patients in type I respiratory failure who remain hypoxaemic despite optimum medical therapy and oxygen, and NIV may be an option for selected patients in type II respiratory failure, especially those with underlying COPD.

Chest wall disorders Pulmonary rehabilitation is indicated in a patient with chest wall deformity from any cause with reduced exercise capacity and/or breathlessness on exertion. The need for ambulatory oxygen or NIV should be assessed before undertaking exercise. Respiratory muscle training may have a role. Work has yet to establish whether breathing or thoracic mobility exercises are helpful in this client group.

Neuromuscular disease and spinal cord injury Respiratory problems are the most common cause of morbidity and mortality for those with respiratory muscle weakness;

physiotherapy therefore provides vital assistance with airway clearance. Difficulty clearing secretions may be due to inspiratory, expiratory and/or bulbar muscle weakness, depending on the underlying condition and stage of disease.

- Regular monitoring of oxygen saturation, vital capacity (VC) and peak cough flow can indicate impending problems with either ventilation or cough effectiveness
- The use of respiratory aids when these measures fall may prevent or reduce complications

Oxygen therapy should be administered with great care in patients with neuromuscular disease because of the risk of increasing ventilation/perfusion mismatch and increasing hypercapnia. In those at risk of developing hypercapnia, NIV should be considered. These are done together with the treating physician.

Traditional physiotherapy techniques are not useful in this group of patients. Strategies to enhance maximal insufflation capacity (MIC) are indicated and include:

- resuscitation bags
- NIV
- mechanical insufflation
- breath stacking *via* the above or
- glossopharyngeal (frog) breathing

The presence of severe bulbar dysfunction or paralysis renders breath stacking ineffective. MIC enhancement, used regularly, is also a means of maintaining range of movement in the lungs and chest wall. These techniques should be used along with strategies to enhance cough effectiveness: manually assisted coughing or mechanical insufflation–exsufflation.

Ventilatory function can be improved with careful positioning to optimise the effect of gravity on weak muscles, as can the use of abdominal binders for those with spinal cord injury (SCI).

In patients with SCI, exercise should be encouraged; respiratory muscle training and functional electrical stimulation may enhance muscle strength or VC. Some patients with early neuromuscular disease may benefit from respiratory muscle training but caution is advised in Duchenne muscular dystrophy.

Patients with critical illness The principles of care remain the same in critically ill patients as in other patients; physiotherapists provide rehabilitation for the prevention and treatment of the common complications associated with prolonged bed rest, immobility and recumbence, including deconditioning, weakness and dyspnoea. Physiotherapy is also used to target specific respiratory problems, such as retained airway secretions, atelectasis and weaning failure.

Further reading

- Bott J, et al. Guidelines for the physiotherapy management of the adult, medical, spontaneously breathing patient. *Thorax* 2009; 64: Suppl. 1, i1– i51. Available from: www.brit-thoracic.org.uk/Guidelines/Physiotherapy-Guideline.aspx.
- Gosselink R, et al. (2008). Physiotherapy for adult patients with critical illness: recommendations of the European Respiratory Society and European Society of Intensive Care Medicine Task Force on Physiotherapy for Critically Ill Patients. *Intensive Care Med*; 34: 1188–1199.
- Langer D, et al. (2009). A clinical practice guideline for physiotherapists treating patients with chronic obstructive pulmonary disease based on a systematic review of available evidence. *Clin Rehabil*; 23: 445–462.
- National Institute for Health and Care Excellence. Critial Illness Rehabilitation. www.nice.org.uk/CG83
- Nici L, et al. (2006). American Thoracic Society/European Respiratory Society Statement on Pulmonary Rehabilitation. *Am J Respir Crit Care Med*; 173: 1390–1413.

Pulmonary rehabilitation

Thierry Troosters, Hans Van Remoortel, Daniel Langer, Marc Decramer and
Rik Gosselink

Definition

Pulmonary rehabilitation is now a recognised therapy for patients with respiratory diseases. Its effectiveness is supported by countless randomised controlled trials. In 2012, the European Respiratory Society (ERS) and American Thoracic Society (ATS) defined pulmonary rehabilitation as 'a comprehensive intervention based on a thorough patient assessment followed by patient-tailored therapies which include, but are not limited to, exercise training, education and behavior change, designed to improve the physical and psychological condition of people with chronic respiratory disease and to promote the long-term adherence to health-enhancing behaviors'. This is definition – although long – identifies the core components of a rehabilitation programme (Spruit et al., 2013). The definition per se is perhaps not as clear as it could be on the expected outcomes of rehabilitation

programmes. The full rehabilitation statement of the ATS and ERS, however, does provide that insight. In an initial phase, a rehabilitation programme aims to map out and restore the nonrespiratory consequences of respiratory diseases (i.e. muscle weakness, depressive symptoms, poor coping with the disease, impaired engagement in physical activities, nutritional deficits, etc.). Subsequently or in parallel, the rehabilitation programme calls for the self-management of patients to engage in a healthy lifestyle in terms of physical activity, nutrition, smoking and coping. The rehabilitation team becomes the patient's coach. In the first phase, exercise training is a crucial part of the rehabilitation programme; later on, the focus can gradually shift towards more lifelong behavioural change. Whereas the science of the former has reached a very high standard, with a clear evidence base, the latter is less well studied but is probably of equal import-ance and it is expected that progress can be made in the years ahead. Here, we will review the different aspects of this definition:

- the evidence base and anticipated effects;
- the selection of patients;
- the individualisation of the programme; and
- the mechanisms through which the programme works (reversing the systemic, extrapulmonary consequences).

Importantly, pulmonary rehabilitation may be an integrated part of other care plans for COPD patients, such as self-management programmes, lung transplant-ation programmes, NIV or smoking cessation programmes.

Key points

- Pulmonary rehabilitation is an evidence-based treatment that improves health-related quality of life and symptoms in COPD.

- Programmes should be tailored to the patient in terms of content, location, duration, frequency and exercise training.

- In order for the effects to be durable, patients' everyday activity should be higher after rehabilitation than before.

The evidence base for pulmonary rehabilitation

Several reviews have summarised the evidence for pulmonary rehabilitation (Lacasse *et al.*, 2006; Troosters *et al.*, 2005) and practice guidelines are available (Ries *et al.*, 2007). Therefore, a comprehensive review of all evidence for the effectiveness of pulmonary rehabilitation is beyond the scope of this short review.

Briefly, in patients with COPD, pulmonary rehabilitation improves health-related quality of life and symptoms unequivocally and clinically significantly. The effect of pulmonary rehabilitation on health-related quality of life is similar or even larger than that obtained by pharmacotherapy in COPD. When exercise training is provided at adequate intensity, exercise tolerance is enhanced and functional exercise capacity improves. These improvements are also clinically relevant if an appropriate exercise stimulus is provided. Other improvements are also important but, to date, are less studied.

Psychological improvements A significant proportion of patients referred for pulmonary rehabilitation suffer from psychiatric morbidity. Anxiety and depression are the most common problems. Recently, depression was identified as a negative prognostic factor in patients with COPD, particularly in patients who suffered from exacerbations. A recent meta-analysis showed the potential small benefit of multidisciplinary pulmonary rehabilitation on mood (Coventry *et al.*, 2007). In patients referred to our rehabilitation programme, depressive symptoms were present in 42% of patients and symptoms compatible with anxiety in 38% of patients (Trappenburg *et al.*, 2005). Clearly, one has to take into account that effects on these variables are only to be expected if patients do have symptoms of depression and/or anxiety. Hence, the relatively small effect size reported in the meta-analysis may be induced by the dilution of the depressed patients in the larger patient pool.

Another, even less studied psychological effect of rehabilitation is the enhanced self efficacy of patients. Self efficacy is the confidence patients have in their ability to carry out a specific task or manage a specific condition (*e.g.* breathlessness). The confidence patients have that they can manage dyspnoea improves after pulmonary rehabilitation and one of the seminal studies in pulmonary rehabilitation also showed an improvement of their self efficacy for walking. It is still unclear to what extent this increased self efficacy contributes to an effective change in behaviour after pulmonary rehabilitation.

Physical activity The amount of activity patients carry out in their daily life is an important outcome for rehabilitation. The 'systemic consequences' of COPD, such as cardiovascular morbidity, muscle weakness and osteoporosis, originate, to a large extent, directly or indirectly from living an inactive lifestyle. When pulmonary rehabilitation aims to achieve a sustained effect, an inactive life style after rehabilitation should be avoided. Currently, it is unclear what effect pulmonary rehabilitation programmes have on physical activity levels. Open studies have reported conflicting results and randomised controlled trials have only studied limited patient numbers in specific situations. Changing physical activity behaviour is challenging and, in general, results are somewhat disappointing. While endurance capacity virtually doubles, physical activity levels increase by about 20% (Troosters *et al.*, 2010a). Our group showed that walking time in daily life only modestly changed after 3 months of pulmonary rehabilitation. After 6 months, there was a more significant improvement in physical activity levels. Changing physical activity may not simply follow the increased exercise capacity. Probst *et al.* (2011) showed that more increased exercise tolerance (by providing higher intensity exercise programmes) did not lead to further enhanced physical activity levels. Indeed, physical activity levels are a complex integration of the exercise capacity of patients and their willingness to use that acquired capacity in a more physically active lifestyle. In recent years, appealing new strategies have been developed that may potentially help to increase the effects of classical rehabilitation on physical activities. First, providing patients real-time feedback on their physical activity levels using pedometers may, along with setting achievable goals, enhance daily activity levels within or without the context of pulmonary rehabilitation. Second, walking at home has been stimulated effectively using group activities, such as Nordic walking, or using modern interfaces, such as mobile phone technology that used walking paced to the rhythm of music adapted to the abilities of the patient. Even more recently, internet-based programmes have become available that may support rehabilitation programmes, but need to be further validated in this context. Future research should focus on further strategies that may help to lead to a sustainable behaviour change.

Utilisation of healthcare resources An important spin-off of pulmonary rehabilitation may be a decrease in the utilisation of healthcare recourses. The most important source of utilisation of healthcare recourses is hospital admissions. In one of the first large randomised controlled trials on pulmonary rehabilitation, there was a trend for a lower number of hospital days and a more recent trial showed a significant reduction in the number of hospital days (Griffiths *et al.*, 2000). In a study from Spain, a similar nonsignificant trend was observed (Guell *et al.*, 2000). Comparable findings were obtained in relatively long open studies comparing utilisation of healthcare recourses before and after taking part in pulmonary rehabilitation. When trials focus on more fragile patients, such as those recently admitted to hospital and at risk for re-admission.

A comprehensive intervention: programme content

As indicated above, programmes need to be individualised, aim to improve the systemic consequences (physiological and psychological) of the underlying respiratory disease, and guide the patients and their families towards a long-term change in physical activity and self-management behaviour. Several options are possible in

terms of the content (the disciplines contributing), location, duration and frequency of the programme. These are summarised in table 1. Studies that compared different modalities of rehabilitation head-to-head are scarce and no unequivocal preference has been reported. Several studies compared hospital-based outpatient rehabilitation to rehabilitation at home and found no differences between them in short-term outcomes. One study compared, in a randomised controlled design, hospital-based outpatient rehabilitation to community-based outpatient rehabilitation and found a trend for a somewhat smaller increase in the exercise tolerance of patients after hospital-based rehabilitation. Effects on health-related quality of life revealed similar nonsignificant trends (Elliott *et al.*, 2004). More research is needed to evaluate the criteria for assigning patients to a specific form of rehabilitation. In addition, it remains unclear to what extent home rehabilitation results in more enduring effects.

The exercise training component is essential, and the programme needs to be individualised in terms of exercise modalities, specificity of the training, the training intensity and specific inspiratory muscle training. In order to obtain significant physiological improvements in skeletal muscle function, it is important to train patients at an intensity that is high relative to the maximum capacity of the patients. Recently, programmes eliciting more significant skeletal muscle fatigue were related to better training effects in terms of functional exercise tolerance and reduction of symptoms (Burtin *et al.*, 2012). In order to combine an effective training programme with patient comfort, clinicians have the choice of several exercise training modalities. These include endurance training, interval training and resistance training. The duration of an exercise training programme is generally believed to be minimally 8 weeks and a minimum of three sessions is needed, although, admittedly, solid evidence as to the optimal duration remains missing (Spruit *et al.*, 2013). One of

Table 1. *Choices to be made when prescribing pulmonary rehabilitation*

Aspects to be individualised	Possible choices or options
Content	Disciplines typically involved are: chest physicians, physiotherapists, nurses, exercise specialists, occupational therapists, psychologists/behavioural coaches, social workers, dieticians, general practitioners
Location	Rehabilitation centre: inpatient, outpatient or home based but with close connection to a specialised centre Community based: outpatient in centre or primary care office Home-based supervised by primary care team
Duration	$\geqslant 8$ weeks, but longer is typically more desirable
Frequency	A minimum of 3 sessions per week of which 2 are supervised
Exercise training component	Exercise modalities (walking, cycling, upper limbs, *etc.*) Exercise intensity Exercise type: interval, endurance, resistance Additional interventions: inspiratory muscle training, oxygen therapy, NIV, neuromuscular electrical stimulation

these sessions can be conducted outside the formally supervised setting, by the patients, provided that the session is comparable in terms of duration and intensity to the supervised sessions.

Maintaining the effects of pulmonary rehabilitation

There has been a lot of debate as to whether the effects of a rehabilitation programme can be maintained or not. From earlier studies, it can be seen that it is indeed difficult to claim enduring effects of short term (6–8 weeks) pulmonary rehabilitation programmes. Older long-term studies (using up to 6 months of rehabilitation) did find more long-term effects.

Our current understanding of the development of systemic consequences of COPD may help to design successful longer term strategies to maintain the effects of pulmonary rehabilitation.

1. All efforts should be made to change the physical activity behaviour of patients. Physical inactivity is likely to be the most important contributor to the development of systemic consequences in COPD. If patients are not more active after the rehabilitation programme than before, it is likely that the effects of rehabilitation on enhanced exercise capacity and skeletal muscle force will be short lived. Efforts should be made to change physical activity behaviour during rehabilitation. We showed that longer programmes were more successful in achieving this goal than short-term programmes (Pitta *et al.*, 2008). However, changes in the programme content, such as providing patients with direct feedback on their physical activity levels or using structured behavioural interventions, may prove to yield results more rapidly.

2. Exercise at home should be facilitated. This can be achieved using feedback on home exercises or incentives. Such exercises need to be individually tailored to achieve effective intensity in order to provide a continued training stimulus. Ideally, the exercises should be regularly supervised.

3. Specific attention should probably be paid to patients who suffer from exacerbations, as these events acutely reduce muscle force and functional exercise capacity. Prevention of such events can be achieved in patients at risk by implementing self-management strategies and a case manager. Although it seems intuitively useful, there is currently little evidence for a short 'booster' programme after a

hospital admission to maintain the benefits of rehabilitation. If these repeated programmes are pre-planned, they seem to contribute little to the overall long-term success of programmes.

Table 2 provides an overview of the different strategies used in the peer-reviewed literature to maintain the benefits of a rehabilitation programme. Many of these studies were relatively small and, as follow-up becomes longer, the drop-out rate is substantial. Altogether, it seems important to achieve an enduring change in physical activity behaviour and patients should continue to carry out planned exercises at high intensity to maintain the physiological benefits of rehabilitation. From table 2, it is clear that interventions that are not regular or are less structured were not successful in maintaining the benefits of rehabilitation. Further evidence suggests that exercise maintenance is important to maintain the benefits of rehabilitation. That study, however, did not find differences between supervised and unsupervised exercise maintenance programmes. Patients were free to choose their preferred form of exercise maintenance strategy, which may have led to selection bias. More research is needed to identify optimal maintenance strategies after pulmonary rehabilitation.

Patient selection: patients with systemic consequences

The 2006 definition of pulmonary rehabilitation included the goals of rehabilitation: pulmonary rehabilitation is 'designed to reduce symptoms, optimize functional status, increase participation, and reduce health care costs through stabilizing or reversing systemic manifestations of the disease' (Nici et al., 2006). From this, it followed that the ideal candidate for rehabilitation is symptomatic, has impaired functional status and participation, high utilisation of healthcare recourses, and should suffer from the 'systemic consequences of COPD'. Hence, the selection of patients should not be performed based on lung function, but rather on the proper assessment of the

extrapulmonary consequences of COPD found to be reversible with rehabilitation, symptoms, functional status, the levels of participation in daily life and health-related quality of life. Other factors, such as age, sex and smoking status, are not important predictors of the outcome of rehabilitation. It is important that patients are screened for pulmonary rehabilitation after establishing optimal pharmacotherapy. While being screened for rehabilitation, patients can also be considered for other programmes, such as lung transplantation or lung volume reduction, NIV support, or oxygen therapy. Such programmes are not exclusion criteria for pulmonary rehabilitation. On the contrary, oftentimes, pulmonary rehabilitation is strongly recommended for these patients. Figure 1 gives an overview of the selection process for patients with COPD and the design of the programme.

Extrapulmonary consequences of COPD In the context of exercise training, the most important systemic consequence of COPD is skeletal muscle dysfunction. In clinical practice, this can be assessed by skeletal muscle force or local skeletal muscle endurance, which is often even more affected. Roughly 70% of patients referred to an outpatient COPD clinic suffer from skeletal muscle weakness and skeletal muscle force is acutely further reduced during acute exacerbations. In patients with less severe, newly detected Global Initiative for Chronic Obstructive Lung Disease (GOLD) stage II COPD, van Wetering et al. (2008) suggested quadriceps weakness occurred in 28% of the patients. In these patients, quadriceps force was related to exercise capacity, as was shown previously in more severe patients. In milder patients (FEV_1 >80% predicted), muscle weakness was actually a predictor of physical activity levels (Shrikrishna et al., 2012). Reversal of skeletal muscle dysfunction is an important goal of the exercise training component of a rehabilitation programme and, hence, patients suffering from skeletal muscle weakness are particularly good candidates for exercise training. Skeletal muscle strength can be improved particularly effectively by including resistance training

Table 2. Different maintenance strategies after outpatient (OP) or inpatient (IP) rehabilitation in randomised controlled trials

	Initial programme	Maintenance strategy	Effect
Moullec et al. (2008)	IP 4 weeks	2 sessions per week of structured exercise (community gymnasium), group interaction, education sessions *versus* usual care	Within group: better preserved performance Between groups: no significant differences
Berry et al. (2003)	OP 12 weeks	15 months continuation of the OP programme	Longer programme more effective
Ries et al. (2003)	OP 8 weeks	Weekly telephone calls and monthly supervised reinforcement sessions	Overall, no major difference between programmes
Brooks et al. (2002)	IP or OP 6–8 weeks	Attend monthly 2-h group sessions and phone call between visits	Overall, no major difference between programmes
Steele et al. (2008)	OP 8 weeks	Weeks 1–4: establishing a home- and community-based exercise programme with emphasis on walking; weeks 5–12: implementing a regular programme of exercise; weekly phone calls and 1 home visit over 3 months	Limited effect for the duration of the intervention; no long-term benefits at 12 weeks
Du Moulin et al. (2009)	OP 3 weeks	Individualised training plan, based on their last 6MWT and monthly phone call	Enhanced 6MWD and health-related QoL until end of follow-up at 6 months

Maintenance strategies were compared with a control group receiving usual care in all studies. 6MWT: 6-min walk test; 6MWD: 6-min walk distance; QoL: quality of life.

exercises in the sessions. When successful muscle force does increase and muscle oxidative capacity is enhanced.

More research is needed on pharmacological interventions that may assist pulmonary rehabilitation in order to restore muscle function more effectively. The short-term benefits of testosterone supplements in selected hypogonadal patients in combination with resistance training is an example of how pharmacotherapy and rehabilitation may have synergistic effects.

Impaired exercise tolerance and functional exercise capacity are the result of the pulmonary and systemic consequences of COPD. In the context of pulmonary rehabilitation, exercise tolerance is best formally assessed before the programme using an incremental exercise test. This will help guide the exercise training programme in terms of its intensity, training modalities and safety. Functional exercise capacity is best assessed using field tests such as the 6-min walk test. For this test, reference values exist, and benchmark improvements to programme quality (Lacasse et al., 2006), and clinical and statistical importance have been reported. When a patient's exercise tolerance is not abnormal, the indication for exercise training is questionable.

Another important extrapulmonary consequence of COPD is the derangement of the body composition. Both obesity, as a consequence of an inactive lifestyle, and cachexia, as observed in other chronic inflammatory disorders, are important to pick up on and treat in pulmonary rehabilitation programmes. Obese patients may experience less dyspnoea for a given oxygen consumption compared to nonobese

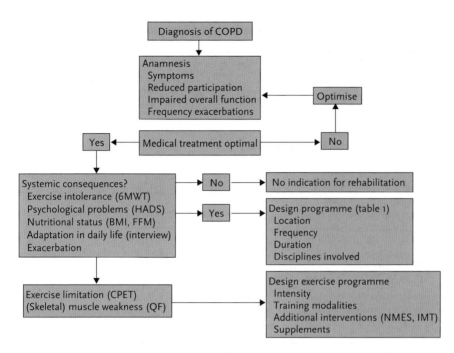

Figure 1. Flow chart for referral to pulmonary rehabilitation programmes. 6MWT: 6-min walk test; HADS: hospital anxiety and depression scale; FFM: fat-free mass; CPET: cardiopulmonary exercise test; QF: quadriceps force; NMES: neuromuscular electrical stimulation; IMT: inspiratory muscle training.

patients due to a favourable mechanical effect of obesity on the operating lung volumes. Nevertheless, obesity (defined as a BMI >30 kg·m⁻²) will limit the functional abilities of patients with limited ventilatory capacity, as it increases the ventilatory need during exercise against gravity. Cachexia, an involuntary loss of fat-free mass, leads inevitably to skeletal muscle weakness. It is a complex problem and its origin is not yet fully understood. Energy imbalance, disuse atrophy, hormonal imbalance, chronic hypoxia, accelerated ageing and systemic inflammation have been discussed as potential factors contributing to cachexia. The treatment of cachexia is an important aspect of rehabilitation in patients with COPD and requires individualised interventions by nutritional specialists. In order to appropriately assess this aspect, body composition should be assessed using dual-energy X-ray absorptiometry (DEXA) or bioelectrical impedance measurements.

Symptoms The most disabling symptom in COPD is clearly shortness of breath. Patients report dyspnoea, particularly during exercise or activity as a significant burden. Another important symptom is fatigue. Symptoms can be assessed during exercise using Borg symptom scores or during activities of daily living using specific questionnaires.

Physical activity The participation of patients in daily activities is not easily assessed. The methodology to assess physical activity was reviewed by Pitta *et al.* (2005). Several questionnaires have been used but, increasingly, activity monitors find their way to the clinical arena and validation studies of several monitors are available (Haskell *et al.*, 2007). In the future, it is likely that benchmark values for physical activity will become available for patients with COPD. As indicated earlier, patients not meeting current guidelines on healthy physical activity (30 min of moderately intense exercise, 5 days per week) can be considered candidates for pulmonary rehabilitation where the focus lies on improving the physical activity lifestyle of the patient.

Severe exacerbations Patients with COPD who have been hospitalised with an acute exacerbation are particularly good candidates for enrolment in pulmonary rehabilitation programmes. Recent narrative (Burtin *et al.*, 2011) and systematic (Reid *et al.*, 2012) reviews exist on the topic. Patients suffering from exacerbations have acutely lost muscle force, functional exercise tolerance and health-related quality of life as the result of an exacerbation. Physical activity levels are also dramatically low during the hospital admission and at least up to 1 month afterwards. That observation prompted investigators to look at the effects of muscle activation during the hospitalisation phase by means of resistance training (Troosters *et al.*, 2010b) or neuromuscular electrical stimulation. In addition, it is well known that patients who had a hospital admission for COPD are very likely to face new hospital admissions in the year following the previous admission, imposing a high burden of healthcare cost. The risk of re-admission is particularly high in patients who remain inactive after a hospitalisation. In these patients, the rehabilitation programme may need significant modification. The emphasis should be on acquiring appropriate self-management skills to prevent subsequent admissions, and the exercise training programme may need to be adapted to more severe ventilatory and/or skeletal muscle limitation, using resistance training or interval training at high intensities. Patients who have experienced an exacerbation are generally excluded from clinical studies. A recent meta-analysis of a handful of studies, however, showed that patients who suffered from exacerbations are very good candidates for pulmonary rehabilitation (Puhan *et al.*, 2011). Clearly, these patients may impose a higher burden on the rehabilitation team and drop-out from the programme is a particularly important problem.

Conclusion

Pulmonary rehabilitation is an evidence-based intervention for patients with COPD. It is individually tailored to the needs of patients, both in terms of the programme structure and its components. The aim of the rehabilitation programme is to lead to an endurable change in physical activity and self-management behaviour. Although the short-term effects of rehabilitation are well known, the long term effects are not always guaranteed. Further research should focus on the strategies to ensure long-term benefits for patients with COPD. Further knowledge on the processes underlying an enduring shift in lifestyle, as well as better understanding of the pathophysiological mechanisms leading to the systemic consequences of COPD and its treatments, may lead to major advances in the future.

Further reading

- Brooks D, *et al.* (2002). The effect of postrehabilitation programmes among individuals with chronic obstructive pulmonary disease. *Eur Respir J*; 20: 20–29.
- Burtin C, *et al.* (2011). Rehabilitation and acute exacerbations. *Eur Respir J*; 38: 702–712.
- Burtin C, *et al.* (2012). Effectiveness of exercise training in patients with COPD: the role of muscle fatigue. *Eur Respir J*; 40: 338–344.
- Coventry PA, *et al.* (2007). Comprehensive pulmonary rehabilitation for anxiety and depression in adults with chronic obstructive pulmonary disease: systematic review and meta-analysis. *J Psychosom Res*; 63: 551–565.
- de Voogd JN, *et al.* (2009). Depressive symptoms as predictors of mortality in patients with COPD. *Chest*; 135: 619–625.
- du Moulin M, *et al.* (2009). Home-based exercise training as maintenance after outpatient pulmonary rehabilitation. *Respiration*; 77: 139–145.
- Elliott M, *et al.* (2004). Short- and long-term hospital and community exercise programmes for patients with chronic obstructive pulmonary disease. *Respirology*; 9: 345–351.

- Garcia-Aymerich J, *et al.* (2003). Risk factors of readmission to hospital for a COPD exacerbation: a prospective study. *Thorax*; 58: 100–105.
- Griffiths TL, *et al.* (2000). Results at 1 year of outpatient multidisciplinary pulmonary rehabilitation: a randomised controlled trial. *Lancet*; 355: 362–368.
- Lacasse Y, *et al.* (2006). Pulmonary rehabilitation for chronic obstructive pulmonary disease. *Cochrane Database Syst Rev*; 4: CD003793.
- Nici L, *et al.* (2006). American Thoracic Society/European Respiratory Society statement on pulmonary rehabilitation. *Am J Respir Crit Care Med*; 173: 1390–1413.
- Pitta F, *et al.* (2005). Activity monitoring for assessment of physical activities in daily life in patients with chronic obstructive pulmonary disease. *Arch Phys Med Rehabil*; 86: 1979–1985.
- Probst VS, *et al.* (2011). Effects of 2 exercise training programs on physical activity in daily life in patients with COPD. *Respir Care*; 56: 1799–1807.
- Puhan MA, *et al.* (2008). Interpretation of treatment changes in 6-minute walk distance in patients with COPD. *Eur Respir J*; 32: 637–643.
- Reid WD, *et al.* (2012). Exercise prescription for hospitalized people with chronic obstructive pulmonary disease and comorbidities: a synthesis of systematic reviews. *Int J Chron Obstruct Pulmon Dis*; 7: 297–320.
- Ries AL, *et al.* (2007). Pulmonary rehabilitation: joint ACCP/AACVPR evidence-based clinical practice guidelines. *Chest*; 131: Suppl., 4S–42S.
- Shrikrishna D, *et al.* (2012). Quadriceps wasting and physical inactivity in patients with COPD. *Eur Respir J*; 40: 1115–1122.
- Spruit MA, *et al.* (2013). An Official American Thoracic Society/European Respiratory Society Statement: Key concepts and advances in pulmonary rehabilitation – an executive summary. *Am J Respir Crit Care Med*; [In press].
- Trappenburg JC, *et al.* (2005). Psychosocial conditions do not affect short-term outcome of multidisciplinary rehabilitation in chronic obstructive pulmonary disease. *Arch Phys Med Rehabil*; 86: 1788–1792.
- Troosters T, *et al.* (2005). Pulmonary rehabilitation in chronic obstructive pulmonary disease. *Am J Respir Crit Care Med*; 172: 19–38.
- Troosters T, *et al.* (2010a). Exercise training and pulmonary rehabilitation: new insights and remaining challenges. *Eur Respir Rev*; 19: 24–29.
- Troosters T, *et al.* (2010b). Resistance training prevents deterioration in quadriceps muscle function during acute exacerbations of chronic obstructive pulmonary disease. *Am J Respir Crit Care Med*; 181: 1072–1077.
- van Wetering CR, *et al.* (2008). Systemic impairment in relation to disease burden in patients with moderate COPD eligible for a lifestyle program. Findings from the INTERCOM trial. *Int J Chron Obstruct Pulmon Dis*; 3: 443–451.
- Van RH, *et al.* (2012). Validity of activity monitors in health and chronic disease: a systematic review. *Int J Behav Nutr Phys Act*; 9: 84.

Palliative care

Sylvia Hartl

Background and definition

Originally, in end-stage diseases, the term 'palliation' was used synonymously with end-of-life support. Today, palliative care is extended to all patients at any stage of chronic disease and their relatives. Palliative care is defined as prevention and relief of symptoms, aiming for improved quality of life with respect to the needs of the patient and their family. It includes all methods to control symptoms like dyspnoea, pain, psychological and spiritual distress, as well as support in the process of dying and bereavement care (table 1).

Implementation

Palliative care is feasible for all progressive chronic diseases or life-threatening diseases where all curative therapies have been applied to maintain quality of life.

For patients who are able to make decisions, it is important to discuss their preferences together with their families at an appropriate time in their disease. Setting up goals of care and empowering the patient and their families to accept or exclude any form of therapy needs sensitive discussion of all symptoms that may cause suffering and disability. The palliative support should start in parallel with the curative approach.

Key point

Palliative care is a multidisciplinary approach and needs teams of specialists with experience and training in palliative care.

The provision of competent caregivers is part of the implementation of palliative care.

The methods of palliative care include the following.

- Medication: opioids and other pain medication, and anxiolytic, antidepressant and sedative drugs
- Psychological counselling, spiritual support
- Dyspnoea management: NIV, oxygen therapy, endoscopic volume reduction
- Withdrawal or withholding of mechanical ventilation
- Bereavement care for the family

Pain relief In chronic or progressive pain, morphine in combination with other pain relievers is effective in the control of pain. In some patients, the risk of sedation or depression of central ventilatory drive has to be discussed and agreed on. In far-advanced disease stages, sedation can be a treatment goal, as end-of-life support.

Dyspnoea management Chronic severe dyspnoea is very frequent in COPD and other respiratory diseases. Medication, besides bronchodilators, does not directly address dyspnoea, but treats anxiety and depression. Pulmonary rehabilitation, endoscopic volume reduction and stenting are used in selected

Table 1. Key processes of palliative care

Pain relief
Dyspnoea control
Psychological and spiritual support
End-of-life support
Bereavement care

cases. Oxygen therapy and NIV are not primarily used for dyspnoea reduction, but some patients feel relieved by the reduction of the work of breathing. It is feasible to have a trial period and select responders. Caregivers have to be trained well for home therapy.

Psychosocial support The burden of symptoms and the fear of dying lead to symptoms of depression and/or anxiety. Frequently used antidepressant drugs are serotonin re-uptake inhibitors and tricyclic antidepressants, whereas tranquilisers are often used as anxiolytic drugs. Effects have to be observed and discussed with the patient. In every case, psychological counselling and coaching must accompany any drug therapy. The aims of these are for the patient to cope with symptoms and accept the dying process at the end of life. Psychological support is also helpful in the creation of advance directives for end-of-life decisions. Spiritual coaching depends on the spiritual background of the patient, and may be helpful for the patient and the family.

Withdrawal or withholding of ventilatory support This is an important goal for life-threatening diseases and is often discussed in the intensive care unit. If an advance directive is available, life support may be withheld or withdrawn, as palliative care does not aim to prolong life. These measures are often difficult to accept for the family, who need enough time for bereavement, especially children.

Bereavement therapy It is important to have clear treatment goals from the beginning, and support the family and the patient in the process of dying before and after death if needed.

Further reading

- Curtis RJ (2008). Palliative and end-of-life care for patients with severe COPD. *Eur Respir J*; 32: 796–803.
- Curtis RJ, *et al.* (2007). Noninvasive positive pressure ventilation in critical and palliative care settings: understanding the goals of therapy. *Crit Care Med*; 35: 932–939.
- Halpin DMG, *et al.* (2009). Palliative and end of life care for patients with respiratory disease. *Eur Respir Monogr*; 43: 327–353.
- Johnson MJ, *et al.* The evidence base for oxygen for chronic refractory breathlessness: issues, gaps, and a future work plan. *J Pain Symptom Manage* 2012; 763–775.
- Lanken PN, *et al.* (2008). An official American Thoracic Society clinical policy statement: Palliative care for patients with respiratory diseases and critical illnesses. *Am J Respir Crit Care Med*; 177: 912–927.

Measuring the occurrence and causation of respiratory diseases

Riccardo Pistelli and Isabella Annesi-Maesano

When reduced to the simplest terms, all medical research may be defined as the study of relationships (differences or associations) between variables. A variable is any quality, constituent or characteristic of a person, animal, thing or environment that can be measured. A variable is, by definition, something that changes and the values associated with its measurements are usually grouped in a set or 'scale'. There are four basic types of scales of which

Key points

- Occurrence of a health outcome is estimated by prevalence (*i.e.* the proportion of subjects affected by the health outcome in the considered population) and/or incidence (*i.e.* the proportion of new cases of the health outcome in the considered population).

- The effect of exposure to a risk factor on the health outcome and the associated risk (*i.e.* the probability that the health outcome will occur following the exposure) is quantified through two measures: the ratio of the measures of disease frequency according to the presence or absence of the exposure to the factor, and the difference between these two measures.

- The existence of a statistically significant association between the exposure to a factor and the health outcome does not imply that the factor is a cause of the health outcome; causation must meet several criteria introduced by Austin Bradford Hill.

definitions and examples are given in table 1.

Any measurement performed by using an interval or a ratio scale (continuous scales) can be translated to a category of an ordinal or nominal scale (categorical scales). For example, body temperature above or below a defined point of the Celsius or Fahrenheit scale can be used to identify subjects affected or not by fever, in this way translating from an interval to a nominal scale. Another example is the use of some values of FEV_1 to identify subjects affected by different levels of severity of COPD according to a conventional ordinal scale. In general, clinical research is mainly involved with patient-centred outcomes that are variables measured using nominal or ordinal scales (*e.g.* dichotomous variables grouping diseased or not diseased, or exposed or not exposed subjects) whereas interval or ratio scales are more frequently used in basic research. However, clinicians should be aware of the basic methods used to study the relationships of variables measured using continuous scales, such as lung function, as well as understanding relationships of nominal or ordinal variables. The aim of this chapter is to provide basic knowledge about measures and methods commonly used to define the occurrence of clinical conditions, and to study the relationships between those variables and other variables that characterise the individual and the environment. These methods have been mainly developed for epidemiological research but they should be the landmark of any clinical reasoning. We hope to improve the skill of readers of this book by

Table 1. Scales grouping measurements of health outcomes and exposure factors

Nominal scale	Uses names or symbols to assign each measurement to a limited number of categories that cannot be ordered one above the other	Race, sex, geographic area, diseased (yes *versus* no)
Ordinal scale	Assigns each measurement to a limited number of categories not equally spaced and ranked in a graded order	Patient status, cancer stage, COPD stage
Interval scale	Assigns each measurement to an unlimited number of categories that are equally spaced without an absolute zero point	Body temperature
Ratio scale	As the interval scale but measurements can be referred to a true zero point	Length, time, mass and all the derived physical units

discussing the relevance of information about the burden of diseases, as assessed by their distribution, the panel of related risk or protective factors, and the evaluation of the effectiveness of preventive measures and therapies in respiratory medicine.

Measuring occurrence

Epidemiology is the study of the distribution and determinants of disease frequency in human populations. The application of this study to determine valid and precise information about the causes, preventions and treatments of disease in order to control health problems is of outstanding clinical relevance. One of the main goals of any epidemiological study is to measure, for instance, the occurrence or frequency of health outcomes, a disease (asthma, COPD, lung cancer, *etc.*) or the intake of a medication. Epidemiological studies allow also estimation of the occurrence of exposure (smoking, air pollution, occupational hazards, *etc.*). Risk, incidence proportion, and incidence and prevalence rates are popular measures of frequency. They all are proportions and rates, and their values are meaningless if the denominator is not clearly and sensibly stated. For example, imagine you read in a newspaper, reported from an important scientific journal, that men who are 40 years old have a >5% risk of developing COPD. Of course, the dimension of this risk changes according to the time interval used in the denominator: the risk is high or low according to short or

long time interval. In many similar cases, the undefined denominator is the entire life span of individuals, but the reader should understand that the life span, which varies between individuals and populations, is not the best denominator to produce a broadly valid measure of risk. Unfortunately, reliable figures of risk are not available for many health problems, including many respiratory diseases.

Incidence and risk Incidence is a measure of the risk of developing a new health condition or outcome within a specified period of time, expressed as a proportion or rate. The risk, or incidence proportion (also known as the cumulative incidence), is the number of new cases within a specified time period divided by the size of the population initially at risk, and can be expressed by the formula

$$\text{Risk} = \text{incidence proportion} = \frac{a}{N} \quad (1)$$

in which a is the number of subjects developing a health outcome out of N people followed for a time period. Of course, any particular noncommunicable disease has a very low risk over a very short time period and the cumulative risk increases with time. However, the risk may change during the lifetime of individuals. As an example, many chronic respiratory diseases are associated with ageing and their risk is clearly increasing from the first to the last decade of life. However, defining risk is not as simple as it may appear from the above formula. Actually, the value of N may decrease over the time period for two main reasons: the competing risk and the loss to follow-up. First, let us consider a study aiming to define the risk of death from lung cancer in a cohort of smokers (*i.e.* a group of individuals sharing a particular demographic characteristic). It is plausible that, during the follow-up period, many subjects in the cohort will die from many different diseases and not from lung cancer. However, some of these subjects may have developed lung cancer but, before clinical manifestation, die of another disease. If we include those subjects in the denominator, the ratio will give an underestimation of the true risk of death from lung cancer. Secondly, suppose that some subjects included in the cohort were lost during the follow-up period (this is usual in cohort studies in which the individuals are followed up for long periods). Those subjects may not develop the outcome we are interested in and their inclusion in the denominator will give an underestimation of risk. In conclusion, it is sensible to pay the same attention to measuring both the numerator and the denominator of a ratio.

Competing risk or loss to follow-up can be managed using a different measure of health outcome occurrence: the incidence rate expressed as the number of new cases during some time period, according to the formula

$$\text{Incidence rate} = \frac{a}{t} \qquad (2)$$

in which a is the number of incident cases in the cohort, as in equation 1, and t is the total time interval experienced by the subjects followed. t is calculated by summing the time for which each subject has been at risk of developing the outcome. For events that may recur during the follow-up period, t is calculated by adding the contribution of each subject according to one of the following options the time experienced up to the first occurrence (in this case, the numerator includes only one occurrence per subject) or all the time intervals the subject was at risk of getting any of these occurrences (in this case the numerator includes all the occurrences experienced by each subject). The exacerbation of COPD is a typical example of

a recurrent event. Readers should be aware that different results may be produced by the different methods of calculating t for this outcome and that, whichever the choice, its rationale should be clearly pre-specified in clinical trials. The interpretation of incidence rate is not as simple as for the incidence proportion. The latter is a probability and is expressed as a number in the range 0–1; however, the incidence rate may assume any value from 0 to infinity. We may represent the incidence rate as the instantaneous velocity of a vehicle and the incidence proportion as the proportion of a journey covered by the same vehicle in a defined time period. Using this representation, we may suggest that incidence rate and risk for a health outcome may be related by the formula

$$\text{Risk} = \text{incidence rate} \times t \qquad (3)$$

We must remember that this formula may hold for short time intervals but not for longer intervals, during which the loss to follow-up and the competing risk will complicate the relationship between the two measures of occurrence. It is possible to find a solution to that complication by dividing a long time into shorter time intervals for which equation 3 may hold, and measuring the risk (or probability) of developing the outcome in each time interval. The overall probability will be equal to the product of probabilities of developing the outcome through all time intervals. This method is what is generally known as a survival analysis, and it can be applied to any outcome with a well-defined time of appearance during the follow-up of a cohort. In respiratory medicine, the results of many trials on chronic disease have been analysed using the survival analysis approach.

Prevalence is the proportion of subjects affected by a disease (or symptom or dysfunction) or, more generally, presenting a health outcome in a defined population. Risk and incidence rate are measures of disease onset. Prevalence is a measure of disease status. The value of prevalence is related not only to disease incidence but also to disease duration. The relationship of prevalence to incidence and duration of disease is expressed by the formula

$$\frac{P}{1-P} = ID \qquad (4)$$

in which P is prevalence, I is incidence and D is the mean duration of the health outcome. The ratio on the left side of equation 4 is known as the prevalence odds (in general, the odds of an event happening is the ratio of the probability that it happens to the probability that it does not). For a low prevalence, equation 4 may be written as

$$P \approx ID \qquad (5)$$

In this case, the prevalence proportion may be considered to approximate to the product of incidence and duration. It is clear that prevalence is a good measure of the burden of a disease and can be quite useful for public health research and decision making. However, prevalence cannot be used for causal inference about risk factors for a disease, except in some rare cases. Factors that may determine a health outcome or may increase its duration can be associated with an increased prevalence. A well-known example of this situation in respiratory medicine is offered by the prevalence studies in asthma published in recent decades. Many factors have been found to be associated with an increased prevalence of asthma but, for most of them, the crucial question 'is it a cause or a factor that increases the duration of asthma and the reporting of symptoms?' is still open. Of course, a reliable prevalence proportion or ratio depends on both a satisfactory measurement of population and prevalent cases. Sometimes, the definition of a prevalent case for a specific health outcome may be different among studies and this may lead to quite different prevalence estimates. Prevalence studies on COPD using different clinical definitions (e.g. diagnosis of chronic bronchitis or emphysema) or, more recently, different cut-off values of spirometric data, are good examples of this situation. Prevalence can be used for causal inference in the case of genetic factors, as genetic background precedes the development of the disease.

Measuring the effects: types of study

The second major goal of epidemiology is to measure the effect of exposure on the health outcome and to estimate the associated risk, i.e. the probability that the health outcome will occur following the exposure. This is obtained through different types of study design, according to the research question. Epidemiological study design is divided into:

- experimental studies, which include clinical or prevention trials (field trials and community trials)
- observational studies, which include cross-sectional studies, cohort studies, case–control studies and panel studies, according to the particular research question (table 2)

In experimental studies, the investigator assigns subjects to treatments (vaccination, treatment, prevention, etc.) and evaluates their effectiveness, whereas in observational studies, the researcher observes subjects and waits for the outcome to happen.

Each type of study design represents a different way of harvesting data and information. In experimental studies, the study population is enrolled on the basis of eligibility criteria that reflect the purpose of the prevention or clinical trial, as well as scientific, safety, ethical and practical considerations. Scientific, safety, ethical and practical considerations are also applied in observational studies. An example of a cross-sectional study is given by the prevalence studies on asthma published in the past few decades, such as ISAAC (International Study of Asthma and Allergies in Childhood). Case–control design was used to find risk factors for lung cancer and for all the diseases with a low occurrence frequency. Cohort studies have provided proof of the cause–effect relationship between tobacco smoking and lung cancer. Another type of study is represented by the panel study. A panel study is defined as an investigation that collects information on the same individuals at different points in time. Panels of asthmatics have been involved in the study of the short-term

Table 2. Main types of epidemiological study

Type of study	Description	Type of estimation
Experimental studies		
Clinical studies	Trial in which subjects are randomly given the treatment or placebo.	Effectiveness of the treatment by comparing the two groups (the treatment and control group, respectively)
Intervention studies	Inference study in which individuals receive an intervention in order to modify a supposed causal factor for disease incidence	Estimation of the effect of the intervention on the health outcome
Observational studies		
Cross-sectional studies	Descriptive study in which health outcome and exposure status are measured simultaneously in a given population It can be thought of as providing a 'snapshot' of the frequency and characteristics of health and exposure in a population at a particular point in time	Prevalence of acute or chronic health outcomes in a population Relationship between exposure and health outcome; however, since exposure and disease status are measured at the same point in time, it may not be possible to distinguish whether the exposure preceded or followed the health outcome and, thus, cause-and-effect relationships cannot be established
Cohort studies	Longitudinal investigation in which the occurrence of a particular health outcome is compared in well-defined groups of people who are alike in most ways but differ in a certain characteristic, such as (but not uniquely) an exposure Cohort studies are both retrospective (backward looking) or prospective (forward looking) In a prospective investigation, at the beginning, the individuals do not present the health outcome The prospective cohort design can establish whether having been exposed is a cause of the disease development	Incidence of health outcome Relationship between exposure and health outcomes Causal relationship (through the relative risk) in the case of prospective cohorts.
Case–control studies	Investigation that compares two groups of people: those with the disease or condition under study (cases) and a very similar group of people who do not have the disease or condition (controls) Medical and lifestyle histories including exposures of the people in each group are analysed to learn what factors may be associated with the disease or condition Case–control studies are usually retrospective but they can be prospective	Relationship between the exposure and the health outcome (through the odds ratio)

effects of air pollution. A panel study is, therefore, a longitudinal study; it differs from other studies that collect information over time, such as time series and cohort studies, in that it studies the same persons longitudinally. All these studies are based on individual data for both health outcomes and exposure. Ecological studies also exist, in which the unit of analysis is a population rather than an individual. For instance, an ecological study may look at the association between smoking and lung cancer deaths in different countries. The geographical information system is a very useful new tool that improves the ability of ecological studies to be able to determine a link between health data and a source of environmental exposure. These ecological studies allow the development of hypotheses that provide limited information.

Quantitative assessment of the relationship between exposure and health outcome There are two ways to quantitatively measure the effect of a factor on the health outcome or the condition of interest: the ratio of the measures of disease frequency according to the presence or absence of the exposure to the factor, and the difference between these two measures. The ratio is the measure of the strength of the association between a factor and the health outcome, whereas the difference is an estimate of the health impact of the factor under the hypothesis that the association is of cause–effect type and of the consequences of avoiding or diminishing the exposure to the factor. Specific statistical tests are necessary to confirm the existence of an effect. In the case that both the health outcome and the exposure are dichotomous variables, their relationship can be quantified and its statistical significance can be established by organising a 2 × 2 (two columns and two rows) contingency table, as represented in table 3.

A visual presentation of the relationship between a factor and a health outcome when both are dichotomous variables is shown in figure 1 where, for instance, the highest number (*a*) is observed for individuals who were exposed to the factor and presented

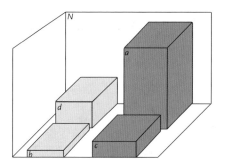

Figure 1. Distribution of the individuals according to the presence or the absence of a health outcome and exposure to a factor. a: number of individuals in the studied sample exposed to the potential risk factor who have experienced the health outcome; b: number of individuals exposed who have not experienced the health outcome; c: number of individuals unexposed who have experienced the health outcome; d: number of individuals unexposed who have not experienced the outcome; N: total number of individuals included in the study.

the health outcome, and the lowest (*b*) for individuals who were exposed to the factor but did not present the health outcome. In addition, the number of unexposed individuals who did not present the health outcome (*d*) is more elevated than the number of unexposed individuals presenting the health outcome (*c*). All these elements support the hypothesis that in this case there is a relationship between the exposure and the health outcome. The statistical significance of the relationship can be determined by applying statistical testing.

Ratio In cohort studies where groups of individuals are identified on the basis of the presence or absence of exposure to a potential risk factor and then followed-up for the appearance of the health outcomes, the relative risk is used to investigate whether such a risk factor is related to the health outcome. Relative risk estimates the ratio of disease occurrence in the exposed group to that in the unexposed group. If it is not possible to find a completely unexposed group to serve as the comparison, then the least exposed group is used.

The principal measure of relative risk is the risk ratio or cumulative incidence ratio, which

Table 3. Contingency table presenting the association data from the case of exposure and disease that are dichotomous variables

	Health outcome		Total
	Yes	No	
Exposure			
Exposed	*a*	*b*	*a+b*
Not exposed	*c*	*d*	*c+d*
Total	*a+c*	*b+d*	*N*

a: number of individuals in the studied sample exposed to the potential risk factor who have experienced the health outcome; b: number of individuals exposed who have not experienced the health outcome; c: number of individuals unexposed who have experienced the health outcome; d: number of individuals unexposed who have not experienced the outcome; N: total number of individuals included in the study.

	Health outcome			Incidence = risk
	Yes	No	Total	
Exposure				
Yes	a	b	$a+b$	$\dfrac{a}{a+b}$ = incidence in exposed
No	c	d	$c+d$	$\dfrac{c}{c+d}$ = incidence in unexposed
Total	$a+c$	$b+d$	N	

a: number of individuals in the studied sample exposed to the potential risk factor who have experienced the health outcome; b: number of individuals exposed who have not experienced the health outcome; c: number of individuals unexposed who have experienced the health outcome; d: number of individuals unexposed who have not experienced the outcome; N: total number of individuals included in the study.

is the ratio of the cumulative incidence in the exposed group ($a/(a+b)$) to that in the unexposed group ($c/(c+d)$) (table 4).

Thereafter, the relative risk is given by the formula

$$RR = \frac{\left(\dfrac{a}{a+b}\right)}{\left(\dfrac{c}{c+d}\right)} \quad (6)$$

A relative risk of 1 means there is no difference in risk between the two groups, a relative risk >1 means the health event is more likely to occur in the exposed group than in the unexposed group and a relative risk <1 means that the health event is less likely to occur in the unexposed group than in the exposed group. To be statistically significantly >1, the RR has to belong to a confidence interval >1. The need to introduce the confidence interval is due to the fact that the studied population is limited and variable due to random errors in selecting it. Similarly, to be statistically significantly <1, the RR has to belong to a confidence interval <1. The method used to calculate the 95% confidence interval for a RR is shown in Appendix 1. The case of a RR >1 with a 95% confidence interval that does not include 1 has to be interpreted as a positive association between the exposure and the health outcome at the 5% significance level, and a RR <1 with a 95% confidence interval that does not include 1

as a negative association between exposure and outcome at the 5% significance level.

In case–control studies in which the subjects are selected on the basis of disease status and the incidence of the health outcome is not available in the exposed and unexposed groups, the effect of the exposure on the health outcome is measured by the ratio of the odds of exposure among the individuals presenting the outcome to that among the individuals not presenting the outcome (the odds of the event is the quotient $p/(1-p)$, in which p is the probability in favour of the event; this value may be regarded as the relative likelihood that the event will happen). This ratio is called the odds ratio and is generally estimated as the ratio between the odds in exposed and nonexposed individuals:

$$OR = \frac{\left(\dfrac{\left(\dfrac{a}{a+b}\right)}{\left(\dfrac{b}{a+b}\right)}\right)}{\left(\dfrac{\left(\dfrac{c}{c+d}\right)}{\left(\dfrac{d}{c+d}\right)}\right)} = \frac{\left(\dfrac{a}{b}\right)}{\left(\dfrac{c}{d}\right)} = \frac{ad}{bc} \quad (7)$$

An odds ratio of 1 indicates that the health event under study is equally likely to occur in both groups. An odds ratio >1 with a 95% confidence interval that does not include 1 indicates that the event is more likely to occur in the exposed group at the 5%

significance level. An odds ratio <1 with a 95% confidence interval that does not include 1 indicates that the condition or event is less likely to occur in the exposed group at the 5% significance level. It can be shown that there is a mathematical relationship between the odds ratio and the relative risk:

$$RR = \frac{1 - \dfrac{a}{a+b}}{1 - \dfrac{c}{c+d}} \times OR \qquad (8)$$

As a consequence, when a disease is rare, a and c are small, and the odds ratio provides a valid estimate of the relative risk.

Table 5. Parameters estimating differences between risks

Measure	Definition	Formula
Attributable risk (AR)	The rate (excess risk) of the outcome in exposed individuals that can be attributed to the exposure It is given by the difference in cumulative incidences or incidence densities of the disease in the exposed (I_E) and the unexposed individuals (I_o) $AR = (I_E \text{-} I_o)$	$AR = \dfrac{a}{a+b} - \dfrac{c}{c+d}$
Preventive fraction (PF)	The attributable risk in the case that the exposure is preventive, so that $a/(a+b) > c/(c+d)$	$PF = \dfrac{\dfrac{c}{c+d} - \dfrac{a}{a+b}}{\dfrac{c}{c+d}}$
Attributable risk percentage or aetiological fraction (AR%)	The attributable risk divided by the rate of disease among the exposed	$AR\% = \dfrac{AR}{\left(\dfrac{a}{a+b}\right)} \times 100$ $= \dfrac{RR - 1}{RR} \times 100$
Population attributable risk (PAR)	The incidence of a disease in a population that is attributable to the exposure Given by the difference between the rate of the disease in the entire population (I_{TOT}) and I_o $PAR = (I_{TOT}) \text{-} (I_o)$ or by multiplying the product of the attributable risk by the proportion of exposed individuals in the population (P_E) $PAR = AR \times P_E$	$PAR = \dfrac{a+c}{a+b+c+d} - \dfrac{c}{c+d} = AR \times \dfrac{a}{a+c}$
Combined PAR	The PAR for a combination of risk factors is the proportion of the disease that can be attributed to any of the risk factors studied	Combined $PAR^{\#} = 1 - (1 - PAR_1)(1 - PAR_2)(1 - PAR_3)...$

a: number of individuals in the studied sample exposed to the potential risk factor who have experienced the health outcome; b: number of individuals exposed who have not experienced the health outcome; c: number of individuals unexposed who have experienced the health outcome; d: number of individuals unexposed who have not experienced the outcome; #: when there is no multiplicative interaction (no departure from multiplicative scale), combined PAR can be manually calculated by this formula

Difference Several types of difference exist between the measures of health outcome frequency according to the presence or the absence of exposure to the factor. They include the attributable risk, preventive fraction and the population attributable risk (table 5). It must be noted that these differences have to be computed under the assumption that the factor is causally related to the health outcome, a condition encountered in prospective cohort studies, having assessed causation and disposing of the entities like incidences and relative risks necessary to compute the differences of risks. These differences can be estimated in several ways, the most used are presented in table 5.

Statistical association between exposure and health outcomes The existence of a significant relationship between exposure and health outcome can be established independently from the estimation of the associated risk (odds ratio, relative risk, *etc.*). The main statistical methods that allow the determination of the existence of a significant statistical association between a factor and the health condition of interest are indicated in Appendix 2. They depend on the type of measurement scales used for the variables.

Causation

The existence of a statistically significant association between the exposure to a factor and the health outcome does not imply that the factor is a cause of the health outcome. Assessing causation implies several criteria introduced by Austin Bradford Hill (table 6). Notably, none of the proposed criteria can bring indisputable evidence for or against the cause-and-effect hypothesis and none can be required *sine qua non*.

Bias and errors

Occurrence of health outcomes and exposure, and measures of associations and causation are challenged by biases and errors. Random error corresponds to imprecision and bias to inaccuracy. Error is defined as the difference between the true value of a measurement and the recorded value of a measurement. There are many sources of error in collecting clinical data. Error can be described as random or systematic. Random error is also known as variability, random variation or 'noise in the system'. Heterogeneity in the human population leads to relatively large random variation in clinical trials. Random error has no preferred direction, so we expect that averaging over a large number of observations will yield a net effect of zero. The estimate may be imprecise but not inaccurate. The impact of random error, imprecision, can be minimised with large sample sizes. Systematic error, or bias, refers to deviations that are not due to chance alone. There are several types of bias:

- recall bias
- selection bias
- information bias
- confounding

Recall bias, selection bias and information bias can be reduced by good protocol. Confounding occurs when a variable is associated with both the exposure and the health outcome that we are studying. When the effect of an exposure is mixed with the effect of another variable (the confounding variable), we may incorrectly conclude that the disease is caused by the exposure. We might then attempt to eliminate the exposure in the hope that the disease could be prevented. If, however, the association between the exposure and the disease is due to confounding and is not causal, elimination of the exposure will have no effect on the incidence of the disease. The existence of confounding variables in smoking studies made it difficult to establish a clear causal link between active smoking and lung cancer, until appropriate methods were used to adjust for the effect of the confounders. An example of confounding variable in the relationship between active smoking and lung cancer is air pollution, which can cause cancer and is also associated with the exposure of interest, smoking. The effect of a confounder can be taken into account by adjusting for it with an appropriate statistical model or matching individuals according to it.

Table 6. Criteria for assessing evidence of causation

1	**Strength** The larger the association, the more likely that it is causal However, a small association does not mean that there is not a causal effect
2	**Consistency** Consistent findings observed by different persons in different places with different samples strengthen the likelihood of an effect
3	**Specificity** The more specific an association between a factor and an effect, the greater the probability of a causal relationship Causation is likely in case of a very specific population at a specific site and disease with no other likely explanation.
4	**Temporality** The effect has to occur after the cause
5	**Biological gradient** Greater exposure should generally lead to greater incidence of the outcome
6	**Plausibility** A plausible mechanism between cause and effect is helpful although, very often, knowledge of the mechanism is limited
7	**Coherence** Coherence between epidemiological and laboratory findings increases the likelihood of an effect of the exposure on the health outcome Notably, sometimes we lack such laboratory evidence
8	**Experiment** 'Occasionally it is possible to appeal to experimental...evidence.'
9	**Analogy** The effect of similar factors may be considered

Information from Hill (1965).

Bias has a net direction and magnitude so averaging over a large number of observations does not eliminate its effect. In fact, bias can be large enough to invalidate any conclusion. Increasing the sample size will not eliminate all bias. In epidemiological and clinical studies, bias can be subtle and difficult to detect. A study can be invalidated by the presence of bias. Thus, the design of clinical or epidemiological trials has to focus on removing known biases. Another important element to be introduced in epidemiological investigations is the effect modifier, a factor that modifies the effect of a putative causal factor under study. Effect modification (also known as statistical interaction) occurs when the effect measure depends on the level of another factor. For example, bacille Calmette–Guérin (BCG) immunisation is an effect modifier for the consequences of exposure to *Mycobacterium tuberculosis* and has to be taken into account when investigating risk factors for TB. Effect modification is detected by varying the selected effect measure for the factor under study across levels of the other factor. In this example, the modification effect of BCG immunisation could be estimated by computing the odds ratio between tobacco smoking and TB according to the presence or absence of BCG immunisation. The effect of a modifier can be taken into account through matching individuals according to different levels of the modifier (stratification).

Table 7. Sensitivity and specificity computation

New criterion results	Reference criterion results	
	Positive	Negative
Positive	TP	FP
Negative	FN	TN

TP: number of true positive specimens; FP: number of false positive specimens; FN: number of false negative specimens; TN: number of true negative specimens.

Sensitivity and specificity

Sensitivity is the probability that the criterion used to define the case will produce a true positive result when used in a population (compared to a reference or 'gold standard'). Specificity is the probability that the criterion will produce a true negative result when used (as determined by a reference or 'gold standard'). Using a contingence table relating reference and new criterion results (table 7), the following formulae are obtained for sensitivity and specificity

$$\text{Sensitivity} = \frac{TP}{TP+FN} \quad (9)$$

$$\text{Specificity} = \frac{TN}{TN+FP} \quad (10)$$

where TP is the number of true positive specimens, FP is the number of false positive specimens, FN is the number of false negative specimens and TN is the number of true negative specimens. An example of an application for sensitivity and specificity calculation is in the validation of biomarkers.

Conclusion

Epidemiology provides methods for measuring the occurrence and the causation of respiratory diseases. In assessing occurrence and relationships between exposure and health outcomes, criteria of relevance should include:

1) the representativeness of the studied samplesm particularly in studies with samples of the general population; and

2) clear definitions of both the health outcome (or dependent variables) and the exposure (or independent variables) to be included in the models.

Further reading

- Hill AB (1965). The environment and disease: association or causation? *Proc R Soc Med*; 58: 295–300.
- Rothman KJ. Epidemiology: An Introduction. New York, Oxford University Press, 2002.
- Swinscow TDV, *et al.* Statistics at Square One. London, BMJ Books, 2002.
- Swinscow TDV, *et al.* Statistics at Square Two. London, BMJ Books, 2002.

Suggested free software

Epi Info. Version 3.5.3 (January 26, 2011). Atlanta, Centers for Disease Control and Prevention, 2011. Available from: wwwn.cdc.gov/epiinfo/

Appendix 1: 95% confidence intervals for the relative risk and the odds ratio

Given the 2×2 contingency table relating exposure to health outcome, a common way to calculate the 95% confidence interval is as follows.

In the case of the relative risk (approximate estimate):

$$\text{Upper limit} = e^{\ln RR + 1.96 \times \sqrt{v\ln RR}} \quad (11)$$

$$\text{Lower limit} = e^{\ln RR - 1.96 \times \sqrt{v\ln RR}} \quad (12)$$

where $\sqrt{v\ln RR}$ represents the square root of the natural log of the risk ratio, defined as

$$\ln RR = \ln\left(\frac{\left(\frac{a}{a+b}\right)}{\left(\frac{c}{c+d}\right)}\right) \quad (13)$$

which is asymptotically normal with variance

$$v\ln RR = \frac{1}{a} - \frac{1}{a+b} + \frac{1}{c} - \frac{1}{c+d} \quad (14)$$

When there are zeros, a common convention is to add 1/2 to each cell.

In the case of the odds ratio:

Table 8. Main statistical methods for assessing the relationship between health outcomes and exposures

Statistical methods	Description
Correlation	A single number that describes the degree of relationship between two continuous variables
Linear regression	Approach to modelling the relationship between a continuous variable y and one or more variables denoted x that may be either continuous or categorical
ANOVA	A statistical test of whether or not the means of several groups are all equal (*i.e.* are not statistically significantly different)
Logistic regression model	Approach to predicting the probability of occurrence of an event by fitting data to a logit function It makes use of several predictor variables that may be either continuous or categorical Usually used to estimate the odds ratio between the exposure and the health outcome after adjustment for potential confounders

Upper limit
$$\ln OR = \ln OR + 1.96 \times SE(\ln OR) \quad (15)$$

Lower limit
$$\ln OR = \ln OR - 1.96 \times SE(\ln OR) \quad (16)$$

which become

$$\text{Upper limit } OR = e^{\text{upper limit } \ln OR} \quad (17)$$

$$\text{Lower limit } OR = e^{\text{lower limit } \ln OR} \quad (18)$$

where $SE(\ln OR)$ is the standard error of the natural log of the odds ratio, which is the variance of $\ln OR$, calculated as $(1/a)+(1/b)+(1/c)+(1/d)$.

Appendix 2: Main methods used to assess the relationship between exposure and health outcome

We have presented how to assess the relationship between the health outcome and exposure in the case where both variables are dichotomous. Table 8 introduces the methods that can be used in other cases.

Index

neuroventilatory dissociation (NVD) 54–55
neutropenia 208, 212
    chemotherapy-induced 461
neutrophils 42
nicotine replacement therapy (NRT) 358, 359
nitric oxide, exhaled fraction see fractional exhaled
nitric oxide measurement
nitrogen dioxide, air pollution 346, 347
nocturnal hypoventilation 503, 504
nocturnal noninvasive ventilation, obesity
hypoventilation syndrome 180, 505
nodular bronchiectasis 252
nodular pattern, high-resolution computed tomography
373, 374
nominal scale 554, 555
nonallergic rhinitis 262
    treatment 263
nonasthmatic eosinophilic bronchitis 395
noninvasive ventilation (NIV) 166–169
    bronchiectasis 167
    chronic obstructive pulmonary disease 540
        acute exacerbations 166–167, 168
        long-term 181
    contraindications 167
    long-term 178–179
    neuromuscular disease patients 167, 179–180,
444–445, 446, 542
    obesity hypoventilation syndrome 167, 180, 505–506
    oxygen therapy and 173
    practicalities of ventilator settings 167
    see also continuous positive airway pressure (CPAP)
therapy
nonsmall cell lung cancer (NSCLC)
    diagnosis 456
    early-stage, definition 467
    staging 153, 457, 467
    treatment
        chemotherapy 462–463, 466, 472
        radiotherapy 466, 472, 473–474, 475
        surgical 466–470
        survival rates and 467, 468, 469–470, 473
    see also lung cancer
nonspecific interstitial pneumonia (NSIP) 386, 387
    diagnosis 116, 388
    high-resolution computed tomography 376–377
    see also idiopathic interstitial pneumonias (IIPs)
nonsteroidal anti-inflammatory drugs (NSAIDs)
    respiratory complications 408
    upper respiratory tract infection management 192
nontuberculous mycobacterial (NTM) infections
251–254
    diagnosis 252, 253
    epidemiology 251
    immunocompromised hosts 207
    pathogenesis 251
    pulmonary disease 251–253
    treatment 253–254
nosocomial pleural infection 215, 216
nosocomial pneumonia see hospital-acquired pneu-

monia (HAP)
nuclear factor-κB 11
nuclear medicine scans 60, 151–153
    see also scintigraphy
nucleic acid amplification tests (NAATs) 184, 187–188
    mycobacterial infections 256
Nuss technique 449
nutritional support, COPD 291

O

obesity
    COPD patients 548–549
    dyspnoea and 56
obesity hypoventilation syndrome (OHS) 167, 180,
505–506, 507
oblique chest radiograph 137
obliterative bronchiolitis, penicillamine-induced 409
obstructive lung disease
    hypoventilation 507–508
    lung volume changes 67, 69
    see also specific diseases
obstructive sleep apnoea/hypopnoea syndrome
(OSAHS) 491–496, 503, 504, 506
    altitude effects 364
    assessment 492
    central sleep apnoea association 492, 498
    consequences 492–493
    definition 491
    pathophysiology 492, 493
    prevalence 492
    symptoms 491
    treatment 493–496
occupational asthma 327–331
    associated occupations/industries 329
    diagnosis 328, 330
    management 330
    sensitising/triggering agents 328, 329
    socioeconomic impact 330–331
    symptoms 328
occurrence, measurement see epidemiological studies
odds ratio 560–561
oesophagus
    cystic fibrosis-related disease 322
    radiotherapy side-effects 476
omalizumab 309
opioid therapy, chronic, central sleep apnoea and 501
opportunistic infections see immunocompromised
hosts, opportunistic infections
opsonins 42
ordinal scale 554, 555
organic dust toxic syndrome (ODTS) 332, 333
    hypersensitivity pneumonitis versus 340
organising pneumonia 377
    cytological findings 34
    drug-induced 406, 408, 409
    see also cryptogenic organising pneumonia (COP)
oseltamivir 224
    resistance 224–225